The
PHYSICIAN
ASSISTANT
SURGICAL
HANDBOOK

The
PHYSICIAN
ASSISTANT
SURGICAL
HANDBOOK

James B. Labus, PA-C

W.B. SAUNDERS COMPANY
A Division of Harcourt Brace & Company
Philadelphia   London   Toronto   Montreal   Sydney   Tokyo

W.B. SAUNDERS COMPANY
A Division of Harcourt Brace & Company

The Curtis Center
Independence Square West
Philadelphia, Pennsylvania 19106

Library of Congress Cataloging-in-Publication Data

Labus, James B.
The physician assistant surgical handbook / James Brox Labus.—
1st ed.

p.   cm.

ISBN 0–7216–6815–1

1. Surgery—Handbooks, manuals, etc.   2. Physicians' assistants—Handbooks,
   manuals, etc.   3. Operating room technicians—Handbooks, manuals,
   etc.   I. Title.
   [DNLM: 1. Surgery—handbooks.   WO 39 L 127p 1998]

RD37.L33 1998   617—dc21

DNLM/DLC   96–49868

THE PHYSICIAN ASSISTANT
SURGICAL HANDBOOK   ISBN 0–7216–6815–1

Printed in the United States of America.

Last digit is the print number: 9   8   7   6   5   4   3   2   1

To Brox and Elise

Don't worry about biting off more than you can chew.
Your mouth is probably a whole lot bigger'n you think.
A Cowboy's Guide to Life—Texas Bix Bender

About the Editor

James B. Labus is a 1986 graduate of the Emory Physician Associate Program. Upon graduation, he was awarded the honor of Who's Who in American Colleges and Universities. He also holds a BS in Health Education from Michigan State University.

As a PA, he worked in the field of neurosurgery for nine years. During that time, he and Patrick Cafferty co-founded the Association of Neurosurgical Physician Assistants (ANSPA). He has been active in teaching and lecturing at the Emory PA program and has given several presentations at meetings of The American Academy of Physician Assistants. He is also the editor of the companion text, The Physician Assistant Medical Handbook.

Mr. Labus currently owns, operates, and works clinically for Mid-Level Temps, Inc., a company that provides corporate services to freelance Physician Assistants and Nurse Practitioners.

Contributors

David A. Adams, PA-C
Gropper Neurosurgical, Atlanta, Georgia
Subarachnoid Hemorrhage

Rita Altman, PA-C, BA, BS
Physician Assistant, Pan Pacific Urology,
    California Pacific Medical Center, San Francisco,
    St. Mary's Medical Center, San Francisco, Seton
    Medical Center, Daly City, California
*Benign Prostatic Hypertrophy; Hydrocele (Newborn
    and Adult) Hypospadias; Prostate Cancer; Testicular
    Torsion; Testicular Tumor; Varicocele*

Nancy Anderson, PA-C
Private Practice
Casting Techniques

Angela Ballard, PA-C, BS
Physician Assistant, Atlanta Plastic Surgery,
    Atlanta, Georgia
Breast Reconstruction; Free Flap

James W. Becker, PA-C
Private Practice
*Abdominal Trauma; Appendicitis;
    Hyperparathyroidism (Primary); Pancreatic Cancer;
    Splenic Rupture*

Clyde Bullion, PA-C, BSN, RN
Physician Assistant in General Surgery and
    Orthopedics, Kaiser Permanente, Richmond,
    California
Anal Fissures; Fistulas; Hemorrhoids

John W. Bullock, PA-C, BA, BS
Program Director, USAF Physician Assistant
    Residency in Orthopaedic Surgery, David Grant
    Medical Center, 60th Medical Operations
    Squadron/SGOSO, Travis AFB, California
*Fractures: Supracondylar Humerus; Sprains:
    Acromioclavicular Injuries; Sprains: Biceps Tendon
    Ruptures; Sprains: Frozen Shoulder; Sprains: Rotator
    Cuff Tears*

Patrick Cafferty, PA-C, BS
Clinical Director, Paducah Medical Pavilion,
   Neurosurgery, and Rehabilitation Medicine,
   Paducah, Kentucky
   *Preoperative and Perioperative Management of the
      Surgical Patient*

Michael E. Champion, PA-C, MMSc, EdM, CCP
Instructor, St. Francis College, Hutchinson;
   Director, Cardiovascular Services, Hutchinson
   Hospital, Hutchinson, Kansas
   Cardiac Contusion; Valvular Heart Disease

Stephen M. Cohen, PA-C, MS
Assistant Professor and Academic Director,
   Physician Assistant Program, Nova Southeastern
   University, Ft. Lauderdale, Florida
   Fractures: Hip

Edward D'Ettorre, PA-C
Physician Assistant, Orthopedic Surgery, Mayo
   Clinic Scottsdale, Scottsdale, Arizona
   *Fractures and Dislocations of the Elbow; Adult
      Reconstructive Surgery*

Richard E. Donnelly, PA-C, BS, BS
Instructor, Kirksville College of Osteopathic
   Medicine, Phoenix; Physician Assistant in
   Orthopedics, Mayo Clinic Scottsdale,
   Scottsdale, Arizona
   *Foot: Clubfoot; Foot: Hallux Valgus; Fractures;
      Fractures: Ankle; Fractures: Distal Radial; Fractures
      and Dislocations of the Elbow; Fractures: Stress;
      Adult Reconstructive Surgery; Strains, Sprains,
      and Tendon Injuries; Sprains: Achilles Tendon
      Rupture; Sprains: Ankle; Sprains: Digits; Sprains:
      Tibialis Posterior*

Joseph Roy Durio, PA-C, MA
Adjunct Associate Professor, Physician Assistant
   Studies, Kirksville College of Osteopathic
   Medicine, Phoenix; Physician Assistant,
   Otorhinolaryngology Department, Mayo Clinic
   Scottsdale, Scottsdale, Arizona
   Nasopharyngeal Carcinoma; Tonsillitis

Bruce Fichandler, PA
Department of Plastic Surgery, Yale University,
   New Haven, Connecticut
   Facial Lacerations; Skin Grafting

Carrie Gunn-Edel, PA-C
Department of Plastic, Reconstructive and Hand
Surgery, Mayo Clinic Scottsdale, Scottsdale,
Arizona
*Carpal Tunnel Syndrome; Sprains: Epicondylitis of the
Elbow; Sprains: Wrist*

J. Jeffrey Heinrich, PA-C, EdD
Department of Plastic Surgery, Yale University,
New Haven, Connecticut
Facial Lacerations; Skin Grafting

Roderick S. Hooker, PA
Adjunct Faculty, University of Washington and
Pacific University, Seattle, Washington;
Department of Rheumatology, Kaiser
Permanente, Portland, Oregon
Percutaneous Muscle Biopsy

James B. Labus, PA-C
President, Mid-Level Temps, Inc., Dunwoody,
Georgia
*Bowel Ischemia; Head Injury; Hydrocephalus;
Meningioma; Metastatic Brain Lesion; Tardy Ulnar
Nerve Palsy; Pituitary Adenoma; Lumbar Puncture*

Demosthenes Y. Lalisan, I, BS, MBA, CPTC
Manager of Organ Recovery Services, Alabama
Organ Center, Birmingham, Alabama
Organ Procurement

Lyle W. Larson, PA-C, MS
Chief Physician Assistant, Cardiothoracic Surgery
Teaching Associate, University of Washington,
Seattle; Chief Physician Assistant,
Cardiothoracic Surgery, Seattle Veterans
Administration Medical Center, Seattle,
Washington
*Cardiac Contusion; Congenital Heart Disease;
Coronary Artery Disease; Cardiac Tamponade;
Valvular Heart Disease; Bronchial Obstruction;
Chest Wall Tumors; Lung Cancer; Pneumothorax;
Pulmonary Contusion*

Susan Lemens, PA-C
Instructor in Neurologic Surgery, Mayo Medical
School, Mayo Clinic Scottsdale; Physician
Assistant, Department of Neurologic Surgery,
Mayo Clinic Scottsdale, Scottsdale, Arizona
*Spine: Cervical and Lumbar Intervertebral Disc
Disease; Lumbar Spinal Stenosis*

Mary Loggins, PA-C, MS, MMSc
Physician Assistant, St. Joseph Hospital, Northside
  Hospital, and Scottish Rite Children's Hospital,
  Atlanta, Georgia
  Glioma

Gerard J. Marciano, RPA-C
Associate Director and Academic Coordinator,
  Physician Assistant Program, Brooklyn Hospital
  Center and Long Island University, Brooklyn,
  New York
  Bladder Carcinoma; Urolithiasis

Robert McNellis, PA-C, MPH
Assistant Professor, The George Washington
  University School of Medicine and Health
  Sciences, Washington, DC
  Prostate Cancer; Stress Urinary Incontinence

Major William A. Mosier, PA-C, EdD, USAF
Chief of Professional Services, 125th Medical
  Squadron, USAF/FLANG; Clinical Director,
  Florida Institute for Neuro-Developmental
  Disorders, Vero Beach, Florida
  Blepharoplasty; Face Lift; Rhinoplasty

Deborah E. Murray, PA-C, BS
Private Practice
  *Bartholin's Cyst/Abscess; Ovarian Cancer;
    Endometriosis; Uterine Cancer*

Karen A. Newell, PA-C
Associate Academic Coordinator, Emory
  University School of Medicine, Atlanta;
  Physician Assistant, Grady Memorial and
  Crawford Long Hospitals, Atlanta, Georgia
  Peptic Ulcer Disease

Judy Nunes, PA-C, BS
Lecturer, Yale University School of Medicine,
  Physician Associate Program, New Haven;
  Adjunct Professor, Quinnipiac College PA
  Program, Hamden; Lecturer, PA Surgical
  Residency Program, Norwalk Hospital, Norwalk;
  Physician Assistant, Division of Neurological
  Surgery, Hospital of St. Raphael, New Haven,
  Connecticut; President, Association of
  Neurosurgical Physician Assistants
  *Epidural Hematoma; Spinal Cord Injury; Subdural
    Hematoma*

Deborah A. Opacic, PA-C, MMS
Instructor, Duquesne University, Department of
   Physician Assistant Studies, Pittsburgh,
   Pennsylvania
   Diseases of the Aorta; Carotid Atherosclerotic Disease;
      Renal Atherosclerotic Disease; Arteriosclerosis
      Obliterans; Acute Arterial Occlusion: Embolism,
      Thrombosis; Thoracic Outlet Syndrome; Varicosities;
      Subclavian Line Insertion

William C. Perry, PA-C
Physician Assistant, Pacific Cosmetic Surgeons,
   Sacramento, California
   Facial/Sinus Fractures; Laryngeal Trauma

Michael G. Phillips, PA-C, BHS, CPTC
Director, Alabama Organ Center, Birmingham,
   Alabama
   Organ Procurement

Jack Pike, PA-C, BS
Adjunct Clinical Assistant Professor, Quinnipiac
   College PA Program, Hamden; Physician
   Assistant, St. Francis Hospital and Medical
   Center, Hartford, Connecticut
   Chest Tube Thoracostomy; Emergency Cricothyrotomy;
      Endotracheal Intubation; Internal Jugular
      Cannulation; Thoracentesis, Saphenous Vein
      Harvesting; Wound Care

Patricia Podres, PA-C
Physician Assistant, Atlanta Plastic Surgery,
   Atlanta, Georgia
   Breast Reconstruction; Free Flap

Carroll F. Poppen, PA-C
Assistant Professor of Otolaryngology,
   Department of Otolaryngology, Mayo Clinic,
   Rochester, Minnesota
   Epistaxis; Sinusitis; Management of Nosebleeds

Karen M. Potts, PA-C
Southeast Gynecologic Oncology, Atlanta,
   Georgia
   Breast Carcinoma; Cholecystitis; Gastric Carcinoma;
      Liver Tumors

Harry F. Randolph, PA-C
Chief Physician Assistant, Chief, Physician
  Extender Section, Green Hospital of Scripps
  Clinic and Scripps Clinic Medical Group, La
  Jolla, California
  Small Bowel Disease

Thomas J. Schymanski, PA-C
Physician Assistant, De Witt Army Community
  Hospital, Fort Belvoir, Virginia
  Adrenal/Renal Neoplasms; Bowel Ischemia;
    Esophageal Disorders

Rhea Sumpter, PA, MMSc
Physician Assistant, St. Joseph's Hospital, Atlanta,
  Georgia
  Anesthesia

Paul Taylor, PA-C, BS
Instructor, Clinical Rotations, Emory University
  PA Program, Atlanta; Physician Assistant,
  Departments of GYN/OB and Neonatology,
  Emory University and Department of Maternal
  and Child Health, Grady Memorial Hospital,
  Atlanta, Georgia
  Ectopic Pregnancy; Urinary Incontinence; Pelvic Organ
    Prolapse; Norplant: Insertion and Removal;
    Intrauterine Devices (IUDs): Insertion and Removal

Frank Trejose, PA-C
Orthopedics/Orthopedic Oncology, Mayo Clinic
  Scottsdale, Scottsdale; Clinical Adjunct Faculty,
  Midwestern University, Glendale, Arizona
  Musculoskeletal Tumors

Kent W. Wallace, PA-C, ARNP
Clinical Instructor, MEDEX Northwest Physician
  Assistant Program, University of Washington,
  Seattle; Washington Orthopedics and Sports
  Medicine Clinic, Kirkland, Washington
  Sprains: Knee; Sprains: Patellofemoral Disorders

Deborah Entrekin Whitehair, PA-C, MS
Physician Assistant, Northeast Georgia Medical
  Center and Northeast Georgia Primary Care
  Network, Gainesville; Baptist North Hospital,
  Cumming, Georgia
  Nasal Polyps; Otitis Media

Preface

The Physician Assistant Surgical Handbook along with the previously published The Physician Assistant Medical Handbook are the first portable, comprehensive reference guides to surgery and medicine for the Physician Assistant profession. This text is designed to present the most commonly encountered conditions in all of the major surgical subspecialties. Additional topics are included to provide a more complete understanding of the role of the PA in a surgical setting. These include preoperative and perioperative management, anesthesia, and organ procurement. A section on procedures commonly performed by the PA has been included. A consistent outline format is utilized when presenting surgical conditions. This format allows for ease of reference when seeking a specific piece of information about a condition.

This text is most useful for PAs who desire information on a disorder outside of their primary specialty. The primary care PA will also find it advantageous in understanding the evaluation and treatment of a surgical disorder in order to counsel patients more effectively.

The goal of this reference guide is to provide the most comprehensive overview of surgery possible. It is not the aim of this text to present the most cost-effective or minimal approach. Evaluation of the patient varies, especially in the surgical subspecialties. Experience with a technique or the development of innovative techniques makes a "cookbook" approach to surgical disease impossible. It is the responsibility of the physician/PA team to decide the most appropriate evaluation and treatment based on the patient's disorder, situation, and desires.

Thanks to all of you who have contributed, offered to contribute, and have purchased this book. I welcome the input of PA professionals as to how to make this guide more useable and beneficial.

James B. Labus

Contents

Chapter **1**

Preoperative and Perioperative Management of the Surgical Patient

Patrick Cafferty, PA-C

The preoperative and perioperative management of the surgical patient can be as important to the overall success of the surgery as the procedure itself. The decision to perform a therapeutic, operative procedure on a patient must be made based on historical data, physical examination, and radiographic findings. Often the determination is quite straightforward, as in the case of an acute abdomen or compound fracture. At other times, surgery may be deferred or performed on an elective basis. In either case, specific information must be gathered whenever possible.

PREOPERATIVE EVALUATION

History of Present Illness. The patient's age and onset, duration, and intensity of symptoms and aggravating, associated, and alleviating factors, along with an appropriate review of the involved system, are initially obtained.

Current Medications. Obtain a list of all medications, prescription, nonprescription, and illicit, including dosage and frequency. Many patients will not think to mention over-the-counter medications such as aspirin and ibuprofen, which may be important due to platelet inhibition.

Allergies. List allergies to medications and the reaction the patient had to the medication. Nausea and diarrhea from an oral antibiotic may not preclude an antibiotic from parenteral administration.

Past Medical History. Include any medical conditions of which the patient is aware. Ask whether the patient is being treated for any problems with the heart, blood pressure, lungs, liver, kidneys, diabetes (if the patient is an insulin-dependent diabetic, it is important to know the degree of control of the glucose level), neurologic system, or thyroid. Also ask if there have been any changes in bowel, bladder, or sexual function. Usually, the patient can inform the clinician if there is a significant medical problem. Also obtain a history of childhood illnesses, past injuries, previous hospitalizations (when, where, and for what purpose), and immunization history.

Review of Systems. In addition to the past medical history, a review of systems is performed to evaluate for any symptoms that may indicate an underlying disorder. Include all major organ systems with the common symptoms and disorders of each system. The patient may not mention certain symptoms or conditions (due to embarrassment or lack of knowledge) if not directly asked.

1

Previous Operations. Obtain a list of all operations the patient has undergone, including the hospital, type of anesthetic used (e.g., general, spinal, or local), and any difficulties the patient might have experienced during or after the surgery. Remember that history often repeats itself!

Social History. Obtain a history of the patient's occupation, which may contain risks for certain conditions (e.g., pulmonary disease in the coal miner). It is important to note any special diet (e.g., diabetic, low salt, vegetarian) in order to continue the diet postoperatively. Obtain a history of exercise habits or lack thereof. History of tobacco use (smoking or chewing) is necessary to note for anesthesia considerations and to counsel the patient postoperatively. A history of alcohol use (quantity and frequency) should be obtained to plan for the possibility of delirium tremens postoperatively. Risk for human immunodeficiency virus (HIV) infection (e.g., intravenous drug users, homosexual men, those who have undergone blood transfusions, and those with multiple sexual partners), despite the controversial nature surrounding the question, should be established. The question should be phrased in a nonthreatening manner. The question should not be used to exclude a patient from surgical treatment, but as a health concern so that additional precautions can be instituted when coming into contact with the patient's blood or serum. The adage that clinicians should take the same precautions regardless of the patient is not entirely true (one tends to drive more cautiously on New Year's Eve than on Sunday mornings).

Family History. A family history should be obtained, including major medical conditions such as diabetes, thyroid disease, neurologic abnormalities, heart disease, liver disease, gastrointestinal disease, bleeding abnormalities, lung disease, kidney disease, hypertension, trouble with anesthetic agents, or unexplained intraoperative death in order to perform any additional screening measures to prevent complications.

PREOPERATIVE ASSESSMENT

LABORATORY

Baseline studies are important to obtain prior to anesthesia and surgery. The specific studies may vary by institutional policy and patient age; however, routine studies would include:

Complete Blood Count. Evaluation for anemia or infectious processes.

PT/PTT. Usually obtained to evaluate clotting mechanism, particularly in patients with hepatic disease. The standard bleeding time, along with history and physical examination, is a much better predictor of bleeding tendency.

Chemistry Panel. A full chemistry profile is obtained, including electrolytes and liver function studies, as a screening measure for any abnormalities.

Urinalysis. Important to rule out an infection that may increase the risk of wound infection or the presence of urinary sediment, which may reveal early renal failure.

Chest X-ray.   Indicated for individuals over the age of 35 or those with significant pulmonary disease, cardiac disease, or a history of trauma.

ECG.   Usually obtained in patients over the age of 35 or performed at a younger age if a history of cardiac disease is noted.

ABG and Screening Pulmonary Function Tests.   FVC and FEV should be obtained on patients with a history of COPD, including responses to bronchodilators. This is especially important in patients undergoing general anesthesia.

PHYSICAL EXAMINATION

The physical examination should be complete and thorough, including inspection, palpation, and auscultation. Although the tendency may be to perform a focused, problem-oriented history and physical examination, remember that the surgical problem for which the patient has sought care may be his or her only medical encounter (particularly for the young or indigent patient, who may not have a regular health care provider). Note the patient's appearance, level of distress, age, sex, affect, and any unusual position or posture. Obtain vital signs including temperature, pulse, respirations, and blood pressure (include orthostatic measurements) and perform a complete and thorough physical examination.

PREOPERATIVE CHARTING

INFORMED CONSENT

With the possible exception of an emergency in which no family member is available, it is imperative that permission be obtained for any surgical procedure. The nature of the procedure and the anticipated results, as well as the possible risks, associated with the operation must be discussed in detail with the patient, family, and/or legal guardian. It is always a good idea to discuss the surgical procedure with a family member, especially in the case of a major operation or trauma when the risk of unfavorable outcome is relatively high.

In addition to the institutional consent form, a note that outlines the history, physical examination and radiologic findings that support the proposed surgery, followed by an explanation of the risks associated with the surgery and the fact that the risks, benefits, and rationale for the procedure have been explained to the patient should be written out. This should then be signed and witnessed by the patient or guardian.

PREOPERATIVE ORDERS

Preoperative orders are written to provide instructions to the medical staff and patient as to what needs to be done in anticipation of surgery.

Frequently, the patient who is scheduled to undergo an elective procedure is seen in an outpatient setting in the hospital several days before surgery to obtain instructions, have the necessary laboratory and radiologic studies performed, and meet with the anesthesiologist. Communication needs to be established so the surgeon's needs and preferences can be addressed in the preoperative setting.

Diet. Standard practice involves a patient being kept NPO after midnight for early morning surgery—clear liquid diet breakfast may be satisfactory for patients who are scheduled for an afternoon surgery. Those patients scheduled for bowel surgery will require low residue and subsequent liquid diet for several days preoperatively.

IV Fluids. Preoperative IV fluids are unnecessary in uncomplicated, elective surgery. In the elderly or diabetic individual, preoperative hydration is indicated.

Bowel Preparation. A 10-mg bisacodyl (Dulcolax) suppository or sodium phosphate (Fleet) enema is given the evening prior to any procedure that may produce an ileus (e.g., abdominal, retroperitoneal, or extensive lumbar procedures). Bowel surgery likely will require more extensive preparation, including oral cathartics and enemas.

Skin Preparation. The past practice of shaving the operative site the evening prior to surgery has fallen into disfavor because this causes microscopic abrasions and is more likely to increase bacterial colony counts. The preparation of the surgical field should be done in the operating room.

Laboratory. Morning laboratory studies on the day of surgery should include electrolytes and glucose in the diabetic patient, as well as a creatinine level in individuals with renal compromise. Other tests may be specific for the patient problem (e.g., PT/PTT for a patient on an anticoagulant).

Urine. For elective procedures of short duration, the patient should void on call to the operating room. As a matter of patient comfort, a urinary catheter can be inserted after the patient is anesthetized, particularly for lengthy surgical procedures, or if an extended period of postoperative bedrest is anticipated.

Blood. The use of blood and blood products has been curtailed intraoperatively in light of patient concerns regarding hepatitis and HIV exposure. Many products, such as 6% hetastarch, are available for use as intraoperative volume expanders. The routine expense of crossmatching blood is unnecessary and should be replaced by a type and screen if a transfusion is believed to be unlikely. For those surgical procedures in which a transfusion is likely to be needed, an autologous donation should be considered. This can be arranged through the American Red Cross with directed donation of one unit of blood per week beginning up to 45 days prior to the proposed surgery. The patient should not donate blood the week prior to the surgery and must be maintained on an iron and folate supplement.

Respiratory. Patients with significant COPD, history of tobacco abuse, obesity, or advanced age are at increased risk for perioperative pulmonary complications such as atelectasis, pneumonia, or respiratory failure. Pulmonary testing should include ABG for hypoxia and CO_2 retention. FVC (forced vital capacity) and FEV_1 (forced expiratory volume in 1 second) should be obtained, and those with significant disease (<50% of predicted) should be started on bronchodilators and incentive spirometry. Marked prevention of respiratory complications can be accomplished with the cessation of smoking 24 to 48 hours prior to surgery.

Medications.   The evening prior to surgery, an anxiolytic agent may be prescribed. Morning medications should include the routine home medications such as antihypertensive agents (particularly the beta blockers, which can be associated with a withdrawal tachycardia). Cardiac medications should be administered in the morning in their usual dose. Intravenous vasodilators such as nitroglycerin (Tridil) or antiarrhythmic agents such as lidocaine can be used in addition to the patient's routine home medication, if necessary. Mild diuretic agents may be held on the morning of surgery.

Diabetics, as a general rule, are given half of their usual dose of NPH and regular insulin on the morning of surgery, provided that their procedure is done early in the day, and they are maintained on a dextrose-containing IV solution. Serial accuchecks are necessary perioperatively. An alternative approach, particularly for lengthy procedures or in brittle diabetics, would be an IV solution of 1 unit of regular insulin per 10 ml of fluid that can be administered continuously. This usually is instituted at 1 unit of insulin per hour and is adjusted based on the results of frequent glucose analysis.

Routine corticosteroid use requires special consideration, given the stress of surgery. An acceptable regimen might include cortisol 100 mg IV preoperatively and 50 mg IV every 6 h during the surgery and during the immediate recovery period. Particular attention is paid to fluid and electrolyte status, as well as the potential for hyperglycemia.

Antibiotics.   The standard for antibiotic use in "clean" surgery would be cefazolin 1 g IV 30 to 60 minutes prior to the incision and repeated approximately 3 to 4 hours later. The use and selection of pre-, intra-, and postoperative antibiotics is somewhat controversial and largely a matter of surgeon preference. Antibiotics can be given at the onset of the procedure, intraoperatively, or continued for a period of time postoperatively.

POSTOPERATIVE NOTE

A postoperative note is written in the progress notes at the conclusion of the procedure to document the diagnosis, intraoperative findings, procedure performed, individuals involved, type of anesthesia used, fluid status, drains placed, any complications encountered, and the patient's disposition. A generally established format is:

Preoperative Diagnosis.   The diagnosis for which the patient was being treated.

Postoperative Diagnosis.   This may be the same as the preoperative diagnosis or may have changed, dependent upon intraoperative findings.

Procedure.   The name of the procedure that was performed.

Surgeon.   The name of the surgeon(s) performing the procedure.

Assistant/Physician Assistant. The names of any assistants who were present (surgeons, residents, interns, PAs).

Anesthesia. The type of anesthesia used (general, regional, or local) and the attending anesthesiologist.

Fluids Administered. A tabulation of intake and output, including blood and blood products.

Estimate of Blood Loss. Include blood in the suction canister as well as blood on any sponges used.

Drains (Size and Location). Any drains remaining in place after the procedure. These may need to be monitored on the floor or in the ICU.

Findings. A brief description of the operative findings, including specimens and preliminary pathology reports.

Complications. Any untoward events encountered during the procedure.

Disposition/Condition. Include a brief description of how the patient responded to the procedure (e.g., stable, critical, guarded). Also include where the patient went after surgery (e.g., patient transferred to the recovery room in stable condition).

POSTOPERATIVE ORDERS

Postoperative orders are written to ensure compliance with all treatments necessary in the postoperative period. Orders should be concise and terms such as "routine vital signs" should be avoided. Every aspect of the patient's care is listed in the postoperative orders (e.g., if a diet is not ordered, the patient does not eat). A common mnemonic (ADD-VAN-DISL) is used when writing these orders so that nothing is omitted.

Admit. To the recovery room, ICU, floor, etc.

Diet. NPO, clear liquids, diabetic, or other special dietary needs.

Diagnosis. The primary diagnosis followed by any secondary diagnoses.

Vital Signs/Monitoring. The frequency that staff will assess blood pressure, pulse, respirations, and temperature (initially, every 15 to 30 minutes for the first 4 to 6 hours after surgery, then periodically thereafter, depending on the complexity of the surgery). Also include specific measurements such as CVP, Swan-Ganz catheters, or ICP monitors. The assessment of neurologic status or extremity pulses would be described here.

Activity. Out of bed as tolerated, bedrest, bathroom privileges, weight bearing status, assistance of therapists or nursing staff.

Nursing. Include patient care items such as surgical drains, Foley catheter, anti-embolic stockings, or sequential compression devices. Make a notation regarding the positioning of the patient or his or her extremity as indicated.

Drugs. All medications that are indicated must be specified on the postoperative orders, including usual home medications that are deemed appropriate. Other agents to order include antinauseants, antipyretics, antibiotics, sedatives, and analgesics (see Pain Management below). Postoperative respiratory medication such as inhaled bronchodilators may be necessary. Remember steroid replacement and sliding scale insulin regimens in steroid-dependent or diabetic patients.

IV Fluids. Postoperative hydration is needed until a patient is able to tolerate oral fluids. Ideal maintenance fluids would be 1.2 to 1.5 ml/kg/hr, with added fluids based on output from surgical drains, nasogastric tubes, and insensible loss from fever or "third spacing."

Special. This is a catch-all category and includes any order that does not fit into the other categories. Special considerations for the specific surgical type are written here. Items include speech therapy, nutritional consult, other specialty consults, informing the primary physician of the patient's room number, etc.

Laboratory/Radiology. Request the needed laboratory studies such as hemoglobin and hematocrit after significant blood loss. Electrolytes, glucose, and renal function tests are ordered for diabetic, renal compromised, or other patients who require serologic monitoring.

Chest x-ray is performed following central line placement or bony evaluation following an orthopedic procedure. Other radiologic studies, as indicated, may be ordered.

POSTANESTHESIA CONSIDERATIONS

After the completion of the surgical procedure, the patient arrives in the recovery room or postoperative holding area. An assessment of the patient's condition is performed and should include the patient's level of consciousness (especially important in neurosurgery), vital signs, and an evaluation of the incision. It is not uncommon for patients to have fluctuations in their vital signs in the postanesthesia period. Hypertension, hypotension, or hypothermia may occur and should be identified and treated as indicated in conjunction with the anesthesia team. The anesthesiologist should be involved in any postanesthesia management in the recovery room, because he or she is familiar with anesthetic agents used during the procedure.

FOLLOW-UP NOTE

It is a good idea to check the patient after the patient has been discharged from the recovery room, to make sure he or she is experiencing a satisfactory recovery. The patient frequently will not recall any discussion attempted in the recovery room and will appreciate the follow-up visit and discussion of the procedure. A progress note is written after this visit and the format is as follows:

Procedure
Level of consciousness
Vital signs
Intake and output (including surgical drains)

Laboratory results

Examination of the chest, heart, abdomen, extremities, level of consciousness, and dressings

Assessment

Plan

DAILY PROGRESS NOTE

The patient is seen daily following a surgical procedure and a note is written to chart the patient's progress. The following information should be included:

General description of the patient's condition, including mental alertness, mood, activity, and pain relief

Vital signs

Physical examination findings

Intake and output measurements, as indicated, which include specifics on tubes and drains

Respiratory status

Intestinal function, especially important in abdominal procedures, should include tolerance of liquid or food, presence of distention, passing flatus or stool, and physical findings

Wounds and dressing description, such as dry and intact, the presence of blood or drainage, etc.

Laboratory evaluation performed as indicated and results charted

Special observations relevant to the procedure

Complications not previously mentioned

Overall assessment and plans for changes in treatment plan

Another method for charting progress is by using the SOAP method (Subjective, Objective, Assessment, and Plan):

S: How the patient describes his or her condition, a direct quote from the patient may be used

O: Any objective data, including laboratory or radiologic results, physical examination findings, etc.

A: Includes diagnosis and an impression of the patient's course

P: What course of action is to be taken; include any orders written to aid in communication with other medical personnel reading the chart.

PAIN MANAGEMENT

In the postoperative period, patients may experience considerable pain. Adequate analgesia should be supplied to patients to lessen discomfort, but in some instances (e.g., neurosurgery) it is important to avoid sedation in order to evaluate the patient for mental status changes. It is also important not to overdose the patient and depress vital signs.

Analgesic dosage should correspond to the level of expected discomfort, the patient's condition, patient age, and the route of delivery. Oral non-narcotic (e.g., nonsteroidal anti-inflammatory drugs or acetaminophen) or narcotic analgesics can be ordered for patients undergoing outpatient procedures, whereas intravenous or intramuscular agents may be used for inpatients. Table 1–1 provides a listing of the pharmacokinetics of common analgesics.

Many oral narcotic analgesics are combined with aspirin or acetaminophen. It is usually necessary to avoid aspirin-containing medications in the postoperative period.

A relatively recent innovation is the use of a patient-controlled analgesia (PCA) pump. As the name implies, the patient is able to control his or her own analgesic dose. The pump itself contains a vial of analgesic (morphine sulfate, hydromorphone, or meperidine) and is programmed to allow delivery of a set dose of analgesic within a specified time frame. When the patient experiences pain, he or she may push a button, which administers a set dose of the analgesic. The pump is programmed not to exceed a maximum dose per hour. A basal rate (continuous infusion) may be ordered, which allows a continuous flow of a small amount of medication. Figure 1–1 is an example of a PCA order sheet. Figure 1–2 provides guidelines in dosing the PCA pump. If the patient is young and healthy, a higher dose and shorter delay may be ordered. Conversely, if the patient is elderly or in poor condition, a lower dose and longer delay is used.

POSTOPERATIVE COMPLICATIONS

FEVER

Fever is a common postoperative occurrence with a lengthy list of possible sources. A helpful thought process for evaluating the source of fever is the five Ws:

Wind: Atelectasis is the most common cause of fever during the first postoperative day. Other causes might include pneumonia (aspiration or bacterial)

Water: Urinary tract infection, particularly associated with indwelling catheters

Wound: Usually occurs 7 to 10 days after surgery, although necrotizing streptococcal infections can occur within hours after closing a wound

Walking: Deep vein thrombophlebitis and catheter-induced infection (line sepsis)

Wonder drugs: Fever associated with medications, particularly perioperative use of atropine

Treatment. Treatment involves identifying the source of the fever and correcting the underlying problem. Cultures of blood, urine, and sputum may be considered for postoperative fever and antibiotics used as appropriate. Incentive spirometry every hour while awake should be considered for those at risk for atelectasis. Removal of urinary catheters as soon as

Text continued on page 14

Table 1–1. Pharmacokinetics (Absorption, Distribution, Metabolism, Elimination)

Drug	Route	Dosing Interval	Onset of Action	Duration of Action	Excreted Unchanged	Elimination Half-life	Route of Elimination
				Narcotic Analgesics			
Butorphanol	IM	3–4 h	10–15 min	3–4 h	<5%	3–4 h	60–80% Renal/11–14% fecal
	IV	3–4 h	1 min	2–4 h			
	Inhal	3–4 h	15 min	4–5 h			
Codeine	PO	4–6 h	15–30 min	4–6 h	7%	2.5–4 h	Renal
	IM, SC	4–6 h	15–30 min	4–6 h			
Dezocine	IM	3–6 h	30 min	2–6 h	1%	—	66% Renal
	IV	2–4 h	15 min				
Fentanyl	IM	1–2 h	7–8 min	1–2 h	<10%	3.6 h	75% Renal/9% fecal
	Patch	48–72 h	24 h	—	92%	—	
Hydrocodone	PO	4–6 h	10–30 min	4–6 h	—	3.8 h	Renal
Hydromorphone	PO	4–6 h	30 min	4–5 h	<10%	1.8–3.5 h	Renal
	IM, SC	4–6 h	15–30 min	4–5 h			
	IV	—	<15 min	4–5 h			
Levorphanol	PO	6–8 h	10–60 min	6–8 h	<10%	11 h	Renal
	SC	6–8 h	60–90 min	6–8 h			
Meperidine	PO	3–4 h	15 min	2–4 h	1–25%	2.4–4 h	Renal
	IM, SC	3–4 h	10–15 min	2–4 h			
	IV	—	1 min	2–4 h			
Morphine	PO	4 h	<60 min	4–5 h	6–10%	1.5–2 h	85–90% Renal/10% fecal
	PO*	8–12 h	<60 min	8–12 h			
	SC	4 h	<50–90 min	4–5 h			
	IM	4 h	<30–60 min	4–5 h			
	IV	—	<20 min	4–5 h			
	Rectal	4 h	<20–60 min	4–5 h			
	IV	3–6 h	2–3 min	3–6 h			

	Route						Biliary/renal
Nalbuphine	IM, SC	3–6 h	<15 min	3–6 h	7%	5 h	
	IV						
Oxycodone	PO	6 h	10–15 min	3–6 h	—	2–3 h	Renal
Oxymorphone	IM, SC	4–6 h	10–15 min	3–6 h	<10%	—	Renal
	IV	4–6 h	5–10 min	3–6 h			
	Rectal	4–6 h	15–30 min	3–6 h			
Pentazocine	PO	4 h	15–30 min	3–4 h	<13%	2–3 h	Renal
	IM, SC	3–4 h	15–20 min	2 h			
	IV	3–4 h	2–3 min	1 h			
Propoxyphene	PO	4 h	15–60 min	4–6 h	25%	6–12 h	Renal

Narcotic Antagonists

Naloxone	IM, SC	2–3 min	>2 min	—	—	—	Renal
	IV		2 min				

Non-Narcotic Analgesics/Nonsteroidal Anti-Inflammatory Agents

Acetaminophen	PO	4–6 h	10–60 min	4–6 h	3%	1.6–2.4 h	Renal
Diclofenac	PO*	12–24 h	2–3 h	10 h	0%	2 h	65% Renal/35% biliary
Diflunisal	PO	8–12 h	1 h	8–12 h	10%	8–12 h	Renal
Etodolac	PO	6–8 h	30 min	4–6 h	1%	—	72% Renal
Fenoprofen	PO	6–8 h	15–30 min	4–6 h	10%	3 h	Renal
Ibuprofen	PO	4–6 h	30 min	4–6 h	<10%	1.8–2 h	Renal
Indomethacin	PO	8–12 h	7–14 days	—	30%	4.5 h	60% Renal/33% fecal
Ketoprofen	PO	6–8 h	—	—	—	2–4 h	60% Renal/40% fecal
Ketorolac	IM	6 h	—	3.8–6.3 h	58%	4.5 h	91% Renal/6% fecal
	PO	4–6 h	10 min	>3 h	—	6 h	91% Renal/6% fecal
Meclofenamate	PO	4–6 h	—	—	<5%	3.3 h	66% Renal/33% fecal
Mefenamic acid	PO	6 h	—	—	67%	2 h	67% Renal/20–25% fecal
Naproxen	PO	12 h	2 h	<7 h	<1%	13 h	Renal

Table continued on following page

Table 1–1. Pharmacokinetics (Absorption, Distribution, Metabolism, Elimination) (*Continued*)

Drug	Route	Dosing Interval	Onset of Action	Duration of Action	Excreted Unchanged	Elimination Half-life	Route of Elimination
Narcotic Analgesics							
Nonnarcotic Analgesics/Nonsteroidal Anti-Inflammatory Agents							
Naproxen sodium	PO	6–8 h	1 h	<7 h	<1%	13 h	Renal
Salicylates	PO	4 h	<30 min	3–6 h	2–80%	2–19 h	Renal
Sedatives							
Butalbital	PO	4 h	—	—	—	—	—
Promethazine	PO	4–6 h	20 min	≤12 h	—	—	Renal
	IM	3–4 h		4–6 h			

*Indicates oral administration of sustained-, controlled-, or extended-release forms.

Data from Compendium of Drug Therapy, Physician Assistant edition, Chapter 3: Analgesics/Antipyretics/Migraine Treatment and Prophylaxis. Secaucus, NJ, Compendium Publications Group, 1995, pp 3.1–11.

SAMPLE PCA PRESCRIPTION

PCA dosing

Mode of operation   PCA/basal

Drug	Morphine 1 mg/ml	_____ml
	Meperidine 10 mg/ml	_____ml
	Hydromorphone 0.2 mg/ml	_____ml

Dose volume   Range 0.1 to 9.9 ml   _____ml

Delay interval   Range 3 to 60 min   _____ml

Basal rate   Range 0 to 10 ml/hour   _____ml

One hour limit   Range 1.0 to 30 ml   _____ml

Bolus loading   Range 0.1 to 9.9 ml   _____ml

Other orders

Consult analgesia support team

PCA flow sheet instructions

IV fluids to be given with analgesic

Narcan ampule (0.4 mg) to be immediately available during PCA therapy

Measures to be taken if the patient continues to complain of pain

Call_____ if respiratory rate is less than 8 per minute
                       inadequate pain relief
                       excessive sedation
                       nausea and vomiting

Hold all orders for hypnotics, sedatives, antiemetics, antipruritics, sleeping
  pills, or other narcotics unless approved by_____and/or
  attending physician

Oxygen 4 liters via nasal cannula or 50% face shield (unless otherwise
  specified) for 24 hours post-op

May give droperidol 0.625 (0.25 ml) IV prn nausea and vomiting. May repeat
  every 15 minutes x 2 for a total of 3 doses

For recurrent nausea and vomiting, may repeat droperidol every 4 to 6 hours

May give Benadryl 25 mg IM every 4 to 6 hours prn itching

For respiratory rate less than or equal to 8 *and* unresponsiveness
                Give Narcan 0.25 ml(0.1 mg) IV every 5 minutes until
                  respiratory rate is greater than 10
                Call_____and/or attending physician STAT

Until PCA is available, may give _____

Change basal rate to 0.0 ml/hour at _____(time/date)
  unless otherwise specified

Figure 1–1. Sample PCA Prescription form. Courtesy of
Fred Yilling, MD, and Brenda Duger, RN.

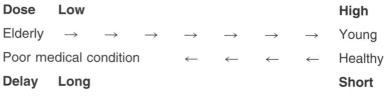

Figure 1–2. Guidelines in dosing the PCA pump.

possible lessens the risk of urinary tract infections. Meticulous attention to sterile technique and wound closure decreases the chance of incisional complications. The use of sequential compression hose for those at risk for deep vein thrombosis (e.g., patients requiring prolonged bedrest) helps prevent thromboembolism. Knowledge of medications used in the operating room also helps the clinician identify the source of a fever. Antipyretics such as acetaminophen (Tylenol) and the use of a cooling blanket may be used to control persistent fever.

ATELECTASIS

Atelectasis is defined as the collapse of pulmonary alveoli, usually occurring in the base segments of the lungs. It is more common following abdominal procedures, in obese patients, or in those individuals who remain at bedrest. It manifests as diminished breath sounds that improve with deeper inspiration.

Treatment. Treatment consists of incentive spirometry and mobilization.

ASPIRATION PNEUMONIA OR PNEUMONITIS

Aspiration pneumonia or pneumonitis, a secondary infection that usually occurs in patients with a diminished level of consciousness, usually follows anesthesia or trauma. Aspiration of gastric contents with a low pH causes an immediate chemical reaction that may subsequently lead to infection.

Treatment. Treatment is primarily aimed at prevention, including proper NPO status, patient positioning, and H_2 blockers (in high-risk patients). Individuals who have aspirated are usually started on IV steroids to reduce the chemical pneumonitis. Prophylactic antibiotics are used, because the majority of these patients subsequently develop a pneumonia.

PNEUMONIA

Pneumonia develops as the result of atelectasis, aspiration, or pre-existing pulmonary disease that does not allow secretions to be cleared. It usually manifests as fever, tachypnea, and localized rales or rhonchi on auscultation. The chest radiograph frequently demonstrates an infiltrate.

Treatment. Treatment consists of incentive spirometry, frequent lavage and suction, and antibiotics, based on the results of bronchotracheal culture and sensitivity testing.

PULMONARY EMBOLISM

Pulmonary embolism is defined as a thrombus that has migrated to the pulmonary vasculature. It usually occurs in postoperative patients who require extended bedrest or in those patients with extensive pelvic or lower extremity surgery. It usually manifests as tachypnea, dyspnea, and tachycardia, and frequently is associated with hypoxia. The clinical diagnosis is confirmed by a lung perfusion (VQ) scan or pulmonary arteriography.

Treatment. Treatment includes supplemental oxygen and analgesia. Heparinization is begun, except in the immediate postoperative period, during which time an inferior vena caval filter can be placed percutaneously. The use of sequential compression devices and early mobilization are important in the prevention of pulmonary emboli.

HYPOTENSION

Hypotension, particularly orthostatic changes with associated tachycardia and low urine output in the immediate postoperative period, is a concern for bleeding. The abdomen, thorax, and the pelvis can accommodate a large amount of blood without obvious clinical signs. Other causes of hypotension include medication effect, allergic reaction, myocardial infarction, dysrhythmia, or pulmonary embolus.

Treatment. Intravenous access and volume replacement is used to maintain blood pressure. Careful evaluation is undertaken to rule out other causes, and re-operation may be necessary for hemodynamically significant postoperative hemorrhage.

HYPERTENSION

Hypertension is aggravated by incisional pain or due to the discontinuance of routine antihypertensive agents.

Treatment. Resume the usual antihypertensive medication. For mild elevations in blood pressure associated with complaints of severe pain, appropriate analgesics may suffice. Oral nifedipine, 10 mg every 4 to 6 hours, or intravenous agents such as nitroprusside can be used for persistent elevations of blood pressure.

MYOCARDIAL INFARCTION

Myocardial infarction may present atypically due to the lingering effects of anesthesia and may manifest simply as hypotension or dysrhythmia. This can be precipitated by periods of hypoxia or hypotension in the perioperative period. The diagnosis is confirmed with electrocardiography and serologic evaluation for cardiac isoenzymes.

Treatment. Treatment consists of continuous ECG monitoring for potential arrhythmia with the cautious use of nitrates and analgesics for chest pain.

VOMITING

Vomiting immediately after surgery is common, and frequently is due to the anesthesia or gastric distention. Later in the postoperative period, vomiting may be related to an ileus or intestinal obstruction.

Treatment. Treatment consists of antiemetic agents or nasogastric drainage. Common antiemetics/antinauseants include:

Prochlorperazine (Compazine), PO, IM, IV
Promethazine (Phenergan), PO, rectally, IV, or IM
Scopolamine (Transderm Scōp), transcutaneous
Trimethobenzamide (Tigan), PO, rectally, or IM

ABDOMINAL DISTENTION

Abdominal distention can be caused by a paralytic ileus, which is frequently seen after trauma or after abdominal, retroperitoneal, or lumbar surgery. The diagnosis is based on the degree of distention, minimal to absent bowel sounds, and the radiographic appearance of diffuse gas in the stomach, small intestine, and colon.

Care must be taken to rule out a gastric or intestinal obstruction, which is associated with cramping pain. Vomiting is common with gastric or small bowel obstruction. Colonic obstruction usually is not a cause for vomiting until very late stages. Radiographs may demonstrate colonic or cecal distention.

Treatment. Treatment includes nasogastric drainage, fluid resuscitation and, in small bowel obstruction, may include a long intestinal tube (e.g., Miller-Abbott tube). Laparotomy may be necessary if the obstruction fails to resolve.

URINARY RETENTION

Urinary retention is a common occurrence after pelvic or perineal surgery, as well as after surgery using a spinal anesthetic. The presence of prostatic hypertrophy is exacerbated by the use of atropine or similar medications perioperatively.

Treatment. Treatment involves intermittent bladder catheterization every 6 hours. Volumes of over 1000 ml indicate the placement of an indwelling catheter for continuous drainage over 2 to 3 days. A catheter should be placed preoperatively in any surgery that is expected to last for greater than 3 hours in order to avoid overdistending the bladder.

RENAL FAILURE/OLIGURIA

Renal failure/oliguria is defined as urine output of less than 20 ml/hour, which can be due to extrinsic or intrinsic factors. Extrinsic causes of oliguria can be broken down into prerenal and postrenal categories. Prerenal causes include decreased intravascular volume secondary to bleeding, hypotension, or dehydration (from vomiting, diarrhea, or third spacing of fluids from surgery or injury). Postrenal causes include a faulty urinary catheter, prostatic hypertrophy, ureteral obstruction, or retroperitoneal pathology.

The intrinsic form of oliguria is acute renal failure, which can occur secondary to renovascular thrombosis, hypotension, sepsis, or nephrotoxins. The differentiating features between the intrinsic and extrinsic causes are that intrinsic factors cause a urine sodium greater than 20 mEq/L and the presence of urinary sediment, including casts.

Treatment. Treatment consists of correcting the underlying cause, particularly the extrinsic causes of oliguria. In intrinsic or acute renal failure, an assessment of overall volume status is necessary. If there is no evidence of a volume overload, then treatment consists of increasing prerenal blood flow, using IV fluids to elevate the central venous pressure (CVP) and a continuous infusion of dopamine at 2 mg/kg/hr. This is followed by diuresis using furosemide (Lasix) or mannitol. Serial blood samples are needed to monitor electrolytes, BUN and creatinine, and an indwelling Foley catheter to monitor the urine output. Dialysis may become necessary in cases of hyperkalemia or significant acidosis.

INCISIONAL SEROMA

Seroma is defined as a fluid collection under the skin edge, particularly with dissection near lymph nodes and under flaps. This subsequently may delay healing and increase the risks of infection.

Treatment. Treatment includes needle aspiration and placement of a compressive dressing. Some instances of persistent seroma require surgical exploration and ligation of a lymphatic duct.

INCISIONAL HEMATOMA

An incisional hematoma is a collection of blood and blood clot underlying the surgical site. This frequently is the result of poor hemostasis of a blood vessel that may have been in spasm during the surgical procedure. This is most critical after procedures on the neck, where an expanding hematoma can cause compromise of the airway. The hematoma can also jeopardize wound flaps and can increase the risk for wound infection.

Treatment. Treatment consists of control of local bleeding either with pressure, cautery, or suture ligation. The expanding hematoma, which is usually seen in the immediate postoperative period, must be surgically drained.

INCISIONAL INFECTION

Incisional infection is usually manifest by the presence of erythema, swelling, pain, and drainage at the surgical site. This usually occurs about 7 to 10 days postoperatively, although it can occur earlier. Many factors contribute to a wound infection, including age, obesity, autoimmune conditions, and medical illnesses, as well as wound characteristics such as a hematoma or seroma, necrosis, wound tension, and the nature of the surgery (e.g., clean vs. contaminated).

Treatment.   Treatment involves opening the wound in order to allow drainage of the purulent material and to determine the depth or extent of the infection. Systemic antibiotics are not always necessary in the superficial infection with the absence of surrounding cellulitis or fever. The infectious organism most often is a gram-positive cocci such as *Staphylococcus* or *Streptococcus,* except in contaminated wounds, where a polymicrobial infection is likely. The recommended antibiotic regimen for a nonseptic patient would include cefazolin 1 to 2 gm IV every 8 h. Specific antibiotic therapy is dependent upon culture and sensitivity results. For those patients who underwent a surgical procedure on the gastrointestinal tract, a regimen of a second- or third-generation cephalosporin along with metronidazole would be recommended.

INCISIONAL DEHISCENCE

Dehiscence usually is evident on examination of the wound. It may take the form of a superficial dehiscence or a complete dehiscence, with or without evisceration. This occurs most frequently at approximately postoperative day 5 to 8, and may be preceded by a bout of coughing or vomiting. An early sign of a superficial wound dehiscence includes serosanguinous drainage. Dehiscence occurs more frequently in older patients with multiple medical illnesses, immunosuppression, or obesity.

Treatment.   For a superficial dehiscence, treatment involves local wound care, including packing with iodophor gauze to allow the wound to heal by secondary intention. A total dehiscence requires a return to the operating room for exploration and the closure of the wound with heavy nylon retention sutures.

Further Reading
The Physician Assistant's Compendium of Drug Therapy. New York, Compendium Publications Group, 1994.

Sanford JP, Gilbert DN, Sande MA: The Sanford Guide to Antimicrobial Therapy, 25th ed. Dallas, Antimicrobial Therapy, Inc., 1995.

Schwartz SI, et al: Principles of Surgery, 6th ed. New York, McGraw-Hill, 1994.

Way LW: Current Surgical Diagnosis and Treatment, 10th ed. Norwalk, CT, Appleton and Lange, 1994.

Chapter **2**
Anesthesia
Rhea Sumpter, PA, MMSc

Anesthesia is defined as that condition in which an individual is rendered insensible to a painful stimulus. Improvements in the delivery of anesthesia over the past 50 years have been most remarkable. Today's pharmacologic agents may be more receptor specific, cause fewer undesirable side effects, and have a shorter duration of action. Technological advances such as pulse oximetry, capnography, and hemodynamic monitoring have resulted in greater safety to a more diverse patient population, as well as accommodate more demanding surgical procedures.

In 1969, specialty-trained PAs employed under the supervision of an anesthesiologist became part of the anesthesia care team. We are now valuable participants in this exciting and challenging profession. The following information is designed for the surgical PA in order that he or she may have a better understanding of how the anesthesia team interacts with the surgical patient.

THE ANESTHESIA CONSULT

An anesthetist's first interaction with the surgical patient is usually initiated after receiving a request from the surgical team for an anesthesia consult. There are three major reasons for participating in an anesthesia consult: (1) to obtain pertinent information in order to develop an anesthetic plan; (2) to establish an anesthetist–patient relationship; and (3) to help allay anxieties that the patient may have about being anesthetized.

A thorough review of the patient's chart, an understanding of the proposed surgical procedure, and the patient interview are major determinants in selecting that most suitable anesthesia technique for the patient. The choices are between a general anesthetic, a regional anesthetic, monitored anesthesia care (MAC) with sedation, or a combination of the above. The patient's chart should contain information as to why the anesthesia consult was requested and the extent of the proposed surgical procedure. When available, important information such as weight, height, vital signs, history and physical, laboratory data, electrocardiogram (ECG), chest x-ray, and previous anesthesia records should be reviewed prior to the patient interview. This preview may help direct questioning into areas that may be of special concern. The patient interview usually begins with an introduction to the patient and with an explanation that an anesthesia consult been requested by the surgeon to provide anesthesia during the surgical procedure. The patient is informed that vital signs will be monitored and every effort to keep him or her safe and comfortable throughout the surgery will be undertaken. After taking a brief history and physical examination, the risks and benefits of the anesthetic options are discussed, and any questions are answered in regard to the anesthetic plan.

PREOPERATIVE HISTORY

The preoperative history usually begins with questions relevant to the proposed surgical procedure. The patient's responses provide insight as to his or her understanding of the procedure and furnish information as to the severity of the problem. The preoperative history includes a review of the major organ systems, the history of previous anesthetics and surgeries, family history of any anesthetic complications, a list of current medications, and a history of any allergies.

Review of Systems

A review of the major organ systems is directed toward areas that are of concern. The following is a typical review of systems that may influence anesthetic management.

Cardiovascular

Angina. The patient with a history of unstable angina has an increased risk of having an intraoperative or perioperative ischemic event. It is important to know what precipitates the angina, the frequency and duration of the attacks, and what relieves the angina (e.g., rest and/or medications). From this information, more advanced cardiovascular monitoring or pharmacologic support or both may be selected. For all cardiac patients, the goal is to increase the oxygen supply to the heart and to avoid situations that increase the oxygen demand by the heart (e.g., tachycardia and hypertension).

Myocardial Infarction. The morbidity and mortality associated with a recent myocardial infarction is greatest within the first 6 months. The extent of myocardial damage and the presence of existing symptoms, such as congestive heart failure (CHF) or exercise intolerance, are major determinants in formulating the anesthetic plan. These patients may also require more hemodynamic monitoring and pharmacologic intevention.

Dysrhythmias. Anesthesia management of the patient with a history of atrial or ventricular dysrhythmias may be challenging, especially if the dysrhythmias are of recent onset and are not well controlled. An unstable condition may cause wide swings in heart rate and blood pressure. The goal is to avoid those anesthetic agents that sensitize the myocardium to dysrhythmias or adversely alter cardiac conduction. Hemodynamics and electrolyte balance must be properly maintained and preparations made to treat malignant dysrhythmias. Patients with an indwelling pacemaker or automatic internal cardioverter defibrillator (AICD) require special consideration.

Heart Murmur. A heart murmur caused by a valvular or septal defect requires special consideration. Murmurs that originate from valvular stenosis or insufficiency require careful control of preload, afterload, and heart rate. A murmur from a septal defect requires similar hemodynamic control, as well as the avoidance of air bubbles in the IV line. If the patient has, or develops, a right-to-left intracardiac shunt, this air may enter the systemic circulation and cause a stroke.

Hypertension. Most of the hypertensive patients encountered have essential hypertension. They are usually hypovolemic and consequently are more susceptible to wide swings in blood pressure during an anesthetic. The goal is to rehydrate those patients preoperatively and intraoperatively in order to maintain a more stable blood pressure. Keeping the blood pressure within the patient's normal range is important in maintaining adequate end organ perfusion.

Peripheral Vascular Disease (PVD).   The patient with PVD from atherosclerosis should also be suspected of having associated cerebral or coronary vascular insufficiency. The objective is to maintain adequate end organ perfusion. The patient with Raynaud's disease is of special concern because the operating room is typically a cold environment and the patient must be kept warm. Insertion of arterial catheters into distal arteries should be avoided, because arterial spasm may lead to ischemia distal to the indwelling catheter.

Endocrine

Diabetes Mellitus.   Diabetes mellitus is the most common endocrinopathy encountered. Insulin-dependent diabetic patients are at increased risk of morbidity because they have a predisposition for coronary, cerebral, and peripheral vascular insufficiency. They may have also developed autonomic and peripheral neuropathies or renal dysfunction. It is important to know if the diabetes mellitus is well controlled, what the patient's insulin protocol is, and the time of the last insulin administration. From this information, glucose- or nonglucose-containing IV fluids may be selected, and decisions made as to whether additional insulin therapy is indicated. Intraoperative blood glucose analysis may be performed to help properly manage the diabetic patient.

Thyroid Disease.   The patient with a history of hyperthyroidism or hypothyroidism may require special consideration if he or she is not rendered euthyroid prior to surgery. The hyperthyroid patient may present with signs and symptoms of tachycardia, heat intolerance, and muscle weakness. The goal is to control the hyperdynamic cardiovascular system, closely monitor temperature, and monitor the level of neuromuscular blockade if muscle relaxants are used. Preparations also are made for the possibility of a thyrotoxicosis (thyroid storm) during surgery or in the immediate postoperative period.

The hypothyroid patient usually has a slow heart rate, cold intolerance, decreased cardiovascular dynamics, decreased intravascular volume, and an overall decreased metabolism. These patients are more sensitive to anesthetic agents and prolonged recovery from anesthetic agents is a possibility.

Gastrointestinal

Hiatal Hernia.   The patient with a hiatal hernia who is symptomatic for esophageal reflux is at increased risk for an aspiration pneumonitis. If the patient is to have a general anesthetic, a rapid-sequence induction is performed. The objective of this procedure is to prevent pulmonary aspiration. During induction of anesthesia, an assistant applies firm, downward cricoid pressure to occlude the esophagus until the trachea is secured with a cuffed endotracheal tube. This maneuver prevents any passive regurgitation of gastric contents from entering the trachea. These patients should not be extubated until they are awake enough to protect their own airways.

Hematologic

Bleeding Disorders. It is important to obtain a history of prolonged bleeding because any invasive procedure, such as performing a spinal or epidural puncture or placement of an arterial or central line, has the potential of causing excessive bleeding from inadvertent puncture of a noncompressible vessel. Coagulation studies may be routinely performed preoperatively or if there is a concern that the patient may have a coagulopathy.

Hepatic

Jaundice/Hepatitis/Cirrhosis. The etiology of the patient's liver dysfunction should be ascertained preoperatively, if possible. The pathology may be due to parenchymal liver disease or cholestasis. Inquiring into alcohol or illegal drug abuse may be helpful in determining possible causative factors and perhaps the extent of the liver damage.

Any patient scheduled for elective surgery who presents with acute hepatitis should be canceled until hepatic function returns to the patient's normal baseline level. Because most anesthetic drugs are biotransformed in the liver, drugs must be carefully selected and dosages moderated in the patient with severe liver dysfunction. Drugs with known or implied hepatotoxicity must be avoided. Oxygen delivery and hepatic perfusion pressure are optimized intraoperatively to prevent additional liver damage.

Immunologic

History of Allergies. A notation of all allergies is documented on the anesthesia consult. If the patient has had an allergic reaction to drugs, it is beneficial to know if it was anaphylactic (immunologic), anaphylactoid (nonimmunologic), or an unpleasant side effect (drug intolerance) that the patient perceives as an allergic reaction. It is also important to know if the patient has an allergic reaction to certain foods (e.g., eggs, soy products, shellfish, or seafood), because some drugs are derived from these products. The patient with a latex allergy will require special considerations. The objective is to avoid those agents that could precipitate an allergic reaction. It may be elected to prophylactically pretreat the suspect patient with steroids, H_1 and H_2 antagonist.

Musculoskeletal

Arthritis. The patient with arthritis may present technical challenges. Management of the airway may be difficult due to a limited range of motion of the cervical spine. Placement of a spinal or epidural catheter may be challenging due to arthritic changes within the spinal column. The goal is to maintain safe positioning for these patients throughout the surgical procedure.

Muscle Weakness. The patient with a history of muscle weakness from such disorders as myasthenia gravis, muscular dystrophy, or a pseudocholinesterase deficiency requires special attention. The objective is to optimize the patient's ventilatory mechanics throughout the procedure and choose anesthetic agents that have the least compromising effect on muscle function.

Neurologic

Seizures. If a patient is currently on anticonvulsant medications, it may be advisable to continue or adjust the dosage during the perioperative period in order to maintain therapeutic levels. Some anesthetic agents are known to lower the threshold for seizure activity and must be avoided. Conversely, other agents may raise the threshold and therefore may be selected as part of the anesthetic plan.

Stroke. Patients with a history of stroke from cerebral vascular insufficiency are at risk during anesthesia, especially if they have experienced transient ischemic attacks. Hypotensive episodes must be avoided and blood pressure maintained within or slightly higher than the normal range in order to provide adequate cerebral perfusion.

Pulmonary

Asthma. The patient with bronchial asthma has a hyperreactive airway that should respond to bronchodilator therapy. The frequency and severity of the asthma attacks and response to bronchodilators should be assessed. Patients may be prophylactically treated with steroids and bronchodilators. Certain anesthetic drugs, such as those that release histamine, should be avoided. If a general endotracheal anesthetic is necessary, the patient must be deeply anesthetized during intubation and extubation to reduce the chances of precipitating an asthmatic attack. Intravenous lidocaine may also be administered to help suppress airway reflexes.

Bronchitis/Emphysema. Cigarette smoking is a major cause of bronchitis and emphysema with the eventual development of chronic obstructive pulmonary disease (COPD). Inquiry into the patient's pack/year history of smoking and exercise intolerance may provide insight into the severity of the disease. COPD patients have a higher incidence of postoperative pulmonary complications. The objective is to keep these patients well ventilated and provide airway humidification during the anesthetic course in order to avoid or minimize atelectasis.

Renal

Renal Disease. The patient with chronic or acute renal dysfunction is at increased risk of developing more advanced renal failure postoperatively. The anesthetized patient is more susceptible to experience a decrease in glomerular filtration rate and renal blood flow during surgery. The objective is to provide proper hydration and maintain adequate renal perfusion pressure. Drugs that are excreted by the kidney need to be avoided or the dosage moderated. The hemodialysis patient obviously requires special consideration.

Reproductive

Pregnancy. Women of childbearing age are asked about their pregnancy status. If the patient could possibly be pregnant, a negative pregnancy test should be confirmed prior to elective surgery. For emergency surgery on the pregnant patient, anesthetic agents must be selected that have the least known teratogenic effects on the developing fetus and are least likely to contribute to premature labor or a spontaneous abortion.

ANESTHETIC HISTORY

During the patient interview, additional questions are asked that concern important considerations in administration of an anesthetic.

History of Previous Anesthetics

The patient is asked if he or she had any problems with a previous anesthetic. If there were any problems, they are most often expressed as complaints of nausea, vomiting, sore throat, pruritus, myalgia, prolonged drowsiness, inadequate preoperative medication, or insufficient postoperative pain control. If available, a review of previous anesthesia records is most valuable. From this information, the goal is to tailor the anesthetic to prevent or minimize the possible causative factors that may have contributed to the complaint. The patient with a known history of a difficult airway, malignant hyperthermia, or a pseudocholinesterase deficiency requires special consideration.

History of Previous Surgeries

Previous surgeries may influence some technical procedures (e.g., for the patient in whom a right radical mastectomy was performed, the left arm would be used for the IV placement and blood pressure monitoring). The nature of the previous surgeries may also provide insight into the extent of any of the patient's coexisting pathologies (e.g., multiple vascular surgeries on a diabetic patient would be indicative of the severity of the endocrinopathy).

Family History of Anesthetic Complications

Inquiry is made as to whether any family member(s) has had a serious complication attributed to an anesthetic. An unexplained death or a sudden and critical elevation in temperature during the course of an anesthetic may be attributed to malignant hyperthermia. A family member who had prolonged muscle weakness following an anesthetic raises the suspicion of a pseudocholinesterase deficiency. Both malignant hyperthermia and pseudocholinesterase deficiency are genetically inherited disorders, and further investigation is prudent in the patient in whom such conditions are suspected.

PREOPERATIVE PHYSICAL EXAMINATION

The physical examination is generally limited to the head, neck, chest, and extremities. Regardless of the anesthesia technique, evaluation of the airway is performed on all patients. Observation is made for abnormalities that would make it difficult to manage the patient's airway with a mask. Presence of a beard, facial deformities, or lack of dentition may make it difficult to obtain a tight face mask seal if positive pressure ventilation is applied. Visible factors that may be indicators of a difficult intubation are small mouth opening, retrognathia, overbite, prominent incisors, loose teeth, large tongue, short neck, or morbid obesity.

There are simple bedside tests that can be performed to evaluate the patient's airway in regard to placement of an endotracheal tube. The range of motion of the patient's cervical spine and temporomandibular joint are tested. A limited range of motion possibly increases the difficulty of endotracheal tube placement. Another test is to measure the distance (in fingerbreadths) between the tip of the mandible to the thyroid cartilage. If the distance is less than three fingerbreadths, a difficult intubation may be encountered. A test described by Mallampati grades, on a scale from I to IV, the varying degree of pharyngeal structures that the examiner visualizes with the patient's mouth opened as widely as possible and the tongue maximally extended. Grade I would be a predictor of an easy intubation, whereas a grade IV may indicate a difficult intubation because fewer pharyngeal structures are visualized during the examination. If placement of a nasotracheal or nasogastric tube is anticipated, the patient is asked to breathe through each nostril to determine the preferred passageway for tube placement. It is important to document the presence of any dental appliances, chipped, loose, or capped teeth during the examination. Dental damage is a known risk of airway management, and this remote possibility is discussed with the patient. The neck is also examined for any abnormalities that may make venous access or regional nerve blocks more difficult. Auscultation is performed for carotid bruits in the patient suspected of having cerebral vascular insufficiency.

The physical examination of the thorax involves observation of chest wall motion during deep breathing and auscultation of the lungs for the quality and distribution of breath sounds. The precordium is auscultated for abnormal heart sounds, the presence of murmurs, or an irregular rhythm.

Examination of the upper and lower extremities entails observation for any gross abnormalities. Palpitation of pulses in the upper extremities is performed to detect any differences in pulse strength. Discrepancies in blood pressure may need further investigation, and the arm with the higher pressure is used for blood pressure measurements.

American Society of Anesthesiologists (ASA) Classification

By using the information derived from the history and physical examination, a physical status classification number is assigned from I to V, with the letter E if the surgical procedure is an emergency. This classification system is a predictor of morbidity and mortality.

- ASA Class I. A normal, healthy patient.
- ASA Class II. A patient with mild systemic disease; no functional limitations.
- ASA Class III. A patient with moderate to severe systemic disease that limits activity but is not incapacitating.
- ASA Class IV. A patient with severe systemic disease that is a constant threat to life and is incapacitating.
- ASA Class V. A moribund patient that is not expected to survive 24 hours with or without surgery.

Clinical Data

Vital Signs. The patient's vital signs are recorded on the anesthesia consult. The patient's age, height, and weight may be used as a general guide to calculate drug dosages, IV fluid infusion rates, ventilator settings, and limitations of acceptable urine output and blood loss.

The patient's blood pressure range gives a guideline as to what level the patient normally functions. The hypertensive patient may require maintenance within the patient's normal blood pressure range in order to adequately perfuse the major end organs.

The source of an abnormally high or low pulse rate needs evaluation prior to surgery because abnormal rates may be exacerbated by some anesthetic agents.

The cause of abnormal respiratory rates or patterns needs to be evaluated prior to the patient being anesthetized.

The patient's temperature is recorded, and if the patient has a fever of unknown origin, elective surgery may require cancellation.

Electrocardiogram (ECG). An ECG on healthy patients under 40 years of age rarely reveals any significant pathology. Any patient with a positive cardiac history or over 40 years old needs a current ECG (recommended age of obtaining an ECG varies within different institutions.)

Chest X-ray. A chest x-ray is not normally required for healthy, asymptomatic patients. If a patient has known pulmonary or cardiac pathology, or if the patient has a coexisting disorder that may impair cardiopulmonary function, a preoperative chest x-ray should be taken.

Pulmonary Function Tests. Pulmonary function tests are reserved for the patient with severe pulmonary dysfunction or for the patient with pre-existing pulmonary disease who is undergoing major thoracic or upper abdominal surgery.

Laboratory Data. The amount of laboratory data required on a patient is usually determined by the nature of the proposed surgical procedure, the patient's age, and the patient's health status. For the healthy, asymptomatic patient, a hemoglobin, glucose, and electrolyte screen may be sufficient. Depending on the information gathered from the history and physical examination, additional testing such as coagulation studies or tests that reflect the patient's liver or renal function may be ordered.

Current Medications. A listing of current medications (scheduled and unscheduled) is important to obtain because of the potential for possible interactions with some of the commonly used anesthetic agents or because of anticoagulant effects. It is important that some scheduled medications are given preoperatively and intraoperatively in order to maintain therapeutic levels. Conversely, those medications that may affect myocardial performance, alter vascular tone, or prolong coagulation may be decreased or discontinued.

THE ANESTHETIC PLAN

To formulate an anesthetic plan for elective surgery, several factors must be considered. These factors are the patient's age, physical status, the type and duration of the proposed surgical procedure, the patient's position during the surgery, the possibility of increased gastric contents, and the patient's preference of anesthesia (if options are available). From this information, an anesthetic technique(s) and the need for additional monitoring is decided upon.

Depending on the type of surgery, the patient may be given an option between general, regional, or MAC sedation. If the patient is to have a regional anesthetic, the possibility is discussed with the patient that if the regional anesthetic is unsatisfactory, a general anesthetic may be required. If indicated, the patient may be given the option for intravenous or continuous epidural patient-controlled analgesia (PCA) for postoperative pain management.

Once an anesthetic plan is devised, the patient is informed as to what to expect, instructed not to eat or drink after midnight, and informed that he or she will be given preoperative medications prior to surgery that will cause drowsiness or relaxation. The need for IV line placement is discussed, and that blood pressure, pulse, respirations, temperatures, and oxygen saturation will be monitored. If invasive monitoring procedures are necessary, this is also explained. It is important to tell the patient what to expect in the postanesthesia care unit or ICU, especially if the patient is to remain intubated.

The patient is further notified that the anesthesia care team will be with him or her throughout the operative procedure, and that the team will be responsible for his or her care until the effects of the anesthetics have worn off. The risks and benefits of the proposed anesthetic plan are explained and questions regarding the anesthetic plan are solicited.

BASICS OF ANESTHESIA

Before discussing the actual administration of anesthesia, it is important to review some of the basics. A brief overview of the anesthesia machine, anesthesia monitors, airway management, and pharmacologic agents should be helpful to the surgical PA in understanding how the anesthesia PA provides care to the patient.

THE ANESTHESIA MACHINE

The primary function of the anesthesia machine is to deliver, with safety and precision, variable concentrations of oxygen and anesthetic gases. Oxygen, air, and N_2O may be supplied to the anesthesia machine either through the hospital gas inlet supply system or by gas cylinders directly attached to the machine. The anesthesia machine has a fail-safe system that is designed to prevent the administration of a hypoxic gas mixture if the oxygen supply pressure drops below a certain level. The whistling sound heard when the machine is turned on and off indicates that the fail-safe valve is functioning properly. All anesthesia machines must have an oxygen analyzer that continuously monitors the fraction of inspired air concentration (FIO_2), an audible low oxygen alarm, and a ventilator disconnect alarm.

The administration of the volatile anesthetic agents halothane, enflurane, isoflurane, desflurane or sevoflurane are delivered through agent-specific, calibrated vaporizers mounted on the anesthesia machine. The most common method of delivering anesthetic gases to the patient is through a semiclosed circle breathing system. This system allows for the partial rebreathing of expired gases after the elimination of CO_2 via the CO_2 absorber.

A collapsible 3-L rebreathing bag is integrated within the circle system. This bag can be used to allow the patient to breathe spontaneously or, by adjusting a pressure limiting valve, the bag can be manually operated to assist or control ventilations. A mechanical ventilator is also available. For the safety of all ancillary personnel, anesthetic gas waste is scavenged into the hospital's vacuum system. All anesthesia machines have an oxygen flush button which, when activated, delivers 100% oxygen at a very high flow rate to the circle system. This flush button is frequently used on the patient who has a significant air leak around the face mask as attempts are made to apply positive pressure ventilation. The oxygen flush button may be repeatedly depressed to rapidly reinflate the rebreathing bag until airway control is obtained. Another use of the oxygen flush button is to rapidly displace any residual anesthetic gases from the breathing system and quickly replace the breathing circuit with 100% oxygen.

For practicality and convenience, a suction apparatus and patient monitors have been incorporated within some machines. Additional hemodynamic monitors or gas analyzers are typically secured on the top of the anesthesia machine. Having everything in one central location makes visual scanning easier for the anesthetist and safer for the patient, because attention is divided between observing the patient, the surgical field, the anesthesia machine, and the patient monitors. Before each case, a detailed anesthesia machine check is performed following a standard protocol established by the American Society of Anesthesiologists.

MONITORING

Technological advances in monitoring have been a major contributing factor in decreasing the morbidity and mortality associated with the administration of an anesthetic. Even so, the practice of "a hand on the pulse and an ear on the chest" should never be abandoned. Visual, tactile, and auditory senses are continually used to evaluate the patient's condition. These observations are enhanced by basic monitoring standards, which have been set forth by the American Academy of Anesthesiologists.

Basic monitoring for all anesthetics includes evaluation of oxygenation, circulation, ventilation, and body temperature. For all of general anesthetics, basic monitoring includes ECG, blood pressure, pulse, respirations, inspired oxygen concentration, oxygen saturation (using pulse oximetry), and end tidal CO_2 ($ETCO_2$) using capnography and temperature. If muscle relaxants are given, the level of neuromuscular block is monitored with a nerve stimulator. During regional or MAC anesthesia, supplemental oxygen is delivered via a face shield or a split nasal O_2, CO_2 sampling cannula.

The decision to use more advanced monitoring is dependent on the patient's physical status and the nature of the surgical procedure. These monitoring devices may include the use of an arterial line, pulmonary artery (PA) catheter, transesophageal echo (TEE) probe, precordial Doppler, electroencephalogram (EEG), an intracranial pressure (ICP) catheter, cerebrospinal fluid (CSF) catheter, or evoked potential (EP) monitor. Even with these sophisticated monitors, the importance of physically observing the skin color, watching chest excursions, palpating the pulse, and auscultating the heart and lungs should not be overlooked.

AIRWAY MANAGEMENT

Management of the patient's airway is one of the most demanding of responsibilities. Regardless of whether the patient is receiving a local or a general anesthetic, untoward events such as partial or complete airway obstruction, laryngospasm, bronchospasm, or pulmonary aspiration may occur. The efficiency of airway management is constantly being monitored by observation of chest excursions, auscultation of breath sounds, pulse oximetry, capnography, and arterial blood gas analysis (as indicated).

During a regional or MAC anesthetic, supplemental oxygen is administered to the patient. This is done because these patients are usually sedated prior to entering the operating room and, with the addition of more intraoperative sedation, a decrease in alveolar ventilation is expected. Delivery of oxygen may either be by insufflation through a face shield, face mask, or nasal O_2 delivering/CO_2 sampling cannula.

As intraoperative IV sedation is given, there may be brief episodes of hypoventilation or upper airway obstruction as the soft tissues relax. This may be resolved by verbally or physically arousing the patient and having him or her take deep breaths. If a partial airway obstruction persists, a simple head tilt/chin lift maneuver is done to regain patency. Additional adjuncts to airway management are described below.

During a general anesthetic, the administration of IV induction agents usually produces profound relaxation of the upper airway soft tissues and usually a decrease in alveolar ventilation to the point of apnea. The following adjuncts are often used for managing the patient's airway.

Anesthesia Face Mask.   With the proper application of the anesthesia face mask and the head tilt/chin lift maneuver, ventilations may be able to be controlled or assisted until efficient spontaneous breathing returns. If there continues to be a partial or complete airway obstruction, an oral or nasal airway may be placed. If the obstruction is relieved, face mask delivery of oxygen or anesthetic gases may be continued. If the airway is unable to be secured with the above methods, the patient may be awoken or more advanced adjuncts are employed.

Laryngeal Mask Airway (LMA).   The LMA is a cuffed tube that is blindly positioned in the hypopharynx. When the LMA is in the correct position, the larynx is isolated from the esophagus. After confirmation (auscultation and $ETCO_2$) of proper LMA positioning, the tube is connected to the anesthetic breathing circuit and the reservoir bag is used to hand control or assist ventilations. The patient may also be allowed to resume spontaneous ventilations.

Endotracheal Tube (ETT). Placement of a cuffed ETT mainly is used to protect the airway from aspiration. An ETT is generally used on patients who are in surgical positions other than supine, in head and neck surgery, in cases of long duration requiring positive pressure ventilation, in patients suspected of having a full stomach or bowel obstruction, in the morbidly obese patient, or in those patients in whom face mask or LMA management is unsatisfactory.

Double-lumen Endotracheal Tube (DLT). The DLT is used in order to periodically administer unilateral lung ventilation during intrathoracic surgery. Collapsing the surgical field lung greatly enhances surgical exposure. There are commercially available left- or right-sided DLTs. The left-sided DLT is discussed below.

Correct placement of the DLT is critical for proper functioning. Position is confirmed by auscultation, fiberoptic bronchoscopy (FOB), and observation of chest excursions. If properly positioned, the left lumen should be in the left main stem bronchus with its cuff just below the carina. The right lumen should be in the trachea just above the carina. When the bronchial and tracheal cuffs are inflated, each lung should be isolated. To check for proper placement, the chest is auscultated for the pressure or absence of breath sounds as alternating lumens are clamped off. FOB via the tracheal lumen is used to confirm that the inflated bronchial cuff is visible in the left main stem bronchus just below the carina, and that the right main stem bronchus is patent. When providing one-lung ventilation, 100% oxygen is used for ventilation. It is essential to recheck the position of the tube any time the patient is repositioned or any time there is a surgical event that may affect the proper functioning of the DLT. If there are dramatic or unsatisfactory changes in SaO_2 or $ETCO_2$ levels, immediate attention is mandatory. If proper tube placement is reconfirmed by FOB and auscultation, and appropriate respiratory care has failed to improve the situation, continuous positive airway pressure (CPAP) may be added to the collapsed lung, or the collapsed lung may be periodically reinflated during the surgical procedure.

THE DIFFICULT AIRWAY

There are basically three situations in which a difficult airway is encountered: (1) the patient with a known history of a difficult airway or intubation, (2) the patient who is suspected of having a difficult airway when evaluated during the physical examination, or (3) the patient with an unsuspected difficult airway.

For the first two situations, there is some advanced warning of the possibility of a difficult airway and an awake intubation may be employed. For the patients with an unsuspected difficult airway, problems may not be recognized until induction or attempted intubation.

The awake intubation procedure begins with preoxygenation. Because the objective is to let the patient maintain his or her own airway until tracheal intubation is successful, caution must be used not to oversedate the patient. As the patient becomes sedated, topical anesthesia is applied to the nasopharynx or oropharynx, depending on the route of intubation. If a nasotracheal tube is to be used, a vasoconstrictive agent such as cocaine or phenylephrine may be topically applied intranasally to prevent or minimize bleeding. A superior laryngeal nerve block or transtracheal administration of lidocaine may also be used to provide localized airway anesthesia. When a satisfactory level of block has been achieved, one of several methods may be used to intubate the patient's trachea:

- A blind approach using the nasal or oral route is performed by listening for the changes in intensity of breath sounds as the tracheal tube is advanced and enters the trachea
- A specially designed lightwand may be blindly manipulated into the trachea; a tracheal tube that has been placed over the lightwand may then be advanced into the trachea
- By direct visualization with a standard laryngoscope and intubating using Magill forceps and/or a styletted tracheal tube
- By direct fiberoptic visualization and intubation using the Bullard scope
- By direct fiberoptic visualization and passage into the trachea a FOB over which a nasal or oral tube may be positioned into the trachea
- By the retrograde wire technique that involves placing a needle through the cricothyroid membrane. A long wire is passed through the needle and threaded retrograde into the hypopharynx. The wire is then retrieved from the mouth and a tube is threaded over the wire and into the trachea.

Once the tube has entered the trachea, the cuff is inflated, tracheal intubation is confirmed by the presence of $ETCO_2$, fiberoptic bronchoscopy, and by watching the patient breathe through the anesthesia reservoir bag. Because the patient is still breathing spontaneously, confirmation by auscultation is not a guarantee that the tube is correctly positioned, so auscultation alone should not be the only source of confirmation. Observing the capnograph for the presence of a CO_2 waveform is the best assurance. Once correct tube placement has been confirmed, general anesthesia can commence. If the trachea is not able to be intubated, elective surgery may be canceled.

For the patient with the unsuspected difficult airway, problems are not apparent until induction or attempted intubation. For these patients, the "difficult airway algorithm" is initiated as established by the American Society of Anesthesiologists.

If at any point the airway is unable to be managed and the situation develops into a life-threatening situation, an emergency cricothyroidotomy or tracheostomy with surgical assistance must be performed. The two key factors in dealing with the difficult airway are: to be prepared and not to hesitate to call for help.

PHARMACOLOGY

Many drugs are administered during the course of an anesthetic. Most of the drugs are chosen because they are fast acting and have a relatively short duration of action. The pharmacokinetics and pharmacodynamics of all the drugs administered must be known, as well as any potential interactions with any of the patient's unscheduled or scheduled medications.

The following is a listing of some of the commonly used drugs given peri- or intraoperatively. This listing is representative but not inclusive, because practitioners and hospitals vary in their selection of drugs kept on their formulary. It must be remembered that drugs have multiple effects and that patient responses may vary. Only the major reason(s) for the drugs' intended use during an anesthetic will be mentioned. A simple MAC with sedation procedure may only require the use of one or two drugs, whereas a more complex procedure (e.g., resection of an abdominal aortic aneurysm) requires the use of multiple drugs.

The patient is potentially exposed to multiple and diverse pharmacologic agents. The objective of the anesthesia plan is to provide a safe anesthetic and maintain homeostasis with the judicious use of these drugs.

ANESTHETIC AGENTS

The ultra–short-acting induction agents propofol, etomidate, thiopental, or ketamine are used to produce unconsciousness. A continuous propofol infusion may also be used as a maintenance agent or for conscious sedation during MAC.

To alleviate pain, the intravenous narcotics morphine, meperidine, fentanyl, sufentanil, alfentanil, remifentanil and the nonsteroidal anti-inflammatory drug (NSAID) ketorolac are used.

The benzodiazepines diazepam, midazolam, and lorazepam are used for their sedative hypnotic effect.

The local anesthetics cocaine, benzocaine, lidocaine, bupivacaine, tetracaine, etidocaine, mepivacaine, chloroprocaine, procaine (Novocain) are used to produce a temporary regional block. Depending on the agent, administration may be used to achieve a topical, local, peripheral, or central neural block.

Oxygen and the inhalational anesthetic agents N_2O, halothane, enflurane, isoflurane, desflurane, and sevoflurane are delivered from the anesthesia machine to the patient. These inhalational anesthetic agents are used to achieve or maintain varying depths of general anesthesia.

CARDIOVASCULAR AGENTS

The administration of anesthetic agents and the stress of surgery disrupt homeostasis. A wide variety of pharmacologic agents are used that can increase or decrease heart rate, myocardial contractility, or vascular tone.

There are many adrenergic agonists: phenylephrine, ephedrine, epinephrine, norepinephrine, isoproterenol, dobutamine, and dopamine. Each agent may be characterized by its varying degree of influence on alpha$_1$, alpha$_2$, beta$_1$, beta$_2$, and/or dopaminergic receptors. Most of these agents have mixed effects. An agent may be selected because of its dominating ability to raise heart rate or improve hemodynamic function. An example might be a situation in which it is necessary to increase both heart rate and myocardial contractility. For this situation, epinephrine may be chosen.

Conversely, in a situation in which it is necessary to increase blood pressure but not increase heart rate, phenylephrine may be the drug of choice. In some cases, a renal dose of dopamine may be used to stimulate dopaminergic receptors and promote diuresis.

Other cardiotonic drugs such as the nonadrenergic sympathomimetics amrinone or milrinone, the cardiac glycoside digitalis, or the hormone glucagon to may be used to enhance myocardial performance. The calcium cation derived from CaCl$_2$ is also used to improve contractility.

There are situations during surgery in which hypertension or tachycardia requires treatment. The adrenergic antagonists esmolol and propranolol are used to decrease heart rate and combat hypertension. Labetalol is also used as an antihypertensive agent.

The vasodilators nitroglycerin, sodium nitroprusside, hydralazine, prostaglandin E$_1$, and nifedipine (oral) are used to decrease vascular resistance, thereby lowering blood pressure. These drugs also have mixed effects and are chosen according to their dominant characteristics. Nitroglycerin dilates coronary arteries, but also causes venodilitation that decreases the preload to the heart (preload reduction). Sodium nitroprusside and hydralazine are arteriolar vasodilators and decrease afterload on the heart (afterload reduction). Both preload and afterload reduction lower systemic blood pressure. Prostaglandin E$_1$ is a potent pulmonary and systemic vasodilator and is generally used to treat the patient with severe pulmonary hypertension. The calcium channel blocker nifedipine relaxes coronary and vascular smooth muscles but must be given orally or through a nasogastric tube.

The anticholinergics atropine, scopolamine, and glycopyrrolate are vagolytic and cause an increase in heart rate. They may also be used as an antisialagogue. Scopolamine may also be used for its amnestic effect.

The antiarrhythmics lidocaine, bretylium, procainamide, verapamil, and adenosine are used to treat various dysrhythmias.

MUSCLE RELAXANTS

Choice of a muscle relaxant generally depends on the duration of action, the length of the surgical procedure, and the patient's ability to metabolize or excrete the drug. The depolarizing muscle relaxant succinylcholine is similar to the neurotransmitter acetylcholine and produces a fast onset and offset of skeletal muscle paralysis. When given in a sufficient dose to help facilitate tracheal intubation, the patient's muscles will fasciculate prior to total paralysis. These fasciculations may appear as mild to severe spasmodic muscle contractions that may result in postoperative myalgia. To prevent or minimize fasciculations, a small dose of a nondepolarizing muscle relaxant such as curare is administered a few minutes prior to giving succinylcholine. However, the pretreatment is not always successful. The nondepolarizing muscle relaxants curare, atracurium, cisatracurium, mivacurium, pancuronium, vecuronium, pipecuronium, and rocuronium produce skeletal muscle paralysis by competing for and blocking acetylcholine receptor sites on skeletal muscle motor end plates. This competitive blockade prevents the neurotransmitter acetylcholine from binding with its receptor site. The resulting skeletal muscle paralysis lasts from a moderate to a long duration, depending on the choice of muscle relaxant and the patient's response to the drug. Some of these agents may require reversal with an anticholinesterase prior to extubation.

ADJUNCTIVE PHARMACOLOGIC AGENTS

The steroid methylprednisolone sodium succinate and the histamine receptor antagonist diphenhydramine, an H_1 blocker, may be used to pretreat the patient who either has the potential for or is presently experiencing an allergic reaction. Famotidine, cimetidine, and ranitidine are H_2 blockers and are used to pretreat the patient suspected of an allergic reaction. These H_2 blockers also decrease gastric acidity and are given preoperatively as prophylaxis to decrease the morbidity associated with an aspiration pneumonitis.

Because nausea is a major complaint following an anesthetic and certain surgical procedures, the antiemetics ondansetron, droperidol, diphenhydramine, or promethazine are used perioperatively or intraoperatively to prevent or relieve nausea.

To promote diuresis, the loop diuretic furosemide or the osmotic diuretic mannitol are commonly used. For bronchodilatation, one of the B_2 adrenergic agonists such as aerosolized albuterol, intramuscular terbutaline, or intravenous ephedrine, epinephrine, or isoproterenol may be selected.

Insulin is used to control hyperglycemia or treat critical hyperkalemia. KCl is employed to treat hypokalemia and $NaHCO_3$ to correct acidosis.

Heparin is used as an anticoagulant during vascular and cardiovascular procedures. The antifibrinolytics aminocaproic acid and aprotinin are used with specific patients to reduce blood loss.

Dantrolene is used in the prevention or treatment of malignant hyperthermia.

Various antibiotics are available to be given as scheduled medications or given upon the surgeon's request.

REVERSAL AGENTS

Several pharmacologic agents are used to counteract certain drug effects. Total reversal of a medication effect is not always possible, and an extended period of time may be necessary for the original drug effect to wear off. The anticholinesterase neostigmine is used to reverse the neuromuscular block caused by nondepolarizing muscle relaxants. Physostigmine crosses the blood–brain barrier and reverses drug-induced anticholinergic central nervous system (CNS) effect.

Naloxone reverses narcotics.
Flumazenil reverses benzodiazepines.
Protamine reverses heparin.

THE ROUTINE ANESTHETIC COURSE

The following describes the responsibilities of the anesthesia care team for the patient who is to undergo a routine, elective surgical procedure.

PREOPERATIVE

Prior to surgery, an anesthesiologist reviews the chart and interviews and examines the patient. An anesthetic plan is formulated and discussed with and agreed upon by the patient. All patients are instructed to remain NPO after midnight the day before surgery. A sedative may be ordered to be taken the night before surgery.

On the day of surgery, preoperative medications are usually given 1 to 2 hours prior to the patient being transported to the operating room. The preoperative medications may include an H_2 antagonist, which decreases gastric acidity. Some practitioners may allow ingestion of clear liquids within 2 to 4 hours of surgery if an H_2 antagonist has been given. An anticholinergic may be prescribed for its vagolytic properties or its anti-sialagogue effect, although dry mouth is a major patient complaint. The patient may be given a narcotic in the preoperative period to reduce pain and a sedative to decrease anxiety. Because narcotics and sedatives may decrease alveolar ventilation, supplemental oxygen may be ordered for the patient with cardiac or pulmonary disease.

When the patient is brought to the surgical area, he or she may first be admitted to the presurgical care unit (PSCU). After proper patient identification and review of the anesthesia consult, the patient's chart is reviewed to evaluate any recent changes in the patient's status or to determine if there have been any new consults that may affect the proposed anesthetic plan. If the anesthetic plan needs to be changed, consent from the unpremedicated patient or the family of the premedicated patient must be obtained.

For the patient who appears to be inadequately sedated upon arrival to the PSCU, reassurance or additional sedation may be given (once IV access has been established). To minimize operating room time, insertion of additional invasive monitoring devices (e.g., arterial line, CVP, continuous epidural catheter, etc.) may be performed in the PSCU.

ENTRANCE INTO THE OPERATING ROOM

When the operating room team is ready, the patient is accompanied from the PSCU to the operating room. Even though the patient may appear to be well sedated, entering the operating room may be a frightening experience. Extraneous noise should be kept to a minimum and reassurance provided. The operating room bed should be kept warm or a warm blanket provided in order to prevent shivering. If the patient is to be supine, he or she is assisted onto the operating table and comfortably positioned prior to being anesthetized. The patient who is to be prone or is in too much pain to be moved may be anesthetized on the stretcher prior to being positioned onto the table.

Before anesthetizing the patient, the patient is connected to the ECG monitor and a blood pressure cuff, pulse oximeter probe, and precordial stethoscope are positioned. If the patient has invasive monitoring lines (e.g., arterial line, CVP, etc.), the lines are connected and calibrated and the vital signs are displayed on the hemodynamic monitor. The patient who is to receive a regional or peripheral nerve block may need to be temporarily repositioned to facilitate administration of the block.

ANESTHETIC TECHNIQUES

Anesthetic techniques may be categorized as general, regional, or MAC. For each of the following techniques, it is assumed that an elective surgical procedure is to be performed on a premedicated patient who has been NPO. The patient is also assumed to be in the supine position, has an IV infusion, and is appropriately monitored. During the surgical procedure, a detailed anesthesia record is maintained, which is a chronological documentation of procedures, events, and patient data. The information collected on the anesthesia record is interpreted and used in management decisions.

GENERAL ANESTHESIA

A general anesthetic is defined as a patient who is rendered unconscious during a surgical procedure. Key determinants in choosing a general anesthetic are the type and duration of surgery, body position, patient's preference to be totally asleep, or a contraindication to alternative anesthetic techniques.

Preinduction. As the patient is being made comfortable on the operating room table and the monitors are being applied, important preinduction procedures are performed. Ideally, the patient should be preoxygenated for several minutes by breathing 100% oxygen through the anesthesia face mask or by taking three to four vital capacity breaths through the mask. This nitrogen-washout procedure fills the lungs with approximately 100% oxygen, which adds a margin of safety if difficulty is encountered during subsequent airway management.

During this time, a small dose of curare may be administered to pretreat the patient if the depolarizing muscle relaxant succinylcholine is to be given. This is done to prevent or mimimize the fasciculations caused by succinylcholine. A small dose of IV lidocaine may be administered to prevent the burning sensation caused by the injection of some of the IV induction agents through small, distal veins.

The course of a general anesthetic may be divided into three major parts: induction, maintenance, and emergence.

Induction. After satisfactory preoxygenation, the patient is again afforded reassurance as he or she is rendered unconscious. Pulse oximetry tones should be audible.

The most commonly used IV induction agents are propofol, etomidate, or barbiturate (e.g., thiopental). When administered as a bolus dose, loss of consciousness usually occurs within 30 to 60 seconds. The patient becomes unresponsive to simple commands such as "open your eyes." For confirmation, the patient's eyelid may be stroked to check for the absence of the lid reflex.

After the patient becomes unconscious, the patient's eyes may be taped closed in order to prevent drying of the cornea or an inadvertent corneal abrasion. Because of patient positioning or the inaccessibility to provide continual monitoring of eye care, special goggles may be applied for additional protection.

As the patient loses consciousness, rapid respiratory and cardiovascular changes must be anticipated. Depending on the dosage of the IV induction agent, there is usually a significant decrease in ventilations, even to the point of apnea. This is attributed to the drug's depressant effect on the cerebellar respiratory center.

This anticipated decrease or absence of ventilations requires immediate attention. At this point, the patient's ventilations are assisted or controlled by using the face mask while hand-squeezing the reservoir bag on the anesthesia machine. In procedures of short duration, the face mask may be used throughout the procedure. In most procedures, an LMA or ETT is used. If an ETT is used, a muscle relaxant is commonly given to help facilitate intubation. To help determine when the patient is sufficiently paralyzed so that a laryngoscopy can be performed, a peripheral nerve stimulator (PNS) may be used to monitor twitch responses as electrical shocks are applied to the side of the face or the forearm.

After intubation and confirmation of correct tube placement, the ETT is taped securely into place. A temperature monitoring esophageal stethoscope may be inserted into a position that maximizes heart and breath sounds. While the patient is still relaxed, a soft bite block may be positioned to prevent dental damage or occlusion of the ETT if the patient were to bite down when muscle tone returns.

While gaining control of the patient's airway, a drop in blood pressure is anticipated. This is caused by a decrease in sympathetic tone or by the myocardial depressant effect of some IV induction agents. This decrease in blood pressure may be more dramatic in the patient who has not been adequately rehydrated preoperatively after being NPO. The hypotensive episode may be treated by giving additional IV fluids, placing the patient into a Trendelenburg position, or by administering a vasopressor or cardiotonic agent. If instrumentation of the airway or surgical stimulation is about to occur, the resulting stimulus may be sufficient to increase the blood pressure.

As the airway is secured and hemodynamics are stabilized, the anesthetic effect of the ultra–short-acting induction agent is rapidly dissipating and the patient will begin to wake up if additional anesthetics are not given. In order to achieve a surgical depth of anesthesia, the IV induction agent must be continued, inhalational anesthetics need to be delivered, or a balanced technique is employed using narcotics, hypnotic sedative, N_2O/O_2, with or without a muscle relaxant. Usually a combination of the above techniques is employed to maintain a general anesthetic.

Maintenance. During the maintenance phase, the depth of anesthesia is controlled and the patient's blood pressure, heart rate, respirations, temperature, skeletal muscle function, intravascular volume status, urine output, glucose, electrolytes, blood gas, and acid–base status are measured and managed. The most common method for maintenance of a general anesthetic is the use of inhalational agents along with the administration of pre-emptive intravenous analgesics. Inhalational anesthetics have the advantage of a quick onset and a rapid rate of elimination. The volatile inhalational agents are enflurane, isoflurane, desflurane, or sevoflurane in combination with O_2, or a mixture of N_2O/O_2. Halothane rarely is used in adults. The inhalational agents in a sufficient concentration cause unconsciousness, analgesia, and amnesia. They are also dose-dependent myocardial and respiratory depressants.

The administration of these volatile inhalational agents may be started as soon as loss of consciousness occurs. Most volatile inhalational agents, except sevoflurane, are upper airway irritants and may cause breath holding, coughing, laryngospasm, or bronchospasm if too high an initial concentration is delivered. The concentration of the inhalational agent is frequently adjusted to achieve or maintain a surgical depth of anesthesia. The depth of anesthesia is assessed by evaluating changes in blood pressure, heart rate, pupil size, ventilation (assisted or spontaneous), and by observing for tearing, sweating, or skeletal muscle movement in response to noxious stimuli.

Since the volatile inhalational agents are dose-dependent myocardial depressants and potent vasodilators, blood pressure tends to drop during the waiting period between induction and the surgical incision. This period of decreasing blood pressure usually coincides with the time that the surgical team is scrubbing. This may be a difficult time, because adequate anesthesia needs to be sustained while maintaining an adequate blood pressure. If the patient becomes hypotensive, it may be elected to increase the blood pressure by placing the patient into a Trendelenburg position, administering additional IV fluids, or administering a vasopressor. If the results are unsatisfactory, the inhalational agent may be decreased or discontinued until blood pressure is restored. Procedures such as prepping the patient or inserting a urinary catheter may be enough to raise the blood pressure.

If the incision is made during the light stage of the anesthesia, the stimulus may result in a significant increase in blood pressure, heart rate, respiratory rate, as well as possible skeletal muscle movement. Once an appropriate level of anesthesia has been achieved, the depth of the anesthesia must be controlled to maintain a quiet surgical field as well as manage homeostasis.

Although not as dramatic as induction or emergence, moderate fluctuations in blood pressure and heart rate are expected. These changes are typically in response to the varying degrees of noxious stimuli. The depth of anesthesia is increased or decreased in anticipation of, or in response to, hemodynamic changes.

Ventilations during maintenance may either be controlled, assisted, or spontaneous. If the patient is paralyzed, breathing is controlled either by using a ventilator or by manual squeezing of the anesthesia reservoir bag. If the patient is breathing but is unable to maintain acceptable respiratory function, respirations may be assisted by squeezing the reservoir bag during patient inspiration. During spontaneous ventilations, the patient is able to self-maintain adequate respiratory functions.

Depth of anesthesia may be judged by observing the ventilatory rate and pattern in patients with assisted or spontaneous respirations. Unexpected, abrupt changes may be indicative of a mechanical airway problem or an untoward pulmonary or neurologic event.

Adequacy of ventilation and respiration is assessed by observation of the patient's color, chest wall excursions, auscultation of breath sounds, and by monitoring SaO_2, $ETCO_2$, respiratory rate, tidal volume (TV) and, if indicated, analysis of arterial blood gases. Intraoperatively, the FIO_2 and minute ventilation (tidal volume × respiratory rate) may be adjusted to optimize pulmonary function.

Temperature is monitored throughout the procedure. General anesthetics are known to inhibit the thermoregulatory response (shivering and peripheral vasoconstriction) to a cold environment. As a result, mild hypothermia is expected.

Heat loss is greatest in the procedure in which there is a large surface area of cutaneous or surgical tissue exposure. The goal is to prevent hypothermia-induced intraoperative complications such as myocardial depression, arrhythmias, or coagulopathies. To keep the patient warm, all nonsurgical cutaneous areas are covered or the patient is actively rewarmed by using circulating water or a forced air heating blanket. Intravenous fluids are warmed, especially during rapid, large volume fluid replacement. Because the delivered anesthetic gases are cool and dry, a heat/moisture exchanger is used during ventilations to retain airway humidity.

Conversely, hyperthermia may result from sepsis, thyrotoxicosis, or overaggressive rewarming. In these situations, the circulating water or air blanket may be used in the cooling mode. Intravenous fluids would not be warmed and more skin surface area is exposed. Malignant hyperthermia is a rare but potentially fatal situation that requires special considerations. If the patient is suspected of having malignant hyperthermia, a standard protocol for management is initiated.

Muscle relaxants may be used as part of the anesthetic plan or administered to provide profound muscle relaxation for special surgical considerations. A peripheral nerve stimulator (PNS) is used to assess the degree of neuromuscular blockade (NMB). Sufficient NMB may be maintained by a continuous infusion or repeat bolus doses of the muscle relaxant. If the surgical team notes that the patient is "too tight" or "pushing," the surgical field is evaluated and findings from the peripheral nerve stimulation help determine if additional muscle relaxant is required. An overdosage of nondepolarizing muscle relaxants near the end of the surgical procedure may be difficult to pharmacologically reverse, and the patient may require postoperative ventilatory support. For this reason, long-acting muscle relaxants are given with prudence at the end of a surgical procedure.

During maintenance, the volume and rate of IV fluid administration is determined by the type of procedure and by the amount of blood loss during surgery. For example, during minor surgery on an extremity, 1 to 2 mL of crystalloid/kg/h may be administered as maintenance. For major abdominal surgery, 10 to 20 mL of crystalloid/kg/h may be necessary to maintain sufficient intravascular volume.

For each mL of blood lost, 3 mL of crystalloid is used as replacement in addition to the calculated maintenance volume. If there has been major blood loss, blood product replacement must be considered. If appropriate, recovery of red blood cells (RBCs) into a cell saver for reinfusion should be considered. Adjustments to these basic guidelines for crystalloid infusion are made if the patient receives colloids and/or blood products. Moderation is also considered for the patient with significant renal or cardiac impairment because these patients may not be able to tolerate a volume overload.

The adequacy of volume replacement is constantly evaluated by interpreting the blood pressure and heart rate changes in response to the administration of IV fluids, administration of anesthetic agents, or changes in table positioning (e.g., Trendelenburg or reverse Trendelenburg position).

If a urinary catheter is inserted, measurement of urine output is an excellent monitor for assessing renal function and intravascular volume status (in the patient with normal renal function). Urine output should be between 0.5 to 1.0 mL/kg/h. If oliguria develops, intravascular volume status and hemodynamics are reassessed. Polyuria develops from overhydration or the administration of a diuretic. If anuria suddenly develops, evaluation is made for mechanical problems (kinked or disconnected urinary catheter) before instituting aggressive fluid or diuretic therapy.

Central venous pressure (CVP) measurements or data derived from the use of a multipurpose pulmonary artery catheter provide very important data in determining intravascular volume status. The CVP and the pulmonary artery occlusion pressure (wedge pressure) are representative of the filling pressures (preload) of the heart.

To help maintain homeostasis, blood may be drawn for STAT analysis of glucose, electrolytes, hemoglobin, blood gas tensions, and acid–base status. Intraoperative coagulation studies may also be performed in the patients with suspected coagulopathy.

Emergence. Emergence from a general anesthetic involves the patient's return to consciousness. The proper timing of emergence is crucial. Early emergence is disruptive to the surgical team and may be detrimental to the outcome. Delayed awakening increases operating room time, delays subsequent surgeries, and raises the possibility of an adverse, intraoperative neurologic event.

As emergence progresses, the central nervous system and peripheral autonomic system become more sensitive to external stimuli. The analgesic effect begins to dissipate and the blood pressure and heart rate tend to increase. Timely administration of pre-emptive analgesics are given to minimize this response.

Plans are made for return of muscle and pulmonary function to a level sufficient to maintain spontaneous ventilations. If the patient is intubated, any residual neuromuscular block must be pharmacologically reversed prior to extubation. The reversal of muscle paralysis is generally timed to occur toward the end of the surgical procedure so that the return of muscle tone does not interfere with surgery.

If sufficient pulmonary function has returned, a deep or an awake extubation is performed. The deep extubation technique is used to prevent the patient from coughing or straining on the ETT. This technique may be used in patients in whom a transient increase in pressure may adversely affect surgical outcome (e.g., hemorrhage, intracranial, intraocular, inner ear, etc.). This technique may also be used in the asthma patient to prevent bronchospasm. During deep extubation, the patient should be breathing spontaneously. Because airway reflexes remain obtunded, the patient should not cough during manipulation of the ETT as it is removed.

During the awake extubation technique, the patient must demonstrate that he or she can maintain and protect his or her own airway after the ETT is removed. The awake technique is used with patients in whom there is a potential for aspiration of gastric contents, with patients who were initially a difficult intubation, or with patients with a potentially compromised airway (secondary to trauma or a surgical procedure that alters airway anatomy). During an awake extubation, coughing during removal of the ETT generally occurs because the airway reflexes are intact. Extubation may be delayed until the patient is able to demonstrate the cough reflex, because this indicates that the patient is able to protect the airway if emesis does occur. If laryngospasm occurs immediately after extubation, the airway must be actively managed by applying continuous positive airway pressure (CPAP) and 100% O_2 through the face mask until the spasm breaks. If hypoxemia or hemodynamic instability occur, more aggressive maneuvers may become necessary.

Before performing a deep or an awake extubation, it must be established that the patient is capable of maintaining adequate pulmonary function while breathing spontaneously after the ETT is removed. To make this determination, multiple parameters are measured and monitored prior to extubation. The SaO_2, $ETCO_2$, respiratory rate, tidal volume, and maximum inspiratory force all are evaluated. In the cooperative awakening patient, measuring vital capacity and having the patient demonstrate a sustained head lift are additional tests used in judging the patient's ability to maintain adequate ventilations after extubation. The patient's response to the PNS is also evaluated on those patients who have received neuromuscular blocking agents. If indicated, arterial blood gas analysis may be helpful. If it is not thought that the patient is ready for extubation, the ETT is left in place until recovery is sufficient for extubation.

Transport. After surgery, it must be determined when the patient has emerged from the general anesthetic to a level sufficient for safe transport from the operating room to the postsurgical or intensive care unit. It must be certain that hemodynamics are controlled, pulmonary function is optimized, and that the patient is comfortable.

When stable, the patient is moved from the operating table onto the stretcher or bed. After the move, the patient's cardiopulmonary status is reassessed, especially if the patient has been in a position other than supine, because intravascular volume shifts may dramatically alter the blood pressure. If not contraindicated, the head of the stretcher or bed is elevated to help improve functional residual capacity (FRC) and reduce the work of breathing. If the patient is at potential risk for aspiration, he or she is placed in a lateral decubitus position to help control emesis. To prevent and minimize shivering, warm blankets are applied. Supplemental O_2 is generally administered during transport to help maintain a satisfactory SaO_2. Continuation of ECG and hemodynamic monitoring during transport is advisable on critically ill patients, especially if their disposition is to another floor or remote recovery area.

On arrival to the PACU or ICU, a pulse oximeter is applied as vital signs are taken and monitoring reestablished. A thorough report is then given to the team who will be monitoring the patient. The anesthesia care team maintains responsibility for the patient until the effects of the anesthetics have worn off and remains immediately available for bedside care.

REGIONAL ANESTHESIA

Regional anesthesia involves selectively anesthetizing a region of the patient's body. A regional anesthetic results from the disposition of a local anesthetic agent adjacent to neuronal membranes. Neural blockade is caused by the ability of the local anesthetic to penetrate the neuronal membrane and temporarily interrupt the transmission of nerve impulses. The term regional anesthetic refers to the centro-neuroaxis blocks (spinal, epidural, and caudal), the peripheral nerve blocks, as well as the head and neck blocks.

The option to use a regional anesthetic technique is made during the preoperative anesthesia consultation. The patient may be the first to ask if the surgeon has discussed any specific anesthetic plan. If a regional anesthetic is suitable for the proposed surgical procedure and there are no contraindications, the risks and benefits are discussed with and agreed upon by the patient for consent. The patient is also informed that if the block fails or becomes inadequate during the procedure, the administration of a general anesthetic may become necessary.

The patient is informed that he or she will be sedated, continuously monitored, and receive supplemental O_2. The goal is to keep the patient safe, comfortable, hemodynamically stable, sedated (yet responsive), and provide a quiet surgical field.

While preparing for a regional anesthetic, the patient is appropriately sedated. Oversedation should be avoided because communication with a cooperative patient is crucial for the administration of safe, effective regional anesthesia. The responsive patient can help with positioning, voice discomfort from paresthesia during needle or catheter placement, announce warning signs of drug-induced toxicity, help describe the degree of neural blockade, or voice any other complaints (e.g., angina pectoris, which may occur in the patient with coronary artery disease who becomes hypotensive).

Centro-neuroaxis Blocks (Spinal, Epidural, and Caudal)

The administration of a spinal, epidural, or caudal anesthetic requires knowledge of the central nervous system, spinal column, spinal cord, and neural structures. Selection of the appropriate neural blocking agent requires a pharmacologic understanding of the local anesthetic agents and adjuvants that may be used to alter the block. Management of a centro-neuroaxis anesthetic requires knowledge of the dermatomal distribution of the spinal nerves, as well as the autonomic, sensory, and motor responses to central neural blockade.

Contraindications to the administration of these blocks include patient refusal, infection at the puncture site, sepsis, coagulopathy, increased intracranial pressure (ICP), uncorrected severe hypovolemia, demyelinating CNS disease, or allergy to the specific class of local anesthetic agent.

Spinal Block. Spinal anesthesia is most suitable for procedures on the lower half of the body and is accomplished by injecting a small volume of a local anesthetic solution through a spinal needle into the subarachnoid space, which contains cerebrospinal fluid (CSF), the spinal cord (which in adults usually terminates at L1), and spinal nerves. To avoid inadvertent needle trauma to the spinal cord, the spinal needle is introduced into the lumbar region at or below the L2–L3 interspace into the subarachnoid space. Proper placement is confirmed by the return of clear CSF. If the patient complains of paresthesia during needle placement or during injection of local anesthetic, the needle must be withdrawn or redirected in order to avoid nerve injury.

The injected local anesthetic mixes with the CSF and bathes the nerve roots, dorsal root ganglia, and possibly the periphery of the spinal cord. The agent causes temporary neural blockade by penetrating the neural membrane and inhibiting the transmission of nerve impulses. The spread of the local anesthetic depends on the amount of agent injected, the baricity of the anesthetic solution, and the position of the patient during and immediately after the injection. Baricity is comparison of the specific gravity of the anesthetic solution in relation to the specific gravity of the CSF.

A hyperbaric solution is heavier, hypobaric lighter, and isobaric being the same specific gravity as CSF. A hyperbaric solution flows downward toward the most dependent portion of the CSF column, a hypobaric solution ascends toward the higher portion of the CSF column, and the isobaric solution remains within the approximate zone of injection. As the agent spreads, the concentration decreases as the drug is absorbed.

The position of the patient during and immediately after the injection is crucial for proper distribution of the anesthetic agent. With the patient in the sitting, lateral decubitus, or prone position, a spinal anesthetic is commonly administered as a single-shot technique (some elect to temporarily place an indwelling subarachnoid catheter for repeated intraoperative dosing). Depending on the intended distribution of anesthetic agent, the patient may remain in the original position for several minutes after injection or be immediately repositioned after injection to achieve the desired effect.

The duration of action of the anesthetic agent is an important consideration. The most commonly used preservative-free agents are procaine, tetracaine, lidocaine, and bupivacaine. Each possesses a diffferent duration of action. Anticipating the length of time to complete a procedure influences the selection of a particular agent. Except for bupivacaine, the duration of action may be extended further by mixing epinephrine or phenylephrine with the local anesthetic prior to injection.

Once the anesthetic agent has been injected into the subarachnoid space, the onset of action is very rapid and evidence of neural blockade may be manifest within 1 to 2 minutes. Because the onset of action is so rapid, the lumbar puncture usually is performed in the operating room. The height of the block should be well established within 15 to 20 minutes.

Because of the differences in nerve size, fiber type, and (un)myelination, some nerves are blocked more easily than others. Consequently, differential zones of neural blockade are expected. The smaller myelinated fibers (sympathetic, pain) are more easily blocked than the larger motor fibers. As a result, the sympathetic block occurs first and is generally two dermatome levels above the sensory block. Motor blockade occurs last and is typically two myotome levels below the level of sensory blockade.

A dermatome's sensory level corresponds to the vertebrae from which the spinal nerve exits the intervertebral foramen. Sensory level T4 (nipple line) and T10 (umbilicus) are good reference points. Immediately after the administration of the local anesthetic, the progression of neural blockade is evaluated by testing successive dermatome levels for a response (or lack of a response) to a stimulus. Touching the skin with an alcohol wipe for sympathetic blockade or pricking the skin with a dull needle for sensory blockade may be used as testing methods. After the block has been established, asking the patient to move his or her lower extremities may be used to assess the degree of motor blockade.

Tracking the level of sensory blockade is very important to ensure adequate anesthesia for the surgical procedure. The level of sympathetic block must be known because resulting cardiovascular effects are proportionate to the degree of neural block. The sympathetic fibers from the T5–L1 distribution help maintain vascular tone (e.g., blood pressure) and cardiac accelerator fibers from T1–T4 help maintain heart rate.

Within the first few minutes after injection of the local anesthetic, a decrease in blood pressure is anticipated. The higher the level of sympathetic block, the greater the drop in blood pressure. A partial sympathectomy at T8–T10 may be well tolerated in the rehydrated patient, because intact baroreceptor activity and the cardiac accelerator fibers provide sufficient input to maintain blood pressure and heart rate. If the sensory level is at or above the T3 level, the patient is considered to have a total sympathectomy. Support of the cardiovascular system with pharmacologic agents, increased IV fluid administration, or Trendelenburg positioning are often necessary to help maintain an acceptable blood pressure and heart rate. If uncorrected, hypoperfusion to the respiratory center in the brain may result in apnea.

The respiratory effect is dependent on the height of the motor block. Effective ventilation results from adequate use of the diaphragm, intercostal, and abdominal muscles. For patients with normal pulmonary mechanics, lower level blocks that paralyze the abdominal muscles should have no effect on ventilations. With higher level thoracic blocks, the intercostal muscles become paralyzed. Because the diaphragm is still functional, these patients should still be able to maintain a normal tidal volume, SaO_2, and $ETCO_2$. With a high-level thoracic block, the patient may complain of dyspnea because of the loss of chest wall sensation. These patients may need to be reassured that they are being monitored and are breathing adequately. The phrenic nerve, which controls the diaphragm, is a large nerve that originates mainly from C4 (with small communicating branches from C3 and C5) and is rarely affected by the administration of a standard spinal anesthetic. If the phrenic nerve does become paralyzed, the patient has a "total spinal" and ventilatory support will be necessary.

The urologic effects may result in an atonic bladder and urinary retention. If the patient has been administered a large volume of IV fluids or is unable to void within a reasonable time after the block has worn off, urinary catheterization may be considered.

The gastrointestinal effect may be beneficial for the surgical team. A sympathetic block of T5–L1 results in unopposed vagal stimulation of the intestine. This results in contracted intestines with active peristalsis. This level of blockade also provides excellent skeletal muscle relaxation for the surgical team. A feeling of nausea may be secondary to the increased vagal tone or hypotension. Administration of an anticholinergic or increasing the blood pressure are standard treatments.

As the surgery progresses, regression of the neural blockade is expected. This regression occurs in the opposite order as the progression of the neural blockade. Although the patient may be able to move his or her legs toward the end of the procedure, there still may be sufficient sensory blockade to complete the case. If the spinal block becomes inadequate, injection of a local anesthetic into the surgical site, a field block, or administration of a general anesthetic may be necessary. If a continuous subarachnoid catheter was placed, a sufficient level of block can be maintained throughout surgery.

Complications attributed to the administration of a spinal anesthetic are uncommon and permanent neurologic deficits are rare. The two most common complications are back pain and spinal headache. The back pain is usually the result of needle instrumentation and should resolve with time. A spinal headache results from the loss of CSF through the dural puncture site. The intensity of the headache is increased when the patient is in the upright position. Conservative therapy includes having the patient remain supine, aggressive hydration, and administration of IV analgesics and caffeine. If this therapy is unsuccessful after 24 hours, an epidural blood patch procedure may be performed. A blood patch procedure involves withdrawing 10 to 15 mL of the patient's blood and immediately administering the blood into the epidural space at the level of the original lumbar puncture. The resulting hemostatic plug should seal the hole in the dura and prevent further leakage of CSF.

Epidural Block. Epidural anesthesia is also indicated for procedures on the lower half of the body, and is more versatile than a spinal anesthetic. A significant advantage is that a continuous catheter may be placed within the epidural space. This catheter is used during obstetrical or surgical procedures to maintain a sufficient level of anesthesia and then may be used postoperatively for pain control with a continuous infusion of a local anesthetic agent or narcotic through the catheter.

An epidural anesthetic is accomplished by injecting a local anesthetic agent into the epidural space. The epidural space extends the length of the vertebral column and contains loose connective tissue, fat, and epidural veins. For surgical procedures, an epidural needle may be placed through the lumbar or thoracic interlaminar space. The needle is advanced midline (to avoid epidural veins) into the firm ligamentum flavum. Needle entrance into the epidural space may be identified by the hanging drop technique or by the loss-of-resistance technique. When performing the loss-of-resistance technique, an air- or saline-filled syringe is attached to the epidural needle after the needle has been positioned in the ligamentum flavum. As the needle is being advanced, continuous or intermittent pressure is applied to the plunger of the syringe. A sudden loss of resistance indicates entry of the needle tip into the epidural space.

If using the hanging drop technique, the epidural needle is placed into the ligamentum flavum. A drop of saline is placed onto the needle hub. As the needle is advanced and enters the epidural space, negative pressure within this space draws the drop inside the needle and indicates proper placement. The epidural space is narrow, so continued advancement of the needle eventually results in inadvertent dural puncture. Return of CSF or blood during needle placement indicates that the dura or an epidural vein has been punctured. If either occurs, the needle must be withdrawn or repositioned.

Regardless of which technique is employed, a 3-mL test dose of local anesthetic with 1 : 200,000 epinephrine first is injected through the epidural needle or epidural catheter. If the dura has been punctured and the local anesthetic enters the subarachnoid space, signs of a spinal anesthetic develop. If the injected dose enters an epidural vein, the epinephrine causes a notable increase in heart rate.

If there is no evidence of blood or CSF return, the needle may be used for a single-dose injection or an epidural catheter may be threaded 2 to 5 cm rostrally into the epidural space. The catheter may be used intraoperatively for anesthetic management as well as postoperatively for pain control.

If there are no adverse reactions to the test dose within 3 to 5 minutes, the calculated dose of local anesthetic is administered slowly in divided doses. After each 5 mL of local anesthetic injection, aspiration is performed to make certain that the epidural needle or indwelling catheter has not migrated into the subarachnoid space or epidural vein.

Because the volume of local anesthetic injected into the epidural space is much greater than that used for a spinal anesthetic, there is a greater risk of systemic or CNS toxicity. Local anesthetic agents such as chloroprocaine, lidocaine, mepivacaine, prilocaine, etidocaine, and bupivacaine are selected because of their characteristic onset of action, intensity of blockade, or duration of action.

After injection, the anesthetic effect results from the absorption of the agent through the dural sheath onto the neural membranes located in the predural space, or possibly by diffusion through the dura into the subarachnoid space. The onset of action is longer than that of a spinal anesthetic, so patience is exercised in waiting for the block to fully develop.

Additives may be used to affect the anesthetic agent. Mixing $NaHCO_3$ decreases the onset of action, adding 1 : 200,000 epinephrine prolongs the duration of action, and mixing narcotics decreases the onset of action and prolongs the duration of action. Adjusting the dosage or concentration of the local anesthetic results in varying degrees of sympathetic, sensory, and motor blockade and can be tailored to match the demands of the surgical procedure. Dosage adjustments are made for patients with spinal deformities, who are morbidly obese, the elderly, or who are pregnant.

Once the epidural anesthetic agent has been administered, the level of the neural blockade must be monitored in the same manner as described for the spinal anesthetic. The level of autonomic and sensory block frequently occurs at the same dermatome level. If motor blockade develops, it may be detected five dermatome levels below the level of the sensory block. Although the neural blockade occurs at a slower rate than that of a spinal anesthetic, preparations for untoward effects must be made.

Complications resulting from an epidural anesthetic are similar to those with a spinal anesthetic. If dural puncture does occur, there is a much greater incidence of the patient developing a spinal headache (for epidurals, a 16- to 18-gauge needle is used; with spinals, a 22- to 25-gauge needle is used). Unintentional injection of a large volume of local anesthetic into the subarachnoid space or an epidural vein results in drug overdosage that may cause CNS or systemic toxicity.

An epidural hematoma is extremely rare. Use of intraoperative heparin or postoperative anticoagulants in patients with indwelling catheters increases the incidence of occurrence. For such patients, normalization of coagulation studies needs to be confirmed prior to withdrawing the catheter. Documentation of an epidural hematoma (by magnetic resonance imaging [MRI]) requires immediate evacuation to relieve pressure on neural structures. Knotting, kinking, or breakage of indwelling epidural catheters has been reported. Also, as with any invasive procedure, infection is a potential risk.

Caudal Block. Caudal anesthesia is most useful during obstetrical or surgical procedures involving the perineal region. A 1 1/2- to 2-inch needle is placed through the sacral hiatus and advanced into the caudal canal until it enters the epidural space. An indwelling catheter may be inserted through the needle. As with an epidural anesthetic, a test dose of local anesthetic is administered to rule out inadvertent subarachnoid or epidural vein puncture. If no adverse effects are detected, the appropriate dosage of local anesthetic is injected into the epidural space as a single-dose technique or through the catheter for repeated dosing. Because the anesthetic agent is introduced into the epidural space, similar physiologic effects and complications as those associated with the administration of a lumbar epidural anesthetic should be considered.

Peripheral Nerve Blocks

Peripheral nerve blocks are chosen for surgical procedures on the upper or lower extremities. The choice to use this block is made in agreement with the patient during the preoperative anesthesia consultation. As with all regional anesthetic procedures, the patient is monitored, provided supplemental O_2, and is appropriately sedated, yet responsive.

Knowledge of neuroanatomy, the actions of the local anesthetic agents, the effects of the resulting neural blockade, and any associated complications resulting from the administration of a peripheral nerve blockade are necessary. Contraindications to this procedure include patient refusal, infection at the proposed puncture site, coagulopathy, or existing neuropathy of the extremity.

An advantage of a peripheral nerve block is that it should have minimal effect on the cardiovascular or pulmonary systems. A disadvantage is that the block may not be completely successful, take a prolonged period to become effective, or require supplementation. In order to allow sufficient time and ensure the adequacy of the neural blockade, the administration of the nerve block may be performed in a "block room" or the PSCU.

Several techniques are employed to favorably position the needle adjacent to the nerve. Identification of bony landmarks, muscle groups, and palpation of arteries are used in selecting the site of needle insertion.

The nerve stimulator technique is a relatively safe method for locating the nerve. With the patient electrically grounded, an insulated needle (except for the blunt tip) is connected to a nerve stimulator and directed toward the nerve. As the needle is advanced, motor or sensory response becomes pronounced. Ideal needle placement is achieved when the maximal neural response is obtained with the lowest current output.

The elicitation of paresthesia technique involves advancing the needle until it comes in direct contact with the nerve. There may be a higher incidence of postblock neuropathy with this procedure. Severe paresthesia during injection of the local anesthetic may indicate intraneural rather than perineural injection. If this occurs, the needle is withdrawn.

The loss-of-resistance technique takes advantage of the fact that some nerves used for neural blockade reside in neurovascular bundles surrounded by a fascial sheath. A blunt, beveled needle is advanced toward the nerve and a loss of resistance is felt as the needle passes through the fascial sheath and enters the neurovascular bundle.

Regardless of the technique employed, a test dose of local anesthetic is injected to rule out inadvertent intravascular, intraneural, or subarachnoid needle placement. If there are no adverse reactions, the local anesthetic is administered in incremental doses with interval pauses. This method of injection is used for large volume dosing because if any adverse effect is noted due to needle malposition, the injection can be terminated prior to administering the full dose.

Upper Extremity Blocks.   For the upper extremity, the brachial plexus block provides the greatest area of blockade. Depending on the proposed surgical site, the interscalene, supraclavicular, or axillary approach to the brachial plexus may be used. The intrascalene approach may provide adequate anesthesia for the shoulder; the supraclavicular approach, for the elbow, forearm, and hand; and the axillary approach for procedures distal to the elbow. Selective blockade of the musculocutaneous, radial, median, ulnar, or digital nerves are employed for anesthetizing more specific regions, or may be used to supplement a brachial plexus block.

Lower Extremity Blocks.   For the lower extremity, the lumbar plexus, sacral plexus, and peripheral nerves are targeted for neural blockade. Because the major nerve plexi are not in close proximity, multiple blocks are necessary to provide sufficient anesthesia for the entire lower extremity. The most commonly performed nerve blocks include the lumbar plexus, femoral nerve, obturator nerve, lateral femoral cutaneous nerve, sciatic nerve, ilioinguinal/iliohypogastric nerves, and popliteal nerve. For an ankle block, the deep peroneal, saphenous, superficial peroneal, posterior tibial, and sural nerves are targeted for blockade.

Complications associated with the administration of peripheral nerve blocks include drug reaction, toxicity, intravascular or subarachnoid injection, neuropathy from needle trauma or intraneural injection, hematoma, or pneumothorax from pleural puncture.

Intravenous Regional Anesthesia (Bier Block)

An intravenous regional anesthesia (Bier block) provides an excellent sensory and motor block for upper and lower extremity surgical procedures of short duration. The technique for this block involves placing a double tourniquet (proximal cuff/distal cuff) around the proximal portion of the surgical extremity. A small-gauge IV line is inserted into the most distal vein. An Esmarch bandage is used to exsanguinate the limb, starting from the most distal portion and continuing up to the base of the double tourniquet. The proximal cuff of the tourniquet is then inflated to occlude blood flow. The Esmarch bandage is removed and the local anesthetic agent is injected through the IV catheter.

The resulting block has a rapid onset and provides excellent anesthesia for approximately 45 to 60 minutes. If the patient begins to complain of tourniquet pain, the distal cuff is inflated. After confirmation that the distal cuff is inflated, the proximal cuff is deflated. The tourniquet pain should then subside.

Upon completion of surgery, the tourniquet is deflated, reinflated, and deflated in timed sequence. This procedure minimizes the possibility of a systemic reaction to the remaining local anesthetic as it returns to the central circulation.

Regional Head and Neck Blocks

Contraindications to and complications associated with the administration of head and neck blocks are the same as those described for centroneuroaxis and peripheral nerve blocks.

Cervical Plexus Blocks.　The cervical plexus blocks are used for procedures on the neck and occipital portion of the scalp. A superficial plexus block is accomplished by injecting a local anesthetic agent along the posterior border of the sternocleidomastoid muscle. A deep cervical block involves individual injections adjacent to transverse process to access C2, C3, and C4 of the cervical plexus.

Superior Laryngeal Nerve Block.　This nerve block anesthetizes the airway between the epiglottis and vocal cords and is used to suppress airway reflexes during laryngoscopy. Bilateral nerve blocks are accomplished by injecting a local anesthetic agent below the greater cornu on each side of the hyoid bone.

Translaryngeal Nerve Block.　This block anesthetizes the airway below the vocal cords and frequently is used in combination with the superior laryngeal nerve block during awake intubations. This block is accomplished by directing a needle through the cricothyroid membrane into the trachea, with subsequent injection of the local anesthetic agent.

Retrobulbar Nerve Blocks.　A retrobulbar block provides excellent anesthesia for corneal, lens, and anterior chamber ocular procedures. This block is accomplished by injecting a local anesthetic agent into the muscle cone behind the globe of the eye.

Facial Nerve Block.　This block frequently is given in combination with the retrobulbar block. Injection of a local anesthetic agent adjacent to the facial nerve causes akinesis of the eyelid and permits placement of the eyelid speculum.

MONITORED ANESTHESIA CARE (MAC)

Some minor surgical procedures are suitable for MAC. MAC means that the anesthesia care team monitors the patient, provides intraoperative sedation, and is prepared to administer a general anesthetic if necessary.

Although these patients are having a minor surgical procedure, their physical status may range from the healthy ASA I to the critically ill ASA V patient. The patient's instructions the night before surgery are the same as if he or she were having a general anesthetic.

The patient is appropriately sedated prior to entering the operating room. Basic monitoring includes ECG, blood pressure, heart rate, respirations, SaO_2, $ETCO_2$, and temperature. Supplemental oxygen is generally administered via a split O_2 delivery/CO_2 sampling nasal cannula. If electrocautery is used during head or neck surgery, a high concentration of O_2 should be avoided because of the danger of fire. Because many of the candidates for MAC are outpatients, IV sedation generally consists of a short-acting analgesic or an ultra–short-acting hypnotic/sedative.

After the patient is monitored and effectively sedated, the surgeon infiltrates a local anesthetic agent around the surgical incision site (field block). Throughout the procedure, it is made certain that the patient remains comfortable, safe, hemodynamically stable, and well oxygenated. If at any point the patient expresses discomfort, additional local anesthetic may be given to extend the field block. To help avoid overdosage, a record is kept of the total anesthetic dose.

The cooperative patient usually does very well with MAC. There are occasions where the anesthetic plan needs to be changed during the surgical procedure. A general anesthetic may become necessary if the surgeon is unable to provide or maintain a field block sufficient enough to keep the patient comfortable. Some patients with sedation become confused and uncooperative, and administration of additional IV sedation may exacerbate the problem. If the patient becomes oversedated, the airway may become difficult to manage. In this situation, reversal of the sedative agent or conversion to a general anesthetic may become necessary.

Overall, MAC is an effective anesthetic plan for minor surgical procedures. The anesthetic agents chosen have a minimal effect on the autonomic nervous system, which is advantageous in the critically ill patient. The rapid recovery from the short-acting agents also allows for a more rapid discharge from the hospital.

CARDIAC ANESTHESIA

Cardiac anesthesia refers to the anesthetic plan or technique that is used during major cardiovascular surgical procedures, particularly for open heart procedures that require cardiopulmonary bypass (CPB). Extensive knowledge of cardiac anatomy, pathophysiology, physiology, pharmacology, surgical routines of the various procedures, and extracorporeal circuitry used during CPB is essential. Once on bypass, there must be an understanding of a patient's physiologic response of suddenly being subjected to abnormal conditions such as nonpulsatile blood flow, hemodilution, hypothermia, and cardioplegic arrest.

Although the commonly performed coronary artery bypass graft (CABG) may be considered routine, an experienced anesthesia care team is essential for maintaining the low morbidity and mortality rates associated with successful heart programs.

THE CARDIOVASCULAR PATIENT

The patient typically consents to elective open heart surgery because symptoms have progressed despite alternative modalities of therapy. The most common cardiovascular pathologies are attributed to coronary artery disease (CAD), valvular heart disease, intracardiac shunts, intracavitary lesions, cardiomyopathies, ascending aortic disease, pulmonary emboli, or acute cardiovascular trauma.

Coronary Artery Disease. Presenting complaints include angina or symptoms of cardiac failure because the oxygen supply to the heart is insufficient to meet demands. Intraoperatively, the oxygen supply is maximized by increasing the FIO_2; administering a coronary vasodilator (e.g., nitroglycerin); maintaining a slow, normal heart rate; and maintaining a normal or slightly elevated mean blood pressure. The goal is to avoid the two major causes of increased oxygen demand, tachycardia and hypertension.

Aortic Stenosis. With aortic stenosis, there is an increased resistance of the ejection of blood during systole. Left ventricular hypertrophy is common. The goal is to maintain a sinus rhythm and avoid hypotension, tachycardia, or bradycardia. During anesthetic induction, a phenylephrine infusion may be carefully titrated to help maintain adequate coronary perfusion pressure to the hypertrophied left ventricle.

Aortic Insufficiency. These patients have an increased left ventricular volume because blood regurgitates back into the left ventricle during diastole. The objective is to maintain a slightly higher than normal heart rate and decrease the systemic vascular resistance.

Mitral Stenosis. There is a reduced flow of blood from the left atrium into the left ventricle. The goal is to avoid tachycardia, maintain intravascular volume, and maintain a sinus rhythm.

Mitral Insufficiency. The patient usually has a dilated left atrium and is in atrial fibrillation. The purpose is to maintain a normal or slightly elevated heart rate and avoid increased systemic vascular resistance.

Atrial-septal/Ventriculoseptal Defects (ASD/VSD). Air should be avoided in all intravascular infusion sites to prevent the possibility of an intra-arterial air embolus if a right-to-left shunt develops.

Idiopathic Hypertrophic Subaortic Stenosis (IHSS). These patients have a hypertrophied interventricular septum and hypertrophied left ventricle. During systole, the left ventricular outflow tract can become obstructed. This obstruction is exacerbated when the heart contracts more vigorously and faster. The goal is to avoid tachycardia, avoid inotropes, and maintain an increased systemic vascular resistance.

Ascending Aortic Aneurysm/Dissection. The pathology may extend up into the innominate artery, so blood pressure measurements in the right arm may be inaccurate or compromised during surgery. If the arch vessels are involved, profound hypothermia, circulatory arrest, and retrograde cerebral perfusion techniques may be used. The goal is to protect the end organs.

End-stage Cardiomyopathy for Heart Transplant. During transplant surgery, strict aseptic technique must be maintained. The patient should receive antibiotics and immunosuppressants according to protocol. The main goal after transplantation is to avoid pulmonary hypertension, which can quickly lead to right ventricular failure in the transplanted heart.

THE CARDIAC ANESTHESIA CONSULT

The surgeon's notes are evaluated to appreciate the nature of the proposed procedure, because this may influence the sites for line placement or the need for additional monitoring. The cardiologist's report is also evaluated for information regarding heart catheterization or ECG. The report on coronary angiography can detail the extent and severity of coronary artery stenosis. Left heart catheterization can reveal aortic valve or mitral valve disease, ASD/VSD, left ventricular aneurysms, left ventricular thrombus, IHSS, left atrial myxoma, and heart wall motion abnormalities.

Left ventricular function can be assessed and the ejection fraction (ratio of blood ejected from the left ventricular cavity [stroke volume] in relation to the total volume of blood in the left ventricle during end diastole [normal, 0.4 to 0.65]) is estimated by the cardiologist. An estimated ejection fraction of less than 0.4 is indicative of left ventricular dysfunction. Measurement of left ventricular end-diastolic pressure (LVEDP) can also be used to evaluate left ventricular function (normal, 2 to 12 mm Hg). LDVEP greater than 18 is indicative of left ventricular dysfunction.

Right heart catheterization can reveal an ASD/VSD, tricuspid or pulmonic valve disease, intracavitary lesions, and pulmonary embolus. Pressure measurements can be used to diagnose pulmonary hypertension and blood gas sampling may be used to calculate intracardiac shunts. Cardiac outputs may also be obtained.

A surface ECG can demonstrate valvular heart disease, intracardiac shunts, cardiomyopathies, intracavitary lesions, pericardial effusion, tamponade, ascending aortic aneurysm/dissection, intracavitary volume status, and wall motion abnormalities. Cardiac function can also be assessed. A TEE is frequently performed intraoperatively.

The ECG is evaluated for abnormalities of heart rate and rhythm. Signs of ischemia, previous myocardial infarction, ventricular hypertrophy, electrolyte imbalance, dysrhythmias, and conduction disorders are noted.

The chest x-ray is viewed for signs of congestive heart failure (CHF), pulmonary disease, pulmonary hypertension, cardiomegaly, pulmonary effusions, and pericardial effusion. Evidence of previous open heart surgery or implantation of a pacemaker or AICD is documented.

Any abnormalities in the laboratory data should be investigated. Of special interest are an increase in potassium, hemoglobin, glucose, creatinine, and bleeding time values.

Vital signs are recorded with an emphasis on blood pressure range and notation of any discrepancies between right and left arm blood pressures.

History and Physical

The patient's cardiac history should be detailed. A history of angina, previous myocardial infarctions, CHF, shortness of breath, palpitations, syncope, and previous open heart surgery is obtained. A positive history of cardiac-related exercise intolerance is especially useful in the prediction of decreased cardiac reserve. A history of coexisting disease, such as hypertension, cerebrovascular insufficiency, peripheral vascular disease, renal insufficiency, insulin-dependent diabetes mellitus, chronic obstructive pulmonary disease (COPD), or bleeding disorders influences anesthetic management. The physical examination should note any abnormalities that may influence airway management, line insertions, or patient positioning.

THE ANESTHESIA PLAN

The anesthetic technique for open heart surgery employs a general anesthetic with endotracheal intubation, mechanical ventilation, and full cardiovascular monitoring. The patient is informed of the necessity of IV lines, arterial line, CVP line and pulmonary artery catheter, and that the ETT may be in place when waking postoperatively.

Preoperative Medication

The patient's scheduled medications are usually continued until the time of surgery, with a few exceptions. Dosages for long-acting antihypertensives, beta blockers, anticoagulants, and glucophages may be moderated or discontinued. Typical preoperative medications include a narcotic, hypnotic sedative, anticholinergic, H_2 blocker, along with supplemental oxygen. Sedation is important because stress and anxiety may result in an increase in heart rate and blood pressure that can precipitate an untoward cardiac event. The narcotic and sedative dosages for patients with marginal cardiac reserve or impaired pulmonary function needs to be appropriately reduced to avoid oversedation.

Intraoperative Considerations

The patient should arrive comfortably sedated, with supplemental oxygen in place. Any complaints such as shortness of breath and chest pain are addressed. The patient's chart is reviewed for any new information that may alter the anesthetic plan. The patient should be kept warm to reduce shivering (which increases oxygen consumption). The patient is positioned and pulse oximetry, ECG leads II and V5, and noninvasive blood pressure monitoring are established and checked for any significant changes from baseline parameters. If the patient is undergoing a repeat open heart surgery, adhesive external defibrillator pads are placed.

Line Insertions

IV. A 16-gauge or larger IV line is started in each arm for fluid administration.

Arterial Line. An arterial line is also inserted into the nondominant arm; however, if there is significant difference in the blood pressures between the arms, the one with the highest pressure is selected. The arterial line is used to continuously monitor blood pressure, measure arterial blood gases, and obtain activated coagulation time (ACT) or other laboratory studies. Observation of abnormal waveform patterns may be suggestive of certain pathologies or altered volume status (e.g., hypovolemia).

Pulmonary Artery Catheter. The pulmonary artery catheter is most useful in the assessment of ventricular function. Direct measurements include pulmonary artery (PA), systolic/diastolic (S/D x), pulmonary capillary wedge pressure (PCWP), CVP, and blood temperature. By using the thermodilution technique, the cardiac output (CO) level is obtained. An additional lumen within the catheter can be used for cardiac pacing or drug infusion. Using CO and pressure measurement data, the peripheral vascular resistance (PVR) can be calculated. Measuring CO and PVR is essential when cardiotonic and vasoactive agents are used to maximize cardiac performance. Filling pressure measurements are also useful in the management of volume replacement. Observations of sudden, abnormal waveform patterns should be investigated. For example, a prominent V wave appearing in the PCWP tracing may be indicative of papillary dysfunction and a failing left ventricle.

After line placements, baseline hemodynamics are recorded, and samples for arterial blood gases (ABGs) and ACT are drawn. Epinephrine, nitroglycerin, and phenylephrine drips are inserted into the sideport for use as needed. An external pacemaker is at the bedside and checked for proper functioning.

INDUCTION OF ANESTHESIA

The patient's nasal oxygen is discontinued and the patient is preoxygenated with 100% oxygen via the face mask. The goal during the induction period is to safely anesthetize the patient, secure the airway, and maintain hemodynamic stability.

For patients who require a normal or higher than normal arterial perfusion pressure (e.g., patients with left main CAD, aortic stenosis, or IHSS), a phenylephrine drip infusion may be started immediately prior to induction to offset the decrease in blood pressure that frequently is encountered during induction.

A typical induction begins with the administration of an ultra–short-acting IV anesthetic agent, a narcotic, and a hypnotic sedative. After loss of consciousness, a muscle relaxant is given. The induction agents are administered in incremental doses so that patient response can be evaluated. The cardiovascular monitor is observed for changes in the ECG, blood pressure, pulmonary artery pressure, and CVP.

The most frequent and noticeable hemodynamic change is a drop in blood pressure as the patient becomes unconscious. If the hypotension is significant, the nonfailing heart may be treated by administering a vasopressor, placing the patient in the Trendelenburg position, or by increasing the IV fluids. If the hypotension is secondary to a failing heart, more aggressive therapy with cardiotonic agents or vasoactive drugs may be necessary.

As the patient loses consciousness, the airway is managed and the adequacy of ventilations assessed. After muscle relaxation has been achieved, endotracheal intubation is performed. This procedure is stimulating and may be timely in helping to restore a decreasing blood pressure after induction. If the patient has good ventricular function, a volatile inhalational anesthetic agent in 100% oxygen is commonly administered to supplement the IV anesthetics. An esophageal stethoscope (or TEE probe) is usually inserted.

The depth of anesthesia is continually assessed by evaluating the patient's blood pressure and heart rate to varying degrees of noxious stimulation. Inadequate sedation may result in hypertension and tachycardia, which can precipitate untoward cardiac events. This is best avoided by adjusting the depth of anesthesia prior to surgical stimulation.

The induction period is a critical time because multiple pharmacologic agents have to be administered, the patient's breathing pattern is changed from spontaneous to controlled, hemodynamics are being stabilized, and the anesthetic level has to be appropriately adjusted. Prior to the incision, antibiotics are routinely administered. Steroids, H_1 antagonists, or diuretics may also be given. Antifibrinolytics may be given to the high-risk patient (e.g., repeat open heart surgery or those who have refused blood transfusions).

SURGERY

Open heart surgery may be divided into the prebypass, bypass, and postbypass periods.

Prebypass

During the prebypass period, a patient's cardiovascular response to surgical stimulation is managed. Patients with limited cardiac reserve are intolerant of large fluctuations in blood pressure and heart rate. When surgery begins, a moderate rise in blood pressure and heart rate are anticipated. As surgery progresses, the patient is subjected to more intense stimulation during median sternotomy, sternal retraction, opening the pericardium, etc. Prior to sternotomy, the lungs are deflated to prevent inadvertent sawing into the pleura, lungs, or myocardium. The depth of anesthesia is increased in anticipation of these events, but increases in blood pressure and heart rate commonly occur. If the patient becomes significantly hypertensive, a vasodilator, additional anesthetics, or a short-acting beta blocker are added. If tachycardia occurs, it needs to be aggressively treated with a short-acting beta blocker or additional anesthetics.

During periods of minimal stimulation, hypotension may occur. In consideration of the patient's cardiovascular pathology, administering vasopressors, increasing IV fluids, or placing the patient into the Trendelenburg position may be used. Acute hypotension may occur secondary to surgical events such as manipulation of the heart (causing dysrhythmias or altering filling pressures). The surgical team must be alerted to cease manipulations until the blood pressure is restored. Hypotension may also occur after intra-arterial injection by the surgeon of the vasodilator papaverine, after harvesting the internal mammary artery. This response may be minimized with the concurrent administration of an IV vasopressor.

The ECG is assessed for signs of acute or progressive ischemia. If this occurs, the oxygen supply–demand ratio is optimized. If life-threatening dysrhythmias occur, the advanced cardiac life support (ACLS) protocol is implemented.

Changes in the SaO_2 and $ETCO_2$ may be reflective of pulmonary or myocardial dysfunction. Arterial blood gases are evaluated as needed.

Urine output should be 1 mL/kg/h. Because the patient is hemodiluted while on bypass, a diuretic is frequently administered to help accommodate the reinfusion of pump blood after bypass.

During the prebypass stage, hypothermia is not treated as patient temperature can be adjusted while on bypass.

Prior to bypass, the patient must be totally heparinized. The calculated dose of heparin is administered through a central line. After 3 minutes, an ACT is drawn to determine the level of anticoagulation.

After the surgeon opens the pericardium, it is important to observe the heart. The right ventricle and right atrium are the most visible. Volume status can be grossly evaluated (empty/full) and contractility assessed (poor/excellent). Direct observation may be helpful in interpreting abnormal rhythms.

When adequate heparinization has been established, the surgeon can cannulate. Prior to placement of the arterial line into the ascending aorta, systolic blood pressure is temporarily decreased to a systolic of 90 to 100 mm Hg. This maneuver may help to minimize the chance for an aortic dissection as the cannula is placed into the aorta. As the arterial line is connected to the pump, the line should be inspected for air bubbles. During venous cannulation(s), hand ventilation may be performed to enhance surgical exposure. For administration of cardioplegia, the surgeon may place a multipurpose cannula into the ascending aorta for antegrade infusion for cardioplegia and for venting blood or air. Another cannula may be placed into the coronary sinus for retrograde infusion for cardioplegia. After confirmation that the ACT is greater than 400 seconds, the patient may be placed on bypass.

Bypass

When going on bypass, frequent inspections are made of the surgical field, the bypass cannulas, the heart–lung machine, the cardiovascular monitors, and the patient. Any abnormalities are brought to the attention of the surgeon and perfusionist.

As the venous line is opened, the blood flows by gravity into the venous reservoir. The heart should empty. When no blood is being ejected from the pulmonary artery, ventilations are discontinued. When full flow is established, there should be little or no pulsatile ejection noted on the arterial waveform. The systemic blood pressure is read as a mean perfusion pressure. The initial mean perfusion pressure typically is low. This mainly is due to hemodilution and decreased viscosity as the patient's blood mixes with the pump prime. If the perfusion pressure remains critically low and shows no signs of improvement, administration of a vasopressor or colloid must be considered. The patient's face is inspected to confirm good venous drainage from the head. Pupils are checked for symmetry to rule out inadvertent cannulation of the innominate artery to an aortic dissection.

Anesthesia, while on bypass, is commonly maintained with the administration of additional IV anesthetic agents and/or the continuation of the inhalational agent through a vaporizer mounted on the heart–lung machine. Additional muscle relaxant may also be given.

The volume status of the heart is continually monitored, especially when the surgeon manipulates the heart. If the patient has aortic insufficiency, overdistention of the left ventricle may rapidly occur if the valve is mechanically distorted while lifting the heart.

Prior to applying the aortic cross clamp, the surgeon may elect to reduce the patient's temperature. The hypothermic patient requires less anesthesia.

When all participants are prepared, the surgeon applies the cross clamp to stop the heart. When the clamp is applied, blood flow to the heart ceases. This is the beginning of the ischemic time. The effective and timely administration of cardioplegia is the single most important factor for preserving myocardial function.

After application of the aortic cross clamp, a cold cardioplegia solution, which has a high potassium content, is administered into the aortic root. It is given in an amount sufficient to arrest the heart in end diastole. This decreases oxygen demand, decreases cellular damage from ischemia, and preserves energy stores of the myocardium.

Throughout the aortic cross-clamp period, the surgeon may periodically administer cardioplegia antegrade through the aortic root, retrograde through the coronary sinus catheter, or directly down the coronary ostia if the aorta is opened. During surgery, cardioplegia is also given through the vein grafts after anastomosis. If electrical activity is noted while the heart should be asystolic, additional cardioplegia is administered as appropriate. Some surgeons prefer to use a continuous warm cardioplegia infusion throughout the cross-clamp period.

The mean arterial blood pressure is typically kept within a range of 50 to 90 mm Hg. The perfusionist ideally maintains a calculated flow rate through the inflow arterial cannula. The mean arterial blood pressure may be increased or decreased by altering the systemic vascular resistance by administering vasopressors or vasodilators or by adjusting the depth of anesthesia. For patients with cerebral vascular occlusive disease or a history of chronic hypertension, the mean arterial blood pressure needs to be maintained in the high range to provide an adequate cerebral perfusion pressure.

During bypass, the volume status of the heart is monitored. The heart should remain empty. If the pulmonary artery pressure or CVP becomes elevated or if the heart appears to be distended, corrective measures must be taken to decompress the heart.

Other physiologic parameters are also monitored and managed. A decrease in urine output is frequently encountered as the patient experiences nonpulsatile flow and hypothermia. If oliguria occurs, perfusion pressure may be increased, a diuretic given, or a renal dose of dopamine administered. Patients with pre-existing renal insufficiency are aggressively treated.

The perfusionist uses ABG results to adjust PaO_2 and $PaCO_2$ levels. If the base excess reveals a metabolic acidosis, the pH is corrected by giving $NaHCO_3$. If acidosis persists, the adequacy of tissue perfusion needs to be re-evaluated.

Anemia is anticipated (acceptable level, 7.0 to 9.0 g/dL) as the patient's blood is diluted with the pump prime. If the hemoglobin becomes critically low, diuretic therapy, extracorporeal hemoconcentration, or the administration of red blood cells (RBCs) must be considered.

The serum potassium level is expected to increase after the administration of cardioplegia. For patients with renal insufficiency, the potassium content of additional cardioplegia may need to be reduced. Dangerously high potassium levels will need to be treated prior to the discontinuation of bypass. Blood glucose levels should be kept within the normal range. Excessively high levels must be treated with regular insulin.

ACTs are monitored and additional heparin administered as needed.

Temperature is monitored at multiple sites and the perfusionist adjusts the temperature by altering the temperature of the blood as it flows through the venous reservoir. If the patient had the temperature reduced during bypass, the perfusionist rewarms the patient at the timely request of the surgeon near the end of the cross-clamp period. Because drug metabolism increases as temperature increases, additional anesthetic agents may be required.

Preparing the patient for release of the cross clamp includes evacuating any air that may have been trapped within the cardiac chambers or aorta. The patient is placed in the Trendelenburg position; ventilated with large tidal volumes, and the table is tilted from side to side as the surgeon assists with the expulsion of air through the vent sites. When air is no longer suspected, the cross clamp is removed.

After removal of the cross clamp, blood flow is re-established to the coronary circulation. If the patient had coronary bypass surgery, air is removed from the vein grafts. As the residual cardioplegia is washed out by the return of blood flow to the myocardium, the heart frequently begins to spontaneously contract. Additional removal of air may be necessary as blood flow returns to the pulmonary circulation and pushes any residual air from the pulmonary veins into the left atrium. The use of the TEE is quite effective in detecting the presence of air within the cardiac chambers.

To prevent ventricular fibrillation, a bolus of lidocaine may be given as the clamp is removed. If this does occur, the heart is defibrillated using internal paddles, starting at 15 to 20 joules. Abnormal heart rates, rhythms, and interventricular conduction patterns are common but typically resolve as the heart is reperfused with warm, oxygenated blood. Temporary arterial or ventricular pacing wires may be placed on the heart to optimize rate and rhythm.

As the heart begins to contract, the rhythm and quality of atrial and ventricular contractions are observed. Myocardial contractility should improve with time as the effects of cardioplegia dissipate.

Prior to coming off CPB, the depth of anesthesia is assessed and monitors recalibrated. Cardiotonic and vasoactive drips are readied for infusion as needed. The external pacemaker's operational status is checked and its settings adjusted for anticipated use. Temperature, hemoglobin, acid–base, potassium, glucose, and calcium abnormalities are treated.

If the heart rate is slow, atrial, ventricular, or atrioventricular sequential pacing is established at 80 to 100 beats per minute. If the contractility appears to be sluggish or the patient has pre-existing myocardial dysfunction, an inotropic infusion is begun to improve contractility before adding volume to the heart. Administration of $CaCL_2$ prior to coming off bypass also helps contractility.

When the surgeon is ready, the lungs are ventilated with 100% oxygen. Bilateral expansion is visually confirmed and atelectasis is eliminated. If the patient has an internal mammary artery bypass graft, care must be taken not to disrupt the anastomosis by hyperexpanding the lung. While hand ventilating, the compliance of the lungs is felt and breath sounds auscultated. If wheezing is present, bronchodilator therapy must be considered.

If cardiotonic or vasoactive agents have already been started, the infusion rates are rechecked. Temporary pacing wires are tested to confirm the ability to capture.

Dependent upon the depth of anesthesia and strength of contractility, delivery of an inhalational agent through the pump vaporizer may be adjusted or discontinued.

When the surgeon, anesthesia team, and perfusionist believe conditions have been optimized, the patient is weaned from bypass. The key for smooth separation from bypass is communication and vigilance.

Discontinuation of Bypass

Weaning the patient from bypass is a systematic process. Ventilation with 100% oxygen is reconfirmed. If the heart appears vigorous, an inhalational anesthetic may be continued to maintain an appropriate depth of anesthesia. The perfusionist slowly allows volume to increase in the right side of the heart by partially occluding the venous return line. As the volume load increases, pulsatile pulmonary artery and arterial pressure waveforms should begin to appear on the cardiovascular monitor. Pressure measurements and direct visualization of the heart are used to judge the appropriate filling pressures. A major goal is not to overload the heart.

The venous line is progressively occluded. The filling pressures (CVP, PCWP, and left arterial pressure) are increased to a volume sufficient to maintain an adequate blood pressure as the arterial flow rate from the pump is decreased.

If the arterial waveform appears dampened or pressure readings inaccurate, the surgeon can temporarily place a needle in the aorta to measure central arterial pressure. If there is a large discrepancy, a femoral line may be inserted for more accurate measurements. Noninvasive blood pressure cuff measurements may also be useful if discrepancies exist.

If hemodynamics are stable, the pump is turned off. After separation from bypass, a cardiac output is obtained and the systemic vascular resistance calculated. This information can be used as a guide to improve cardiac performance and adjust blood pressure. Inotropes, vasodilators, vasopressors, or temporary pacing are frequently used to optimize cardiovascular dynamics.

If, during the weaning process, there are signs of heart failure, acute ECG ischemic changes, or significant dysrhythmia, the patient is maintained on bypass until the possible causes are identified and corrected.

Inotropic support needs to be instituted or increased if the heart appears to be sluggish. It is important to discern if the patient has left- or right-sided ventricular failure. The use of the TEE is beneficial in assessing the overall contractility, regional wall motion abnormalities, valve function, volume status, or presence of retained air.

If acute ECG changes occur, coronary grafts must be rechecked for patency, kinking, spasm, or air embolus.

Dysrhythmias may be caused by ischemia, electrolyte imbalance, or a malpositioned pulmonary artery catheter. Corrective measures must be taken to eliminate the cause. Lidocaine is administered for ventricular ectopy. Tachydysrhythmia and bradydysrhythmia are treated per ACLS protocol.

When contractility has sufficiently improved and cardiac stability achieved, the weaning process is repeated.

If evidence of failure reoccurs, the patient is maintained on bypass while the use of an intra-aortic balloon pump (IABP) is considered. The IABP typically is inserted via the femoral artery and positioned in the descending aorta just distal to the left subclavian artery. When properly timed, the balloon inflates during diastole. This results in increased coronary artery perfusion pressure and blood flow. The balloon is deflated just prior to left ventricular ejection. This reduces afterload, which results in decreased oxygen consumption. When proper timing of the IABP has been achieved, the patient is weaned from bypass. If the patient is still unable to be weaned, a left (or right) ventricular assist device may be temporarily used until the heart recovers or the patient becomes a candidate for a heart transplant.

Postbypass Period

After the patient has been successfully weaned from bypass and is hemodynamically stable, the venous cannula may be removed. Any blood left in the pump is reinfused back into the patient through the arterial cannula. If there is a large volume to be infused and the patient has good myocardial and renal function, the preload is intentionally reduced by placing the patient in the reverse Trendelenburg position and administering vasodilators. The residual pump blood is then reinfused through the aortic cannula. The rate of infusion is guided by visual observation of the heart and changes in PCWP and arterial blood pressure. If the heart cannot tolerate all of the volume, the perfusionist bags the blood for subsequent IV infusion. If a cell saver is being used, the remaining blood may be hemoconcentrated before infusion. When the surgeon is ready to decannulate the aorta, the arterial pressure is lowered to approximately 100 mm Hg to avoid tearing the aorta as the aortotomy is closed after decannulation.

Protamine is administered to neutralize the anticoagulant effect of heparin. Adverse reactions are rare but may be seen in patients with previous exposure to protamine (e.g., previous open heart patients, diabetic patients taking protamine-containing insulin preparations) or shellfish allergy. The high-risk patient may be pretreated with steroids or H_1 and H_2 antagonists to minimize an anaphylactic reaction. These patients are administered a test dose of protamine before administering a full reversal dose. Although the protamine is administered slowly, a decrease in blood pressure may be seen secondary to vasodilation. If pulmonary artery pressure suddenly increases and arterial blood pressure decreases, a protamine reaction must be considered along with other causes of cardiac failure.

After the protamine is given, an ACT and ABGs are drawn. If the ACT has returned to normal, evidence of coagulation should become evident on the surgical field. If heparinized pump blood is administered after the initial reversal, additional protamine must be administered to neutralize the pump blood.

The ABGs are evaluated and abnormalities corrected. The hemoglobin level should increase as diuresis continues, provided that the patient is not actively bleeding. The serum potassium level typically decreases after bypass, especially if the patient has responded well to diuretic therapy. KCl may be added to the carrier solution to prevent or correct hypokalemia. The blood glucose level generally increases in response to the stress of surgery and if an adrenergic agonist (e.g., epinephrine) is being infused. The calcium level should be adequate if $CaCL_2$ was administered while weaning from bypass. Urine output should be sufficient for the reasons described above. Oliguria may persist in patients with renal insufficiency or occur in patients on high-dose norepinephrine infusion or patients in cardiogenic shock. Temperature typically decreases despite warming the IV fluids, increasing room temperature, and using a heat–moisture exchanger and a heating mattress.

As the surgical team continues to establish hemostasis, the heart may be manipulated to check for bleeding. This may result in a decreased blood pressure or dysrhythmia. If the cardiac output drops too low, manipulations are discontinued or altered until output returns to an acceptable level.

The surgical team then positions mediastinal or pleural tubes and begins to close the sternum. Drainage tubes are connected to suction.

Sternal Closure

When the chest is closed, the ability to visually inspect the heart and lungs is lost. Prior to closure, bilateral expansion of the lungs should be documented. Any fluid in an open pleural cavity should be removed by suctioning. If the patient has significant pleural effusions, the pleura should be opened to remove the fluid. Pneumothorax should be appropriately treated. Poor pulmonary compliance secondary to bronchospasm is treated with bronchodilator therapy.

A dynamic heart with normal filling pressures should easily tolerate chest closure. As the sternum is reapproximated, any vein grafts are observed for kinking. After closure, the temporary pacing wires should be tested to ensure capture.

For the patient with marginal myocardial function and increased filling pressures, chest closure may not be well tolerated. Cardiac output and filling pressures are evaluated preclosure and postclosure. Adjustments in pharmacologic support and filling pressures are made to allow the patient to tolerate closure. In rare circumstances, the patient does not tolerate closure and the chest is left open and covered with a rubber dam.

Cardiorespiratory parameters continue to be monitored after closure. If acute ECG changes develop, the possibility of a kinked or compressed coronary graft must be considered. If ECG changes are consistent with increasing ischemia, the chest may be reopened to examine the grafts.

The remaining portion of the surgical procedure should have little influence on anesthetic management.

Preparations are made for the safe transport of the patient to the ICU. The patient's cardiorespiratory status must be stable. The goal of the anesthesia team is to have the patient come out of anesthesia comfortable and extubatable within the first few hours after surgery. If an inhalational agent was used as the primary anesthetic, additional narcotic is administered because the analgesic effect diminishes fairly quickly after the vaporizer is turned off.

Transport to the ICU

When the patient is transferred from the operating table to the bed, changes in pressures sometimes occur. The transport bed should be equipped with a transport monitor, a self-inflating breathing bag, and a full oxygen tank. An anesthesia face mask and resuscitative drugs are placed on the bed for emergency use. Upon arrival in the ICU, cardiovascular monitoring is re-established and the patient is connected to a mechanical ventilator. Pertinent information is transmitted to the staff regarding the patient's ideal filling pressures, blood pressure range, review of any drips, the patient's underlying rhythm (if paced), and the most recent cardiac output, hemoglobin, base excess, potassium, and glucose. Plans are also made for extubation. Periodic visits are made throughout the day to evaluate progress. Any complications are noted and follow-up care is provided.

NEUROANESTHESIA

The administration of anesthesia for neurosurgical procedures requires knowledge of neuroanatomy, neurophysiology, and neuropathophysiology. An understanding of the patient's disease process and proposed surgical procedure is essential. Anesthesia management by a skilled neuroanesthesia care team plays a critical role in optimizing patient outcome.

CEREBRAL PHYSIOLOGY

Normal cerebral function depends on having a constant supply of oxygen and glucose available to meet the high metabolic demand for substrate of the brain. When a region of the brain is stimulated, the cerebral metabolic rate (CMR) of oxygen and glucose consumption increases. To meet this increase in demand, the cerebral blood flow (CBF) to the region of the brain stimulated also increases. The neuroanesthesia team must understand how this coupled relationship between CMR and CBF may be altered during neurologic disease or manipulated during anesthesia management.

Cerebral Blood Flow

CBF is calculated by dividing the cerebral perfusion pressure (CPP) by the cerebral vascular resistance (CVR). The CPP is the difference between the mean arterial pressure (MAP) and the intracranial pressure (ICP) or, if greater, the central venous pressure (CVP).

$$CBF = \frac{CPP}{CVR} = \frac{MAP\text{-}ICP \text{ (or CVP if } >ICP)}{CVR}$$

The CBF in normal adults is approximately 50 ml/100 g brain tissue/minute. If flow rates become diminished, cerebral dysfunction occurs. Depending on the duration and severity of low flow, cerebral impairment may be temporary or result in irreversible brain damage.

Major physiologic determinants of CBF are cerebral autoregulation, $PaCO_2$, and PO_2. Cerebral autoregulation refers to the ability of the cerebral vasculature to maintain a near constant CBF when the MAP is between 50 to 150 torr. If the MAP is outside of this range, the CBF becomes pressure dependent. If the pressure falls below 50 torr, hypoperfusion results in cerebral dysfunction. If the MAP exceeds 150 torr, disruption of the blood–brain barrier may occur and cause hemorrhage and cerebral edema.

Changes in $PaCO_2$ values have a major effect on altering CBF. The CBF varies directly with $PaCO_2$ values between 20 to 80 torr. For each 1 torr change in $PaCO_2$, the CBF changes 1 to 2 ml/100 g/min. Because CBF influences cerebral blood volume, control of $PaCO_2$ levels are critical, especially in patients with increased ICP. Changes in Pao_2 have little effect on CBF unless the patient becomes severely hypoxic. When the PaO_2 falls below 60 torr, CBF rapidly increases.

Cerebral Metabolic Rate

Normally, CMR is coupled with CBF. An increase or decrease in CMR is associated with a corresponding increase or decrease in CBF. During anesthesia, CMR or CBF may be altered by the administration of anesthetic agents, changes in temperature, or seizure activity.

Multiple pharmacologic agents are administered during a neurosurgical procedure. Most anesthetizing agents decrease or have little effect on CMR. Knowledge of which agents increase CBF is essential, because the effect may have deleterious effects on patients with increased ICP.

Changes in temperature alter CMR. For each 1°C change in temperature, there is a 7% change in CMR O_2. Consequently, mild hypothermia may be beneficial in some neurosurgical procedures.

Increased CMR during seizure activity may be precipitated by the use of certain anesthetic agents and should be avoided in patients predisposed to seizures.

Intracranial Pressure
The intracranial contents by volume consist of brain tissue (80%), blood (12%), and CSF (8%). The ICP reflects the relationship between these relatively incompressible components within the rigid intracranial vault. Normal ICP is between 5 to 15 torr. If there is an increase in volume in one compartment, a reciprocal change in one or both of the other compartments must occur to maintain a normal ICP (e.g., a neoplasm increasing in size displaces CSF to the more distensible subarachnoid space). The ICP may remain normal until this compensatory mechanism can no longer accommodate an additional increase in the size of the neoplasm. As compliance decreases, any small increase in volume results in a large increase in ICP.

Intracranial hypertension is defined as a sustained ICP greater than 15 torr. Signs of intracranial hypertension include headache, nausea, vomiting, papilledema, focal neurologic deficits, and altered consciousness. Moderate to severe increases in ICP may significantly decrease CPP, especially if the MAP is decreased. If uncorrected, permanent neurologic deficit will occur.

ANESTHESIA CONSIDERATIONS
Preoperative
Preoperative evaluation for the surgical patient is addressed above. Coexisting disease processes that may affect anesthesia management are addressed. Documentation of existing neurologic deficits is important, because this information is useful as a reference during the postoperative assessment. The patient should be evaluated for any skeletal, neural, or vascular pathology that may influence airway management or surgical positioning.

Attention is given to the patient with decreased intracranial compliance or documented intracranial hypertension, because this is the major determinant that influences anesthesia management. Preoperative medications may be given in a routine fashion except to patients with increased ICP. For these patients, narcotics and other CNS depressants should be avoided because the resulting respiratory depression results in an increase in $PaCO_2$, which subsequently increases the ICP.

Monitoring
Determinants of how the patient will be monitored depends on the type of procedure, the surgical position, anticipated duration of surgery, the potential for major blood loss, and any coexisting diseases. More advanced hemodynamic monitoring may include the use of intra-arterial, central venous, or a pulmonary artery catheter. ICP may be measured via a ventriculostomy catheter or a subarachnoid bolt. CSF pressure may be measured after the placement of a lumbar subarachnoid catheter. Electrophysiologic monitoring may include the use of an electroencephalogram (EEG) during neurovascular surgery or evoked potential (EP) monitoring during spinal cord or craniotomy procedures. Doppler ultrasound and TEE are used as indicated for the detection of air embolism.

ANESTHETIC AGENTS
Pharmacologic agents must be chosen carefully. Selections of intravenous and inhalational agents are based on the presence or absence of an elevated ICP, spinal cord injury, degenerative or demyelinating disease, seizure disorder, or cerebrovascular insufficiency. If EPs are to be monitored, a special drug protocol must be followed intraoperatively.

Most intravenous anesthetizing agents decrease CMR and CBF. Ketamine is the exception, because it increases CBF. The inhalational agents decrease CMR, but cause cerebral vasodilatation. This vasodilating effect results in an increased CBF, which increases cerebral blood volume with a subsequent increase in ICP. Because this effect may be attenuated by hyperventilating the patient, an agent such as isoflurane may be given in a concentration of less than or equal to 1 MAC during craniotomy procedures after hypocapnia has been established.

Muscle Relaxants
Muscle relaxants have no direct cerebral effect. The choice of which agent to administer is based on which agent has the least adverse effect on ICP or cardiovascular dynamics. The administration of the depolarizing agent succinylcholine may result in a mild, temporary increase in ICP, but this effect may be minimized by pretreatment with a defasciculating dose of nondepolarizing muscle relaxant and with mild hyperventilation. For patients with spinal cord injury or other denervating disorders, succinylcholine must be avoided because of the potential for acute, life-threatening hyperkalemia as potassium is released from extrajunctional receptors.

Selection of nondepolarizing agents is important if the patient has increased ICP. Nondepolarizing agents that cause histamine release should be avoided because the resulting vasodilatation may cause an increase in ICP as well as a decrease in MAP.

Vasoactive Agents

Vasoactive agents are frequently administered during a general anesthetic to normalize blood pressure. If cerebral autoregulation is intact, the administration of a vasopressor has little effect on CBF if the MAP is between 50 to 150 torr. If the patient becomes hypotensive, the administration of a vasopressor should increase CPP and help improve CBF. For patients with decreased intracranial compliance or elevated ICP, administration of vasodilators (except trimethaphan) should be avoided because the resulting increase in CBF further increases ICP.

Diuretic Therapy

The administration of mannitol and furosemide is most frequently employed to rapidly reduce ICP. Mannitol is an osmotic diuretic which, when administered, produces a hyperosmolar state. Because mannitol does not cross the blood–brain barrier, the resulting osmotic diffusion gradient rapidly removes water from the brain. This results in a transient increase in intravascular volume, which may increase blood pressure as diuresis begins. Because of this temporary increase in filling pressure, care must be exercised in patients with limited cardiac reserve.

Furosemide is a loop diuretic that decreases ICP by promoting diuresis, decreasing production of CSF, and promoting transport of intracellular water.

Steroid Therapy

Steroids are effective in reducing cerebral edema in patients with mass lesions (e.g., hematoma, abscess, brain tumors) and should be administered preoperatively because the effect is of slow onset. High-dose steroid therapy for acute head or spinal cord injury or ischemia from cardiac arrest or stroke remains controversial.

INTRAVENOUS FLUID MANAGEMENT

IV fluid management is crucial for the patient with increased ICP or the patient with a potential for cerebral vasospasm following rupture of a cerebral aneurysm. For patients with increased ICP, administration of hyposmolar and iso-osmotic glucose solutions should be avoided because such solutions promote transfer of free water into the brain. Additionally, an elevated serum glucose prior to an ischemic event is known to aggravate neurologic outcome. The administration of isotonic saline frequently is used on patients with increased ICP. Baseline fluid replenishment is normally 1 to 3 ml/kg/h. Additional isotonic crystalloid or colloid solutions may be administered in consideration of excessive urine output or blood loss. Monitoring CVP or pulmonary artery pressures are useful guides in fluid replacement.

PREOPERATIVE MEDICATIONS

Preoperative medication may be given in a routine fashion except to patients with increased ICP or decreased intracranial compliance. For these patients, CNS depressants (e.g., narcotics) should be avoided because the resulting decrease in minute ventilations causes the $PaCO_2$ to increase, with a subsequent rise in the ICP. Patients receiving anticonvulsants or steroids should continue on schedule in order to maintain therapeutic drug levels. For patients with a cerebral aneurysm and normal ICP, generous sedation may be appropriate to help avoid a hypertensive episode.

ANESTHETIC MANAGEMENT

The following briefly describes anesthetic management for the patient scheduled for intracranial and cerebrovascular surgery.

INTRACRANIAL SURGERY

Intracranial surgery commonly is performed on patients for removal of mass lesions or clipping of cerebral aneurysms. Anesthetic management for patients with mass lesions mainly is focused on control of ICP, because these patients probably have decreased intracranial compliance or documented intracranial hypertension.

Mass Lesions

Typical measures employed include supplemental O_2 for transport to the operating room, elevation of the head of the bed (to facilitate cerebral venous drainage, which decreases central venous pressure), documentation of the preoperative neurologic examination, and placement of intra-arterial and central venous pressure lines. If a ventriculostomy catheter is used for measurement of ICP, the level of the transducer should be placed at the level of the external auditory meatus.

Intraoperative administration of steroid and diuretic therapy and parameters for $PaCO_2$ levels should be confirmed with the surgeon. Prior to induction, the cooperative patient is asked to hyperventilate. This maneuver is performed to prevent a significant increase in $PaCO_2$ if difficulty is encountered during induction and airway management.

After satisfactory preoxygenation and hyperventilation, an ultra–short-acting induction agent such as thiopental (which decreases ICP and lowers CMR) is given to produce unconsciousness. Hyperventilation is continued. Prior to laryngoscopy, a narcotic or beta blocker may be administered to prevent hypertension secondary to manipulation of the airway. To facilitate tracheal intubation, a rapid-onset, nonhistamine-releasing, nondepolarizing muscle relaxant may be given. After the airway is secured and mild hypocapnia confirmed by capnography, administration of inhalational anesthetic agents may be used to help maintain a surgical depth of anesthesia. If the patient's blood pressure and heart rate increase during laryngoscopy, additional narcotic administration may be appropriate to blunt the sympathetic response to pin fixation of the head or the surgical incision. Once the airway is secured, the surgical team may insert a urinary drainage catheter. The volume of urine output is monitored throughout the procedure to evaluate the efficiency of diuretic therapy and to help guide intravascular volume replacement.

Surgical positioning is performed after the patient is determined to be stable. Because neurosurgery may take several hours, extreme hyperflexion or hyperextension of the head should be avoided because this may hinder cerebral vascular return, compromise arterial perfusion, or compress neural structures. The arms and legs should be placed in neutral positions and all pressure points well padded. To help prevent thromboembolism from the lower extremities, the legs should be wrapped or fitted with pneumatic intermittent compression hose. The eyes should be taped closed and protected with eye goggles, if appropriate.

During the maintenance phase of neuroanesthesia, the goal is to maintain a quiet surgical field, provide a "relaxed" brain, control ICP, and ensure sufficient CPP. Hyperventilation is continued to achieve a $PaCO_2$ of 25 to 30 torr. Mannitol and furosemide are administered in a timely fashion in order to maximize cerebral dehydration prior to opening the dura. When the dura is exposed, the surgeon will be able to tell if the brain is relaxed or tight. If the dura is bulging, opening must be delayed until a further reduction in ICP is achieved. If there is a ventriculostomy or lumbar subarachnoid drainage catheter in place, CSF may be withdrawn to help reduce ICP. An additional bolus dose of thiopental or elevation of the head may also help reduce ICP.

Once optimal surgical conditions have been achieved, the dura is opened and the intracranial procedure performed. Intracranial complications may occur. If sudden, unexpected changes in hemodynamics and/or cardiac rhythm occur, the surgeon must be notified immediately because the changes may be directly attributable to surgical manipulation, retraction, blood loss, or from venous air embolism. Any adverse effect on the respiratory center will go undetected if these patients are completely paralyzed by neuromuscular blocking agents. If the adverse changes are related to manipulation or retraction, discontinuation of the offending stimulus usually results in restoration of pre-event blood pressure and cardiac rhythm.

Venous air embolism occurs when there is a venous opening above the level of the heart and room air is entrained through the vein into the heart. The TEE and Doppler ultrasound are the most sensitive monitors for detecting air emboli and should be used in high-risk procedures (e.g., posterior fossa procedures performed in the sitting position). If these monitors are not being used, air embolism may be suspected if there is an unexplained, precipitous decrease in $ETCO_2$ and the appearance of end tidal nitrogen (ETN_2). The $ETCO_2$ drops when a large amount of air enters the pulmonary circulation and increases dead space. The ETN_2 is detected because room air has entered the pulmonary circulation. Stethoscope detection of a mill-wheel murmur is the least sensitive monitor and is indicative of a large volume air embolus. If air embolus is suspected, the surgeon floods the field with saline, packs the wound, or applies bone wax to the edges of the cranium. N_2O, if utilized, is discontinued. The operating table is manipulated so that the level of the patient's head may be at or slightly below the level of the heart. Aspiration of air is attempted via the CVP catheter. Temporary, bilateral jugular venous compression may be applied to help identify an open venous sinus. If the patient is hypovolemic, fluid is given to achieve euvolemia. If air embolism persists, a more pronounced Trendelenburg position, with the table tilted to the left, may trap the air in the right atrium and make air aspiration through the CVP catheter possible. If the cardiorespiratory system becomes severely compromised, resuscitative efforts may become necessary.

Hemostasis is necessary to control significant bleeding and isotonic crystalloid or colloid volume replacement may be necessary to maintain hemodynamics. Care must be taken not to overinfuse, because this may promote cerebral edema if the blood–brain barrier has been interrupted.

After successful removal of the intracranial mass, the $PaCO_2$ is gradually allowed to normalize as the surgeon closes. The depth of anesthesia is decreased to allow for a smooth, rapid awakening. During emergence, hypertension, coughing, and straining must be avoided so as not to precipitate an acute cerebral hemorrhage or intracranial hypertension.

When the patient awakens in the operating room, a neurologic evaluation is performed to rule out any new deficits. Delayed awakening is troublesome and may result from anesthetic overdosage, acute intracranial hemorrhage, elevated ICP, or pneumocephalus. If anesthetic overdosage has been ruled out, an emergency computed tomography (CT) scan or rapid re-exploration may be necessary to evaluate the cause. After satisfactory neurologic recovery has been demonstrated, the patient is transported to the PACU. Frequent neurologic checks are performed. Any sign of neurologic deterioration requires immediate attention.

Cerebral Aneurysm

The approach to anesthetic management for the patient with cerebral aneurysm depends on whether or not the aneurysm has ruptured and if the patient has elevated ICP. If the aneurysm has not ruptured, the goal of the anesthetic is to prevent pre- or intraoperative events that could potentially cause the aneurysm to burst. Avoiding hypertension is the major goal. ICP is generally normal.

Preoperatively, patients with normal ICP are heavily premedicated. Additional anxiolytics may be given as needed. An arterial line, CVP catheter, and large-bore IV catheter are inserted after anesthetizing the puncture site with a local anesthetic. During induction and maintenance, pre-emptive analgesics or beta blockers are given before stimulating events (laryngoscopy, intubation, head pinning, incision, etc.) in order to prevent a hypertensive response.

During the clipping or ligation of the aneurysm, the surgeon may request a brief period of controlled hypotension (MAP, 60 to 70 torr). To avoid wide swings in blood pressure, appropriate hydration prior to administering vasodilator therapy is helpful. The MAP is gradually reduced by giving a potent vasodilator (e.g., sodium nitroprusside). When the MAP has been sufficiently lowered, the aneurysm is clipped. If there is no bleeding, the

MAP is allowed to gradually increase to normal levels. As the surgeon closes, the depth of anesthesia is adjusted so the patient will awaken and be extubated in the operating room. This allows for rapid assessment of neurologic function.

If the aneurysm has ruptured, surgery may be performed early or in a delayed fashion, depending on the patient's clinical status (see Chapter 7, Neurosurgery: Subarachnoid Hemorrhage).

Preoperative pharmacologic therapy for a patient with a ruptured aneurysm may include the use of aminocaproic acid, an antifibrinolytic (to retard clot dissolution), and nimodipine (calcium channel blocker to reduce cerebral vasospasm). Preoperative evaluation should document existing neurologic deficit and evidence of intracranial hypertension. Considerations for the administration of preoperative medication are the same as described in craniotomy for a nonruptured aneurysm.

The major goal pre- and intraoperatively is to maintain CPP, avoid hypertension, and prevent or manage cerebral vasospasm. Treatment of vasospasm includes expanding intravascular volume and augmenting blood pressure. This therapy must be used cautiously prior to clipping, because overzealous treatment may result in rerupture of the aneurysm. Hyperventilation should be avoided because it promotes cerebral vasoconstriction. If necessary, intraoperative reduction in ICP must be coordinated with the surgeon because premature, rapid reduction in ICP may negate the tamponade effect on the aneurysm and result in rerupture.

After completion of surgery, a smooth, rapid emergence from anesthesia should be attempted in order to allow for early assessment of neurologic function. Postoperative management includes prevention and management of vasospasm and close observation for neurologic deterioration.

SUMMARY

The anesthesia team works in concert with the surgical team to provide the best possible outcome for the surgical patient. Communication and understanding of the procedure and techniques employed by various surgeons is essential in order to prevent complications. The PA anesthetist plays a vital role on the anesthesia care team in both general and specialized procedures.

A comparison often is made between the administration of a general anesthetic and the flying of an airplane. The induction and emergence is analogous to the take off and landing. The maintenance phase may be like that of cruising, fewer adjustments need to be made, but vigilance needs to be maintained as turbulence may occur when it is least expected.

Further Reading

Davison JK, Eckhardt WF, Perese DA (eds): Clinical Anesthesia Procedures of the Massachusetts General Hospital, 4th ed. Boston, Little, Brown, 1993.

Kaplan JA (ed): Cardiac Anesthesia, vol. 2. Orlando, Grune and Stratton, 1983.

Miller RD (ed): Anesthesia, 3rd ed. New York, Churchill Livingstone, 1990.

Morgan GE, Mikhail MS: Clinical Anesthesiology. Norwalk, CT, Appleton and Lange, 1992.

Stoelting RK, Dierdorf SF (eds): Handbook for Anesthesia and Co-Existing Disease. New York, Churchill Livingstone, 1993.

Chapter **3**

Cardiovascular Surgery
Cardiac Contusion
Michael E. Champion, PA-C, MMSc, EdM, CCP, and Lyle W. Larson, PA-C, MS

DEFINITION

Blunt, nonpenetrating trauma to the anterior chest wall sufficient to compress the heart between the sternum and vertebral bodies produces a contusion to the heart, as does rapid deceleration injuries where the heart is thrust forward into the sternum. The size of the contusion is directly related to the amount of hemorrhage into the myocardium.

HISTORY

Symptoms.   The patient may present with no symptoms, or with tachycardia, arrhythmias, precordial pain, or symptoms indistinguishable from angina pectoris.

General.   Any patient presenting with blunt trauma to the thoracic area or rapid deceleration injury (e.g., auto accident, sports injury, etc.) should raise the suspicion of cardiac contusion.

Age.   Any.

Onset.   May be immediate to delayed (12 to 24 hours), depending on extent of myocardial damage.

Duration.   Variable; symptoms usually last 1 to 3 weeks if treated with bedrest.

Intensity.   May be asymptomatic or present with the same intensity as a myocardial infarction.

Aggravating Factors.   Other underlying cardiac problems (e.g., preexisting coronary disease, aneurysm, valvular disease, etc.). Anticoagulants (e.g., aspirin, warfarin [Coumadin], ticlopidine HCl) may increase contusion area.

Alleviating Factors.   Rest.

Associated Factors.   With cardiac contusion, the following potential complications should be ruled out: myocardial infarction, rupture of the free cardiac wall, rupture of the septum, aortic aneurysm, and myocardial laceration. Also consider associated pericardial injury, other myocardial injury, arrhythmias, valvular injury, coronary artery injury, and great vessel injury.

PHYSICAL EXAMINATION

General.   Patients with cardiac contusions are trauma patients; and as such they should undergo a rapid trauma evaluation to rule out trauma to other organ systems. The patient may be asymptomatic or present with dyspnea and hypotension.

Cardiovascular.   Cardiac contusion may mimic myocardial infarction. Strong suspicion of ventricular septal rupture, valvular rupture, or hemopericardium must be considered during evaluation. Careful auscultation should be performed to assess for murmurs, muffled heart sounds, and arrhythmias. The vascular examination should be directed to assess for jugular venous distention, diminished or absent peripheral pulses, and bruits.

    Musculoskeletal.   Careful evaluation for fractured ribs or sternum, flail chest, or costochondral dislocation is performed.

    Pulmonary.   Auscultation and percussion are performed to rule out associated pulmonary contusion, pneumothorax, hemothorax, or tracheal or bronchial compromise.

PATHOPHYSIOLOGY

Cardiac contusion may take the form of small petechial lesions progressing to ecchymotic lesions, which may be subepicardial, subendocardial, or full thickness. Major coronary arteries remain patent, whereas small vessels are disrupted. This leads to extravasation of red blood cells into the interstitial spaces. Myocardial cells become fragmented and edematous. As inflammatory cells infiltrate into the affected areas, scar tissue forms. Of note, the right ventricle is more often involved than the left ventricle, probably as a result of its more anterior location.

DIAGNOSTIC STUDIES

    Laboratory.   Cardiac isoenzymes may suggest myocardial infarction (MI). Check creatinine kinase isoenzyme (CK-MB) levels as well as lactate dehydrogenase (LDH)–cardiac-specific levels when ruling out MI.

    Radiology.   Chest x-ray may show fractures of the bony skeleton, or a "water bottle" heart, suggestive of pericardial fluid. An echocardiogram (ECG) is useful in defining valvular function and identifying wall motion abnormalities.

    Other.   Although a relatively insensitive and nonspecific indicator, the ECG may show nonspecific ST and T-wave abnormalities, or Q waves similar to that of an acute MI. Sinus tachycardia is the most frequent finding. Other rhythm disturbances may include right bundle branch block, left bundle branch block, unifascicular block, or second- or third-degree atrioventricular block.

The radionucleotide ventriculogram (RNVG) is a relatively sensitive indicator of right and left ventricular function. It is well suited for assessing ejection fraction and segmental wall motion abnormalities, which may help locate and quantitate the contusion.

DIFFERENTIAL DIAGNOSIS

    Traumatic.   Blunt vs. penetrating injury, including rib or sternal fracture; costochondral separation seen on chest x-ray.

Infectious. Pericarditis, demonstrated by nonspecific ST and T-wave changes, without cardiac enzyme elevation.

Metabolic. Not applicable.

Neoplastic. Not applicable.

Vascular. Occult, pre-existing MI. With or without cardiac enzyme elevations, ECG with changes in a characteristic pattern.

Congenital. Pre-existing cardiac abnormalities such as valvular, septal disorders are demonstrated by a known murmur; no elevation in cardiac enzymes. Other cardiac arrhythmias, aneurysms, or congestive heart failure (CHF) may also be pre-existing.

Acquired. Not applicable.

TREATMENT

Medical. Rest, supportive treatment, treatment of dysrhythmias, monitor arrhythmias. Sinus tachycardia, right bundle branch block, left bundle branch block, and unifascicular block do not generally require intervention. Second- or third-degree heart block may require temporary pacing, but is usually transient.

Surgical. Surgical intervention for complications of cardiac contusion is often performed emergently. Cardiopulmonary bypass should be readily available, and the femoral artery and vein should be isolated for cannulation.

Indications. Valvular or septal rupture are true surgical emergencies and usually present with profound hypotension, acute pulmonary edema, or cardiogenic shock.

Contraindications. Surgical intervention is contraindicated for cardiac contusion. Surgery is indicated only in the areas noted above and as a salvage for cardiac rupture.

TECHNIQUE OF SURGICAL ASSISTING

The PA, when assisting with opening the chest, must be prepared to encounter adhesions (as seen with pericarditis), hemopericardium, pulmonary lacerations, and injury to the great vessels (e.g., aortic dissection). The role of the assistant is focused primarily on providing exposure, which may be quite difficult.

PEDIATRIC CONSIDERATIONS

Pediatric patients may present with similar complaints as adults. Because these injuries are related to blunt trauma, other, more serious injury patterns, including fractured spleen or pulmonary contusion, may accompany this condition.

OBSTETRICAL CONSIDERATIONS

Cardiac contusion may mimic symptoms of an MI. As a result of an expanded intravascular volume during pregnancy, severe myocardial injury may be more likely to occur, and as such, may place the pregnancy at risk or cause greater physiological stress on the mother.

PEARLS FOR THE PA

Always take a good history of injury and maintain a high degree of suspicion.

Cardiac contusion may occur more frequently than realized and should be included in the differential diagnosis with all patients subjected to major trauma or rapid deceleration.

The RNVG is a good indicator for quantitating the degree of contusion.

Frequent follow-up is recommended.

Congenital Heart Disease
Lyle W. Larson, PA-C, MS

DEFINITION

Congenital heart disease may be described as a malformation of the heart or great vessels that occurs during fetal development with cardiac and pulmonary consequences that may present from birth to adulthood. A wide spectrum of anatomic variation exists, making classification of these anomalies confusing and cumbersome. Congenital heart disease may be thought of as structural (stenosis, left-to-right shunt, right-to-left shunt), functional (cyanotic, noncyanotic), or as a result of the symptoms it produces (CHF, cyanosis, pulmonary disease, or arrhythmias).

HISTORY

Three major presentations of critical heart disease occur in infancy: severe cyanosis, low output state, and pulmonary edema. In childhood, the most common presentation is that of the asymptomatic murmur. The adult population generally presents with an asymptomatic murmur that becomes symptomatic or with progression of previously known congenital disease that may or may not have been surgically corrected in childhood.

Symptoms. Symptoms are variable, depending on the cause of the underlying disorder and age of presentation. They may be absent (benign atrial septal defect), or present over a wide range, culminating with defects incompatible with life if not recognized immediately at birth (complete transposition of the great vessels). The four basic symptomatic presentations include (1) cyanosis (severe hypoxia in the absence of respiratory distress), (2) CHF (manifest by tachypnea, tachycardia, grunting respirations, pallor, diaphoresis, nasal flaring, failure to thrive, poor feeding), (3) pulmonary disease (increased pulmonary blood flow resulting in edematous, poorly compliant lung parenchyma, increased infection rate, pulmonary hypertension), and (4) arrhythmias (paroxysmal atrial tachycardia, atrial flutter and fibrillation, reciprocating tachycardia from Wolff-Parkinson-White syndrome, and heart block). A representation of the more common congenital anomalies follows.

General. The most common stenotic lesions are coarctation of the aorta, congenital pulmonary stenosis, and congenital aortic stenosis.

Common left-to-right shunts include patent ductus arteriosus, atrial-septal defect, and ventricular septal defect.

The most common right-to-left shunt is the tetralogy of Fallot.

The most common congenital arrhythmia is the Wolff-Parkinson-White syndrome.

Coarctation of the Aorta (CA). Characterized by a fibromembranous ledge along the outer curvature of the aorta at the level of the ligamentum arteriosus.

Congenital Pulmonary Stenosis (CPS). Stenosis of the pulmonary valve; may range from minimal stenosis to dysplasia to atresia. This is the most common form of congenital right ventricular outflow tract obstruction.

Congenital Aortic Stenosis (CAS). Stenosis of the aortic valve, the most common congenital cause of left ventricular outflow tract obstruction. Bicuspid valve is the most common aortic valve anomaly.

Patent Ductus Arteriosus (PDA). Failure of ductus arteriosus to close; usually closes within the first day of life to become the ligamentum arteriosus. Comprises 10% of all congenital heart disease.

Atrial Septal Defect (ASD). An opening of the atrial septum, allowing blood flow between the left and right atria. Four types include ostium secundum, ostium primum, sinus venosus, and patent foramen ovale. Flow is left to right, because the right ventricle fills more than the left ventricle at a similar pressure, producing a higher pressure gradient in the left heart.

Ventricular Septal Defect (VSD). An opening in the ventricular septum, allowing an abnormal connection between the systemic and pulmonary circulation. Varies in size and location; small defects with low gradients may be asymptomatic. Most common of all forms of congenital heart disease with the exception of bicuspid aortic valve. Occurs in 20% of all cases of congenital disease.

Tetralogy of Fallot (TF). Consists of four components: ventricular septal defect, pulmonary stenosis, dextroposed (over-riding) aorta, and right ventricular hypertrophy. Although the dextroposed aorta rarely has functional importance, patients who exhibit severe obstruction to the right ventricular outflow tract develop a true right-to-left shunt through the ventricular septal defect and have significant reduction of blood flow to the pulmonary vascular bed.

Wolff-Parkinson-White Syndrome (WPW). One or more anatomical accessory pathways providing conduction of electrical impulses between the atria and ventricles that do not include native conduction tissue.

Age

CA. Infancy; 2:1 male-to-female ratio.

CPS. Infancy.

CAS. Infancy throughout adult life; 4:1 male-to-female ratio.

PDA. Birth; 2:1 female-to-male ratio.

ASD. Present at birth; extends into late adulthood (with surgical intervention reported on septuagenarians).

VSD. Prenatal (septum usually closes by third month of gestation); 1:1 male-to-female ratio.

TF. Infancy to adulthood, although most commonly seen and corrected in early childhood.

WPW. Present at birth.

Onset

CA. Not usually noted until closure of ductus arteriosus; may not present until teenage years or early adulthood (usually with upper extremity hypertension).

CPS. At birth.

CAS. Varies, ranging from less than 1 year of age with atretic valve or unicuspid or dome-shaped valve, to middle adulthood (30 to 45 years) in patients with bicuspid aortic valve.

PDA. Within first 48 hours of life.

ASD. Most common appearance is in children 3 to 5 years of age as the right ventricle becomes more compliant; if asymptomatic through childhood, adults in their 20s and 30s present with increasing exercise intolerance. Those presenting in their 50s to 60s present with CHF.

VSD. At birth.

TF. Variable, depending on degree of right ventricular outflow tract obstruction. In severe cases, the patient may present in the early neonatal period with profound hypoxia concomitant with closure of the ductus arteriosus. In more mild forms, the young child may present with a gradual progression of cyanosis, progressing to cyanosis at rest.

WPW. Variable; most common onset in mid-teens to mid 20s.

Duration

CA. Present at birth; until corrected, average life expectancy without correction is 35 years.

CPS. Present until corrected; most progress to adulthood, natural history variable.

CAS/PDA/ASD/TF. Present until corrected.

VSD. Present until corrected (evidence that some defects may close spontaneously).

WPW. Present throughout life; arrhythmias (reciprocating tachycardia) most common in early adult life.

Intensity

CA. Ranges from asymptomatic in early years; may present with moderate CHF or severe shock that may ensue following ductus closure.

CPS. Asymptomatic with minimal stenosis to severe cyanosis with atretic valve.

CAS. Ranges from asymptomatic to low cardiac output state with cyanosis from excessive oxygen extraction; dependent on degree of stenosis of the valve.

PDA. Variable, depending on size of defect. If small, patient may be asymptomatic throughout adult life; otherwise, if left untreated, transmission of systemic pressures to the pulmonary vascular bed results in pulmonary vascular obstruction (Eisenmenger's syndrome).

ASD. Varies from asymptomatic to symptoms of CHF, depending on size and location of defect, as well as status of pulmonary pressures.

VSD. Variable, depending on size of defect. If small, patient may be asymptomatic throughout adult life; otherwise, if left untreated, transmission of systemic pressures to the pulmonary vascular bed results in pulmonary vascular obstruction (Eisenmenger's syndrome) similar to that of patent ductus arteriosus.

TF. Variable from life threatening in neonatal period to progressive during childhood. The hallmark of the intensity and severity of tetralogy of Fallot is cyanosis.

WPW. Dependent on direction of conduction through pathway. Antidromic reciprocating tachycardia (re-entrant loop antegrade down the accessory pathway and retrograde back to the atrium via the His bundle and atrioventricular node) may be life threatening, because pathway does not have decrementing properties.

Aggravating Factors

CA. Closure of ductus arteriosus.

CPS. Reduced preload (volume depletion), atrial arrhythmias preventing adequate filling of the right ventricle.

CAS. Mitral insufficiency leading to pulmonary edema. Decreased preload may produce angina or syncope; left atrial overload may produce atrial arrhythmias.

PDA. Pulmonary congestion, systemic hypertension, respiratory tract infections.

ASD. Any pulmonary disorder that produces elevated pulmonary artery pressures (which, if high enough, can reverse the shunt), right ventricular failure or infarct, arrhythmias (atrioventricular node often malpositioned in ostium primum defects).

VSD. Pulmonary congestion, respiratory infections, systemic hypertension.

TF. Increased respiratory stress or requirements (crying, feeding), endocarditis, respiratory tract infection.

WPW. Atrial fibrillation (may produce ventricular tachycardia or fibrillation if conduction down accessory pathway is antegrade).

Alleviating Factors

CA. Formation of collateral vessels supplying distal aorta.

CPS. Optimal management of preload, correction of arrhythmias.

CAS. Increased preload (volume), decreased afterload (arterial vasodilators), correction of arrhythmias.

PDA. Aggressive control of systemic hypertension, prostaglandin infusion to stimulate closure of patent ductus arteriosus.

ASD. Control of pulmonary artery pressures, optimization of volume status.

VSD. Control of systemic hypertension, spontaneous closure.

TF. Squatting, knee-chest position, alleviation of respiratory stresses.

WPW. Atrioventricular node blocking agents (digoxin, beta blockers, calcium channel blockers) may be helpful in orthodromic reciprocating tachycardia (conduction down normal conduction pathway and retrograde back up to the atria via the accessory pathway) but are **contraindicated** in antidromic reciprocating tachycardia.

Associated Factors

CA. Failure to thrive (weight greater than height), decreased urine output, exercise intolerance, abdominal pain.

CPS. Right ventricular hypertrophy, tricuspid regurgitation; with atretic valve, patients may develop supra-systemic right ventricular pressures.

CAS. Left ventricular hypertrophy, dyspnea on exertion; if associated with hypoplastic left heart syndrome, prognosis is poor.

PDA. Failure to thrive, dyspnea at rest, recurrent respiratory tract infections (atelectasis and bronchopneumonia common with minor respiratory infections during first year of life), increased incidence with maternal rubella.

ASD. Atrial arrhythmias (atrial fibrillation, flutter) from atrial overload and distention, sick sinus syndrome, pulmonary congestion in advanced ages.

VSD. Maternal alcohol consumption, can accompany other congenital anomalies, presence increases chances of having other defects.

TF. "Tet spells" include paroxysmal episodes of dyspnea occurring with minimal provocation and resulting in profound cyanosis. Thought to be produced as a result of right ventricular infundibular spasm, it is often relieved with squatting.

WPW. Ebstein anomaly.

PHYSICAL EXAMINATION

General. Patients presenting with CHF may be irritable or anxious, with tachycardia and tachypnea. Those with cyanosis may present with an ashened or blue appearance to the mucosa, lips, or nail beds, and may show clubbing if cyanosis has been present for an extended period.

Cardiovascular. Physical findings vary widely, depending on the underlying anomaly. The following physical findings are present in the more commonly encountered anomalies listed above.

CA. Differential pulses and blood pressure between upper and lower extremities, bounding carotid pulses with a palpable thrill in the suprasternal notch; a gallop rhythm may be present, a cardiac murmur may not be present (if present, may be associated bicuspid aortic valve), whereas the murmur from the coarctation may range from a short, nonspecific systolic murmur to a continuous murmur with maximum intensity in the left infraclavicular area, or over the back or axilla.

CPS. Typically a long systolic murmur peaking late in systole and extending into or beyond A_2, with a palpable thrill in the left second intercostal space, presence or absence of an ejection click, prominent "a" wave on jugular venous pulse, and a prominent fourth heart sound.

CAS. Manifest by a harsh, loud systolic ejection murmur heard at the base that radiates to the neck, with associated left ventricular lift; a systolic thrill at the right upper sternal border, suprasternal notch, and carotid arteries, a systolic ejection click, and an audible fourth heart sound.

PDA. Classic early onset systolic murmur with crescendo up to the second heart sound followed by a decrescendo murmur through diastole (the so-called "machinery" murmur), best heard at the second left intercostal space.

VSD. Early onset, high-pitched blowing pansystolic murmur with maximum intensity between the apex and left lower sternal border; an early systolic click may be present.

TF. Loud systolic murmur heard in the left cardiac base, transmitted to the back, with a wide split second heart sound and a soft pulmonary closure.

WPW. Paroxysmal onset of narrow complex tachycardia, with regular rhythm and rates from 100 (uncommon) to greater than 180 (common) beats per minute.

Gastrointestinal. Hepatomegaly or splenomegaly may be present in those patients with right-sided obstruction.

Neurologic. Careful assessment of cranial nerve function, as well as sensory and motor function, is essential to rule out occult stroke from brain abscess (cyanotic heart disease).

Pulmonary. Patients with right-to-left shunts or communication between systemic and pulmonary circulation may present with pulmonary edema, effusions, infiltrates, or consolidation.

PATHOPHYSIOLOGY

Several mechanisms exist to account for the pathophysiology of congenital heart disease. It is important to note that congenital anomalies may be isolated or mixed. Effective treatment is targeted toward a specific cause, thus making identification of the mechanism of the anomalies paramount. Mechanisms of congenital disorders include excessive blood flow, obstruction to forward flow, primary myocardial failure, inadequate pulmonary blood flow, intracardiac mixing of systemic and pulmonary venous blood, complete diversion of systemic venous blood into the aorta without passage through the lungs, low cardiac output states, combinations, and arrhythmias.

Excessive Blood Flow.   These are the left-to-right shunts, which place a higher volume of blood throughout the pulmonary vasculature, resulting in an engorged pulmonary bed, increased pulmonary vascular resistance, and decreased compliance of the pulmonary parenchyma. Anomalies include atrial and ventricular septal defects, patent ductus arteriosus, aorto-pulmonary window, and truncus arteriosus.

Obstruction to Forward Flow.   These are anomalies with stenoses or atresia, including coarctation of the aorta, hypoplastic left heart syndrome, aortic stenosis or atresia, mitral stenosis or atresia, and cor triatriatum.

Primary Myocardial Failure.   Due to defects in blood supply to the myocardium (anomalous coronary artery) or defects in the myocardium (endocardial fibroelastosis).

Inadequate Pulmonary Blood Flow.   These include the right-to-left shunts, whereby blood passes from the right heart to the left heart through a septal defect or patent ductus arteriosus. This results in obstruction of desaturated venous blood to the pulmonary vascular bed, resulting in systemic atrial desaturation. The tetralogy of Fallot is included in this group.

Intracardiac Mixing of Systemic and Pulmonary Venous Blood.   Resulting in a mixture of varying proportions of well-oxygenated blood leaving the heart into the aorta. Both right-to-left and left-to-right shunts fall into this category.

Complete Diversion of Systemic Venous Blood into the Aorta Without Passage Through the Lungs.   Is incompatible with life unless another defect (atrial or ventricular septal defect, patent ductus arteriosus) that allows mixing within the heart exists. Transposition of the great vessels is classic for this group.

Low Cardiac Output States.   Cyanosis as a result of excessive oxygen extraction at the tissue level, represented by aortic atresia, hypoplastic left heart syndrome, pulmonary atresia.

Combinations.   Pulmonary vascular obstruction, increased pulmonary blood flow, and cyanosis may occur with total anomalous pulmonary venous return. Defects causing increased pulmonary blood flow and intracardiac mixing (transposition of the great vessels with a septal defect, truncus arteriosus, complete atrioventricular canal defect) cause varying degrees of CHF and cyanosis.

Arrhythmias.   May occur as result of anomalous conduction tissue (Wolff-Parkinson-White syndrome), hypoxia, or treatment of underlying disease (digoxin).

DIAGNOSTIC STUDIES

Laboratory
CBC.   To rule out polycythemia (common in cyanotic heart disease) or infection.

PT, PTT, Platelet Count. As early indicator for hepatic congestion, and to assess extrinsic and intrinsic pathways during planning stages for surgery.

Electrolytes. To rule out metabolic imbalance, acidosis, blood urea nitrogen (BUN) and creatinine to assess renal function preoperatively or during diuresis, glucose to rule out diabetes mellitus.

Drug Levels. As indicated to assess for toxicity (e.g., digoxin).

Urinalysis. To assess renal function and rule out infection.

Nutrition Panel. To assess nutritional status prior to surgical intervention.

Radiology

Chest X-ray. To evaluate for cardiac size (cardiomegaly) and location (dextrocardia), presence or absence of anomalous vasculature (persistent left superior vena cava, anomalous pulmonary venous return, location of aorta), rib notching from collateral circulation from coarctation of aorta, assessment of pulmonary vasculature, infiltrates, congestion, effusions, and to rule out visceral situs inversus.

Other

ECG. May be diagnostic, or may show atrial or ventricular hypertrophy (right ventricular hypertrophy [RVH] with transposition of great vessels, left ventricular hypertrophy [LVH] with aortic stenosis), presence of infarction (anomalous coronary artery), extrasystoles (PACs, PVCs), short PR intervals with or without delta waves (Wolff-Parkinson-White syndrome), or various degrees of heart block.

Echocardiogram. Essential to identify the presence, location, position, and size of shunts or defects, to define principal cardiac anatomy, evaluate valves and valvular annulus, identify source of blood flow, identify pulmonary venous anatomy, and quantitate flow across gradients.

Cardiac Catheterization. Used to define atrial, ventricular, and coronary artery anatomy, measure pressures, assess pulmonary flow and resistance, rule out multiple septal defects, define relationship of structures, measure oxygen saturations across gradients, and confirm echocardiographic findings.

Cardiac Magnetic Resonance Imaging (MRI). Gated studies are not affected by absorption from lungs or reflection on bone (limitation of echocardiogram) and can be useful after specific areas are targeted.

DIFFERENTIAL DIAGNOSIS

The following diagnoses must be considered and ruled out when approaching the patient with cyanosis.

Traumatic. Stricture from traumatic or prolonged intubation for related or unrelated disease.

Infectious. Bacterial endocarditis.

Metabolic. Thyrotoxicosis.

Neoplastic. Not applicable.

Vascular. Persistent fetal circulation (neonates).

Congenital. Diaphragmatic hernia, pulmonary parenchymal disease (cystic fibrosis).

Acquired. Asthma.

Other. Airway obstruction from foreign body.

TREATMENT

Medical. An accurate diagnosis is essential to providing optimal medical management. For those conditions not considered life threatening (e.g., transposition of the great vessels), management is directed toward the symptoms. For acute exacerbations, patients may be treated with volume restriction, including concentration of all intravenous drips and caloric sources, diuresis (furosemide, bumetanide), inotropic support as required (digoxin, epinephrine, norepinephrine), and supplemental oxygen. All patients with shunts should receive subacute bacterial endocarditis (SBE) prophylaxis, and those with right-to-left shunts should be considered candidates for anticoagulation with heparin or warfarin.

Surgical. Surgical intervention may be broken down into five primary goals: to patch an undesirable connection between two chambers, to increase pulmonary blood flow, to decrease pulmonary blood flow, to relieve obstruction or restriction, or to remove an undesirable conduction circuit. Obviously, the goal is dependent upon the congenital anomaly. Examples of each are listed below.

Procedures to Patch Undesirable Connections Between Two Chambers

Atrioseptal and Ventriculoseptal Defect. Closed primarily or with pericardial or Dacron patch.

Procedures to Increase Pulmonary Blood Flow

Pott's Procedure. Graft of descending thoracic aorta to left pulmonary artery.

Blalock-Taussig. End-to-side anastomosis of subclavian vein to pulmonary artery.

Modified Blalock. Use of Gore-Tex tube interpositioned between innominate or subclavian artery and main branch of pulmonary artery.

Fontan. Consists of superior vena cava to right pulmonary artery anastomosis, right atrial appendage to proximal stump of right pulmonary artery anastomosis with homograft valve prosthesis, closure of the interatrial communication, and ligation of the proximal pulmonary artery. Many modifications to this original procedure are known.

Glenn. Anastomosis of superior vena cava to right pulmonary artery.

Rastelli. Conduit to create a new outflow channel from the right ventricle to the main pulmonary artery.

Procedures to Decrease Pulmonary Blood Flow

Patent Ductus Arteriosus. Ligature with or without transection.

Rashkind. Balloon atrial septostomy (in neonates with transposition of great vessels).

Pulmonary Artery Banding. Placement of restrictive band to selectively reduce flow.

Mustard. Rerouting systemic and pulmonary venous return within the atria ("venous switch") by performing atrial septostomy and use of pericardial patch to form intra-atrial baffle.

Senning. Similar to a Mustard procedure, except uses own atrial wall instead of pericardial patch for baffle.

Arterial Switch. Surgical transposition of aorta and main pulmonary artery to correct systemic and pulmonary ventricle.

Procedures to Relieve Obstruction or Restriction

Balloon Valvotomy. To relieve pulmonic or aortic stenosis.

Septal Myoplasty. To remove subaortic stenosis.

Valvular Repair or Replacement. Using bioprosthetic, mechanical, or homografts.

Coarctation of Aorta. Resection with end-to-end anastomosis, patch aortoplasty, Dacron tube interposition graft, subclavian flap.

Removal of Undesirable Conduction Circuit

Wolff-Parkinson-White Syndrome. Catheter or open ablation of accessory pathway(s).

Indications. The decision to proceed with surgery depends on the nature of the underlying defect and its effect both "upstream" and "downstream." Cyanosis is the most frequent condition that warrants intervention, with protection of the pulmonary vascular bed as a primary goal. Although one procedure may be definitive and curative (arterial switch for transposition of the great vessels, pathway ablation for Wolff-Parkinson-White syndrome), others may be only staging procedures to allow the patient to grow before a more definitive procedure is performed (balloon valvotomy prior to valvular replacement). However, a definitive open repair that can be performed at low risk is preferable to an interventional repair for early palliation followed by later open heart surgery.

Contraindications. Although some procedures (transposition of the great vessels, severe tetralogy of Fallot) are designed to palliate otherwise life-threatening cardiac disease, others (atrial septal defect, mild aortic stenosis) do not require immediate intervention. The decision to postpone surgery, and for how long, should be a joint decision involving the surgeon, the cardiologist, and the patient.

TECHNIQUE OF SURGICAL ASSISTING

Familiarization with median sternotomy and thoracotomy approaches, as well as standard techniques of cardiopulmonary bypass, is necessary in order to function as an effective assistant. Because of the wide variety of anomalies possible with congenital heart disease, a myriad of variations from the basic tasks such as placement of lines and cannulae, initiation of cardiopulmonary bypass, cardioplegia, circulatory arrest, and cooling (including deep hypothermic circulatory arrest) is possible. Even the most seasoned cardiothoracic PA can become overwhelmed if he or she is not familiar with congenital surgery. Therefore, a thorough understanding of the underlying pathophysiology by the surgeon and the assistant and a review of the surgical plans prior to surgical intervention is paramount to a successful outcome.

PEDIATRIC CONSIDERATIONS

Cyanosis is a sure sign of cardiac abnormality. Patent ductus arteriosus may resolve spontaneously, as may closure of the foramen ovale, although surgery may be necessary later in life. All other lesions most likely require surgical intervention to improve cardiac function. With few exceptions (ablation of an accessory pathway in Wolff-Parkinson-White syndrome, arterial switch, and closure of patent ductus, atrial or ventricular septal defect), surgery is usually palliative and not curative.

OBSTETRICAL CONSIDERATIONS

Good prenatal care and screening are essential in order to assess the risk for congenital heart disease. Rubella and alcohol consumption have a positive correlation with some forms of congenital heart disease (patent ductus arteriosus, ventricular septal defect), and viral infections during the first trimester have been implicated as well.

PEARLS FOR THE PA

Volume status is the most important postoperative parameter to watch.

The younger and smaller the patient, the less risk for error in management exists.

Counseling for school, career selection, hobbies and recreation, marriage, and plans to raise a family must begin at an early age and continue throughout life.

Although many of these procedures (e.g., Glenn) are seldom used, many patients who have undergone the procedure have reached adulthood and require close follow-up, because many will require further surgical intervention.

Antibiotic prophylaxis and other endocarditis precautions are critical in all patients with shunts.

Any patient with suspected congenital disease should be referred to an appropriate center for work-up and intervention.

Patients with cyanotic heart disease have an increased incidence of brain abscesses from occult or known endocarditis and may present first with a cerebrovascular accident.

The risk of mortality in pregnant women with congenital heart disease is low in conditions of mild or surgically corrected atrial or ventricular septal defect, patent ductus arteriosus, pulmonary valvular stenosis, or tetralogy of Fallot. The risk of mortality in moderate or severe mitral stenosis, aortic stenosis, coarctation of the aorta, or Marfan's syndrome (with a normal aorta) is much higher. The mortality in those women with primary pulmonary hypertension, Eisenmenger's syndrome, or Marfan's syndrome with aortic involvement may reach 50%.

Coronary Artery Disease
Lyle W. Larson, PA-C, MS

DEFINITION

Coronary artery disease (CAD) involves partial or total occlusion of one or more coronary arteries. Angina pectoris and MI are intimately associated with coronary artery disease.

HISTORY

Symptoms. Although the first presentation of CAD may be infarction or survival from sudden death, CAD is most often diagnosed after the patient experiences symptoms of angina or heart failure that produce ischemic changes on the ECG and prompt invasive procedures (e.g., coronary angiography). However, patients may have significant disease without anginal symptoms.

General. Risk factors that should be elicited in the interview include smoking, hypertension, hyperlipidemia, diabetes mellitus, obesity, age, male sex, and a positive family history.

Age. Variable; risk increases with age (direct correlation).

Onset. Angina may be insidious, intermittent, precipitated with exercise or at rest. Patients may present with acute myocardial infarction, cardiogenic shock, or aborted sudden death.

Duration. Anginal symptoms may occur predictably with exertion, emotions, cold weather, or other factors that increase myocardial oxygen demand; sporadically with or without exercise, or at rest. Coronary atherosclerosis is continuous and progressive if untreated. Whether atherosclerotic lesions are reversible remains controversial.

Intensity. The symptoms of angina range from retrosternal dullness, pressure, heaviness, and radiation to the neck or arm, to frank pain. Intensity is typically graded on a scale of one to ten, with ten considered the most severe pain.

Aggravating Factors. Any activity or condition in which myocardial oxygen demand exceeds supply will precipitate symptoms. Myocardial oxygen demand may increase with conditions such as smoking or large body habitus. Supply may also be compromised in conditions of coronary atherosclerosis, diabetes, and anatomical variation.

Alleviating Factors.   Alleviating factors include those that serve to normalize the mismatch between oxygen supply and demand.

Associated Factors.   Atherosclerotic disease beyond the heart including carotid artery stenosis, aortic sclerosis, renal artery stenosis, and femoral artery sclerosis may accompany CAD and should be excluded.

PHYSICAL EXAMINATION

General.   The physical examination for patients with known CAD presenting for interventional treatment (cardiac catheterization, angioplasty, or bypass surgery) should be directed yet thorough. In addition to vital signs, an accurate height and weight are important to calculate the body surface area (necessary for implementing extracorporeal circulation). It is important also to note the overall nutritional status of the patient.

Cardiovascular.   Evaluate for jugular venous distention, quality of S1 and S2, presence or absence of S3 and S4, murmurs, displaced point of maximal intensity, rhythm, presence of rubs, heaves, or gallops. Peripheral vascular system should be examined for the presence, absence, and quantitation of peripheral pulses, presence of varicose or saphenous veins, or prior venous stripping. The carotid arteries, abdominal aorta, and femoral arteries should be auscultated for bruits.

Neurologic.   Evaluation of cranial nerves, gait, judgment, and reflexes, and to quantitate residual deficits from prior neurologic events.

Skin.   To rule out infectious lesions or evaluate for evidence of vascular insufficiency (e.g., venous stasis, arterial insufficiency).

Thorax.   Evaluate sternum for prior sternotomy; identify structural anomalies such as pectus that could complicate surgical approach. Auscultation of the lung for crackles that may suggest cardiac failure.

PATHOPHYSIOLOGY

Interruption of flow through a coronary artery may occur by one of three mechanisms (plaque formation, embolus, or spasm) or combination thereof.

Atherosclerotic Plaque.   Begins as chronic injury to the vascular endothelium by stimuli such as elevated cholesterol, hypertension, infection, or noxious stimuli (e.g., tobacco). Low-density lipoproteins (LDLs) then enter the vessel wall through these injured sites, become oxidized, and form a "fatty streak." The fatty streak attracts monocytes, which in turn enter the vessel wall, convert LDLs to their highly oxidized form, and form foam cells. Lesions are formed as foam cells grow and generate byproducts including cholesterol esters, and subsequently rupture and contribute to the atheromatous lesion. Clinical events occur when these lesions fissure and disrupt the plaque.

Embolus Formation.　May occur as a result of thrombus generated by a disrupted plaque or as a result of dislodgment of thrombus proximally. Embolus may occur spontaneously or from iatrogenic reasons (e.g., catheter manipulation).

Focal Spasm.　Is known to occur or without an underlying substrate. Powerful vasoconstrictors such as cocaine are often responsible. Spasm is difficult to diagnose unless it is observed during catheterization.

DIAGNOSTIC STUDIES

Laboratory

Full Chemistry Profile.　To rule out baseline electrolyte abnormalities, establish baseline renal function, and assess serum glucose levels.

CBC.　To rule out infection, and document baseline hemoglobin and hematocrit.

Coagulation Studies.　To evaluate extrinsic and intrinsic coagulation pathways preoperatively in anticipation of perioperative bleeding.

Serum Cholesterol and Triglyceride Levels.　To document baseline.

Type and Cross Match.　For blood replacement during the perioperative period.

Identification of Cold Agglutinins.　If cardiopulmonary bypass is considered.

Radiology

Chest X-ray.　To assess heart size; lung edema and consolidation; location and size of great vessels; and presence of indwelling devices such as pacemakers, defibrillators, and prosthetic valves.

Other

ECG.　To identify conduction disorders, presence of hypertrophy, presence and location of current anginal symptoms, or prior infarct.

Echocardiography.　To evaluate global left ventricular function, structure and function of heart valves, presence or absence of septal defects, or other congenital defects.

Radionuclide Scanning.　To identify areas of "hibernating" myocardium.

Cardiac Catheterization.　To provide an accurate map of the coronary arteries, and to identify location(s) of lesions and quantitate their size and effect on flow distal to the obstruction.

DIFFERENTIAL DIAGNOSIS

Traumatic.　Not applicable.

Infectious

Pericarditis.　Pain usually continuous, not precipitated by stress, not relieved by pharmacological intervention or rest, nonspecific ECG changes in all leads.

Endocarditis.　Presence of fever, chills, bacteremia, new murmur; ECG changes usually not present.

Metabolic

Esophageal Reflux. No ECG changes; symptoms precipitated by meals.

Peptic Ulcer Disease. No ECG changes, relieved with H_2 blockers, proton pump inhibitors, or antacids.

Neoplastic

Esophageal, Gastric, Pancreatic, or Hepatic Cancers. Symptoms nonspecific, no ECG changes.

Vascular

Aortic Aneurysm. "Tearing" pain in back or shoulders, acute onset, associated with hypertension or Marfan's syndrome.

Valvular Heart Disease. Presence of murmurs, syncope or near-syncope, arrhythmias.

Congenital. Not applicable.

Acquired. Not applicable.

TREATMENT

Medical. Antianginal therapy is instituted using nitrates, beta-adrenergic blocking agents, calcium channel blockers. Nitrates (nitroglycerin, isosorbide dinitrate) redistribute blood flow along collateral channels from epicardial to endocardial regions and relieve coronary spasm. They act by venodilation and relief of coronary spasm.

Beta blockers (atenolol, metoprolol, propanolol) reduce oxygen demand, control heart rate, and treat hypertension.

Calcium channel blockers (verapamil, nifedipine, diltiazem) reduce afterload, control heart rate, and treat hypertension.

Antithrombotic treatment is begun with aspirin, heparin, warfarin, or ticlopidine hydrochloride.

Cholesterol and triglyceride lowering agents are ordered as indicated. These include bile acid sequestrants (cholestyramine, colestipol) that bind irreversibly with bile acids; nicotinic acid (niacin), which decreases esterification of hepatic triglycerides; fibric acid derivatives (gemfibrozil, clofibrate) that reduce triglyceride rich VLDL fractions; and HMG-CoA reductase inhibitors (fluvastatin, lovastatin, pravastatin, simvastatin) that reduce production of LDL by acting competitively with HMG-CoA reductase.

Diet is modified to a low-salt (for hypertension) and a low-fat diet to lessen the progression of the stenotic lesion.

An exercise program (which may require close supervision) is begun if surgery is not required or in the postoperative period.

Smoking cessation is strongly encouraged. Nicotine gum or patches may be used to help with this process.

Diabetes mellitus, when present, is monitored for optimal control.

Surgical. Coronary artery bypass grafting (CABG) is one of the most common major operations performed on adults in the United States. There are many variations in the procedure, which are surgeon dependent. A brief description follows.

The patient is prepped and draped in the supine position. The chest is entered via a median sternotomy. If an internal thoracic artery and/or radial artery will be used for conduit, they are harvested at this time. Simultaneously, greater or lesser saphenous vein is harvested from the lower extremity with sufficient length taken to provide conduit for other vessels. The lower extremity incision is closed in a manner dictated by the surgeon.

Following acquisition of adequate conduit, the pericardium is opened and sutured to drapes to produce a pericardial sling. The right atria and ascending aorta are cannulated, and catheters for venting and administration of cardioplegia are inserted. Heparin is given, cardiopulmonary bypass is initiated, the aortic cross clamp is applied, and cardioplegia (antegrade via the ascending aorta, retrograde via a coronary sinus cannula, or both) is instituted to arrest the heart.

The coronary arteries are inspected to confirm the location of stenoses. Following completion of both distal and proximal anastomoses on all grafts, the heart is rewarmed and allowed to eject. The patient is then weaned from cardiopulmonary bypass, heparin is reversed with protamine, cannulae are removed, bleeding is controlled, and the chest is closed in a routine manner.

Indications. Unstable angina pectoris.

Contraindications. Contraindications to medical treatment include sensitivity or allergies to pharmacological agents, rapid progression of disease, significant left main coronary artery disease, or "left main equivalent" (proximal left anterior descending and circumflex artery disease).

TECHNIQUE OF SURGICAL ASSISTING

The physician assistant is an ideal choice for harvesting greater and lesser saphenous vein and radial artery, as well as first and second assisting. A thorough knowledge of both anatomy and the multitude of specialized instruments is necessary. It is essential that the assistant be comfortable with suturing, knot tying, and recognition of potential complications.

PEDIATRIC CONSIDERATIONS

Not applicable.

OBSTETRICAL CONSIDERATIONS

Not applicable.

PEARLS FOR THE PA

Patients with anginal symptoms may have mixed coronary artery and valvular heart disease.

The goal in surgical intervention is to supply sufficient oxygenated blood to all areas of the ischemic bed, including "hibernating myocardium."

Patients may have significant CAD without angina.

Cardiac Tamponade
Lyle W. Larson, PA-C, MS

DEFINITION

Tamponade is a syndrome of cardiac compression caused by an accumulation of fluid in the pericardial space. This raises the intrapericardial pressure high enough to impede venous return to the heart and negatively influence the hemodynamic state of the patient. The term tamponade is used for all degrees of cardiac compression, whereas "decompensated" or "critical" tamponade may be used to describe a hypotensive, shock-like condition.

HISTORY

Symptoms. Exercise intolerance, dyspnea, tachycardia, tachypnea, anxiety, or shock leading to profound circulatory collapse.

General. The patient may have a history of penetrating or blunt trauma to the chest or recent MI. Hemodynamic compromise may have been present during or following invasive cardiac procedures, in a patient with a known pericardial disorder as a result of infection (bacterial, fungal, tuberculosis), secondary neoplasm (e.g., metastatic carcinoma from lung or breast), idiopathic pericarditis, radiation pericarditis following radiation therapy, uremia from volume overload, or rheumatic disease.

Age. Variable.

Onset. Acute, due to sudden accumulation of blood in pericardial space, or insidious from a gradual accumulation of fluid or blood in the pericardial space.

Duration. Constant and persistent, with eventual circulatory collapse if left untreated.

Intensity. May range from hemodynamically stable to complete circulatory collapse.

Aggravating Factors. Volume depletion, pericarditis, pericardial thickening, progression of underlying cause (neoplasm, infection, bleeding, etc.).

Alleviating Factors. Often only temporizing, but involves improving right-sided filling pressures and cardiac output.

Associated Factors. Postoperative (coronary artery bypass graft, valve, etc.), pleural effusions, metastatic disease, aortic dissection, aortic valve insufficiency, MI, myocardial perforation or rupture, iatrogenic (coronary artery perforation, dissection), infection (viral, bacterial, fungal), and use of anticoagulants (warfarin, aspirin, anti-inflammatory agents).

PHYSICAL EXAMINATION

General. Vital signs may reveal a paradoxical pulse (greater than 10 mm Hg decrease in systolic blood pressure between inspiration and expiration) and a narrow pulse pressure.

The patient may present with dyspnea, tachycardia, tachypnea, anxiety, or symptoms of shock that suggest profound circulatory collapse.

Cardiovascular. Beck's triad of distant heart sounds, hypotension, and jugular venous distention are classically present with tamponade. Jugular venous distention is present with a rapid X descent.

Kussmaul's sign (a rise in the level of venous pressure with inspiration) occurs only in cases of tamponade associated with constriction.

If a Swan-Ganz catheter is in place, elevated venous pressure (CVP) may be seen, as well as equalization of right atrial, pulmonary artery, pulmonary wedge, left atrial, and left ventricular end diastolic pressure.

PATHOPHYSIOLOGY

The normal pericardial space occupies less than 5 mm and contains less than 20 ml of fluid. The presence of fluid in larger amounts indicates the existence of underlying disease. As fluid accumulates, blood return to the heart decreases as a result of compression on the atria and ventricles. If this occurs rapidly, the compliant pericardium cannot expand, and accumulations of greater than 100 ml can cause symptoms. If allowed to expand over time, the pericardium expands to accommodate the fluid and, as such, chronic accumulations of greater than 2000 ml have been reported without symptoms. Tamponade physiology occurs when systemic venous return falls, cardiac output and blood pressure decrease, and the CVP increases. Tachycardia ensues to compensate for a falling cardiac output, but fails to succeed due to the decreased filling times that accompany a shorter diastole. As a result, circulatory collapse ensues as systolic and diastolic pressures equilibrate.

DIAGNOSTIC STUDIES

Laboratory
Cardiac Enzymes. To rule out MI.

Rheumatologic Studies (ANA, Rheumatoid Factor). To rule out auto-immune process.

Effusion Fluid. Laboratory diagnosis often is made at the same time as the therapeutic removal of fluid. The clinical setting of effusion dictates type of analysis performed, but may include Gram stain for bacteria, acid-fast bacilli, and fungi, as well as protein content, cytology, white blood cell count with differential, and blood cultures.

Radiology
Chest X-ray. May show enlarged cardiac silhouette with "water bottle" appearance, normal or enlarged pulmonary vasculature, and enlarged superior vena cava.

Computed Tomography (CT) of the Chest. Will show pericardial fluid; may show atrial or ventricular compression.

Other
ECG. May show ST segment elevation or depression, flat T waves, low voltages, or electrical alternans.

Echocardiography. Is the most reliable clinical method to detect tamponade. The M mode is adequate but 2-D is more definitive. The study demonstrates presence of fluid but only gives indirect clues of physiology. An echo-free space of 1 cm gives confident diagnosis of tamponade.

Hemodynamic Studies. CVP is always elevated (unless severely volume depleted), the right atrial and pulmonary artery wedge pressures are equal, and the left ventricular end-diastolic pressure is equal to the right ventricular end-diastolic pressure.

DIFFERENTIAL DIAGNOSIS

Traumatic
Acute, Catastrophic Blood Loss (e.g., Aortic Transection). Profound circulatory collapse.

Infectious
Endocarditis with Large, Right-Sided Vegetations. Bacteremia, sepsis, new murmur; differentiated by echocardiography.

Metabolic. Not applicable.

Neoplastic
Atrial Myxoma. Arrhythmia, isolated (right or left) inflow or outflow obstruction; differentiated by echocardiography.

Vascular
Acute Cor Pulmonale. Diffuse inspiratory rhonchi, wheezes, elevated pulmonary artery pressures.

Superior Vena Cava Obstruction. Evidenced by nystagmus, visual changes, venous congestion of face, neck, upper extremities.

Right Ventricular Infarct. Differentiated by ECG, echocardiography (hypokinetic or akinetic right ventricle).

Acute Tricuspid Valve Obstruction (Thromboembolism or Tumor). Differentiated by echocardiography.

Congenital. Not applicable.
Acquired. Not applicable.

TREATMENT

Medical. Pericardial effusions without hypotension or tamponade physiology may be managed conservatively while the underlying condition is treated. At best, medical treatment is only temporizing and should not delay the definitive intervention (e.g., removal of pericardial fluid).

Systemic circulation should be supported by using isoproterenol to stimulate cardiac contractile forces and increase cardiac output, pressors such as norepinephrine to constrict resistance arterioles, and vasodilators to reduce peripheral resistance.

Augment right-sided filling pressures with fluid by using crystalloid such as normal saline or lactated Ringer's solution.

Surgical

Pericardiocentesis. Pericardiocentesis is the quickest, most convenient method to remove pericardial fluid and reduce intrapericardial pressure. It is done most easily and safely under fluoroscopic control in the cardiac catheterization laboratory of ICU. The patient is placed supine with 30 degrees of head elevation in order to allow fluid to settle to the level of the diaphragm. ECG monitoring (with audible tone) and sedation are advised. Vasodepressor reactions are not uncommon, and premedication with atropine is recommended. The chest and abdomen are prepped and draped, and 1% lidocaine is instilled into the subxiphoid area beginning at the skin and progressing into the deeper tissues beneath the xiphoid in a line directed toward the left scapula. Following small stab wound in the skin, an 18-gauge needle with plastic catheter is advanced in similar fashion while aspirating. Needle advancement is stopped and redirected if an arrhythmia is observed. If grossly bloody fluid is aspirated, 5 ml is withdrawn and allowed to stand for a few minutes to assess its ability to clot (nonclotting blood represents hemorrhagic pericardial effusion, whereas the presence of clot represents blood taken from a cardiac chamber, usually the right ventricle). When the pericardial space is entered, the catheter is advanced over the needle, and fluid is removed. Clear or straw-colored fluid is removed easily, whereas more viscous fluid (old blood, pyogenic effusion) may require a larger bore catheter.

Subxiphoid Pericardiostomy. Following general anesthesia, the patient is prepped and draped in the supine position. A subxiphoid incision is performed, and dissection is carried superiorly beneath the xiphoid process until the pericardium is identified. The pericardium is then entered (often with a brisk release of fluid). A catheter may then be placed, or a "window" of pericardium may be excised to allow further pericardial contents to drain into the pleural space, where it may be more readily absorbed and not reaccumulate within the pericardial space.

Indications. Threatened or actual hemodynamic compromise or cardiovascular collapse. A true emergency exists when systolic pressure is less than 100 mm Hg and arterial pulse pressure is less than 30 mm Hg.

   Contraindications.   In the setting of hemodynamic compromise or collapse: none. Documented organized clot or pyogenic effusion are relative contraindications to pericardiocentesis and may require more aggressive surgical management.

TECHNIQUE OF SURGICAL ASSISTING

Pericardiocentesis is usually performed without a surgical assistant. For pericardiostomies, assistance is limited to retraction, suction, and assistance with visualization.

PEDIATRIC CONSIDERATIONS

Causes and treatment are similar to adults.

OBSTETRICAL CONSIDERATIONS

Not applicable.

PEARLS FOR THE PA

The effects of pericardial effusion on intrapericardial pressure and hemodynamics are highly dependent on the rate of fluid accumulation.

No consistent or constant correlation exists between the volume of pericardial fluid, intrapericardial pressure, and symptoms.

Tamponade should be viewed as a spectrum of hemodynamic changes rather than an all-or-none condition.

Although the central venous pressure is almost always elevated, cardiovascular collapse may occur in patients who are intravascularly volume depleted.

Volume loading or pharmacological maneuvers do not have a dramatic effect on the relief of tamponade; therefore, a thoracentesis or more definitive procedure should be performed as soon as possible.

Valvular Heart Disease

Lyle W. Larson, PA-C, MS, and
Michael E. Champion, PA-C, MMSc, EdM, CCP

DEFINITION

Stenosis, insufficiency (regurgitation), or a combination of each in any of the four heart valves results in valvular heart disease. The most common causes include calcification, rheumatic heart disease, chordal rupture, myxomatous degeneration, and endocarditis.

HISTORY

Symptoms. Patients with valvular heart disease may present with a host of symptoms, including chest pain, syncope, arrhythmias, exercise intolerance, orthopnea, or CHF with jugular venous distention, peripheral edema, and pulmonary or hepatic congestion. A description of the various valvular diseases follows, with specific considerations listed when applicable.

Aortic Stenosis (AS). Classic triad of angina, syncope, and CHF; sudden cardiac death is a catastrophic complication.

Aortic Insufficiency (AI). Acute insufficiency may progress quickly from dyspnea at rest to frank pulmonary edema, whereas symptoms of chronic insufficiency occur late in the time course of the disease with exertional dyspnea, palpitations, angina, dull substernal discomfort and, rarely, abdominal pain from splanchnic ischemia.

Mitral Stenosis (MS). Dyspnea on exertion, easy fatigability, palpitations, irregular heart rhythm, hemoptysis with pulmonary hypertension.

Mitral Regurgitation (MR). Slow, progressive dyspnea on exertion, fatigue, palpitations.

Pulmonic Stenosis (PS). Pulmonic stenosis is a congenital anomaly and is the most common form of right ventricular outflow tract obstruction (see section on Congenital Heart Disease).

Pulmonic Insufficiency (PI). Pulmonic insufficiency occurs not only in patients with pulmonary hypertension, but also in a mild degree in up to 75% of normal individuals. As such, it should not be regarded as pathologic without other evidence of heart disease. Management then becomes focused on the underlying disease.

Tricuspid Stenosis (TS). There is no particular symptom or complex of symptoms that are unique for tricuspid stenosis. Rheumatic tricuspid stenosis almost always occurs in a multivalvular pattern and management is focused on the other valve(s).

Tricuspid Insufficiency (TI). Functional tricuspid insufficiency is common, reversible, and difficult to evaluate, even at the time of surgery.

Rheumatic tricuspid insufficiency, like stenosis, is part of a multivalvular pattern, and management is similar. Isolated tricuspid insufficiency may be present in the setting of infective endocarditis, carcinoid, or congenital lesions.

General

AS. Male-to-female ratio of 3:1; causes include deterioration of congenital bicuspid valve, calcification, or valvular scarring from rheumatic heart disease.

AI. Acute insufficiency may be a result of ascending aortic aneurysm or dissection, Marfan's syndrome, or trauma; chronic causes include aortic root dilatation from long-standing hypertension, rheumatic changes, or Ehlers-Danlos syndrome.

MS. It is generally accepted that mitral stenosis is of rheumatic origin, whether or not the patient has a history of rheumatic fever. Patients with similar degrees of stenosis may have very different symptoms, physical findings, and prognosis.

MR. Causes include rheumatic heart disease, rupture of chordae tendineae, papillary muscle dysfunction or rupture, physiologic mitral valve prolapse, endocarditis.

Age

AS. Throughout adult life, bicuspid stenosis presents in the age group of 30 to 50 years; after 50 to 60 years, calcific causes are most common. Aortic stenosis from endocarditis can occur at any age.

AI. Throughout adult life.

MS. Symptoms generally do not appear until the third or fourth decade of life.

MR. Onset usually in fourth to sixth decade of life.

Onset

AS. Usually long latent period followed by progressive exercise intolerance that leads to the cardinal symptoms of angina, syncope, and heart failure.

AI. Sudden, as with acute aortic dissection, or gradual over years as result of aortic root dilatation or valve leaflet degeneration.

MS. Slow and subtle. The exception is in patients from third-world countries with high incidence of rheumatic fever, who may become symptomatic early in life during periods of physiologic stress (e.g., exertion, febrile illness, pregnancy).

MR. Sudden onset with chordal or papillary muscle rupture; otherwise, slow and insidious.

Duration

AS. Progressive and ultimately fatal without surgical intervention.

AI. Progressive; may be fatal in acute cases of wide open aortic insufficiency.

MS. Chronic; progressive unless corrected.

MR. Progressive unless corrected.

Intensity

AS. Ranges from mild exertional intolerance to New York Heart functional class IV symptoms.

AI. Mild if chronic; life threatening if acute.

MS. From insidious to mild symptoms that progress with advancement of disease.

MR. Mild onset and slow progression of symptoms (unless chordal rupture occurs).

Aggravating Factors

AS. Atrial or ventricular arrhythmias, reduced preload.

AI. Hypertension, exercise, tachyarrhythmias, anemia, volume overload.

MS. Increased preload, respiratory infections, arrhythmias, myocardial infarction.

MR. New-onset atrial fibrillation, volume overload, myocardial infarction, increased preload or afterload.

Alleviating Factors

AS. Rest, aggressive afterload reduction.

AI. Tight control of hypertension, rest, alleviation of arrhythmias, afterload reduction.

MS. Mitral valvuloplasty, correction of atrial fibrillation, reduction in preload and pulmonary filling pressures.

MR. Reduced afterload, correction of atrial fibrillation to allow for greater "atrial kick," diuresis.

Associated Factors

AS. Compensatory left ventricular hypertrophy, higher risk for endocarditis.

AI. Coexisting aortic stenosis, aortic root dilatation, CHF, predisposing condition for endocarditis.

MS. Left atrial enlargement, atrial fibrillation, increased risk for embolic events, pulmonary hypertension, bacterial endocarditis.

MR. Decreased left ventricular contractile state, atrial fibrillation (becomes chronic), pulmonary edema, CHF.

PHYSICAL EXAMINATION

General. The patient undergoing consideration for valvular replacement should have a careful physical inspection to rule out occult infection, including a complete examination of the mouth to rule out dental caries or abscesses. If present, these should be addressed preoperatively to reduce the risk of prosthetic valve seeding postoperatively.

Cardiovascular

AS. Identified by a harsh systolic crescendo-decrescendo murmur, loudest at the right second intercostal space, with a palpable thrill, often audible at the apex, which decreases with premature beats. Associated findings include a fourth heart sound, paradoxical splitting of the second heart sound, and delayed carotid upstrokes.

AI. Identified by a high-pitched, diastolic decrescendo murmur beginning with the second heart sound, best heard along the left sternal border during expiration with the patient sitting. Maneuvers that increase afterload (squatting, handgrip, phenylephrine) accentuate the murmur. A characteristic Austin Flint murmur (apical mid-diastolic rumble) is usually present with severe aortic insufficiency. Associated findings include a sharp carotid pulse with rapid upstrokes and collapse, pistol-shot sounds, Quincke's sign (capillary pulsations), and head-bobbing in synchrony with the heart beat.

MS.   Identified by three classic signs: a loud first heart sound, an opening snap, and a diastolic rumble murmur heard in the apex with the patient lying on the left side, increasing with maneuvers that increase flow across the mitral valve (exercise, vigorous coughing). Associated signs include prominent right ventricular impulse, a Graham Steell murmur (of functional pulmonary insufficiency), pulmonary rales, and atrial fibrillation.

MR.   Identified by a holosystolic murmur loudest at the apex, with radiation to the left axilla (may be mid to late systolic with papillary muscle dysfunction) with an S_3 gallop.

PS.   Identified by a systolic murmur present at birth, loudest at the left upper sternal border, ejection in quality, occurring early in systole in mild disease, and pansystolic in severe disease. Associated symptoms include failure to thrive, small body habitus, and cyanosis (including clubbing).

PI.   Characterized by a soft, early diastolic murmur best heard at the right upper sternal border; accentuated in pulmonary hypertension.

TS.   Characterized by an early diastolic murmur, loudest at the left sternal border, with radiation to the upper sternal border or apex. Absence of a right ventricular lift differentiates tricuspid stenosis from mitral stenosis. Associated findings include a prominent A wave with a slow Y descent of the jugular venous pulse.

TI.   Characterized by a holosystolic murmur at the left lower sternal border that increases with inspiration or maneuvers that increase venous return (e.g., leg raising, liver compression). Associated findings include a prominent jugular V wave and a distended, pulsatile liver.

Neurologic.   Examination should be performed to document pre-existing disease prior to surgery because perioperative embolic phenomenon may adversely affect the overall outcome of the patient.

DIAGNOSTIC STUDIES

Laboratory

Full Chemistry Profile.   To rule out volume overload (hyponatremia), acidosis, and hypo- or hyperkalemia as a source for arrhythmias. BUN and creatinine and liver function tests are used to assess preoperative renal function and hepatic status respectively. Glucose is used to rule out underlying diabetes mellitus.

PT, PTT, and Platelets.   To assess baseline coagulation status (especially if patients are to be anticoagulated postoperatively).

Type and Cross Match.   In preparation for surgery.

Radiology

Chest X-ray (Posteroanterior and Lateral).   To evaluate cardiac chamber enlargement, size and condition of aorta, identify calcific aortic or mitral annulus, presence or absence of prominent pulmonary vasculature (which may be indicative of pulmonary hypertension), and determine presence of pulmonary congestion or effusions.

Other

ECG. To determine rhythm (sinus or atrial fibrillation), intervals, presence of bundle branch block (unifascicular or bifascicular block), presence of MI, and presence of atrial or ventricular hypertrophy.

Echocardiogram. Quantitates the degree of valvular stenosis or insufficiency, evaluates valve structure and motion of leaflets, quantitates gradient across the valve, and evaluates chamber size and function (ejection fraction, wall motion abnormalities).

Cardiac Catheterization. To rule out associated CHF, measure pressures proximal and distal to the diseased valve to determine transvalvular gradient, and evaluate chamber size and function.

DIFFERENTIAL DIAGNOSIS

Traumatic

Chest or General Trauma. May cause ruptured chordae tendineae; may present in trauma cases.

Infectious

Rheumatic History. Must be ruled out preoperatively.

Endocarditis with Valvular Vegetations or Intracardiac Abscess. Differentiated on echocardiogram.

Metabolic

Thyrotoxicosis. May be manifested by a hyperdynamic heart with an ejection murmur.

Neoplastic

Intracardiac Myxoma. Differentiated on echocardiogram.

Vascular

Arteriovenous Fistula of Coronary Artery or Coronary Sinus/Pulmonary Arteriovenous Fistula. Rare; identified on cardiac catheterization.

Congenital. See section on congenital heart disease.

Acquired. Not applicable.

Other

Invasive Catheterization Procedures. Resulting in iatrogenic trauma; may cause ruptured chordae tendineae.

Indwelling Pacemaker Defibrillator Leads, Pulmonary Artery Catheter. Seen on chest x-ray.

TREATMENT

Medical. In general, patients may be followed for extended periods of time with periodic echocardiograms to document progression of disease before surgical intervention is required. Treatment consists of modification of lifestyle, diuretics (furosemide, bumetanide, thiazides), inotropic support (digoxin), control of hypertension with beta blockers (atenolol, metoprolol) and calcium channel blockers (nifedipine, diltiazem), anticoagulation (heparin, warfarin) for chronic or recurrent atrial fibrillation, and careful management of angina, especially with aortic stenosis (venous vasodilators such as nitroglycerin may decrease preload and actually exacerbate angina across a tight stenotic valve and induce life-threatening ventricular tachycardia or fibrillation).

The decision to proceed with surgery is made when the patient has a marked increase in symptoms, documentation of more rapid acceleration of disease occurs, or specific criteria are reached (see below).

Surgical. Indications for replacement:

Aortic Valve. Peak systolic gradient greater than 50 mm Hg, valve area less than 0.5 to 0.9 cm^2 (varies with institution), progressive ventricular enlargement, acute severe aortic insufficiency, endocarditis, aortic dissection with involvement of the aortic valvular annulus.

Mitral Valve. Gradient greater than 10 to 15 mm Hg, valve area less than 1.0 to 1.5 cm^2 (varies with institution), ventricular dilatation with signs of failure, acute MI with papillary muscle enlargement, endocarditis.

Pulmonic Valve. Generally not necessary unless congenital defect or endocarditis is present (see section on Congenital Heart Disease).

Tricuspid Valve. Gradient greater than 5 mm Hg (controversial), severe right ventricular failure, endocarditis with involvement of valve leaflets.

Endocarditis. Seventy percent of cases are localized to a congenital cardiac defect or acquired valvular abnormality. The left heart is more often affected than the right, with the exception of tricuspid valve involvement in intravenous drug users. Causes include dental procedures (including cleaning), instrumentation of the respiratory, genitourinary, or gastrointestinal system, or other invasive medical procedures. The most common organisms include non–group A streptococci, *Staphylococcus aureus, S. epidermidis,* and gram-negative bacilli. Fungi may also produce endocarditis and may be difficult to diagnose. Surgical intervention requires complete resection of the infected valve, which may not always be possible.

Valve Choices. In general, the choice of valve for replacement is individualized and decided on by the surgeon and the patient. Choices include

1. Mechanical valve (St. Jude, Medtronic-Hall, Duromedics): Advantages include long life; disadvantages include small risk of embolization (approximately 1% per year) that requires lifelong anticoagulation (may be contraindicated in young women who wish to become pregnant, known coagulopathies, unreliable patient, and those with dangerous vocations).

2. Xenografts (porcine, bovine, pericardial): Advantages include brief postoperative need for anticoagulation (ranging from none to 4 to 6 weeks); disadvantages include short life span of valve (typically 5 to 10 years), requiring reoperation.

3. Allograft (homograft [e.g., human cadaver valve]): Advantages include lack of need for anticoagulation, longer lifetime than xenograft; disadvantages include availability and sizes available.

4. Autograft (patient's own valve): Typically involves the Ross procedure, where the patient's pulmonary valve is moved to the aortic valve position, and a homograft is then used to replace the pulmonary valve. Advantages include lack of need for anticoagulation, autograft should have longer lifespan than xenograft or allograft in high-pressure position, homograft in low-pressure position should last longer than in high-pressure position; disadvantages include longer time on bypass, multiple valve procedure, higher technical expertise required, availability of homograft for pulmonic position.

Indications. See above.

Contraindications. See above.

TECHNIQUE OF SURGICAL ASSISTING

The PA should be familiar with the fundamentals of chest opening via a median sternotomy, assisting with cannulation, and initiation of cardiopulmonary bypass. In the patient with critical aortic stenosis, the surgeon and assistant should be scrubbed at the time of induction and ready to initiate bypass (femoral artery, vein) should ventricular fibrillation occur as a result of a drop in blood pressure.

For valvular replacement, assistance with exposure is essential as the surgeon excises the valve and prepares the annulus. During this time, it is critical to watch for extraneous valve leaflet or calcific material left behind, because this may produce a catastrophic embolus. As the valve is sutured in place, care must be taken to avoid inadvertent damage to the sewing ring or leaflets, or tangling or twisting the anchoring sutures. The valve must be seated on the annulus without tilting, and suture knots must not interfere with the valve leaflet function. Careful closure of the aortotomy (aortic valve) or atriotomy (mitral valve) is critical to avoid postoperative bleeding. Upon termination of bypass, the left ventricular function should be carefully observed, particularly with mitral valve repair or replacement for mitral insufficiency. If valvular repair (typically mitral) is performed, exposure is essential (and often difficult) to ensure a successful chordal shortening or quadrangular resection (essentially placing a "dart" in the posterior valve leaflet). If an annuloplasty is performed, care must be taken to prevent tangling of the sutures while they are placed. Closure of the chest is routine.

PEDIATRIC CONSIDERATIONS

See section on Congenital Heart Disease.

OBSTETRICAL CONSIDERATIONS

Because of an effective hypervolemic state during pregnancy, valvular heart diseases affected by volume status (mitral or aortic insufficiency, mitral stenosis) must be followed closely to prevent occurrence of CHF or pulmonary edema. At term, patients with moderate to severe aortic stenosis should be delivered in the operating room with surgical back-up, as a sudden drop in pressures may lead to life-threatening ventricular tachycardia or fibrillation unless prompt cardiopulmonary bypass is initiated.

PEARLS FOR THE PA

The most severe valvular dysfunction is often accompanied by the softest murmur.

In the preoperative setting, the patient with critical aortic stenosis should be watched very carefully, because any drop in preload (volume depletion, venous dilatation) may precipitate angina and arrhythmias. VT or VF is almost always fatal, as no amount of CPR can generate sufficient flow across a tightly stenotic valve.

Postoperatively, these patients do well, because the left ventricle no longer has to work against a high resistance.

In the postoperative setting, the patient with previously moderate to severe mitral insufficiency is at greatest risk for left ventricular failure. A left ventricle squeezing against a combination of systemic pressure and a low left atrial pressure now has to work harder, and as such is more prone to failure.

Antibiotic prophylaxis against endocarditis is necessary postoperatively and throughout life in all valve repairs and replacements.

Further Reading

Baue AE: Glenn's Thoracic and Cardiovascular Surgery, ed. 5. Norwalk, CT, Appleton & Lange, 1991.

Bojar RM: Adult Cardiac Surgery. London, Blackwell Scientific Publications, 1992.

Bojar RM: Manual of Perioperative Care in Cardiac and Thoracic Surgery. London, Blackwell Scientific Publications, 1992.

Eagle KA: The Practice of Cardiology, ed. 2. Boston, Little, Brown, 1989.

Hurst JW: The Heart, ed. 6. New York, McGraw Hill, 1985.

Kirklin JW: Cardiac Surgery. New York, Wiley, 1986.

Moller JH, Neal WA: Heart Disease in Infancy. Norwalk, CT, Appleton-Century-Crofts, 1981.

Norton LW, Steele G Jr, Eiseman B: Surgical Decision Making, ed. 3. Philadelphia, W.B. Saunders, 1993.

Parmley WW: Cardiology. Philadelphia, J.B. Lippincott, 1993.

Chapter 4

General Surgery
Abdominal Trauma
James W. Becker, PA-C

DEFINITION

Injury inflicted on the abdomen, which can be subdivided into either penetrating injury (when the abdominal cavity is perforated) or blunt injury (no penetration).

HISTORY

Symptoms. Range from an acute abdomen to relatively little pain.

General. Often in the rush to care for a serious trauma patient, the abdomen is not given the full attention it requires. Valuable information must be obtained from witnesses and the first responder team upon arrival. The nature of the trauma can give needed information regarding potential injury. The severity of the motor vehicle accident, the height of the fall, the caliber and distance of the gunshot wound, etc., can supply valuable information about the injury. For example, in the instance of a motor vehicle accident, one must determine such information as whether or not the patient was restrained, if the patient was conscious at the time of initial assessment, and the condition of the vehicle and steering wheel. This helps direct the evaluation of potential injury sites that may have otherwise been missed. If any family members are available, additional information regarding past medical history may be obtained. Do not forget to look for a medical alert tag on the wrist and check for a medical information card in the patient's wallet (with appropriate documentation of the contents).

Age. Any, but the elderly patient is less tolerant of major trauma.

Onset. Obtained from the patient or the responding medical personnel. The "golden hour" for major trauma needs to be considered.

Duration. Acute.

Intensity. Can be life-threatening with intra-abdominal hemorrhage, or benign with low-impact trauma.

Aggravating Factors. Do not apply to the trauma patient.

Alleviating Factors. Prompt recognition and appropriate treatment.

Associated Factors. Multisystem trauma.

PHYSICAL EXAMINATION

General. Airway, breathing, and circulation require immediate attention before any abdominal assessment is initiated. After these crucial functions are established, a quick assessment of the central nervous system should be performed.

Gastrointestinal. A full inspection of the abdomen is required. Check for signs of abdominal wall trauma. Note any lacerations, abrasions, contusions, or structural deformities. Inspect the umbilicus for a bluish discoloration (Cullen's sign), which may indicate intra-abdominal bleeding. Any evidence of a shearing force on the abdominal wall may indicate similar severe forces on the abdominal contents, which may indicate tears of the mesentery, pancreas, liver, or spleen. Auscultation of the abdomen may yield rare bowel sounds. Crepitus may indicate associated rib or pelvic fracture. Palpation may reveal areas of tenderness or deformity (from organ disruption or hematoma formation). Rectal examination for blood or structural deformity must also be performed. Examination of the back is frequently overlooked. Palpation of the flanks, spine, and buttocks should also be performed in the trauma setting.

PATHOPHYSIOLOGY

Abdominal trauma can be divided into two classifications: solid and hollow organ trauma.

Solid Organs. Include the spleen, liver, and pancreas. These organs can sustain significant injury from what may have been considered minor trauma; significant hemorrhage can occur in a short period of time.

Hollow Organs. Include the stomach, colon, and intestines. Trauma to these organs may lead to infectious problems when penetration occurs.

Injury to the mesentery may not be initially evident but can lead to ischemia over several hours (see the topic Bowel Ischemia).

The degree of trauma sustained is a combination of the masses of the objects that collided and the speed at which the collision took place. Therefore, the severity of a gunshot wound is related to the size and speed of the projectile. The direction of the projectile may be altered by deflection from internal structures and fragmentation of the bullet. Likewise, shotgun injuries are notoriously serious due to the number of involved sites of injury. Overall, motor vehicle injuries can be decreased by the use of seatbelts, airbags, and energy-absorbing steering columns.

DIAGNOSTIC STUDIES

Laboratory

Complete Blood Count (CBC). To evaluate for anemia due to blood loss. Include crossmatch and transfuse as indicated.

Coagulation Profile (PT, PTT, Bleeding Time). Performed to rule out coagulation defects and as a preoperative screening tool.

Chemistry Profile. To evaluate for electrolyte abnormalities. Liver enzyme abnormalities may indicate developing liver injury or ischemia.

Amylase. Increased from absorption of duodenal secretions in peritoneum after perforation. Used to rule out associated pancreatitis from trauma.

Lipase (Serum). Elevation may suggest pancreatic injury.

Urinalysis. The presence of hematuria may indicate direct renal injury or pelvic fracture involving ureter disruption or bladder injury.

Toxicology Screen. Including blood alcohol. To rule out coexisting toxicity or intoxication.

Arterial Blood Gas. To evaluate for hypoxemia, especially in the setting of multitrauma or chest injury.

Radiology

Chest X-ray. Posteroanterior (PA) and lateral. Used as routine preoperative study and to rule out chest/lung/heart structural abnormalities that may impact on general anesthesia.

Abdominal Films. Flat and upright (if possible) to evaluate for free air under the diaphragm, which may indicate hollow organ penetration. If no free air is seen, perforation may still exist, especially if it leads to the retroperitoneum or has been sealed by the omentum. Check for the gastric air bubble, which is normally located in the left upper quadrant. If it is displaced medially, an enlarging splenic hematoma may be present. Air in the biliary tree indicates a duodenal injury.

Intravenous Pyelogram (IVP). Indicated when pelvic trauma is present.

Abdominal Ultrasound. Used to evaluate solid organ disruption. This noninvasive test can be performed in the trauma unit.

Abdominal CT Scan. The definitive test for abdominal trauma, because all organs can be viewed simultaneously.

Arteriogram. Indicated for suspected vascular disruption.

Other

Paracentesis. Performed when abdominal hemorrhage is suspected. A positive paracentesis warrants surgical exploration.

DIFFERENTIAL DIAGNOSIS

Not applicable to the trauma patient.

TREATMENT

Medical. If there is no evidence of abdominal perforation or organ disruption, the patient may be hospitalized and observed.

Surgical. When preparing the patient for laparotomy, a generous abdominal prep from the clavicular area to the groin is performed. A solution of "weak tea" (70% alcohol and tincture of iodine) or an iodine-impregnated surgical drape is used. A midline incision from the xiphoid to the umbilicus is appropriate and provides adequate initial visualization. All four quadrants should be quickly assessed and packs placed to control any venous bleeding encountered. Direct pressure to major arterial bleeds allows time for resuscitative measures to be performed and stabilization to occur. Once the bleeding sources have been controlled, attention can then be directed to the intestinal contents. A systematic examination of the stomach, duodenum, small intestine, colon, and rectum (including the mesentery) should be accomplished. The solid organs should be likewise evaluated with inspection for hematomas of the liver, spleen, and pancreas.

If abdominal exploration is indicated, a broad-spectrum antibiotic is essential (penicillin or cephalosporin). Hollow organ injuries require the addition of an aminoglycoside or metronidazole.

Indications.   Any evidence of penetration of the abdominal wall into the peritoneum indicates immediate surgical exploration.

Contraindications.   Bleeding dyscrasia, inability of the patient to undergo anesthesia (dependent on the severity of the trauma). Abdominal exploration may be deferred (if not immediately life-threatening) pending treatments to other organ systems in the multitrauma patient.

TECHNIQUE OF SURGICAL ASSISTING

Approach to the duodenum or stomach is through a midline or left paramedian incision. The PA assists with retraction during opening, using caution not to grasp any bowel underlying the tissue being opened. Retraction and assistance with hemostasis, anastomosis, or resection are provided throughout the procedure. The PA assists with closure (with a ribbon or malleable retractor placed into the incision to prevent inadvertent suturing of bowel), placement of dressings, and postoperative care.

PEDIATRIC CONSIDERATIONS

Children between the ages of 6 and 8 years have the highest incidence of abdominal trauma (usually blunt), which may be due to pedestrian-versus-automobile accidents, motor vehicle accidents, or falls. Solid organs are more frequently involved. Adolescents between the ages of 15 and 18 years suffer more abdominal injuries, usually of the penetrating type. Essentials of trauma management apply to the pediatric and adolescent populations.

OBSTETRICAL CONSIDERATIONS

Serum hCG is indicated in all trauma patients with the potential to be pregnant. Gynecology consultation is required to evaluate for fetal trauma in the patient with abdominal trauma. Anesthetic agents and medications that may be harmful or teratogenic should be avoided.

PEARLS FOR THE PA

Obtain a history from rescue personnel, family, and friends regarding the mechanism of injury.

Remember the ABCs (Airway, Breathing, Circulation).

Include a quick examination of the back in the setting of abdominal trauma.

Adrenal/Renal Neoplasms

Thomas J. Schymanski, PA-C

DEFINITION

Adrenal Adenoma. Neoplasm of the adrenal gland that may cause excessive concentrations of cortisol or other glucocorticoid hormones in the circulation, resulting in Cushing's syndrome.

Pheochromocytoma. Tumors of the adrenal medulla and related chromaffin tissues elsewhere in the body that secrete dopamine, epinephrine, or norepinephrine, resulting in sustained or episodic hypertension and other symptoms of excess catecholamine.

Nephroblastoma (Wilms' Tumor). A malignant tumor of the kidney that originates in immature neural crest tissue; most often encountered in childhood.

Renal Cell Carcinoma. The most common solid renal tumor of adults. Arises from the cells of the convoluted tubule.

HISTORY

Symptoms

Adrenal Adenoma. Muscle weakness, obesity/weight gain, easy bruising, growth retardation in children.

Pheochromocytoma. The manifestations of pheochromocytomas are caused by increased levels of circulating catecholamines and include hypertension, headache, sweating, palpitations, weight loss, nervousness, and tremor. Other features may include hyperglycemia, hypermetabolism, and postural hypotension in a hypertensive patient.

Nephroblastoma. Symptoms consist of abdominal enlargement (flank mass) in 60% of cases; pain in 20%; hematuria in 15%; malaise, weakness, anorexia, and weight loss in 10%; and fever in 3%. Hypertension, noted in over half of patients, may cause congestive heart failure.

Renal Cell Carcinoma. Asymptomatic, or the patient may present with classic hematuria, flank pain, and renal mass. Weight loss, fever, malaise, night sweats, or anemia may also be present.

General

Adrenal Adenoma. Most patients (50% to 60%) presenting with Cushing's syndrome have a pituitary adenoma (see Pituitary Adenoma, Chapter 7). Ectopic adrenocorticotropic hormone (ACTH) production may occur secondary to neoplasms elsewhere in the body (see differential diagnosis below). To diagnose this condition, the patient should have hypertension, hypokalemia (nondiuretic induced), high aldosterone output with a high sodium intake, and reduced serum renin levels that do not rise with a sodium-restricted diet.

Pheochromocytoma. A rare condition that is suspected far more often than it is diagnosed.

Nephroblastoma. Comprises approximately 95% of malignancies of the urinary tract in children. May metastasize to the lung, liver, bone, or brain.

Renal Cell Carcinoma. May metastasize to the lung, bone, brain, and subcutaneous tissue.

Age

Adrenal Adenoma. Third and fourth decades; females more frequently than males.

Pheochromocytoma. Any, with 20% occurring in children; maximum incidence is between the fifth and sixth decades.

Nephroblastoma. Approximately 90% present in children less than 7 years of age.

Renal Cell Carcinoma. Primarily a tumor of adults (60 to 80 years of age), with a 3:1 male predominance.

Onset

Adrenal Adenoma. May be sudden, particularly in patients with oat cell carcinoma of the lung.

Pheochromocytoma. May be quite rapid, with sustained hypertension.

Nephroblastoma. Insidious, with an enlarging, unilateral abdominal mass.

Renal Cell Carcinoma. Insidious, and may be an incidental finding on radiographic procedures.

Duration. Progressive. With pheochromocytoma, paroxysmal hypertension lasts 15 to 30 minutes and the frequency of bouts varies.

Intensity. The patient may be relatively asymptomatic until the disease is more advanced.

Aggravating Factors

Pheochromocytoma. Precipitated by maneuvers that disturb the abdominal contents such as exercise, bending, palpation of the abdomen, urination, or defecation.

Alleviating Factors. Prompt identification, appropriate diagnosis, and definitive treatment.

Associated Factors

Nephroblastoma. May be allied with other congenital abnormalities.

Renal Cell Carcinoma. May have associated liver dysfunction in the absence of hepatic metastases. The lesion may produce hormones that result in symptoms of hypercalcemia, galactorrhea, hypertension, Cushing's syndrome, or virilization. Patients with Hippel-Lindau disease have a high incidence of developing renal cell carcinoma.

PHYSICAL EXAMINATION

General

Adrenal Adenoma. The patient may exhibit central obesity with moon facies, a cervical fat pad (buffalo hump), purple striae, supraclavicular fat pads, and hypertension.

Pheochromocytoma. Orthostatic hypertension may be a prominent finding.

Nephroblastoma. Hypertension may be present.

Renal Cell Carcinoma. Hypertension may be present. Weight loss suggests advanced, metastatic disease. Perform a full and complete survey of all systems to evaluate for metastases.

Abdominal. Palpate the abdomen and kidneys for masses. Check for costrovertebral angle tenderness.

Nephroblastoma. An abdominal mass, palpable in almost all cases, is usually very large, firm, and smooth; does not ordinarily extend across the midline.

PATHOPHYSIOLOGY

Adrenal Adenoma. The adenoma secretes cortisol with an associated low serum ACTH.

Pheochromocytoma. The majority (80%) are single tumors of the adrenal medulla. However, 10% to 20% are located outside of the adrenal gland, and 1% to 3% are in the chest and neck. About 20% are multiple and 10% are malignant.

Nephroblastoma. The tumor is composed of embryonic, nephrogenic tissue that enlarges and invades renal tissue, lymphatics, and vasculature.

Renal Cell Carcinoma. There are no known etiologic factors associated with the development of these tumors. The lesion extends locally and often causes thrombus of the renal vein.

DIAGNOSTIC STUDIES

Laboratory

Full Chemistry Profile. May show electrolyte or liver function abnormalities with renal disease. Hypokalemia is present with Cushing's syndrome. Alkaline phosphatase is increased with renal cell carcinomas (produced in the tumor).

Dexamethasone Suppression Test. Used when Cushing's disease is apparent in order to identify the source. Urine and plasma free cortisol are normally suppressed with low-dose dexamethasone (0.5 mg every 6 hours). Levels are also suppressed with high-dose dexamethasone (2 mg every 6 hours) in pituitary-dependent Cushing's disease. There is no suppression of levels in nonpituitary Cushing's disease.

24-Hour Urinary Free Cortisol. May be elevated with adrenal Cushing's syndrome.

Renin Level. Reduced with Cushing's syndrome. The level does not rise with restricted sodium intake.

Urine Catecholamines and Their Metabolites. Elevated in most confirmed cases of pheochromocytoma. The 24-hour urinary metanephrine excretion rate may be the most useful screening test, but tests of urinary free catecholamine (e.g., epinephrine and norepinephrine) and vanillyl-mandelic acid concentrations are also of value.

Serum Catecholamine Levels. Are quite variable and are more difficult to interpret than the 24-hour urine measurements.

Clonidine Suppression Test. Useful in patients with mild catecholamine elevation.

Radiology

CT/MRI of the Abdomen (with Contrast). Detects most renal and adrenal neoplasms and may allow differentiation of types of lesions. May show metastases.

Intravenous Pyelogram. To fully evaluate the upper and lower urinary tract. Nonopacification on the study indicates tumor extension into the ureter or renal vessels. Shows distortion of the calices and kidney with nephroblastoma.

Adrenal Venography. Performed in conjunction with venous sampling studies to diagnose adrenal lesions.

Selective Renal Angiography. Primarily reserved for patients with solitary kidneys to gain knowledge of the vascular anatomy for planning a conservative surgical excision.

Ultrasound. May confirm the lesion as being cystic or solid.

Metastatic Work-up. Including chest x-ray, radionuclide bone scans, abdominal CT scan, isotope liver scans, and brain MRI to evaluate for metastatic lesions.

DIFFERENTIAL DIAGNOSIS

Traumatic

Renal Contusion. May cause hematuria and flank pain. History of trauma.

Infectious

Pyelonephritis. May cause hematuria and acute flank pain. Usually associated with fever; urine culture positive.

Metabolic

Splenomegaly. May be confused with a large renal mass on physical examination. CT of the abdomen differentiates.

Kidney Stones. May cause hematuria and flank pain. IVP positive.

Neoplastic

Oat Cell Carcinoma of the Lung, Carcinoma of the Pancreas, Bronchial Carcinoid Tumors. May be the cause of ectopic ACTH production and Cushing's syndrome. Knowledge and suspicion of these lesions, coupled with appropriate diagnostic studies differentiates.

Pituitary Adenoma. May be the cause of Cushing's syndrome. Knowledge and suspicion of this condition, coupled with appropriate diagnostic studies differentiates.

Other Renal Tumors. Include renal hamartoma, renal sarcoma, lipoma, leiomyoma, angioma, lymphoma, mesenteric cysts, and are differentiated by radiographic appearance or by histologic confirmation.

Adrenal Lesions. Such as cysts and carcinomas are rare. Ganglioneuromas are benign lesions, usually seen in children, differentiated on CT and ultrasound, and may require surgical removal. Adrenal carcinomas are usually functional, present with Cushing's syndrome or virilization, and metastasize.

Pseudotumor. May appear as a renal mass, but is a normal variant comprised of functional renal tissue. Differentiated on DMSA renal scan.

Vascular

Hemangiopericytoma. A vascular renal mass which may be malignant. Treated with nephrectomy.

Acute Renal Artery Occlusion. Causes renal failure. Occlusion diagnosed on renal angiogram or renal artery Doppler/ultrasound.

Congenital

Polycystic Kidney Disease. Can cause renal failure. Multiple cysts seen on CT/ultrasound. May have a positive family history of polycystic disease.

Acquired

Medications. Such as chronic analgesic or nonsteroidal anti-inflammatory drugs (NSAIDs) may cause interstitial nephritis and chronic renal failure.

Other

Hydronephrosis. Kidney may be palpable if hydronephrosis is severe. Differentiated on CT/ultrasound.

TREATMENT

Medical

Adrenal Adenoma. Treatment initially consists of controlling the symptoms of Cushing's syndrome (hypokalemia, hypertension, elevated aldosterone). The patient is initially given a trial of spironolactone and placed on a sodium-restricted diet. If the patient fails to respond or if a lesion is identified, surgery is indicated.

Pituitary irradiation may be given, although this is more effective in children than adults. If the pituitary is the source, a transphenoidal adenomectomy is performed (see Pituitary Adenoma, Chapter 7). If the source is an adrenal adenoma, the treatment is surgical, because some tumors (adenocarcinoma) may be insensitive to radiation and chemotherapy.

Pheochromocytoma. Alpha- and beta-adrenergic blocking agents are used in preparation for surgery and for inoperable tumors.

Nephroblastoma. Treatment is surgical, although it may be elected to reduce the size of large tumors with radiation or chemotherapy preoperatively. Postoperatively, chemotherapy (double agent) and radiation therapy are given. Irradiation of the tumor bed is indicated if the tumor has extended beyond the capsule of the kidney to involve adjacent organs or lymph nodes. Specific treatments vary, depending on histologic type.

Renal Cell Carcinoma. Radiation therapy has limited value. Chemotherapy is relatively ineffective, with transient tumor regression occurring in less than 5% of patients. Immunotherapy may be attempted for advanced disease.

Surgical

Adrenal Adenoma. A radical adrenalectomy and lymphadenectomy is performed. The contralateral adrenal should be evaluated for hyperplasia. Most lesions are encountered in the left adrenal.

Pheochromocytoma. Surgical removal of the pheochromocytoma is the treatment of choice. Careful exploration of the adrenal gland and the periaortic sympathetic chain should be performed.

Nephroblastoma. The preferred treatment is immediate nephrectomy, inspection of the other kidney, and excision of all surrounding tissues within Gerota's fascia (the perirenal fascia), including retroperitoneal lymphadenectomy.

Renal Cell Carcinoma. The tumor is staged based on regional or distant spread. In stage I, the tumor is confined to the kidney; stage II, the tumor involves Gerota's fascia; stage III, the regional lymph nodes, renal vein, or vena cava are affected; and stage IV refers to disseminated disease or metastases. Radical nephrectomy with lymph node dissection is the treatment of choice for stage I, II, and III lesions. Nephrectomy should also be considered for patients with disseminated disease to relieve hematuria and flank pain. Radical nephrectomy results in a 5-year survival rate of 75% of patients with localized tumors.

Indications. If a symptomatic lesion is identified, surgery is indicated. For nephroblastoma, the survival rate is improved with prompt diagnosis and excision. For renal cell carcinoma, prompt surgical intervention is indicated to prevent disease spread, because adjunctive therapies are of limited value.

Contraindications. Coagulopathy, inability to tolerate anesthesia.

TECHNIQUE OF SURGICAL ASSISTING

The PA assists with opening, closing, and retraction for visualization of the kidney and adrenal gland. Careful attention to technique must be maintained to prevent tumor spillage and potential subsequent metastases with some lesions. Attention to pre- and postoperative electrolyte balance and renal function are important aspects of care. Coordinating ancillary services and patient and family counseling are also key roles of the PA.

PEDIATRIC CONSIDERATIONS

Nephroblastoma. Renal neoplasms account for about 10% of malignant tumors in children. Eighty percent of patients are under 4 years of age at the time of diagnosis. A high degree of suspicion, prompt identification, and appropriate treatment result in a relatively favorable prognosis.

Other conditions which affect the kidney and adrenal glands of children include ganglioneuromas, polycystic kidney disease, hydronephrosis, neuroblastoma, and lymphoma.

OBSTETRICAL CONSIDERATIONS

General concerns in operative intervention during pregnancy include avoidance of x-rays and teratogenic drugs; adequate oxygenation; fluid, electrolyte, and blood volume normalization; appropriate sedation (to minimize the risk of premature labor); gastric decompression; treatment of urinary retention; measures to reduce the risk of deep vein thrombosis (antiembolism stockings or pneumatic compression hose); rest; and avoidance of antibiotic prophylaxis as indicated.

PEARLS FOR THE PA

Urinalysis is the single most useful screening device available to the primary care provider for evaluation of renal disease.

Cushing's syndrome is localized as being of adrenal origin by using the dexamethasone suppression test.

Pheochromocytoma is suspected more often than diagnosed.

A high index of suspicion should be maintained for nephroblastoma in children, because prompt identification and treatment result in a relatively favorable prognosis.

The patient with renal cell carcinoma is frequently asymptomatic, but work-up is indicated if there is a suspicion of a lesion, because these tumors are resistant to adjunctive therapies (radiation/chemotherapy).

Anal Fissures
Clyde Bullion, PA-C, BSN, RN

DEFINITION

A longitudinal laceration in the squamous epithelium of the anal canal, most often in the posterior canal, leaving the internal sphincter muscle exposed.

HISTORY

Symptoms. A new fissure usually presents with an abrupt onset of tearing or sharp pain, and bright red drops of blood on the stool, on toilet paper, or in the toilet water. Chronic fissure(s) present with either burning or no pain and blood streaks on the stool or toilet paper, in underwear, or in the toilet water.

General.   The diagnosis is made largely by history. History should include questions that cover the entire gastrointestinal system, to include changes in stool color, consistency, and caliber; problems with constipation or diarrhea; previous history of the same complaint; pain and bleeding; and a sexual history (e.g., herpes, syphilis, anal intercourse).

Age.   Any age, including infants. Most common between 20 and 40 years of age, with a mean of 36 to 39 years of age.

Onset.   Abrupt. Most patients present with pain, bleeding, or both.

Duration.   Pain may last 3 to 4 days or, with chronic fissures, weeks.

Intensity.   Initially severe. As the fissure becomes a chronic problem, the pain decreases to burning or no pain, flaring up occasionally to a severe tearing or sharp pain.

Aggravating Factors.   Any problems related to diet that cause hard stool, such as dehydration, or severe diarrhea.

Alleviating Factors.   Increasing fiber in the diet, psyllium (e.g., Metamucil), or through the use of stool softeners (e.g., docusate sodium). Local measures aimed at reducing the pain include sitz or warm baths and compresses and possibly hydrocortisone creams.

Associated Factors.   Basically, a benign condition. However, without proper evaluation of change in stool habits, bleeding, weight change, and proper physical examination, a cancer may be diagnosed as a fissure.

PHYSICAL EXAMINATION

General.   With new onset, a fissure may not be visualized, partly due to patient discomfort, and in part to extra folds of tissue that may cover over the area. In a chronic fissure, look for a skin tag (otherwise called a sentinel tag) that forms external to the canal.

Gastrointestinal.   Listen for bowel sounds, and then check for pain or tenderness, guarding, rigidity, masses, and organomegaly.

Rectal.   Have patient lie on left side, left leg straight, right leg bent. Have patient take right hand and pull right buttock away from left, gently, exposing the anus to direct view. Look for bleeding, skin tags, or piles. Use a Q-tip to gently open the anus, looking posterior, anterior, and then right and left lateral, for any signs of laceration. If possible, a well-lubricated gloved finger may then be inserted to check for masses, stool guaiac, stool consistency and, in males, the prostate.

PATHOPHYSIOLOGY

The exact cause is unknown, but most persons who have tears have a higher anal pressure in the internal sphincter muscle, which is measured by a manometer. When a large, hard stool is passed, the internal sphincter should relax, but appears to contract very strongly, resulting in a tear. Conversely, with diarrhea, the strong alkalinity of the stool results in a breakdown of the anal canal lining. The result of both is severe pain as the highly innervated squamous epithelium parts, revealing the internal sphincter muscle.

DIAGNOSTIC STUDIES

No tests are usually indicated, unless one suspects other contributing conditions.

Laboratory

Human Immunodeficiency Virus (HIV) Testing. As indicated if acquired immunodeficiency syndrome (AIDS) is suspected.

Radiology

Barium Enema. If Crohn's disease or other pathology needs to be excluded.

CT Scan of the Abdomen. Important for diagnosing extramural complications of Crohn's disease or other pathologies.

Other

Endoscopy. Used as a complement to radiographic procedures and useful for biopsy of strictures, mass lesions, or filling defects seen on barium enema.

DIFFERENTIAL DIAGNOSIS

Traumatic

Rape, Intercourse. Positive history.

Infectious

Abscess. May be missed because history is the same, but the patient is too tender to examine.

Herpes Simplex. Painful, with small amounts of blood. Usually has prodromal pain 1 to 3 days before lesion occurs. If suspected, also suspect HIV. Herpes simplex virus culture should be done.

HIV or AIDS. May present with same symptoms, but laceration may be in an unusual position, lateral rather than posterior or anterior.

Leukemia. Excessive bleeding tendencies occur with this disease, and hard stool tearing the anus can lead to prolonged bleeding. The gastrointestinal (GI) system is one of the three common sites for bleeding that leads to death.

Syphilis. May present as an ulceration after sexual contact. It is actually a chancre, usually painless. Inguinal lymphadenopathy is notable. If anal condylomata are noted, there is a discharge from the lesion, or if there are two lesions on opposite sides, cultures for syphilis should be taken.

Tuberculosis. The initial ulceration may appear similar to a fissure, but fails to heal with normal therapy. It progresses to several ulcers, the edges appear to be undermined, and eventually destroys the sphincter muscle. Sigmoidoscopy, purified protein derivative (PPD), and cultures are required for diagnosis.

Metabolic.   Not applicable.

Neoplastic

Colorectal Tumors.   Usually painless. Seen on flexible sigmoidoscopy, colonoscopy, barium enema, transrectal ultrasound, CT, or MRI.

Lymphoma.   May present as an ulcerated mass. Digital examination is the key to differentiating.

Vascular

Hemorrhoid.   May present with same history. Visualization is the key.

Congenital.   Not applicable.

Acquired

Crohn's Disease.   Diarrhea and rectal bleeding. If patient has persistent rectal fissures, he or she should be checked for Crohn's. Ulcer is usually painless.

Pruritus Ani.   A patient may come in complaining of itching. Fissures tend to occur superficially and there is usually more than one, all radiating like spokes from the anus out to the perineal skin.

Ulcerative Colitis.   Constipation and rectal bleeding, but may have diarrhea as well. Recurrence may be best key to diagnosis. Fissure is very painful.

TREATMENT

Medical.   In many cases, eating a proper diet with high fiber and plenty of fluids is all that is required. Psyllium-containing preparations, stool softeners like docusate sodium, sitz baths, compresses, and hydrocortisone ointments or creams all help alleviate symptoms.

Bulk-Forming/Stool-Softening Agents
- Citrucel powder: 1 tablespoon 1 to 3 times per day in 8 oz water
- Colace capsule: 50 mg; 1 to 6 capsules per day
- Effer-syllium powder: 1 teaspoon 1 to 3 times per day in 8 oz water
- Fiberall: 1 chewable tablet 1 to 4 times per day with 8 oz water
- Fibercon: 2 to 4 tablets 1 to 4 times per day with 8 oz water
- Maalox powder: 1 teaspoon up to 3 times per day in 8 oz water
- Maltsupex: 4 tablets 4 times per day
- Metamucil: 1 teaspoon 1 to 3 times per day in 8 oz water, followed by 8 oz water
- Mitrolan: 3 chewable tablets 4 times per day, up to 12 per 24 hours
- Modane: 1 teaspoon 1 to 3 times per day in 8 oz water
- Mylanta fiber: 1 tablespoon in 8 oz water, 1 to 3 times per day
- Perdiem fiber powder: 1 to 2 teaspoons swallowed with 8 oz cool fluid in the evening and before breakfast
- Serutan: 1 teaspoon in 8 oz water, 1 to 3 times per day
- Syllact: 1 teaspoon in 8 oz water, 1 to 3 times per day

Anti-Inflammatory Creams/Ointments
- Americaine ointment: apply up to 6 times per day

- Anusol-HC 1: apply 3 to 4 times per day
- Corticaine 0.5%: apply 3 to 4 times per day
- Preparation H (hydrocortisone) 1% cream: apply 3 to 4 times per day
- Proctofoam 1%: apply with tissue up to 5 times per day

Mineral oil preparations should not be used, because of the difficulty in keeping the area clean and irritation to the rectum. Suppositories should not be used because of pain and increasing tears and spasms. The use of highly concentrated nitroglycerin paste or botulinum toxin is still in the early stages of study, but may prove to be beneficial in the future.

Surgical. There are two methods: anal dilatation and internal sphincterotomy. Many surgeons have tended to prefer dilatation because the method does not involve cutting and thus creates fewer problems for those with AIDS or Crohn's disease. Internal sphincterotomies tend to have a slightly better success rate, with less recurrence. The major risk with all of the surgical procedures is postoperative fecal incontinence.

Anal Dilatation

Finger Method. With patient in the left lateral position, under general, spinal, or local anesthesia, insert one well-lubricated index finger into the anus. Follow with another finger. Then insert the other index finger, followed by another finger. With all four in place, stretch the rectum for several seconds. In a female patient, stretch right to left, or transversely. In a male, stretch anterior-posteriorly.

Balloon Method. Insert a rectosigmoid balloon into the canal, inflate, and maintain for 5 minutes.

Lateral Internal Sphincterotomy

Open. A small incision is made through the fissure to expose the internal sphincter. This sphincter is cut and the area closed.

Closed. A knife blade is passed parallel to the sphincter, rotated 90 degrees, then levered toward the internal sphincter. An incision in the sphincter is made, the blade is rotated back 90 degrees and removed. If bleeding occurs, stop with pressure or a single suture.

Indications. If diet, bulk-forming/stool-softening agents, and local measures fail, then surgical therapy becomes a necessity.

Contraindications. Dilatation has a higher incidence of fecal incontinence in patients over 60 years old.

TECHNIQUE OF SURGICAL ASSISTING

Other than retraction, no assistance is usually required for these procedures.

PEDIATRIC CONSIDERATIONS

Because anal fissures are the most common cause of infant rectal bleeding, all of these procedures have been tested on children (although anal dilatation may be one to two fingers) and have been found to be effective.

OBSTETRICAL CONSIDERATIONS

Because these procedures can be performed under local anesthesia, if medical measures fail, then dilatation should be attempted to alleviate symptoms.

PEARLS FOR THE PA

Any unusual presentation of fissures, such as multiple fissures or those on lateral sides, should caution one to look further for another diagnosis.

The use of suppositories and mineral oil preparations should be avoided.

Medical treatments are usually very effective, and patients should not be referred to surgeons until these measures have been tried for 6 to 8 weeks, dependent on the level of patient discomfort.

Appendicitis

James W. Becker, PA-C

DEFINITION

Acute inflammation of the appendix due to obstruction or infection.

HISTORY

Symptoms. Sequential onset of abdominal pain, initially periumbilical that localizes to the right lower quadrant. Frequently associated with nausea and vomiting.

General. Appendicitis is the most common cause of acute abdominal pain in the young, healthy patient.

Age. Most common in ages 10 to 30 years, but may occur at any age.

Onset. May be rapid, over a few hours, or insidious, over several days.

Duration. Progressing to possible rupture if left untreated.

Intensity: Usually mild to moderate peri-umbilical pain progressing over 12 to 18 hours into moderately severe right lower quadrant pain.

Aggravating Factors. Sudden movements such as going over bumps in a car or stretcher, signifying peritoneal irritation.

Alleviating Factors. Lying in the fetal position (knees flexed).

Associated Factors. None.

PHYSICAL EXAMINATION

General. The patient may appear ill, but usually not in acute distress when lying still. Temperature may be elevated, especially if the patient is dehydrated (>100°F).

Gastrointestinal. The abdomen appears nondistended, with guarding in the lower quadrants with right lower quadrant tenderness and rebound tenderness, usually graded at 2 to 3 (range, 1 to 4) on palpation. The point of maximum tenderness is usually over McBurney's point (1/3 of the distance from the right iliac crest to the umbilicus). Pain is usually present on percussion of the right lower quadrant. Bowel sounds are diminished. With perforation of the appendix, positive perineal signs may be found. These are the psoas sign (hyperextension of the hip joint causes pain) and obturator sign (flexion and internal rotation of the thigh causes pain).

PATHOPHYSIOLOGY

The appendix is most commonly found in the right lower quadrant at the origin of the cecum. It may be flipped into the retrocecal space, where the point of tenderness may be more lateral and posterior. Appendicitis is caused by obliteration of the lumen of the appendix by either a fecalith or fibrous tissue. The most common organisms that cause infection are the enteric pathogens *Escherichia coli* and *Klebsiella*. Amebic pathogens have also been implicated. Cases of chronic appendicitis with repeated episodes of smoldering abdominal pain have also been reported.

DIAGNOSTIC STUDIES

Laboratory

CBC. WBC is frequently but not always elevated (>10,000/mm^3). WBC differential may show a left shift.

Urinalysis. May reveal a leukocytosis (>10 WBC/HPF).

Erythrocyte Sedimentation Rate (Westergren). May be elevated (>20).

Human Chorionic Gonadotrophin (hCG). Should be performed in the patient with potential ectopic pregnancy.

Radiology

Flat/Upright Abdominal Films. To evaluate for fecalith (rare) and to rule out other pathologies (e.g., free air, ileus).

Pelvic Ultrasound. Used to rule out tubo-ovarian process or evaluate for abscess or free fluid in the pelvis.

Abdominal or Pelvic Computed Tomography (CT) Scan. May reveal cecal inflammation, phlegmon, or abscess.

Other

Diagnostic Laparoscopy. Used if the diagnosis of appendicitis versus tubo-ovarian process is in doubt.

DIFFERENTIAL DIAGNOSIS

Traumatic.   Not applicable.

Infectious

Colitis.   May be due to a variety of organisms. The parasitic infection *Giardia* can mimic acute appendicitis. The patient may have a history of drinking contaminated water 1 to 2 weeks prior to presentation.

Urinary Tract Infection.   Usually presents with an elevated temperature ($>101°F$) and raised leukocytes in the urine, along with symptoms of urgency and dysuria.

Tubo-ovarian Infection.   Tenderness of the adnexa present on examination.

Metabolic

Acute Cholelithiasis.   May have elevated liver enzymes and a tender right upper quadrant on examination. Gallbladder ultrasound may reveal cholelithiasis or gallbladder edema.

Crohn's Disease.   Usually more insidious in presentation. May have a history of previous, less acute episodes.

Renal Calculi.   May have an elevated erythrocyte count on urinalysis. Calculi may be seen on radiograph. Intravenous pyelogram is positive.

Ectopic Pregnancy.   hCG positive.

Ruptured Diverticulum.   Free air may be seen on radiograph or CT.

Perforated Duodenal Ulcer.   May have positive occult blood on rectal examination and free air seen on radiograph or CT.

Neoplastic

Ovarian Cyst Rupture.   May be seen on pelvic ultrasound or be diagnosed with laparoscopy.

Vascular.   Not applicable.

Congenital.   Not applicable.

Acquired.   Not applicable.

TREATMENT

Medical.   Upon diagnosis, begin intravenous hydration with lactated Ringer's solution or 5% dextrose in normal saline and obtain surgical consultation for appendectomy. In the male patient, the diagnosis is usually more concise, because there are no ovarian pathologies to consider. In the female patient, laparoscopy may be considered to differentiate appendicitis from an ovarian disorder.

Surgical.   Under a general anesthetic, the laparoscope can be introduced and, if the diagnosis of acute appendicitis is confirmed, the appendix may be safely removed through the scope, thereby avoiding a larger incision. Likewise, if the diagnosis proves to be of a tubo-ovarian process (e.g., ectopic pregnancy or ovarian cyst), then appropriate treatment can be performed using the scope. If the patient is diabetic, on chronic steroid therapy, or immunocompromised, the incidence of postoperative abscess complication is higher with laparoscopic therapy. If the appendix has ruptured, then conversion to an open procedure should be undertaken.

The use of the laparoscope should be determined by the health status of the patient, along with the patient's size and history of previous surgeries. The laparoscopic experience of the surgeon should be taken into account.

Before any surgery, the patient should be given a broad-spectrum antibiotic such as a penicillin derivative or a second- or third-generation cephalosporin. Anaerobic coverage with an aminoglycoside or metronidazole should be used in those patients with suspected rupture.

If appendiceal abscess is discovered on CT scanning and the patient is stable, CT-guided drainage with adequate antibiotic coverage may be performed. If the patient remains stable, he or she may then be converted to an oral antibiotic and discharged. A semielective appendectomy may then be performed in 6 weeks without the added trauma of a large incision that will require the secondary healing of a packed, open wound.

TECHNIQUE OF SURGICAL ASSISTING

The PA assists with manipulation of the scope during laparoscopic procedures. With the open procedure, the assistant provides retraction, helps with opening, closing, and stapling or suturing of intra-abdominal contents, as indicated.

PEDIATRIC CONSIDERATIONS

Appendicitis is most commonly encountered between the ages of 15 to 30 years, but may be present in any age, including infancy. There is a relatively high incidence of perforation in children. Infants may present with signs and symptoms of peritonitis from a ruptured appendix. Presentation may be atypical (e.g., afebrile, normal WBC, umbilical pain, diarrhea). Chest x-ray and pulmonary examination are indicated, because referred pain from pneumonia can mimic appendicitis.

OBSTETRICAL CONSIDERATIONS

The location of the appendix changes with uterine expansion in the pregnant woman (e.g., right upper quadrant by 9 months). Symptoms of pain, nausea, or vomiting should not be casually discounted, because they may be due to the pregnancy or from intra-abdominal pathology. A normally elevated WBC in pregnancy may be confusing.

General concerns in operative intervention during pregnancy include avoidance of x-rays and teratogenic drugs; adequate oxygenation; fluid, electrolyte, and blood volume normalization; appropriate sedation (to minimize the risk of premature labor); gastric decompression; treatment of urinary retention; measures to reduce the risk of deep vein thrombosis (antiembolism stockings or pneumatic compression hose); rest; and avoidance of antibiotic prophylaxis as indicated.

PEARLS FOR THE PA

Appendicitis is the most common cause of acute abdominal pain in the young, healthy patient.

Leukocytosis may not always be present.

Bowel Ischemia
Thomas J. Schymanski, PA-C, and
James B. Labus, PA-C

DEFINITION

The term *ischemia* means to suppress or withhold blood flow. Bowel ischemia is that which pertains to an interrupted blood flow to the large or small intestines. It may be of a primary vascular cause (e.g., atherosclerosis, embolus, vasculitis) or secondary to mechanical lesions (e.g., volvulus). Sudden vascular occlusion produces an acute abdomen that requires rapid diagnosis and intervention to prevent the development of an infarct.

HISTORY

Symptoms. Weight loss is a common complaint with chronic ischemia. This is due to the fact that pain is increased after meals and eating is avoided. Vomiting, diarrhea, or "gut emptying" occur with vascular obstruction. The presence of melena suggests peritonitis and potential septic shock. These patients may be hypotensive and present with heart failure, shock, or vasoconstriction.

In vasculitis, the presenting manifestation is usually perforation with peritonitis or intraluminal bleeding.

With volvulus, patients present with colicky abdominal pain, usually with persistence of pain between spasms, abdominal distention, and vomiting. The patient with a sigmoid volvulus presents with progressive abdominal distention, anorexia, and constipation that has been present for several days. Cramping lower abdominal pain may or may not accompany the illness. With a cecal volvulus, the patient presents with a rapid onset of colicky or continuous abdominal pain in the mid- or right abdomen followed by nausea and vomiting, and distention with obstipation completes the clinical picture. The majority of patients may have a history of similar but milder attacks.

General. In patients with suspected primary vascular disease, obtain a history of systemic vascular disease such as coronary artery, cerebrovascular, or peripheral vascular disease. Determine the patient's eating habits. If pain is increased after meals (postprandial pain), the patient may avoid food or eat smaller meals. Pain will be relieved between meals, but the pain-free interval gradually decreases as ischemia worsens, leading to potential infarction.

With volvulus, the patient may have a history of previous episodes of abdominal distention that have been relieved by the passage of large amounts of flatus and stool after the administration of enemas.

Age. Vascular obstruction and mechanical lesions are usually encountered in the older age groups, although infants also may be affected.

Onset. May be acute with bowel infarction, or chronic with ischemia.

Duration. May be chronic with mild ischemia. Progressively worsens as ischemia increases.

Intensity. May be relatively insidious or life-threatening with sepsis, perforation, or shock.

Aggravating Factors. Pain is increased after eating meals with ischemic disease.

Alleviating Factors. Avoidance of food initially allows the patient to remain pain free.

Associated Factors. Peripheral vascular disease, coronary or cerebrovascular disease with vascular obstruction. With volvulus, the patient may reveal a history of chronic constipation and laxative abuse. Vasculitis may be caused by systemic disease such as polyarteritis nodosa, systemic lupus erythematosus, or rheumatoid arthritis.

PHYSICAL EXAMINATION

General. The patient may appear thin or cachectic with weight loss (the only consistent physical finding with intestinal vascular disease). Patients may present with septic shock when a segment of bowel has become gangrenous.

Cardiovascular. A full cardiac examination should be performed to rule out coexisting cardiac disease in patients with vascular obstruction, which may impact on the surgical decision and anesthetic management. Patients may have diminished peripheral pulses. Auscultation may reveal bruits of the carotid artery, abdominal aorta, or femoral arteries. An epigastric bruit may be heard in patients with celiac artery disease.

Gastrointestinal. With vascular disease, symptoms may be much worse than clinical findings suggest. Check for occult blood, which may or may not be present.

The characteristic findings with volvulus of the colon are massive abdominal distention and tympany with mild or absent tenderness. Bowel sounds vary from hypo- to hyperactive. Rectal examination reveals an empty vault or a rectum filled with liquid stool. With a cecal volvulus, abdominal distention, hyperperistalsis, and mild to moderate palpation tenderness over the distended loop may be present and may be found in any quadrant.

PATHOPHYSIOLOGY

The two main causes of bowel ischemia are vascular obstruction and hypotension. Most ischemic lesions are the result of these factors acting together. Vascular obstruction of large arteries usually is caused by atherosclerosis near the aorta with or without thrombosis or emboli. Complete obstruction of the artery is not necessary to produce ischemia. Arterial occlusion of one or two mesenteric arteries may not produce symptoms, because there is good collateral blood supply.

As the intestine contracts during peristalsis, blood flow decreases. When the vascular supply is compromised, this leads to ischemia and subsequent spasm. Symptoms of abdominal pain or cramping are due to intestinal spasm. Septic shock may occur, because ischemia allows infiltration of the intestinal mucosa by bacteria.

Venous compression is usually a result of external pressure from a volvulus or hernia or from internal pressure due to a thrombosis or infection. Disorders affecting mural vessels include vasculitis and intravascular coagulation.

Vasculitis is an inflammation of the small arteries that occurs in a variety of diseases. Vascular lesions result that may cause patchy infarction on the small intestine and which mimic arterial embolization.

Volvulus of the colon is defined as a twisting or rotation of a mobile segment of the colon about its mesentery. It involves either the sigmoid colon (most common) or the cecal region. Cecal volvulus involves not only the cecum but also the terminal ileum in rotation, so the symptoms also include those of a distal small bowel obstruction.

DIAGNOSTIC STUDIES

Laboratory
CBC. The leukocyte count may be normal or moderately elevated in cases without strangulation. When strangulation is present, the white count is usually elevated, often above 20,000 cells/mm^3 with a left shift.

Chemistry Profile. As a routine preoperative screen and to evaluate for electrolyte or other disorders.

Radiology
Plain Films of the Abdomen. Supine and upright films with volvulus show the characteristic bent inner tube or omega sign created by the markedly distended loop of sigmoid colon that arises from the pelvis and frequently fills most of the abdominal cavity. Upright examination is diagnostic in about 90% of cases of cecal volvulus. Findings include a

characteristically dilated cecum, usually with a single, large air–fluid level. Additional contributory findings include associated small bowel gas (indicating obstruction of the terminal ileum, especially if the small bowel gas is to the right of the cecum), indentation of the ileocecal valve on the right of the cecum, and an empty distal colon.

Ultrasound. Noninvasive examination used in evaluation of the intestinal vessels. May be limited due to the presence of gas.

Angiography. Used to establish the diagnosis of intestinal vascular disease.

Barium Enema. Can also be used only if sigmoidoscopy fails to confirm the diagnosis of volvulus. The characteristic "bird's beak" deformity is seen. Examination of the colon is pathognomonic of cecal volvulus (although rarely required).

CT Scan of the Abdomen. Is used to rule out other conditions that may cause similar symptoms (e.g., neoplastic disease).

Other

Endoscopy. May show superficial ulceration in the stomach or duodenum with ischemia.

Colonoscopy. Can be used to reduce a cecal volvulus. If the findings of colonic gangrene are present or the volvulus cannot be reduced, then emergent surgery is required.

Sigmoidoscopy. In volvulus, may reveal a characteristic twist or obstruction encountered by the release of large amounts of stool and flatus on advancement of the sigmoidoscope.

DIFFERENTIAL DIAGNOSIS

Traumatic

Head Injury. May lead to vasoconstriction and bowel ischemia. Treatment is aimed at the underlying cause.

Infectious

Sepsis. May lead to vasoconstriction and bowel ischemia. Treatment is aimed at the underlying cause.

Metabolic

Peptic Ulcer Disease. May cause similar symptoms. Differentiated on endoscopy; pain is usually relieved with meals rather than exacerbated.

Neoplastic

Gastric, Pancreatic, Intestinal Cancer. May present with weight loss and similar symptoms. Differentiated on CT of the abdomen, endoscopy, or barium studies.

Vascular

Cardiac Failure, Aortic Valve Insufficiency. May lead to vascular insufficiency of the bowel. Treatment is aimed at the underlying cause.

Acquired

Amphetamine Abuse. May cause arteritis; history of abuse.

Oral Contraceptive Use and Heavy Smoking. May cause vascular thrombosis.

TREATMENT

Medical. Colonoscopy may be used to reduce a cecal volvulus. Otherwise, surgery is required to prevent bowel infarction or to remove infarcted bowel to prevent sepsis.

Surgical. There are many different techniques employed in the treatment of intestinal vascular disease. The prognosis depends on the underlying pathologic process and the severity of peritoneal contamination.

Endarterectomy. Is an open procedure that removes atherosclerotic plaque from the lumen of the vessel. This procedure requires cross clamping of the aorta.

Embolectomy. May be performed with superior mesenteric artery occlusion in the attempt to save bowel from becoming infarcted. Postembolectomy, it is important to make sure that the tissue is viable before closing.

Bypass. Of diseased vessels via the supra- or infrarenal aorta or iliac artery to the visceral arteries using autologous or prosthetic grafts. Preferred over endarterectomy.

Arterial Reconstruction or Reimplantation. Of diseased vessels. Multiple reconstructions are favorable.

Bowel Resection. If the bowel has infarcted, the segment may be removed. Resection of the gangrenous loop and colostomy may be necessary with volvulus.

Indications. With vascular conditions, surgery is required for acute infarction, or for angiographically or ultrasonically apparent symptomatic ischemia to avoid infarction. Surgery is indicated for volvulus if signs of strangulation are present on sigmoidoscopy.

Contraindications. Inability of the patient to undergo anesthesia.

TECHNIQUE OF SURGICAL ASSISTING

The PA assists with opening, closing, reanastomosing of vessels or bowel, performing a colostomy, and retraction of abdominal contents. The assistant plays a role in the inspection and identification of ischemic areas following vascular procedures.

PEDIATRIC CONSIDERATIONS

Necrotizing enterocolitis may be caused by an infectious illness in the premature infant, infants given excessive fluids or feeding concentrations, and patients with patent ductus arteriosis. Surgery is usually required. Volvulus may occur in the pediatric patient. Diagnosis is made by plain abdominal x-ray with findings consistent with intestinal obstruction. Vomitus associated with bile is indicative of an obstruction.

OBSTETRICAL CONSIDERATIONS

General concerns in operative intervention during pregnancy include avoidance of x-rays and teratogenic drugs; adequate oxygenation; fluid, electrolyte, and blood volume normalization; appropriate sedation (to minimize the risk of premature labor); gastric decompression; treatment of urinary retention; measures to reduce the risk of deep vein thrombosis (antiembolism stockings or pneumatic compression hose); rest; and avoidance of antibiotic prophylaxis is indicated.

PEARLS FOR THE PA

Key symptoms of bowel ischemia include postprandial pain and weight loss.

Intestinal infarction may lead to sepsis, shock, and death.

Diagnosis is confirmed by angiography.

Mechanical lesions such as volvulus (twisting or rotation of a mobile segment of the colon) may lead to intestinal infarction.

Breast Carcinoma
Karen M. Potts, PA-C

DEFINITION

Malignancy originating in the ducts, lobules, or supporting stroma of the breast, including the nipple. May be confined to the epithelium of the ducts or lobules, without crossing the basement membrane (*in situ* carcinoma), or extend beyond the basement membrane into the surrounding stroma (invasive carcinoma), which is associated with tumor formation and systemic spread.

HISTORY

Symptoms.   Often asymptomatic. Lesions are found on routine mammography, palpable mass by the patient self-examination, or during routine physical examination. May have associated local skin changes with more advanced or aggressive involvement.

General.   The upper, outer quadrant is most frequently involved. Women are by far the more affected sex.

Age.   Women over age 50 years are at higher risk, although the disease has been documented in women as young as the teenage years.

Onset.   Insidious.

Duration.   Variable.

Intensity.   Variable, often depends on degree of involvement.

Aggravating Factors.   Not applicable.

Alleviating Factors.   Not applicable.

Associated Factors.   A family history of breast cancer, especially in a mother, daughter, or sibling, indicates a higher risk. Other risk factors may include early menarche and late menopause, nulliparity or late onset (after age 30 years) of pregnancy, and obesity. A diet high in fat may slightly increase the risk of breast cancer.

PHYSICAL EXAMINATION

General.   Patient is usually in no distress, although many are anxious.

Breast.   Careful examination may reveal a mass, with or without tenderness. Note any skin changes, such as retractions or erythema, and check for nipple discharge.

Cardiopulmonary.   Routine for potential surgical candidate. Auscultate for rales or rhonchi that may indicate fluid associated with metastasis.

Extremities.   Evaluate for upper extremity edema associated with lymphatic blockage.

Lymphatic.   Palpate the axillary, cervical, supraclavicular, inguinal, and epitrochlear nodes for evidence of metastasis.

Neurologic.   Evaluate for changes in strength or sensation associated with nervous system involvement with metastatic lesions.

PATHOPHYSIOLOGY

Ductal Carcinoma *In Situ* (DCIS) or Intraductal Carcinoma.   Originates in and is confined to the ducts of the breast, without invasion of the basement membrane, and has a more favorable prognosis. Although DCIS can cause enlargement of the ducts themselves, it does not usually produce a palpable mass. DCIS may or may not produce calcifications to be seen on mammography. Histological examination often reveals DCIS associated with invasive carcinoma.

Invasive or Infiltrating Ductal Carcinoma (IDC).   The most common type of tumor identified. Its origin is within the ducts, but the disease is no longer confined to the ducts, and has spread into the surrounding stroma. IDC usually presents as a mass by physical examination or as a density, with or without calcifications, by mammography.

Lobular Carcinoma *In Situ.*   Originates in the breast lobules, or acini, and has a more benign course. It can progress to invasive lobular carcinoma, forming a tumor, and is treated in much the same way as IDC, although it has a better prognosis.

Paget's Disease of the Nipple. A noninvasive or minimally invasive tumor on the undersurface of the nipple that usually presents with a crusting, scaling areola or nipple.

DIAGNOSTIC STUDIES

Laboratory
CBC, Electrolytes, PT, PTT. Used as preoperative screening studies and to evaluate for systemic conditions.
Liver Function Tests. May be elevated in liver or bone metastasis.
CA 15-3 Antigen. For following progress in treatment of metastatic lesions.
Radiology
Mammography. Recommended at yearly intervals starting at age 50 years, with routine screening starting earlier for patients at higher risk.
Ultrasonography of the Breast. Useful in differentiating cystic from solid lesions.
Ultrasound, CT of the Abdomen, Chest X-ray, Bone Scan. May be helpful in determining presence of metastatic lesions.
Other
Biopsy. Usually done in an outpatient setting. Needle-aspiration biopsy is performed if the mass is clinically palpable. Radiographically assisted core biopsy or excisional biopsy are used for lesions detected by mammogram. A nonpalpable lesion can be localized radiographically or by ultrasound prior to excisional biopsy.

DIFFERENTIAL DIAGNOSIS

Traumatic. Hematoma, scar tissue from previous trauma or surgery.
Infectious. Mastitis, infected cyst, or frank abscess.
Metabolic. Gynecomastia or fibrocystic, often affected by hormonal status.
Neoplastic. Not otherwise applicable.
Vascular. Not applicable.
Congenital. Fibrous tissue, fibroadenoma.
Acquired. Not applicable.

TREATMENT

Medical. Conservative therapy does not apply.
Surgical
Partial Mastectomy. Of the involved area with removal of a portion of surrounding healthy tissue (also called quadrant resection or lumpectomy).
Partial Mastectomy with Axillary Lymph Node Dissection. Essential for the evaluation of lymph nodes and the potential for metastasis.

Modified Radical Mastectomy. Removal of the breast in its entirety along with the axillary lymph nodes. Often necessary for larger lesions or when complete surgical excision with breast preservation is not feasible.

Additional Therapy. Includes chemotherapy or radiation therapy, with total treatment being tailored to the specific patient in conjunction with an oncologist. Reconstruction procedures can be performed after the mastectomy (see Plastic and Reconstructive Surgery).

Indications. Histologic confirmation should be made on any suspicious breast mass. The type of procedure used depends on the tumor type, spread, and (to some degree) patient preference.

Contraindications. Essentially none, but patients with bleeding dyscrasias, inability to tolerate anesthesia, and those with disseminated disease may require less aggressive procedures.

TECHNIQUE OF SURGICAL ASSISTING

Depending on the type of procedure, surgical assisting may include retraction, assistance with hemostasis, and resection. For less involved procedures, an assistant may not be required. Other important roles of the PA include (but are not limited to) preoperative evaluation and work-up, patient education and counseling about disease and surgical options, and postoperative management.

PEDIATRIC CONSIDERATIONS

Not applicable.

OBSTETRICAL CONSIDERATIONS

For the pregnant patient with a breast lump, biopsy may be chosen in order to confirm or rule out the presence of a breast cancer. If the biopsy is positive, the risks and benefits of treatment on the mother and fetus must be carefully weighed.

PEARLS FOR THE PA

A negative mammogram should NEVER delay biopsy of a clinically suspicious lesion.

The type of surgical treatment is ultimately the choice of a well-informed patient.

Cholecystitis
Karen M. Potts, PA-C

DEFINITION

Cholecystitis is a chemical or bacterial inflammation of the gallbladder. It may be acute or chronic, associated with gallstones (calculous—95%), or without gallstones (acalculias—5%). Cholecystitis is usually precipitated by an attack of biliary colic involving a stone that creates blockage of bile drainage.

HISTORY

Symptoms. Most prominent feature is pain in the epigastrium or right upper quadrant, often radiating around the right side to the right scapula or shoulder. Nausea and vomiting (60% to 70%), fever or chills may be present.

General. Many patients with gallstones are asymptomatic (20% to 40%). Often, patients with gallstones relate a history of epigastric fullness, flatulence, belching, and dyspepsia, especially after a fatty meal.

Age. Female to male ratio 3:1 under age 50 years, then nearly equal between males and females after age 50 years.

Onset. Often quite sudden, occurring especially after meals, with large meals or those high in fat content being more precipitous.

Duration. Biliary colic usually lasts for 1 to 4 hours, although a soreness in the right upper quadrant may persist for as long as 24 hours or more. Acute cholecystitis persists, with other systemic symptoms developing as well.

Intensity. May be severe.

Aggravating Factors. Large meal or high-fat meal.

Alleviating Factors. Time, in some instances, relieves acute symptoms but not the cause. Recurrent symptoms may be prevented for the short term with clear liquids and a low-fat diet.

Associated Factors. Obesity, high-calorie diet, diet high in polyunsaturated fats, oral contraceptives and estrogens, pregnancy, diabetes mellitus, chronic biliary tract infection, alcoholic cirrhosis, and some drugs. Complications of untreated cholecystitis include rupture of gallbladder and bile peritonitis, pancreatitis, sepsis, fistula, and death.

PHYSICAL EXAMINATION

General. Patient may be in distress due to severe pain. Temperature may be elevated (80%) due to inflammatory nature of the attack or to infectious process; 10% of patients have evidence of mild jaundice, which may be due to cholangitis, but choledocholithiasis must be ruled out.

Gastrointestinal. Auscultate for bowel sounds, which are usually present. Percuss for fullness in the right upper quadrant. Check for rebound tenderness and mass in the right upper quadrant. Check for Murphy's sign (pain in the right upper quadrant that intensifies with simultaneous palpation and deep inspiration).

Head, Eyes, Ears, Nose, and Throat (HEENT). Check for icterus associated with elevated serum bilirubin.

Skin. Observe for evidence of jaundice.

PATHOPHYSIOLOGY

Normal bile acids are synthesized from cholesterol in the liver and travel through interlobular and septal bile ducts into the right and left hepatic ducts, which join to form the common hepatic duct and, once united with the cystic duct, becomes the common bile duct. Due to the resistance of the sphincter of Oddi, bile refluxes upward through the cystic duct into the gallbladder, where it is stored until needed. The hormone cholecystokinin is largely responsible for triggering the dilatation of the sphincter and the contraction of the gallbladder in response to dietary intake. Gallstone formation is a concretion of normal and abnormal bile components, usually due to an increase in biliary secretion of cholesterol. There are three main types of gallstones: cholesterol, pigment, and mixed variety. The cholesterol and mixed types predominate. Gallstones may be present for long periods of time without significant problems; however, a stone may cause obstruction of the cystic duct or the junction of the cystic duct and gallbladder, causing severe pain upon contraction of the gallbladder. Secondary to the obstruction is the formation of gallbladder distention, irritation and erosion of the mucosal lining of the gallbladder, with subsequent inflammation, edema, and venous and lymphatic blockage. This is known as acute cholecystitis. Empyema and perforation may occur. The presence of a markedly distended gallbladder due to obstruction and without concomitant inflammatory reactions or sepsis is referred to as *hydrops* of the gallbladder. Chronic inflammation causes fibrosis of the gallbladder wall, mucosal thickening, and inflammatory cell changes.

DIAGNOSTIC STUDIES

Laboratory
CBC. WBC count may be elevated.
Bilirubin, Amylase, Alkaline Phosphatase and Liver Function Studies. To evaluate for possible choledocholithiasis.
Electrolytes. To evaluate for pancreatic involvement (glucose) or dehydration (creatinine).

Radiology

Gallbladder Ultrasound. Is recommended because it is noninvasive, highly sensitive to the imaging of stones, gallbladder and duct dilatation, and gallbladder wall thickening. It may also be used to evaluate the liver for abnormalities.

Abdominal X-ray. Is relatively unreliable in the diagnosis of gallstones, because most stones are not calcified. May show calcified stones, porcelain gallbladder, or emphysematous cholecystitis, as well as other findings associated with intra-abdominal abnormalities. Recommended as a cost-effective, first-line test if diagnosis is uncertain.

Oral Cholecystogram. Is also accurate (90% to 95%) in identifying stones, but it requires the ingestion of oral medication, which may not be tolerated by the patient.

Radioisotope Scans (e.g., HIDA). Are very useful in confirming suspected cholecystitis.

Other

Endoscopic Retrograde Cholangiopancreatography (ERCP). Is useful in removing stones from the common bile or cystic ducts.

Intraoperative Cholangiogram. An injection of radiopaque dye into the cystic duct; is of great benefit to establish the presence of stones within the cystic or common bile ducts, as well as confirming the anatomy of the ducts.

DIFFERENTIAL DIAGNOSIS

Traumatic. Not applicable.

Infectious

Viral Hepatitis. Positive hepatitis profile.

Metabolic

Acute Pancreatitis. Usually has an insidious onset, frequently associated with alcohol abuse, dull epigastric pain, often referred to the back, nausea, vomiting, and physical examination findings on palpation of the epigastric area. Laboratory findings of leukocytosis and elevated serum amylase and lipase.

Perforated or Penetrating Gastric or Duodenal Ulcer. Positive guaiac, visualized on endoscopy.

Acalculias Cholecystitis. No stones visualized.

Acute Appendicitis. Negative ERCP or oral cholecystogram (see topic Appendicitis).

Neoplastic

Hepatic Lesion. Seen on CT/MRI of the abdomen.

Vascular. Not applicable.

Congenital. Not applicable.

Acquired.

Drug-Induced Hepatitis. History of ingestion of hepatotoxic drug.

Other

Intestinal Obstruction. Obstruction may be suspected based on plain abdominal films.

TREATMENT

Medical. Gallstone dissolution with oral agents is available but is rapidly becoming obsolete with the improvement of laparoscopic surgical techniques. Overall, there is a long-term commitment to the use of oral agents (1 to 3 years) and low success rate in dissolving pigment stones, stones larger than 1.5 cm, or radiopaque or calcified stones. Gallstone lithotripsy has been performed as well, but the possibility of stones reforming is ever present. ERCP may be used to remove stones in choledocholithiasis.

Surgical. Cholecystectomy is the procedure of choice and should be performed in patients with cholecystitis unless the patient is clearly unstable for surgery. Cholecystectomy may be performed through an open incision or may be performed laparoscopically. It may be delayed until the acute episode of inflammation is over or may need to be done at the time of presentation to prevent complications associated with delayed treatment (perforated gallbladder, bile peritonitis, fistula, sepsis). The decision to delay surgical treatment should be based on the severity of the patient's condition and the degree of improvement during the period of hospital observation. The procedure involves decompression of the gallbladder, if needed, followed by careful dissection and identification of the cystic duct and cystic artery. Intraoperative cholangiogram is used if the anatomy is unclear. The cystic duct and artery are then ligated and divided and the gallbladder is dissected away from the undersurface of the liver, where it is attached by adhesions. The gallbladder and stones are then removed. The patient is given intravenous antibiotics, and postsurgical care is given based on the type of procedure performed.

For patients too unstable to undergo a formal surgical procedure, a cholecystostomy may be performed to insert a drainage tube into the gallblader percutaneously and provide temporary decompression until cholecystectomy can be performed.

Indications. Acute cholecystitis, with or without stones, or chronic, recurrent episodes of biliary colic due to stones.

Contraindications. Unstable condition due to other factors, such as cardiac, severe pulmonary problems, or hemodynamics. Every effort should be made to correct any underlying problem in order to make the patient stable for surgery, and care should be aggressive postsurgically for the prevention of complications associated with underlying problems.

TECHNIQUE OF SURGICAL ASSISTING

With open procedures, the PA assists with opening, closing, and retraction for visualization of the gallbladder, cystic duct, and cystic artery. For laparoscopic procedures, the PA assists with manipulation of the scope and closing.

PEDIATRIC CONSIDERATIONS

A history of hemolytic disorders (e.g., sickle cell anemia) should be obtained, because the incidence of cholelithiasis is increased in this patient population. Other systemic disorders, such as typhoid or scarlet fever, measles, or obstruction, are associated with cholecystitis without stones. In the pregnant or obese adolescent or teen, there is increased risk of gallstones. Treatment is by cholecystectomy.

OBSTETRICAL CONSIDERATIONS

Symptoms suggesting cholecystitis should not be discounted as being due to the pregnancy. Symptoms and work-up are the same, with the use of x-rays only when necessary.

General concerns in operative intervention during pregnancy include avoidance of x-rays and teratogenic drugs; adequate oxygenation; fluid, electrolyte, and blood volume normalization; appropriate sedation (to minimize the risk of premature labor); gastric decompression; treatment of urinary retention; measures to reduce the risk of deep vein thrombosis (antiembolism stockings or pneumatic compression hose); rest; and avoidance of antibiotic prophylaxis as indicated.

PEARLS FOR THE PA

The classic symptom of cholecystitis is pain in the epigastrium or right upper quadrant, often radiating around the right side to the right scapula or shoulder, usually following a meal high in fat content.

Murphy's sign is pain in the right upper quadrant that intensifies with simultaneous palpation and deep inspiration.

Cholecystectomy can be performed through a laparoscopic approach.

Esophageal Disorders
Thomas J. Schymanski, PA-C

DEFINITION

Surgical disease of the esophagus consists of motility disorders (achalasia [failure of the lower esophageal sphincter to open] and gastroesophageal reflux [GER]), obstructive conditions (esophageal stricture, neoplasm, webs, and rings), tears, and hernia.

HISTORY

Symptoms
Motility Disorders. Progressive dysphagia, heartburn, regurgitation, noncardiac chest pain, or weight loss.

Obstructive Conditions. With benign esophageal stricture, symptoms of heartburn may initially be present but lessen as solid food dysphagia worsens due to the progression of the stricture. Neoplasms present with progressive dysphagia, initially to solid foods, then to liquids as the lesion expands. Esophageal web presents with symptoms of dysphagia. Esophageal rings present with dysphagia for solids that is often intermittent, especially if the narrowest point of the esophagus measures between 1.2 cm and 2.0 cm.

Tears. Esophageal tears are seen most commonly after vomiting (75% of cases), straining, and coughing. A mucosal tear (Mallory-Weiss syndrome) produces a significant hematemesis after an initial, nonbloody vomitus.

Hernia. Chest pain, upper gastrointestinal bleeding, dysphagia, and ischemia.

General. Obtain a history of what foods or liquids the patient has difficulty swallowing, the presence of halitosis or heartburn, odynophagia (discomfort with swallowing), coughing after attempts at swallowing, progressive or intermittent nature of the dysphagia, accidental ingestion of toxins, and current medications (e.g., antacids). Chest pain may be the presenting feature, and a detailed history, physical examination, and diagnostic studies are performed as indicated to rule out a primary cardiac source.

Age. Any, but more common early and late in life.

Onset. Usually slow and insidious. If rapid onset, suspect neoplasm. The sudden onset of odynophagia suggests trauma, infection, or foreign body reaction. Noncardiac chest pain is usually sudden.

Duration. Progressive, although noncardiac chest pain, odynophagia, and hematemesis may be intermittent. Rapidly progressive dysphagia suggests the presence of a neoplasm.

Intensity. Varies from mild symptoms to severe dysphagia.

Aggravating Factors. Ingestion of solid, acidic, or spicy foods or hot or cold liquids; tight fitting clothes or neckwear; recumbent position; obesity; and smoking.

Alleviating Factors. Appropriate identification and treatment. Dysphagia, hematemesis, and noncardiac chest pain are relatively resistant to nonmedical intervention.

Associated Factors. Nasal speech, dysarthria, hoarseness, sore throat, aspiration, and pneumonia. Esophageal neoplasms are associated with alcohol abuse and smoking. Dysphagia may be a symptom of a systemic connective tissue disorder. Esophageal webs may be associated with iron deficiency anemia in Plummer-Vinson syndrome. Esophageal tears are associated with alcohol abuse and post-binge drinking.

PHYSICAL EXAMINATION

General. The patient may appear in no acute distress, or have overt signs of dysphagia such as the inability to swallow secretions. The patient may present with hemorrhagic shock due to blood loss from hematemesis. The patient may have a nasal quality to speech, hoarseness, or dysarthria.

Cardiovascular. A full and complete evaluation is warranted to rule out primary cardiac disease in any patient presenting with chest pain.

Gastrointestinal. Palpate for tenderness of the epigastric region. Perform a rectal examination and perform guaiac testing for occult blood. A mediastinal mass may be felt with an incarcerated paraesophageal hernia.

Head, Eyes, Ears, Nose, and Throat (HEENT). Examine the teeth for enamel loss. Halitosis may be present. Evaluate the nasopharynx for lesions, burns, and tonsillar hypertrophy. Palpate the neck for adenopathy.

Neurologic. Perform a complete evaluation, with attention to the cranial nerves to evaluate for a neurogenic source.

Pulmonary. Auscultate for signs of aspiration. Rales or rhonchi may be heard.

PATHOPHYSIOLOGY

The esophagus is adjacent to the trachea, left pulmonary bronchus, aortic arch, descending aorta, and left atrium. Due to the location and lack of serosa, the esophagus is difficult to manipulate, remove, replace, and reconstruct. Unlike the intestine, there is nothing to spare.

Motility Disorders. There is no clearly defined cause for achalasia, although heredity or infection are suspected. The disorder is due to a loss or diminution of myenteric neurons. GER is due to incompetence of saliva, gastric acid, and pepsin production, inadequate peristalsis or lower esophageal sphincter tone, or delay in gastric emptying.

Obstructive Conditions. Benign esophageal stricture and rings may be a sequelae of prolonged reflux esophagitis. Squamous cell carcinoma (66%) and adenocarcinoma (33%) are the most common esophageal neoplasms. Esophageal web is an obstructive condition seen in the upper third of the esophagus that may be due to failure of complete embryonic recanalization. Esophageal rings most commonly occur at the squamocolumnar junction and are called Schatzki's rings. Both rings and webs are comprised of mucosa and, if long standing, contain muscle tissue.

Tears. A rupture of the esophagus (Boerhaave's syndrome) usually occurs above the esophagogastric junction.

Hernia. Unlike the much more common and clinically insignificant hiatal hernia, a paraesophageal hernia may lead to gastric vascular compromise. The esophagogastric junction is noted to traverse the diaphragm in the appropriate location. The body of the stomach then travels above the diaphragm, and gastric volvulus with incarceration may occur.

DIAGNOSTIC STUDIES

Laboratory
CBC. Decreased hemoglobin and hematocrit associated with hemorrhage.
Serum Electrolytes. May be abnormal with dehydration or systemic conditions.
Liver Function Profile. To rule out hepatic disease.
Radiology
Bolus Barium Swallow. For diagnosis of benign esophageal stricture.
Chest X-ray. Air in the left mediastinal region suggests an esophageal tear and immediate surgical intervention is necessary for any chance of survival. Also used to evaluate for primary chest pathology.
Other
Endoscopy. Performed emergently with esophageal burns to assess the extent of the damage. Benign esophageal stricture can be visualized.
Esophageal Manometry. Used to measure esophageal sphincter and peristaltic pressure. Useful in motility disorders.
Electrocardiogram (ECG). To rule out myocardial infarction.

DIFFERENTIAL DIAGNOSIS

Traumatic
Esophageal Injury. History of trauma; may have associated laryngeal or cervical spine injury.
Esophageal Burns. The ingestion of cardiac agents (e.g., strong alkali or acid) can cause serious esophageal injury. Esophageal burns that occur after ingestion of lye or detergents (e.g., chlorine bleach) are a common suicidal gesture in adults and a common accident in children.
Costochondritis. May cause chest pain. Chest wall palpation reveals tenderness.
Infectious
Herpes Zoster. Usually encountered in immunosuppressed patients. Herpetic eruption may be seen on the lips. Odynophagia and dysphagia may be presenting symptoms.
Oral and Pharyngeal Infections. Such as tonsillitis, tuberculosis, abscess, diphtheria, etc., may cause dysphagia. Lesions or infections may be visualized on physical examination. WBC may be elevated; viral titers as indicated may be positive.
Metabolic
Nutcracker Esophagus. A nonsurgical esophageal motility condition associated with high-amplitude peristaltic contractions. Frequently presents with noncardiac chest pain. Differentiated on manometry.

Esophageal Spasm. An uncommon motility disorder. Differentiated on barium swallow, endoscopy, and motility studies.

Conditions Affecting the Muscular System. Such as scleroderma, myasthenia gravis, amyloidosis, etc., may present with swallowing disorders.

Cholelithiasis. May have elevated liver enzymes and a tender right upper quadrant on examination. Gallbladder ultrasound may reveal cholelithiasis or edema.

Ruptured Diverticulum. Free air may be seen on radiograph or CT.

Peptic Ulcer Disease. Identified on endoscopy of the stomach and duodenum.

Neoplastic

Other Esophageal Neoplasms. Such as metastatic lesions, lymphoma, melanoma, leiomyoma, or fibroadenoma, may be seen on endoscopy or radiographic studies. Biopsy is performed to differentiate from primary esophageal lesion.

Vascular

Angina Pectoris. Pain may be referred upward into the neck, shoulders, or arms. Differentiated by ECG and cardiac isoenzymes.

Pericardial Tamponade/Mitral Valve Prolapse/Aortic Dissection/Hypertensive Crisis/Pulmonary Hypertension. All may cause chest pain that may mimic esophageal disease. Physical examination and appropriate diagnostic studies differentiate from esophageal disease.

Congenital

Esophageal Atresia. Symptoms are present at birth and include persistent drooling, coughing, gagging, or aspiration pneumonia.

Tracheal Esophageal Fistula. Presentation is dramatic with achalasia, reflux, gagging, choking.

Pathologic Acid GER. Presents with recurrent pneumonia, nocturnal apnea, night cough, and may cause sudden infant death syndrome (SIDS).

Acquired

Esophageal Foreign Body. Visualized on endoscopy, physical examination, or other radiographic studies.

Cervical Disc Disease. Anterior disc herniations or postoperative swelling may cause dysphagia. Differentiated on MRI or plain film of the cervical spine, respectively.

Exposure to Toxins. Such as arsenic, lead, tetanus, *Clostridium botulinum,* or mercury, may result in difficulty in swallowing.

Other

Psychogenic. Conditions such as depression, anxiety, or panic disorders may present with esophageal symptoms or a feeling of a lump in the throat (globus hystericus). A negative work-up and a thorough psychosocial history may reveal the cause.

Neurologic Disease. Any condition (e.g., stroke, multiple sclerosis) that affects the brainstem or cranial nerves V, VII, IX, X, XI, and XII may result in swallowing problems.

TREATMENT

Medical

Motility Disorders.   Achalasia initially may be treated with calcium channel blockers (e.g., nifedipine) in an attempt to reduce the tone of the smooth muscle. For GER, initial therapy involves reducing aggravating factors such as smoking, avoidance of certain foods, weight reduction, no lying down after meals, and head elevation while sleeping. Medications such as antacids, H_2 blockers, metoclopramide or bethanechol, or omeprazole may reduce symptoms.

Obstructive Conditions.   Neoplasms must be histologically identified as being malignant or benign. If lesions are metastatic or nonresectable, irradiation or chemotherapy are given as indicated, depending on the histological type. Attention is given to the patient's nutritional requirements. Parenteral nutrition or a gastric tube may be required temporarily or permanently, depending on esophageal patency. Benign esophageal stricture may initially be treated with calcium channel blockers (e.g., nifedipine). For esophageal webs, iron is administered if there is associated anemia.

Tears.   There may be significant blood loss with an esophageal tear. Vital signs are stabilized and transfusions are given as indicated.

Paraesophageal Hernia.   Symptomatic treatment for small defects and uncomplicated conditions.

Surgical

Motility Disorders.   If medical therapy is unsuccessful for achalasia, pneumatic (balloon) dilatation is performed to open the lower esophageal sphincter. This procedure may be repeated; if subsequent attempts are unsuccessful, surgery may be required. The Heller myotomy procedure is performed to open the lower esophageal sphincter by creating an incision at the gastroesophageal junction. A fundoplication or Nissen procedure is performed for GER only if symptoms are debilitating, if erosive esophagitis develops, and if medical treatment has failed.

Obstructive Conditions.   Esophageal stricture, rings, and webs are generally treated with a tapered bougienage or with pneumatic (balloon) dilatation. If this treatment is unsuccessful for esophageal rings, surgical rupture of the rings may be required. This is generally coupled with repair of a hiatal hernia as indicated.

Benign neoplasms may be resected or, if causing significant dysphagia, may be treated with tapered bougienage or with pneumatic (balloon) dilatation. Malignant tumors are surgically resected or vaporized with an endoscopic laser. This may be followed by esophageal stent placement.

Tears.   Minor tears tend to spontaneously resolve. Surgery is required in less than 10% of cases. The tear may be repaired endoscopically or via open approach, as indicated.

Paraesophageal Hernia.   Surgery may be required for refractory pain, upper gastrointestinal bleeding, or large defects. Immediate surgical intervention is required for ischemic or incarcerated hernias.

Indications. For motility disorders, surgery may be indicated if medical therapy is unsuccessful. For symptomatic obstruction, dilatation procedures are usually indicated. For neoplasms, biopsy is required for diagnosis and subsequent surgery, performed depending on the type of lesion and resectability. Continued bleeding from tears requires intervention. For hernias, surgery is performed urgently if ischemia is present.

Contraindications. Inadequate medical trial for motility disorders.

TECHNIQUE OF SURGICAL ASSISTING

The PA assists with manipulation of the scope during endoscopic procedures. With the open procedure, the assistant provides retraction, helps with opening, closing, and suturing of esophageal or intra-abdominal contents, as indicated.

PEDIATRIC CONSIDERATIONS

Infants presenting with gagging, coughing, choking, wheezing, or with recurrent aspiration pneumonia should be evaluated for esophageal disease. Pathologic acid GER must be suspected in children with recurrent pneumonia, nocturnal apnea, and night cough, because this has been associated with sudden infant death syndrome (SIDS).

Tracheoesophageal fistula, with or without esophageal atresia, is considered a surgical emergency once diagnosed.

OBSTETRICAL CONSIDERATIONS

General concerns in operative intervention during pregnancy include avoidance of x-rays and teratogenic drugs; adequate oxygenation; fluid,

---

PEARLS FOR THE PA

Dysphagia is aggravated by ingestion of solid, acidic, or spicy foods or hot or cold liquids; tight-fitting clothes or neckwear; recumbent position; obesity, and smoking.

Physical examination may be normal in uncomplicated disease.

Rapidly progressive dysphagia or weight loss indicates neoplastic or complicated disease.

Always rule out cardiac disease in patients complaining of chest pain.

electrolyte, and blood volume normalization; appropriate sedation (to minimize the risk of premature labor); gastric decompression; treatment of urinary retention; measures to reduce the risk of deep vein thrombosis (antiembolism stockings or pneumatic compression hose); rest; and avoidance of antibiotic prophylaxis as indicated.

Fistulas

Clyde Bullion, PA-C, BSN, RN

DEFINITION

Sinus tracts that lead from the anorectum (or hollow organ) to the perineal area or skin. *Fistula* is Latin for pipe or reed.

HISTORY

Symptoms. Many patients first present with pain and swelling. If an anal abscess has formed, resulting in pain and occasionally fever, the area is swollen, and only gradually begins to open and drain.

General. A thorough history of gastrointestinal symptoms and prior anal abscesses or fistulas is highly suggestive. There are a number of other colorectal problems that must be distinguished from fistulas (e.g., suppurative hidradenitis and pilonidal cysts).

Age. Most patients present between 30 and 50 years of age, and occurrence is very uncommon after 60 years. Most are males.

Onset. Sudden. Usually begins after an abscess drains spontaneously or is drained in the office.

Duration. Indefinite. Fistulas remain until treated.

Intensity. Many cases present with severe pain, then gradually decrease to dull or no pain. Drainage and recurrent abscesss with pain become the standard over time.

Aggravating Factors. Poor hygiene may cause many of the initial abscesses, leading to a sinus tract. Diet, fissures, infections following surgery for hemorrhoids or on the sphincter muscle may also aggravate symptoms.

Alleviating Factors. Good personal hygiene.

Associated Factors. Diabetes, anal intercourse, and hypertension have been noticed as concurrent conditions in many of those with fistulas.

PHYSICAL EXAMINATION

General. An exit site, or hole, may be noted around the anus. This may be filled with fecal material. Using hydrogen peroxide to flush it out, while having an anoscope in the rectum, allows for visualization of the internal entrance site, but should be reserved for the specialist.

Rectal. Place the patient in the left lateral position, right knee to chest, left leg straight. Examine the area around the anus first. A good light assists greatly. If an external site is found, insert a finger into the anus and palpate for the tract, swelling, and an entrance. If not palpable, insert an anoscope and either insert a malleable probe very gently (never force it) to track the sinus, or try using hydrogen peroxide to flush through the site.

PATHOPHYSIOLOGY

Currently, it is believed that an infection in an anal gland leads to an anal fistula. The gland develops an abscess, which may either resolve or begin draining into the anal canal. If no opening occurs, the infection tends to travel along the points of least resistance, along the intersphincteric plane, until reaching the skin of the perineum. At this point, it can open and drain, or form a larger, painful abscess. Sinus tracts may go in all directions, double back on themselves (horseshoe shape), or lead into multiple branches, some of which may not lead out to the skin.

DIAGNOSTIC STUDIES

Laboratory
CBC. To check for signs of infection.
Gram Stain and Acid-Fast Stain for Actinomyces. Are helpful for diagnosis and appropriate treatment.
Radiology
Barium Enema. To evaluate for ulcerative colitis.
Other
PPD. To check for tuberculosis.

DIFFERENTIAL DIAGNOSIS

Traumatic
Rape, Intercourse, Falling on Sharp Objects. Can be elicited in the history.
Infectious
Actinomycosis. Gram positive. Commonly seen with pelvic infections and use of intrauterine devices.
Bartholin's Cyst. May be chronically infected, leading to a sinus tract.
Hydradenitis. May be seen as multiple fistulas. Care is the same.
Pilonidal Cyst. If it occurs near the anus, it may be mistaken for a fistula.
Sexually Transmitted Diseases. Occur from rape or intercourse. If this

is suspected, cultures should be performed and laboratory tests for HIV, hepatitis, syphilis, and *Chlamydia* should be done. A viral culture for herpes simplex is also indicated.

Tuberculosis.   Rare now. Most often seen in East Indian population.

Metabolic.   Not applicable.

Neoplastic

Perirectal Dermoid Cyst.   After opening/excision, may develop sinus.

Rectal Cancer.   Should always be considered, because it can develop in an established fistula or create a fistula. Seen with barium enema and endoscopy.

Sacrococcygeal Teratoma.   May form sinus after drainage.

Vascular.   Not applicable.

Congenital

Congenital Fistula Tracts.   Present at birth or in infancy. Treatment is the same.

Acquired

Crohn's Disease.   May occur, usually several at a time. Usually few symptoms, and patient is known to have Crohn's.

Ulcerative Colitis.   Does not often occur, but may ulcerate through to perineum. Patient has had long history of GI complaints.

TREATMENT

Medical.   Medical treatment is generally ineffective, and if a perirectal abscess is suspected, the patient should be referred for incision and drainage. Antibiotics may be employed initially to treat the abscess. Culture and sensitivity should guide therapy. Diet and personal hygiene should be stressed. High-fiber, low-fat diets promote rapid transit times and decrease the amount of stool remaining in the colon. Washing after defecation may help.

Bulk-Forming/Stool-Softening Agents
- Citrucel powder: 1 tablespoon 1 to 3 times per day in 8 oz water
- Colace capsule: 50 mg; 1 to 6 capsules per day
- Effer-Syllium powder: 1 teaspoon 1 to 3 times per day in 8 oz water
- Fiberall: 1 chewable tablet 1 to 4 times per day with 8 oz water
- Fibercon: 2 to 4 tablets 1 to 4 times per day with 8 oz water
- Maalox powder: 1 teaspoon up to 3 times per day in 8 oz water
- Maltsupex: 4 tablets 4 times per day
- Metamucil: 1 teaspoon 1 to 3 times per day in 8 oz water, followed by 8 oz water
- Mitrolan: 3 chewable tablets 4 times per day, up to 12 per 24 hours
- Modane: 1 teaspoon 1 to 3 times per day in 8 oz water
- Mylanta fiber: 1 tablespoon in 8 oz water, 1 to 3 times per day
- Perdiem fiber powder: 1 to 2 teaspoons swallowed with 8 oz cool fluid in the evening and before breakfast
- Serutan: 1 teaspoon in 8 oz water, 1 to 3 times per day
- Syllact: 1 teaspoon in 8 oz water, 1 to 3 times per day

Anti-Inflammatory Creams/Ointments
- Americaine ointment: apply up to 6 times per day
- Anusol-HC 1: apply 3 to 4 times per day
- Corticaine 0.5%: apply 3 to 4 times per day
- Preparation H (hydrocortisone) 1% cream: apply 3 to 4 times per day
- Proctofoam 1%: apply with tissue up to 5 times per day

Mineral oil preparations should not be used, because of difficulty keeping the area clean and irritation to rectum. Suppositories should not be used because of pain and increasing tears and spasms.

Surgical

Fistulotomy. A probe is placed through the sinus tract, pulled to tense the tissue, and then cut open to release the probe and expose the tract. This is allowed to heal as is.

Fistulectomy. The opening is elevated with an instrument, and the entire tract is followed and completely excised. Depending on the direction of the fistula path, the remaining tissue may be used as a flap to cover the excision site, or cut open to heal.

Seton. Depending on the type of fistula and any underlying diseases, a seton suture, either cutting or noncutting, is placed through the tract and tied tightly to itself. As the tissue heals, it pushes the seton suture up and out, over time pulling entirely through the skin and leaving only scar tissue behind.

Indications. All fistulas that do not heal rapidly or that recur.

Contraindications. High-risk patients unable to withstand anesthesia.

TECHNIQUE OF SURGICAL ASSISTING

Use an enema to cleanse the lower bowel for the procedure. Identification of each tract is essential, so exposure is essential.

PEDIATRIC CONSIDERATIONS

Some infants are born with fistulas. Treatment is the same in pediatrics. Most heal rapidly after surgery.

OBSTETRICAL CONSIDERATIONS

The largest consideration is the choice of anesthesia. Regional anesthesia is preferred in fistulectomies. Patient comfort in positioning is important, because visualization is the key to success with these procedures.

PEARLS FOR THE PA

Get a thorough history, consider all of the differentials, and refer quickly.

Mineral oil preparations and suppositories should be avoided.

Gastric Carcinoma
Karen M. Potts, PA-C

DEFINITION

Carcinoma of the stomach may involve any aspect of the stomach, but especially the pyloric and antral regions. There are several types, but the main classification includes a diffuse type and an intestinal type. Diffuse tumors are more widely spread, decrease the distensibility of the stomach wall due to its invasive nature, and have a poorer prognosis. Intestinal tumors are associated with a prolonged precancerous process (such as ulceration), and more commonly involve the antrum and lesser curvature.

HISTORY

Symptoms.   Usually nonspecific or absent in the early stage. May have weakness, anorexia, weight loss, and/or fatigue. Gastrointestinal symptoms include indigestion, postprandial fullness, loss of appetite, heartburn, vomiting, and/or dyspepsia. Pain may be intermittent with lesions, especially of an ulcerative nature, and may present like benign peptic ulcer disease. Metastatic or associated symptoms include peritonitis from perforating lesion, hematemesis from bleeding lesion, abdominal swelling with ascites from hepatic or peritoneal metastasis, dyspnea from pulmonary metastasis and plural effusion, weakness of chronic anemia in slowly bleeding lesions, or continuous pain from extension of tumor to intra-abdominal organs.

General.   Symptoms may be related to fullness of the stomach from tumor enlargement, decreased motility due to large area of invasion of the wall of the stomach, or extension of the tumor to other organs outside the stomach. Higher incidence in Japan, Chile, Colombia, China, and Ireland.

Age.   Higher in males than females; incidence increases with age.

Onset.   Initially insidious, then progressively worsening symptoms.

Duration.   Variable.

Intensity.   Variable.

Aggravating Factors. In certain instances, meals can initiate symptoms such as postprandial fullness, vomiting, indigestion, heartburn.

Alleviating Factors. Food or antacids may initially alleviate pain associated with ulcerative lesions, similar to peptic ulcer disease.

Associated Factors. Incidence increases with lower socioeconomic groups. Pernicious anemia may increase risk, but is not proven. Adenomatous polyps may be the precursor in certain tumors. Chronic atrophic gastritis, any chronic hypo- or achlorhydric state, or Ménétrier's disease may increase risk. Dietary factors such as starch; pickled vegetables; salted, dried, or smoked foods high in nitrates or which can be converted to nitrites by bacteria increase the risk. Previous gastric surgery may increase incidence by two to six times.

PHYSICAL EXAMINATION

General. Check for evidence of weight loss, chronic illness.

Extremities. Evaluate for lymph node enlargement—supraclavicular (Virchow's sentinel node), inguinal, axillary, etc.

Gastrointestinal. Bowel sounds are usually present unless an acute process (e.g., peritonitis) is associated with perforation. Palpate and percuss for epigastric mass or fullness, hepatomegaly or ascites associated with metastasis. Examine umbilicus for evidence of infiltration (Sister Mary Joseph node). Palpate for Krukenberg's tumor (metastasis to the ovary).

Genitourinary. Usually unremarkable unless there are metastases.

Pulmonary. Auscultate and percuss for mass, pleural effusion associated with metastasis. Otherwise, routine preoperative evaluation.

PATHOPHYSIOLOGY

Ninety percent of gastric cancer is of the adenocarcinoma variety. The other 10% includes non-Hodgkin's lymphoma and leiomyosarcoma. Adenocarcinoma develops from mucosal cells in the stomach. The most common areas are the pyloric and antral regions. The tumors can take on many different characteristics and can include multiple characteristics within the same tumor. There are several different classification systems of gastric tumors based on predominant component, basic structure, and biological behavior. Tumor cells can spread diffusely and infiltrate the wall of the stomach, causing decreased distensibility of the stomach. Expanding tumors take a more nodular form, and can cause obstructing symptoms, especially if located in the pyloric region.

DIAGNOSTIC STUDIES

Laboratory

CBC. To evaluate for anemia.

Liver Function Tests. Abnormal with metastases.

Serum Pepsinogen I Levels, Gastric Secretory Studies, Carcinoembry-onic Antigen (CEA), Fetal Sulfoglycoprotein Antigens. As serological screening measures if cancer is suspected.

Guaiac. Check stool for occult blood that may suggest cancer.

Radiology

Barium Upper GI Radiograph. With double contrast, helps identify polypoid masses, ulcerative lesions, and nondistendible stomach.

CT Scan of the Abdomen. Is performed to look for nodal involvement, liver metastasis, extragastric extension.

Other

Endoscopic Ultrasound. Is used to identify tumor infiltration and lymph node involvement.

Gastroscopy. Performed by experienced endoscopist; is the procedure of choice for diagnosis. Allows direct visualization of the stomach. Multiple biopsies can be obtained, as can brushings and irrigation aspirate for cytologic evaluation.

DIFFERENTIAL DIAGNOSIS

Traumatic. Not applicable.

Infectious

Gastroenteritis. Usually a transient course and related to a noxious agent (e.g., food poisoning).

Metabolic

Benign Peptic Ulcer Disease. Ulcer visualized on endoscopy; resolves with appropriate treatment.

Hypertrophic Gastropathy. Visualized on endoscopy.

Neoplastic

Benign Gastric Polyp. Visualized on endoscopy; differentiated histologically.

Adenomatous Polyp. Visualized on endoscopy; differentiated histologically.

Vascular. Not applicable.

Congenital. Not applicable.

Acquired. Not applicable.

TREATMENT

Medical. Except for adjuvant chemotherapy, not applicable for gastric cancer.

Surgical. Surgical resection is the only chance for cure in the treatment of gastric carcinoma.

Exploratory Laparotomy. Is beneficial to examine the stomach, regional lymph nodes, and evaluate for evidence of extragastric extension and metastasis.

Subtotal Gastrectomy. Is indicated in distal lesions, which are the most common. This involves resecting the greater and lesser omenta, the duodenum distal to the pylorus, and the stomach at the lesser curvature adjacent to the esophogogastric junction and the greater curvature at the vasa brevia. A gastroduodenostomy (Billroth I) or a gastrojejunostomy (Billroth II) is performed to reconnect the stomach to the intestine.

Total Gastrectomy. Is indicated if the carcinoma is the remaining section following previous subtotal resection, or if the cancer is diffuse or in the proximal portion of the stomach, with a Roux-en-Y esophagojejunostomy to help prevent bile reflux.

Palliative Procedures. Can be performed for tumors that have evidence of distant metastasis and obstruction.

Indications. Gastric carcinoma by biopsy, or radiographic or clinical suspicion.

Contraindications. Obvious and histologically proven distant metastasis without obstructive symptoms.

TECHNIQUE OF SURGICAL ASSISTING

The PA assists with opening, closing, reanastomosis, retraction for visualization, hemostasis, and excision of the stomach.

PEDIATRIC CONSIDERATIONS

Rare in children.

OBSTETRICAL CONSIDERATIONS

Do not discount symptoms as being due to the pregnancy. General concerns in operative intervention during pregnancy include avoidance of x-rays and teratogenic drugs; adequate oxygenation; fluid, electrolyte, and blood volume normalization; appropriate sedation (to minimize the risk of premature labor); gastric decompression; treatment of urinary retention;

PEARLS FOR THE PA

The patient is usually asymptomatic in the early stages.

Food or antacids may initially alleviate pain associated with ulcerative lesions, similar to peptic ulcer disease.

Surgical resection is the only chance for cure in the treatment of gastric carcinoma.

measures to reduce the risk of deep vein thrombosis (antiembolism stockings or pneumatic compression hose); rest; and avoidance of antibiotic prophylaxis as indicated.

Hemorrhoids
Clyde Bullion, PA-C, BSN, RN

DEFINITION

Varicosed veins of the anus. Classified anatomically as internal or external. Internal hemorrhoids form from the superficial superior hemorrhoid veins above the dentate line (mucocutaneous juncture), whereas the external hemorrhoids arise from the inferior hemorrhoidal veins, distal to the dentate line. Internal hemorrhoidal veins lie under the rectal mucosa, which is poorly innervated, and therefore are less likely to have associated pain. Inferior hemorrhoidal veins lie in external anal skin, are innervated by somatic nerves, and thus are more apt to respond to stimuli with pain.

HISTORY

Symptoms. Bleeding is most common and the earliest symptom most patients note. Pruritus, feelings of discomfort or dull pain with straining or defecation, an obvious mass or edema, discharge, underwear soiling and other hygiene problems may be present. Severe or sharp pain (other than with strangulated hemorrhoids) should suggest another diagnosis.

General. Although the history is helpful, many other conditions are commonly called hemorrhoids, and often turn out to be something different. A complete GI history is essential, including length of time on toilet, fluid intake, and stool caliber, color, and consistency. Hemorrhoids tend to occur more frequently in whites than blacks, and in those with a higher socioeconomic situation.

Age. Occur mostly in adults, more often 50 years of age or older, and pregnant females of any age.

Onset. Gradual. Most patients note either bleeding, pain, or protrusion, and come in with a complaint of a flare-up of symptoms.

Duration. Bleeding may occur only with defecation and be minimal. Protrusion can occur with straining and defecation, and can reduce spontaneously or with finger pressure. All of the symptoms last until treated, whether medically or surgically, except pruritus. This is a separate problem and is not resolved by treating the hemorrhoids.

Intensity. Varies from minimal spotting to heavy bleeding with each bowel movement. Protrusion can be minor and reducible, or painful and irreducible.

Aggravating Factors. Any of the following can cause or exacerbate hemorrhoids: diet, anatomy, drugs, constipation or diarrhea, straining, vomiting, coughing, infection, pregnancy, hormonal change, and heavy exercise.

Alleviating Factors. High-fiber diet, adequate water intake, and short length of time on toilet.

Associated Factors. There may be a familial component, diet, personal occupation, environment, climate, depression and other emotional conflict, and possibly decreased mentation in the elderly.

PHYSICAL EXAMINATION

General. Hemorrhoids are classified by grades.

First Degree. Symptomatic, usually bleeding; when straining, no hemorrhoidal tissue protrudes past the dentate line.

Second Degree. Symptomatic; when straining, hemorrhoid appears distal to the dentate line. When straining is stopped, the pile returns above the dentate line.

Third Degree. Same as second degree, but the hemorrhoid needs to be pushed up after straining or a bowel movement.

Fourth Degree. Same as third degree that remains distal to dentate line, and protrudes back out after manipulation, without straining or a bowel movement.

Rectal. Have patient lie in left lateral position, holding right buttock apart from left. Inspect the external area for skin tags, protruding piles, or fistulas. Next, insert anoscope and check in all four quadrants for hemorrhoids, signs of active bleeding, fissures, or fistulas. After identifying the cause, if apparent, examine the prostate in males and, if there are no signs of active bleeding, a stool guaiac may be indicated.

PATHOPHYSIOLOGY

During a bowel movement, vascular cushions formed from a direct artery-to-vein connection fill and empty rapidly. By straining, the hemorrhoid complexes fill with blood but cannot empty. This causes an enlargement of the area and a protrusion of the cushion, or pile. When exposed to air, the high pressures in the arteries cause bright red bleeding. Over time, these get larger and often become symptomatic.

DIAGNOSTIC STUDIES

Laboratory

CBC. Is useful to identify anemia if the patient has a history of a high level of blood loss.

Carcinoembryonic Antigen (CEA). May be quite useful if there is a concern of colon cancer.

Radiology
Barium Enema (BE).   Is helpful to outline the rectum and colon if a diagnosis other than, or in addition to, hemorrhoids is suspected.
Other
Anoscopy.   Necessary to identify the presence of internal hemorrhoids.
Endoscopy.   The sigmoidoscope may demonstrate rectal ulcers, polyps, or even lesions that are cancerous and is useful for all patients with rectal bleeding. Anal pressures can be measured in the GI laboratory before trying anal dilatation. Otherwise, this is rarely used.

DIFFERENTIAL DIAGNOSIS

Traumatic
Rape, Intercourse.   Positive history.
Infectious
Abscess.   May be missed because history is same, but patient is too tender to examine.
Herpes Simplex.   Painful, with small amounts of blood. Usually has prodromal pain 1 to 3 days before lesion occurs. If suspected, also suspect HIV. Herpes simplex virus culture should be done.
AIDS.   May present with symptoms of hemorrhoids, history of anal sex, frequent symptoms and possibly infections. Should always be considered.
Leukemia.   Excessive bleeding tendencies occur with this disease, and thrombosed hemorrhoids can lead to prolonged bleeding. The GI system is one of the three common sites for bleeding that leads to death.
Tuberculosis.   May present with bleeding. An ulceration may be found on examination, which may appear to be similar to a fissure, but fails to heal with normal therapy. It progresses to several ulcers, the edges appear to be undermined, and eventually destroys the sphincter muscle. Sigmoidoscopy, PPD, and cultures are required for diagnosis.
Metabolic.   Not applicable.
Neoplastic
Colorectal Tumors.   Are usually painless. Seen on flexible sigmoidoscopy, colonoscopy, barium enema, transrectal ultrasound, CT, or MRI.
Lymphoma.   May present as an ulcerated mass. Digital examination and direct visualization are the keys to differentiating.
Vascular.   Not applicable.
Congenital.   Not applicable.
Acquired
Anal Fissures and Fistulas.   May present with same history. Visualization is the key.
Crohn's Disease.   Diarrhea and rectal bleeding. If patient has persistent hemorrhoids, he or she should be evaluated for Crohn's.
Pruritus Ani.   A patient complains of itching. Although hemorrhoids may be noted and treated, the pruritus does not resolve.
Ulcerative Colitis.   Commonly presents with constipation and rectal

bleeding, but may have diarrhea as well. Recurrence may be the best key to diagnosis. On examination, fissure rather than hemorrhoid is most often found.

TREATMENT

Medical. First begin with stool softening, bulk-forming, and high-fiber agents; increase the oral water intake; careful personal hygiene; and possibly suppositories for rectal lubrication. If this fails, sclerotherapy with 5% phenol in almond oil, injected directly into each pile, is helpful. This may be repeated once a week for 2 weeks, then about 1 month later, with good results.

Rubber band ligation of internal hemorrhoids can be done in the office by using a special instrument to grasp and place two rubber bands around the pile. If pain or discomfort occurs, the rubber bands must be removed and placed higher on the hemorrhoid. After about 8 to 10 days, the hemorrhoid resolves, leaving a raw spot that heals quickly. Two other office procedures, cryosurgery and infrared coagulation, are being studied with varying results.

Bulk-Forming/Stool-Softening Agents
- Citrucel powder: 1 tablespoon 1 to 3 times per day in 8 oz water
- Colace capsule: 50 mg; 1 to 6 capsules per day
- Effer-Syllium powder: 1 teaspoon 1 to 3 times per day in 8 oz water
- Fiberall: 1 chewable tablet 1 to 4 times per day with 8 oz water
- Fibercon: 2 to 4 tablets 1 to 4 times per day with 8 oz water
- Maalox powder: 1 teaspoon up to 3 times per day in 8 oz water
- Maltsupex: 4 tablets 4 times per day
- Metamucil: 1 teaspoon 1 to 3 times per day in 8 oz water, followed by 8 oz water
- Mitrolan: 3 chewable tablets 4 times per day, up to 12 per 24 hours
- Modane: 1 teaspoon 1 to 3 times per day in 8 oz water
- Mylanta fiber: 1 tablespoon in 8 oz water, 1 to 3 times per day
- Perdiem fiber powder: 1 to 2 teaspoons swallowed with 8 oz cool fluid in the evening and before breakfast
- Serutan: 1 teaspoon in 8 oz water, 1 to 3 times per day
- Syllact: 1 teaspoon in 8 oz water, 1 to 3 times per day

Anti-Inflammatory Creams/Ointments
- Americaine ointment: apply up to 6 times per day
- Anusol-HC 1: apply 3 to 4 times per day
- Corticaine 0.5%: apply 3 to 4 times per day
- Preparation H (hydrocortisone) 1% cream: apply 3 to 4 times per day
- Proctofoam 1%: apply with tissue up to 5 times per day

Mineral oil preparations shoud not be used, because of difficulty keeping the area clean and irritation to rectum. Suppositories should not be used because of pain and increasing tears and spasms.

Surgical

Closed Hemorrhoidectomy. Used for mixed internal and external hemorrhoids. May be done under local with sedation or regional anesthesia, in the left lateral position, or in a jackknife position. A V-shaped incision is made over the external hemorrhoids, so they can be dissected off the external sphincter. Then, the internal hemorrhoids are dissected off the internal sphincter. The tissue left is clamped, excised, and sewn, each quadrant necessitating a different incision.

Indications. Third- and fourth-degree hemorrhoids, and piles not responsive to medical management.

Contraindications. Inflammatory bowel disease, Crohn's disease; any patient with bleeding disorders such as leukemia or lymphoma; and patients who may be at risk for any operation (e.g., severe coronary artery disease).

TECHNIQUE OF SURGICAL ASSISTING

Exposure is the most important aspect of this case. The Hill-Ferguson retractor makes the operation much easier.

PEDIATRIC CONSIDERATIONS

None.

OBSTETRICAL CONSIDERATIONS

Under local anesthesia, this operation has proven to be safe and effective in all three trimesters. Only the symptomatic hemorrhoids are removed.

PEARLS FOR THE PA

Do everything medically possible before sending off for a surgical consult.

It takes very little for the PA to learn how to rubberband ligate hemorrhoids in the family practice setting. Find a local specialist to teach you.

Rectal bleeding with hemorrhoids, a fissure, or fistula may come from another source. Always consider cancer.

Hyperparathyroidism (Primary)
James W. Becker, PA-C

DEFINITION
Increased amount of parathyroid hormone, either from a single enlarged parathyroid gland or from multiple hyperplastic parathyroid glands, resulting in a condition of hypercalcemia.

HISTORY
Symptoms. Most patients have minimal symptoms.

Mild Hypercalcemic Syndrome. Vague reports of abdominal pain, bone pain, mental disorientation, mood swings, and general fatigue are often seen. Frequently, patients deny any symptoms until the hypercalcemia is corrected; and then, after recovery, report an overall improvement of their feeling of well-being. After several years of persistent hypercalcemia, complications including osteoporosis with multiple fractures and repeated bouts of renal calculi may occur.

Acute Hypercalcemic Crisis. Is a medical emergency. Serum calcium levels greater than 15 mg/dl (normal, 8 to 10 mg/dl), can result in a patient with severe muscle weakness, dehydration, tachycardia, various cardiac arrhythmias, oliguria, coma, and sudden death. Persistent calcium levels in that range may also lead to serious episodes of pancreatitis.

General. In the past, hyperparathyroidism was investigated only after the development of the complications of this disease. However, with the increased usage of screening laboratory evaluation and routine physical examinations and health fairs, asymptomatic patients with hypercalcemia are being detected and treated. Think of primary hyperparathyroidism in the patient who keeps returning to the hospital with fractures following minimal trauma. Determine if the patient is taking exogenous calcium supplements or diuretics.

Age. Usually found after the third decade; more common in females.

Onset. Gradual, with the exception of acute hypercalcemic crisis (rare).

Duration. Until corrected.

Intensity. The patient may have very mild symptoms, or the condition may be life-threatening with acute hypercalcemic crisis (rare).

Aggravating Factors. Use of thiazide medications, calcium supplements, high vitamin D supplements.

Alleviating Factors. None.

Associated Factors. Look for evidence of multiple endocrine neoplasm (MEN) syndromes either in the form of pheochromocytoma, islet cell tumors of the pancreas, thyroid cancers, or pituitary adenomas. Other studies suggest an increase in the incidence of peptic ulcer disease and pancreatitis with hyperparathyroid patients.

PHYSICAL EXAMINATION

General.   The patient usually appears quite healthy. Check vital signs for corresponding fever, hypertension, or tachycardia.

Extremities.   Evaluate for evidence of old or new fractures.

HEENT.   Normally, the parathyroid glands are soft and nonpalpable, even when five to ten times the normal size.

Neurologic.   For preoperative screening, check for a positive Chvostek sign. This is elicited by briskly tapping on the facial nerve root as it exits in front of the ear. A positive sign is when it triggers a twitch of the upper, ipsilateral lip and is found in about 10% of the population with a normal calcium level. This sign becomes more evident in the hypocalcemic patient, especially as the calcium level drops below 7 mg/dl. Therefore, it is important to identify those individuals with a positive Chvostek sign without hypocalcemia so as not to be misled during postoperative management.

PATHOPHYSIOLOGY

The anatomy of parathyroid glands can be quite variable. Although most patients have four glands, there have been cases reported of only three being detected or as many as five glands detected. The normal parathyroid gland is about the size of a pea and has an orange/yellow color. They have a soft consistency and are usually found dangling from their slender blood supply. Normally located two on each side of the thyroid, they can also be found down within the mediastinum and sometimes within the lobe of the thyroid itself. Primary hypercalcemia can be brought about by three separate causes. The first and rarest is parathyroid carcinoma, with an incidence of less than 1%. A single gland benign adenoma accounts for about 80% of cases, and multiple gland hyperplasia makes up the remaining 20%.

DIAGNOSTIC STUDIES

Laboratory

Serum Calcium.   The initial screening test and indicator of potential primary hyperparathyroidism. If the serum calcium is elevated, the patient should be interviewed to determine if there are any external factors that could be contributing. Patients who have been taking high doses of calcium supplements may elevate their serum calcium level. Patients on diuretic therapy may also have an elevated value.

Serum Albumin.   Serum calcium is bound to albumin, so that the patient with a low albumin level and normal calcium level may actually be hypercalcemic if adjustments are made for the low albumin.

Serum Parathyroid (normal 0 to 40 µl Eq/ml). Performed if repeat calcium levels are consistently elevated. When plotted along with serum calcium levels, a nomograph can be created to indicate a positive association diagnostic of primary hyperparathyroidism. If parathyroid hormone levels are consistently normal, other diagnostic tests should be performed to elicit the cause (see Differential Diagnosis).

Radiology

Sestamibi Scan. A nuclear medicine scan that visualizes the parathyroid glands and reveal areas of increased parathyroid activity (Fig. 4–1). Thyroid cancer may also be detected. This scan is highly recommended for any patient who has had prior neck surgery or has other existing medical problems that would be potential risks for prolonged anesthetic.

Selective Angiogram. For localization and imaging of the parathyroid glands. Largely supplanted by the Sestamibi scan.

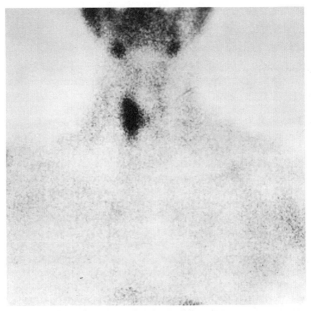

Figure 4–1. Sestamibi scan revealing increased uptake of isotope in the right inferior parathyroid gland, consistent with a parathyroid adenoma. (Courtesy of Andrew Jacoby, CNMT, Director of Nuclear Medicine, Northside Hospital, Atlanta, GA.)

Other
Selective Thyroid Venous Sampling. Invasive; used in sampling for excessive parathyroid hormone concentration. Largely supplanted by the Sestamibi scan.

DIFFERENTIAL DIAGNOSIS

Traumatic
Trauma Patient with Multiple Fractures. May exhibit hypercalcemia but have normal parathyroid levels.
Infectious. Not applicable.
Metabolic
Multiple Endocrine Neoplasia. May be associated with hyperparathyroidism with associated pheochromocytoma, islet cell tumors of the pancreas, thyroid cancers, or pituitary adenomas.
Neoplastic
Extensive Malignant Disease. Hypercalcemia may be evident.
Vascular. Not applicable.
Congenital. Not applicable.
Acquired
Excessive Calcium Intake. Hypercalcemia evident; history of taking calcium supplements.
Diuretic Therapy. Hypercalcemia present due to electrolyte imbalance.

TREATMENT

Medical. In the patient with acute hypercalcemic crisis, the initial therapy is medical while the search for the cause begins. Those patients with calcium levels approaching 15 mg/dl should be hospitalized in a telemetry setting. All calcium supplements should be discontinued. The primary goal is to enhance calcium secretion by hydration and diuresis. Hydration is provided by using normal saline at rates of 5 to 10 liters every 24 hours and diuretic therapy of furosemide (Lasix) 100 mg IV every 2 hours. If hydration and diuresis are required, central venous pressure (CVP) monitoring is indicated with frequent laboratory evaluation and potassium supplementation as needed. If this regimen is not successful, dialysis can be used.

Surgical. Neck exploration is carried out under adequate general anesthesia. Initially, all of the parathyroid glands should be identified and examined closely. If a single parathyroid gland is found to be enlarged and the remaining glands are normal in appearance, then the adenoma is removed and pathological examination by frozen sectioning is performed. If this confirms the presence of an adenoma, then the remaining glands are inspected again prior to closure of the neck. If there is any evidence of imminent ischemia of any of the remaining glands, it should be harvested and reimplanted (see complications).

In the patient with parathyroid hyperplasia, three glands are excised and sent for pathological examination by frozen section. The remaining gland is examined to ensure survivability. Frequently, in order to guarantee that some parathyroid tissue will continue to function, a segment of the remaining gland is sectioned off and reimplanted in the neck. In those patients who may be a difficult surgical risk or have had numerous neck explorations in the past, the parathyroid segments can be reimplanted into other parts of the body. Traditionally, the muscle of the nondominant forearm has been used. In the event that the patient continues to have persistent hypercalcemia, the implanted tissue in the arm can easily be removed without requiring a general anesthetic and additional neck exploration.

For the extremely rare patient with parathyroid cancer, the malignant gland is removed, along with any associated lymph nodes.

Complications. There are two major risks for parathyroid surgery; laryngeal nerve injury and permanent hypoparathyroidism. Upon initial neck exploration, the laryngeal nerves must be identified. If this is a repeat neck exploration, that task may be difficult. Care must be taken to identify any structure before it is ligated. In the event of unilateral nerve trauma, the nerve can be repaired using 7-0 prolene suture, although the patient will have significant hoarseness that may not fully recover. In the event that both nerves are injured, the surgical team should be prepared to perform a tracheostomy if true vocal cord paralysis has occurred.

In the event that all of the existing parathyroid tissue is removed, the patient becomes permanently hypoparathyroid; therefore, every effort must be taken to preserve some viable parathyroid tissue. When a parathyroid gland is becoming ischemic, it is removed and placed on a cold surface (prepared by placing frozen slush or frozen IV fluids in a sterile bowl and inverting another sterile bowl on top of the frozen material to create a workspace) and sectioned into pieces approximately 2 to 3 mm in size. These pieces are then reimplanted into the muscle beds of the sternocleidomastoid muscle of the neck or the muscle bed of any donor site outside of the neck. In patients with parathyroid hyperplasia, these segments of gland can be marked with small surgical clips so that in the event that the patient needs further tissue removed, they can be identified again.

In cases where the cause of the hyperparathyroidism is not found after a thorough neck exploration, a search for the pathology outside the neck must be done. If a Sestamibi scan was not performed initially, it should be ordered and, if necessary, a repeat surgical exploration, including mediastinal exploration, is required.

In all patients with hyperparathyroidism, be prepared to treat for sudden hypoparathyroidism postoperatively. Serial calcium levels need to be monitored and the development of paraesthesia, especially around the face and mouth, may indicate low serum calcium levels. If the patient did not have a Chvostek sign prior to surgery and exhibits one postoperatively, then the serum calcium level needs to be rechecked. It may require 4 to 6 weeks for any reimplanted parathyroid segments to begin producing hormone again.

As with any neck exploration, observe for the development of any hematomas that may cause airway restriction and require evacuation and control of bleeding. Tracheostomies, because of airway restriction due to hematoma formation, should never be required.

Indications. Patients with elevated serum parathyroid, positive Sestamibi scan, or other diagnostic evidence of a parathyroid adenoma may require surgical exploration. After medical stabilization, the patient presenting with acute hypercalcemic crisis may require surgical exploration.

Contraindications. Surgery may be deferred and the patient medically managed if there are significant medical conditions that would prohibit the use of anesthesia, such as bleeding dyscrasias.

TECHNIQUE OF SURGICAL ASSISTING

The role of the assistant in this form of neck exploration is primarily to aid in the identification of all required structures. The point of observation of the assistant can be crucial to visualizing different areas of the anatomy that are not within the field of the surgeon's view. Frequently, the keen assistant will note the location of the laryngeal nerve or parathyroid gland. Adequate exposure of the underside of the thyroid is essential for the discovery of many parathyroid adenomas. The preparation of any parathyroid gland for reimplantation is also an important role of the assistant.

PEDIATRIC CONSIDERATIONS

Children with adrenocortical insufficiency may have an associated autoimmune hypoparathyroidism. Patients with DiGeorge's syndrome may have a congenital absence of the parathyroids associated with absence of the thymus, cardiovascular, cerebral, and ocular defects.

OBSTETRICAL CONSIDERATIONS

Transient newborn hypoparathyroidism may be due to fetal asphyxia, maternal diabetes mellitus, or maternal hyperparathyroidism.

PEARLS FOR THE PA

Think primary hyperparathyroidism with any patient who presents with elevated calcium on screening blood work.

Screen patients for a Chvostek sign prior to surgery.

Liver Tumors
Karen M. Potts, PA-C

DEFINITION

Carcinoma arising in the hepatocytes (hepatocellular carcinoma) of the liver (80% to 90% of liver malignancies), or in the bile duct cells (cholangio-carcinoma), or a combination. Many other, much less common tumors are documented as well. Because of its vascularity and physiologic functions, the liver is frequently a site of metastasis from bronchogenic, colon, pancreas, breast, and stomach cancers, among many others.

HISTORY

Symptoms. Variable. Patients usually present with a combination of weakness, malaise, and weight loss. May have vague or upper abdominal pain or discomfort with or without radiation to the shoulder. In more advanced disease, the patient may have dyspnea, asthenia, pruritus, and may have underlying chronic liver disease and associated symptoms.

General. Fatal if untreated. Patients often have underlying liver disease such as cirrhosis that may complicate or delay diagnosis. Incidence much higher and occurs much earlier in Africa and Asia.

Age. Males are four times more likely to be affected than females; peaks at fifth and sixth decades in western countries.

Onset. May be quite rapid, or unrecognized if associated with chronic underlying liver disease.

Duration. Often rapid course (3 to 6 months).

Intensity. Variable, depends on degree and location of involvement.

Aggravating Factors. Progressive.

Alleviating Factors. None.

Associated Factors. Any chronic liver disease, especially hepatitis B virus and chronic alcoholic cirrhosis. Many lesser associated causes, such as smoking, oral contraceptives, exposure to vinyl chloride or organochloride pesticides, androgens and anabolic steroids and parasitic infection.

PHYSICAL EXAMINATION

General. May show signs of chronic illness or underlying liver disease.
Extremities. Check for muscle wasting, peripheral edema.
Gastrointestinal. Inspect the abdomen for tortuous vasculature associated with collateral circulation. Auscultate for friction rub or arterial bruit over the liver. Percuss for liver border and spleen, and ascites. Palpate for hepatomegaly, masses, and tenderness.
HEENT. Examine the sclera for icterus.
Neurologic. Test for asterixis (flapping), rigidity, hyperreflexia. Mental status examination for changes associated with hepatic encephalopathy (late finding with severe destruction of the liver).
Pulmonary. Auscultate for rales or rhonchi associated with metastasis; percuss for dullness, suggesting metastatic lesions.
Skin. Look for jaundice, spider angiomas, and bruising.

PATHOPHYSIOLOGY

The liver is divided into the right and left lobe, with the left lobe divided into medial and lateral segments separated by the falciform ligament. The main lobes are further divided into segments based on bile duct and hepatic vessel distribution. Blood supply is from the hepatic artery and the portal vein. Biliary fluid drains from the liver into the hepatic duct, then common bile duct, with retrograde flow into the gallbladder, which is located on the visceral surface of the liver.

Hepatic carcinoma may develop in the hepatocytes, the bile ducts, or a combination. There are multiple types, with varying degrees of prognosis. Liver tumors most commonly metastasize to the lung. Multiple sites of carcinoma can metastasize to the liver. Hepatic adenomas are benign lesions, but can transform into malignant lesions in some patients. Most hepatic carcinoma is precipitated by chronic insult to the liver, especially with the hepatitis B virus and alcoholic cirrhosis.

DIAGNOSTIC STUDIES

Laboratory
CBC. To evaluate for anemia.
Alpha Fetoprotein (AFP), Alkaline Phosphatase. Will be abnormal with hepatic involvement.
Radiology
Ultrasound of the Liver. Used for screening and identifying tumor location.
Abdominal CT Scan. Performed to identify tumor location and distant metastasis.
Hepatic Arteriography. To determine tumor location, vascularization, major arterial pattern.

Other
Intraoperative Ultrasonography. For tumor location and to rule out diffuse hepatic involvement.

DIFFERENTIAL DIAGNOSIS

Traumatic
Hematoma or Hemoperitoneum. History of trauma that causes discomfort.
Infectious
Parasitic Abscess. Mass lesion may be present on radiographic studies. Differentiated on biopsy.
Hepatitis. Positive hepatitis profile, negative radiographic studies.
Metabolic
Focal Nodular Hyperplasia, Nodular Regenerative Hyperplasia. Biopsy to differentiate if necessary.
Neoplastic
Hepatic Adenoma. Biopsy to differentiate if necessary.
Cystic Lesion. Biopsy to differentiate if necessary.
Other Solid Benign Tumors. Biopsy to differentiate if necessary.
Vascular
Cavernous Hemangioma. Diagnosis can be made from CT scan. Biopsy of vascular hemangiomas can cause significant bleeding and should be avoided if possible or performed under controlled conditions.
Congenital. Not applicable.
Acquired
Alcoholic Cirrhosis. History of alcohol abuse, abnormal liver function studies, negative radiographic studies for lesion.
Drug-Induced Hepatitis. History of ingestion of hepatotoxic drug, negative radiographic studies for lesion.

TREATMENT

Medical. Intra-arterial chemotherapy, hepatic artery ligation, arterial embolization, targeting chemotherapy or radiation therapy, direct tumor injection, and implantable pump for direct hepatic artery infusion of chemotherapeutic agents are all used in the management of hepatic cancer. Some may be used as adjuvant therapy to surgery.
Surgical. Surgical resection remains the treatment of choice when possible.
Lobectomy. Resection of an entire lobe of the liver.
Segmentectomy. Resection of a segment of the liver.
Wedge Resection. Resection of portion of liver with tumor involvement, without formal lobectomy or segmentectomy. The use of the CUSA, a special surgical instrument used to dissect through the liver parenchyma

while leaving the vessels intact, has made wedge resections, multiple resections, and medial left lobe resections much more common and safer.

Indications. Hepatic tumor or tumors present without total liver involvement or distant metastasis.

Contraindications. Total hepatic involvement, distant metastasis, advanced cirrhosis.

TECHNIQUE OF SURGICAL ASSISTING

The PA assists with opening, closing, and retraction of intra-abdominal contents. Careful attention must be paid to hemostasis when assisting with a procedure on this vascular organ.

PEDIATRIC CONSIDERATIONS

Hepatic cancer is one of the most common malignancies encountered in the newborn patient. The incidence peaks in the first year of life and again in adolescence. Physical findings include a firm, nontender liver mass, failure to thrive, and fever. Jaundice is rare and its absence should not be used to rule out liver disease.

OBSTETRICAL CONSIDERATIONS

General concerns in operative intervention during pregnancy include avoidance of x-rays and teratogenic drugs; adequate oxygenation; fluid, electrolyte, and blood volume normalization; appropriate sedation (to minimize the risk of premature labor); gastric decompression; treatment of urinary retention; measures to reduce the risk of deep vein thrombosis (antiembolism stockings or pneumatic compression hose); rest; and avoidance of antibiotic prophylaxis as indicated.

PEARLS FOR THE PA

The liver is a frequent site of metastases from other primary sources.

Liver tumors most commonly metastasize to the lung.

Most hepatic carcinoma is precipitated by chronic insult to the liver, especially with the hepatitis B virus and alcoholic cirrhosis.

Jaundice is rarely seen in the pediatric patient.

Pancreatic Cancer

James W. Becker, PA-C

DEFINITION

Surgery performed on the pancreas either for cancer, pseudocyst, or insulinoma. Unfortunately, the majority of surgical cases are for pancreatic cancer and the prognosis is frequently poor.

HISTORY

Symptoms. Patient typically presents with an insidious onset of painless jaundice and weight loss. Some patients may initially report only weight loss and back pain, with jaundice developing at a later time.

General. Painless jaundice, instead of the painful biliary colic of choledocholithiasis, usually indicates an obstructive neoplasm of the bile duct, ampulla, or pancreas.

Age. Most frequently noted in the fifth and sixth decades.

Onset. Retrospectively, patients may report noting gradual weight loss and vague symptoms of malaise or back discomfort over several weeks or months.

Intensity. The pain is usually mild to moderate and radiating into the back.

Aggravating Factors. None.

Alleviating Factors. None.

Associated Factors. As with many cases of obstructing jaundice, the patient commonly has intense pruritus. This may also be the presenting symptom at which time the patient is found to be jaundiced.

PHYSICAL EXAMINATION

General. The patient may appear quite healthy in early cases, or cachectic and jaundiced when the disease is advanced.

Gastrointestinal. If the patient is thin, the gallbladder may be visibly distended. A palpable, nontender, distended gallbladder in a jaundiced patient suggests a neoplastic obstruction of the common bile duct (Courvoisier's law). An epigastric fullness or mass may be palpable. Palpable liver mass may be noted in advanced metastatic cases.

HEENT. Facial muscle wasting may be noted. Scleral icterus usually presents if the total bilirubin is greater than 3 mg/dl.

PATHOPHYSIOLOGY

The pancreas is both an exocrine and an endocrine organ. The exocrine function is to produce the enzymes that break down proteins and lipids. The islet cells of the endocrine pancreas produce insulin and glucagon.

DIAGNOSTIC STUDIES

Laboratory
Chemistry Profile. Elevated liver enzymes, especially alkaline phosphatase and GGTP, indicate probable obstruction. The transaminases (SGOT and SGPT) may also be elevated. Total bilirubin increases as obstruction occurs, with clinical jaundice becoming evident. Total bilirubin is frequently over 10 mg/dl at time of diagnosis.

CA 19-9. This relatively new tumor marker is frequently elevated with pancreatic cancer.

Radiology. Unfortunately, most radiographic studies fail to diagnose early pancreatic cancer.

Ultrasound and Abdominal CT Scan. Confirms the presence of dilated bile ducts. Sometimes a pancreatic mass is identified and possible CT-guided biopsy makes the diagnosis. In advanced cases, evidence of metastatic disease may be seen in surrounding lymph nodes and the liver.

Endoscopic Retrograde Cholangiopancreatography (ERCP). Is indicated with evidence of a dilated common bile duct without obvious cholelithiasis. This examination may indicate the source of the obstruction and biopsy-proven evidence obtained.

Mesenteric Arteriogram. Obtained in the patient with suspected pancreatic cancer who appears to be a candidate for curative surgery. This allows examination of the arterial supply and portal venous drainage of the surgical site. Tumor encasement of any of these vessels would make surgical removal unlikely and a less invasive course of therapy may be considered.

DIFFERENTIAL DIAGNOSIS

Traumatic. Not applicable.
Infectious. Not applicable.
Metabolic
Chronic Pancreatitis. With or without the formation of pancreatic pseudocyst, may present with similar weight loss and discomfort of pancreatic neoplasm. Radiographic studies of the pancreas in this situation would also be more difficult to interpret.

Choledocholithiasis. May present with elevated liver enzymes and jaundice, but usually is associated with biliary colic and should be excluded by radiographic studies.

Vascular. Not applicable.

Congenital. Not applicable.
Acquired. Not applicable.

TREATMENT

Medical. Essentially none, as the lesion will need at least a biopsy for histological confirmation.

Surgical. Surgical treatment for pancreatic cancer includes palliative procedures for biopsy-proven cases that cannot be resected either due to evidence of metastatic disease or massive bulk tumor involvement of the superior mesenteric vessels or portal vein (may not be evident until surgical exploration takes place). In these cases, the pancreatic cancer is functionally bypassed by creating a choledochojejunostomy (or similar anastomosis using the gallbladder or duodenum) to relieve the bile duct obstruction and a gastrojejunostomy to prevent small bowel obstruction as the tumor enlarges. Some advanced disease patients can avoid surgery if a biliary stent can be placed during ERCP, thereby relieving the bile duct. Life expectancy for pancreatic cancer patients with metastatic disease is frequently less than 1 year. Postbypass patients are treated with external beam radiation, and cases of a longer period of quality function have been reported. Some centers have also considered resection of the primary tumor after completion of radiation and are reporting favorable outcomes.

In the pancreatic cancer patient who presents with a small tumor in the head of the gland and has no evidence of metastatic disease, primary resection is performed. A pancreaticoduodenectomy (Whipple) is the most complicated general surgical procedure that can be performed. The resection includes the antrum of the stomach, the entire duodenum, head of the pancreas, segment of the common bile duct, and the gallbladder. There are variations on the reconstruction of these structures, but essentially the pancreas is anastomosed to the jejunum, as is the common bile duct and the stomach. Upon initial surgical exploration, any evidence of metastatic disease must be ruled out because involvement of the liver or lymph nodes would mean that a surgical cure is not possible and the patient should not be subjected to a complicated procedure.

Indications. For histological confirmation, palliative, or for attempts at complete resection.

Contraindications. Essentially none, because the lesion will need at least a biopsy for histological confirmation.

TECHNIQUE OF SURGICAL ASSISTING

The PA assists with opening, closing, retraction of abdominal contents for exposure of vital structures, and reanastomosing. The duration of the Whipple procedure requires an assistant to help with all aspects of the procedure.

PEDIATRIC CONSIDERATIONS

Not applicable.

OBSTETRICAL CONSIDERATIONS

General concerns in operative intervention during pregnancy include avoidance of x-rays and teratogenic drugs; adequate oxygenation; fluid, electrolyte, and blood volume normalization; appropriate sedation (to minimize the risk of premature labor); gastric decompression; treatment of urinary retention; measures to reduce the risk of deep vein thrombosis (antiembolism stockings or pneumatic compression hose); rest; and avoidance of antibiotic prophylaxis is indicated.

PEARLS FOR THE PA

A high index of suspicion is required for diagnosing early pancreatic cancer in patients presenting with persistent back pain, weight loss, or jaundice.

Peptic Ulcer Disease
Karen A. Newell, PA-C

DEFINITION

Peptic ulcer disease (PUD) includes both duodenal and gastric ulcers that result from the corrosive action of gastric acid on weakened gastrointestinal epithelium. May be associated with infection with *Helicobacter pylori*.

HISTORY

Symptoms.   Most patients report epigastric pain described variably as aching, burning, gnawing, or hunger-like. Patients describe characteristic pain cycle beginning early morning (empty stomach) with recurrence 1 to 2 hours after meals, temporarily relieved by eating and antacids. When compared with duodenal ulcer, pain from gastric ulcer tends to occur earlier after eating (often within 30 minutes). Occasionally, nausea and vomiting, anorexia, weight loss, weight gain, and arousal from sleep occur secondary to pain. Occasionally, if the ulcer erodes through head of pancreas (posteriorly), patients can present with back pain that is more constant with less relief from food and antacids. With perforation, the patient may or may not have chronic symptoms of PUD preceding the event. The classic presentation is sudden, severe upper abdominal pain.

General. Patients may have symptoms attributable to occult blood loss. PUD causes 50% to 70% of upper gastrointestinal (UGI) hemorrhages. If hemorrhage has occurred, it is important to estimate the amount and rate of bleeding. Hematemesis is present unless blood loss is minimal. Coffee-ground emesis occurs if blood is in the stomach long enough for gastric acid to convert hemoglobin to methemoglobin. Patients may present with melena, because the most common cause of lower GI blood is upper GI bleeding. Hematochezia may occur due to the rapid transit of a massive upper GI bleed.

Age
Duodenal. More likely in the age range of 20 to 45 years. Males affected more often than females.

Gastric. Usually 40 to 60 years of age and older.

Onset. PUD may be insidious or acute (with hemorrhage or perforation). Stress ulcers can occur as early as 72 hours after a major stressful event (e.g., trauma, unrelated surgery).

Duration. Continue until treated.

Intensity. Symptoms may be relatively minor or life-threatening.

Aggravating Factors. Empty stomach, certain foods.

Alleviating Factors. Antacids, H_2 blockers, food intake.

Associated Factors. Compulsive (type A) personality, cigarette smoking, alcohol use, excessive caffeine use, NSAIDs, genetic predisposition, certain disease states (gastrinomas, Zollinger-Ellison syndrome, hyperparathyroidism). Infection with *Helicobacter pylori*.

Gastric. Six times increased risk for neoplastic changes.

PHYSICAL EXAMINATION

General. The patient may appear in no acute distress, in shock due to blood loss, or septic if perforation has occurred. With perforation, the patient appears severely distressed, often with knees drawn up to chest, breathing shallow, attempting to lie motionless.

Gastrointestinal. May have localized epigastric tenderness; many have a normal abdominal examination. With obstruction, bowel sounds are usually diminished, occasionally succussion splash early, or totally absent. Percussion may reveal tympany with distention. Diffuse pain with palpation and peritoneal signs of rigidity, guarding and rebound, or decreased or absent bowel sounds may occur with perforation. Rectal examination may be guaiac positive with associated bleeding.

PATHOPHYSIOLOGY

The body of the stomach contains parietal cells (HCl), zymogen or chief cells (pepsinogen + acid = pepsin, the principal enzyme in gastric juice), and mucous cells (mucus and bicarbonate). The antrum contains G cells (gastrin) under vagal control, which causes stimulation of parietal and chief cells. Mast cells release histamine and the vagal nerve releases acetylcholine. Intrinsic factor is secreted by parietal cells, and binds with dietary vitamin B_{12}, enhancing absorption in the terminal ileum, important in total gastrectomy, because patients become dependent on parenteral administration of vitamin B_{12}.

Stimulation of Acid Secretion
Cephalic Phase.   Acid production via vagal stimulation from sight, smell, taste, or thought of food.

Gastric Phase.   Presence of protein, distention, alkalinization causes gastrin release.

Intestinal Phase.   Presence of acid in duodenum and secretin cause release of biliary and pancreatic secretions and decrease of gastrin and HCl.

Duodenal.   Ninety percent of patients have evidence of *H. pylori* infection, which breaks down the mucosal barrier and makes gastric epithelium vulnerable to ulceration. The other 10% are often associated with the use of NSAIDs or other agents. About 95% of ulcers are found within 2 cm of the pylorus in the duodenal bulb and infrequently are associated with malignancy. Duodenal ulcers located posteriorly in duodenal bulb can erode the GI wall, exposing and eroding into gastroduodenal artery. Risk of rebleeding is three to one (gastric to duodenal).

Gastric.   Most common are individuals with no clinical or radiographic evidence of previous duodenal ulcer disease; gastric output is low or normal; ulcers are usually located within the pyloric mucosa and are associated with antral gastritis and *H. pylori.* Ulcers are located close to the pylorus, closely associated with duodenal ulcers, and those that occur in the antrum usually result from chronic NSAIDs use. Risk of carcinoma is low; acid secretion is normal or increased.

Perforated Peptic Ulcer.   Most located anteriorly (these tend to perforate rather than bleed, because no major vessels are located here). Once perforated, gastroduodenal secretions enter the peritoneum and peritonitis develops over the next 12 to 24 hours (presents as abrupt severe pain, followed by a period of relief, then gradual worsening).

Pyloric Obstruction.   Secondary to PUD may occur due to repetitive cycles of inflammation and repair, which may cause edema, muscle spasm, and scarring. It is important to rule out malignancy with obstruction.

Stress Ulcers.   Stress gastroduodenitis are shallow, discrete ulcers with edema and congestion. Most associated with shock, sepsis, burns, central nervous system (CNS) tumor or trauma, major surgical procedure.

DIAGNOSTIC STUDIES

Laboratory
Full Chemistry Profile, PT, PTT.   As a routine preoperative evaluation in those that have a surgical abdomen.

CBC.   Used as part of the routine preoperative evaluation. May have a low hemoglobin or hematocrit with hemorrhage or mild leuko-cytosis (12,000/μl) with perforation; after 12 to 24 hours, increases to 20,000/μl range. CBC is frequently normal in those who are not actively bleeding or are bleeding slowly.

Serum Gastrin.   Average, 50 to 100 pg/ml. If greater than 200 pg/ml, is considered elevated.

Clo Test.   To assess for *H. pylori*.

Amylase.   Increased from absorption of duodenal secretions in perito-neum after perforation.

Radiology

Upper Gastrointestinal Series.   May visualize inflammation/scarring with distortion of duodenal bulb; 50% false-negative rate. Often confirms the ulcer. Can detect malignancies.

Plain Abdominal X-ray.   With pyloric obstruction, demonstrates large gastric fluid level when correlated with timing of normal gastric emptying.

Supine and Upright Abdominal X-rays.   With perforation, demon-strates subdiaphragmatic free air in 85% of patients. In those who are unable to be positioned properly, a left lateral decubitus film may be helpful. In those who are clinically suspicious with questionable initial results, consider injecting 400 ml of air through the NG tube and repeating the films. Water-soluble contrast media can be swallowed or placed into the NG.

Saline Load Test.   Performed if pyloric obstruction is suspected.

Other

Gastric Analysis.   Measures acid production by an unstimulated stom-ach under basal fasting conditions during stimulation by histamine (maxi-mal acid output or MAO). May have normal or increased gastric acid se-cretion.

Endoscopy.   Gastroduodenoscopy useful for uncertain diagnosis, those with bleeding or obstruction, those with nonresolution of symptoms after medical trial, and as a periodic evaluation during therapy. During early endoscopy, epinephrine, sclerosing agents, cautery, or lasers may be used to stop active bleeding in a visible vessel. Biopsy may also be performed on suspicious lesions.

Stool Guaiac.   Can detect between 10 and 50 ml/day. False positives include hemoglobin and myoglobin (found in meat) and plant peroxidase (turnip, cauliflower, broccoli, cantaloupe, horseradish, and parsnip); iron does not give positive results.

DIFFERENTIAL DIAGNOSIS

Traumatic.   Not applicable.

Infectious.   Not applicable.

Metabolic

Acute Pancreatitis.   Usually has an insidious onset, frequently associ-ated with alcohol abuse, dull epigastric pain, often referred to the back, nausea, vomiting, and physical examination findings on palpation of the epigastric area. Laboratory findings of leukocytosis and elevated serum amylase and lipase.

Cholecystitis. Location of pain is usually in the right upper quadrant, often referred to the right scapula; associated with nausea and vomiting more frequently. Physical examination findings on palpation of the right upper quadrant.

Neoplastic

Gastric or Intestinal Cancer. May present with hemorrhage. Will not respond to usual ulcer therapy; differentiated on diagnostic studies and biopsy.

Vascular. Not applicable.

Congenital

Pyloric Stenosis. Seen in newborns; associated with abdominal distention and projectile vomiting. May present as failure to thrive. Palpation in the right upper quadrant may reveal a mass.

Duodenal Atresia. Usually associated with bilious vomiting, abdominal distention, and failure to pass meconium; may be associated with prematurity.

Acquired. Not applicable.

Other

Reflux Esophagitis. Associated with postprandial epigastric burning and regurgitation, worse when supine.

Hiatal Hernia. Associated with postprandial epigastric burning and regurgitation, worse when supine.

Irritable Bowel Syndrome. Pain described as crampy and located in the lower abdomen. Often associated with abdominal distention, increased frequency of bowel movements, loose stools, and pain often alleviated after bowel movement.

Intestinal Obstruction. Usually has a gradual onset, more crampy, and associated with vomiting.

TREATMENT

Medical. H_2 receptor antagonists (cimetidine, ranitidine, famotidine, nizatidine) are used to decrease secretion of acid and heal 80% of ulcers within 6 weeks. Afterward, a single dose at bedtime decreases the recurrence rate (of approximately 80%) within 1 year. If the ulcer recurs, the medication is changed or the dosage increased. Repeat endoscopy may be required to document resolution of the ulcer.

Proton pump blockers (omeprazole) are reserved for those refractory to H_2 receptor antagonists or those with Zollinger-Ellison syndrome (pancreatic tumor that produces gastrin, which causes hydrochloric acid and pepsin to be secreted by the stomach [60% are malignant]).

Antacids are used to buffer acid. These include magnesium-based medications (Maalox, Mylanta), and aluminum-based (Amphojel) and calcium-based (Tums) compounds.

Prostaglandin analogues (misoprostol) increase the mucus–bicarbonate barrier.

Exogenous barriers (sucralfate, colloidal bismuth) may be used in conjunction with the above medications.

Counsel patients to decrease risk factors (e.g., smoking, alcohol, caffeine, NSAIDs). Special diets have never been shown to be of benefit.

To eradicate *H. pylori*, many combinations of acceptable therapy (e.g., bismuth subsalicylate 2 tablets orally four times a day with meals for 2 to 3 weeks and tetracycline 500 mg orally four times a day with meals for 2 to 3 weeks and metronidazole 250 mg orally three times a day with meals for 2 to 3 weeks) is greater than 85% to 90% effective. Use serologic testing to confirm eradication of the organism.

Hemorrhage. For acute hemorrhage, obtain hematocrit, hemoglobin, liver function studies, blood type and crossmatch. Place an IV and a 16 Fr or larger NG tube for iced normal saline lavage and clot aspiration until the aspirate is clear. Give H_2 receptor antagonist or omeprazole. Monitor closely for hemorrhagic shock (tachycardia/hypotension). Consider placing a urinary catheter to monitor urine output if shock is a possibility. Consider oxygen 5 to 10 l/min by nasal cannula. If hematocrit is low but there is no evidence of shock, then the bleed is probably slow. The hematocrit, however, is not a reliable indicator of status.

Once the patient is stable, obtain endoscopy within 24 hours to identify the source of bleeding, obtain upper gastrointestinal (UGI) series if endoscopy is equivocal or unavailable, and consider transfusion based on hemodynamic measurements and the estimated amount of blood loss. Follow the hematocrit serially to assess progress (each transfused unit of packed cells increases the hematocrit two to three points and three points are dropped for every 500 ml of blood lost).

Patients can be fed after 12 to 24 hours, if hungry, once bleeding has stopped.

Guaiac all stools, but this test is unreliable as the sole indicator of hemorrhage, as it may persist for days after bleeding has stopped.

Patients should not smoke, as this can cause rebleeding.

Perforation. Use a nasogastric tube to remove secretions, allowing less to traverse into the peritoneum; IV antibiotics (cefazolin, cefoxitin) to treat peritonitis; IV fluids for hydration.

Stress Ulcers. Prevention is preferred over treatment. Use H_2 receptor antagonists prophylactically in all perioperative and critically ill patients.

Surgical. Surgery is required less commonly due to the widespread acceptance and treatment of *H. pylori*. Excision of ulcer itself is not sufficient, because recurrence is inevitable. Procedures include:

Truncal Vagotomy. Decreases acetylcholine (cephalic phase). Each vagal trunk (left found anterior/right found posterior) can be resected at the level of the distal esophagus; but then, because of delayed emptying by stomach into duodenum, a pyloroplasty must also be performed (drainage procedures are the Heineke-Mikulicz/Finney/Jaboulay). Patients can be left with dumping syndrome or diarrhea.

Vagal Denervation. Of specific sites includes (a) parietal cell portion of the stomach, known as parietal cell vagotomy/proximal gastric vagotomy/or superselective vagotomy (only those branches to upper 2/3 of the stomach are affected), decreasing or eliminating the need for a drainage procedure; (b) selective vagotomy (both main branches of nerve transected below celiac and hepatic branches).

Antrectomy and Vagotomy. Decreases gastrin and acetylcholine.

Billroth I. The pylorus is excised and the upper stomach is reattached to the duodenum; used in those with bleeding.

Billroth II. Subtotal excision of the stomach with closure of proximal duodenum and side-to-side anastomosis of jejunum to remaining stomach; used in those with obstruction.

Surgical Hemigastrectomy (Including the Ulcer), Vagotomy/Pyloroplasty. Prior to identification of *H. pylori* was the preferred method of treatment for gastric ulcers. Currently, most patients are medically treated and surgery is reserved only for those with complications.

Postsurgical Complications. Early complications include anastomotic leakage, gastric retention, and hemorrhage. Late complications include recurrent ulcer, gastrojejunocolic and gastrocolic fistula (between stomach and colon), dumping syndrome, alkaline gastritis, iron deficiency anemia, and postvagotomy diarrhea.

Perforation. Laparoscopy or laparotomy are performed to identify and close the perforated area and for removal of spilled contents from peritoneal cavity. Prior to *H. pylori* recognition, aggressive consideration to surgically correct initial cause was also employed (e.g., parietal cell vagotomy or truncal vagotomy and pyloroplasty). Current thought indicates simple surgical closure and eradication of *H. pylori* with additional surgery in only the most severe cases.

Indications. Bleeding, perforation, or obstruction. Bleeding from a gastric ulcer is considered more serious than gastritis or duodenal ulcer; therefore, surgery is considered earlier.

Contraindications. Inadequate medical trial (relative, depending on the extent and type of ulcer), inability of the patient to undergo anesthesia.

TECHNIQUE OF SURGICAL ASSISTING

Approach to the duodenum or stomach is through a midline or left paramedian incision. The PA assists with retraction during opening, using caution not to grasp any bowel underlying the tissue being opened. Retraction and assistance with hemostasis, anastomosis, and resection are provided throughout the procedure. The PA assists with closure (with a ribbon or malleable retractor placed into the incision to prevent inadvertent suturing of bowel), placement of dressings, and postoperative care.

PEDIATRIC CONSIDERATIONS

In the pediatric age group, males are more affected than females. The age group most affected is the 12- to 18-year-old. There tends to be a strong family association, relationship to aspirin and NSAIDs, hypoxia, hypotension, burns, central nervous system injury, or other critical illness. There is no evidence to currently suggest an association to *H. pylori*.

Suggested treatment is liquid antacids 0.5 to 2.5 ml/kg, every 1 to 2 hours or 1 to 3 hours after meals and at bedtime; cimetidine 5 mg/kg orally before meals and at bedtime, or ranitidine 2.5 mg/kg orally every 12 hours for 4 to 8 weeks. Avoid caffeine, aspirin, and NSAIDs. Surgery is performed only in refractory cases.

OBSTETRICAL CONSIDERATIONS

Careful consideration must be given to both the life of the mother and fetus when evaluating for the possibility of surgical intervention in the pregnant woman. Medications often used to treat patients for PUD must be carefully evaluated in the pregnant patient. Cimetidine should not be used unless the benefit outweighs potential fetal risk. No nursing should be done while taking this medication.

Ranitidine, nizatidine, famotidine, omeprazole, sucralfate: risk during pregnancy is unknown; therefore, use only if the potential benefit outweighs fetal risk. Use caution when nursing.

Misoprostol is associated with spontaneous abortion. No nursing should be done while taking this medication.

Tetracycline is associated with retarded fetal skeletal development and, in the later portion of pregnancy, may cause permanent tooth discoloration of the fetus. No nursing should be done while taking this medication.

Metronidazole is contraindicated, especially in the first trimester. Do not use during pregnancy or while nursing.

PEARLS FOR THE PA

Peptic ulcer disease may be associated with Helicobacter pylori *infection.*

The characteristic symptom is that of burning, gnawing pain in the early morning and 1 to 2 hours after meals.

The most common cause of lower GI blood is upper GI bleeding.

Ulcer prophylaxis may be indicated for patients under extreme physiologic stress (e.g., major trauma).

Small Bowel Disease
Harry F. Randolph, PA-C

DEFINITION

Most small bowel pathology necessitating surgical intervention is caused by varying degrees of obstruction (intrinsic or extrinsic), perforation, or vascular compromise.

HISTORY

Symptoms.   Generally include a colicky abdominal pain that comes in waves. Bloating and anorexia are often seen and, in cases of partial or complete obstruction, nausea and bilious vomiting are common. Occasionally, diarrhea is noted and, as disease severity increases, cessation of bowel movements, fever, severe abdominal pain, prostration and dehydration, hematochezia, or frank rectal bleeding can occur.

Age.   Generally adulthood, with increasing incidence over the age of 50.

Onset.   Chronic conditions are insidious, but most requiring surgery are relatively acute and progressive.

Duration.   Acute conditions develop over 12 to 24 hours prior to presentation.

Intensity.   May be mild at first and progress steadily in intensity to severe pain and inability to sustain oral intake. Occasionally, acute and intense at outset. Abrupt cessation of pain may indicate bowel infarction.

Aggravating Factors.   Oral intake, sitting, and movement.

Alleviating Factors.   Bowel rest (NPO), emesis.

Associated Factors.   Prior history of abdominal or pelvic surgery, Crohn's disease, ulcerative colitis, or radiation therapy to abdomen or pelvis.

PHYSICAL EXAMINATION

General.   The patient may be in moderate to severe distress from pain. Tachycardia, dry mucous membranes, hypotension, or diaphoresis occur from dehydration. A mass representing an incarcerated hernia may be found in the abdominal wall or inguinal region.

Gastrointestinal.   Abdominal distention. Bowel sounds are usually diminished; occasionally, succussion splash early, or totally absent with complete obstruction. Percussion may reveal tympany with distention. Diffuse pain with palpation to peritoneal signs of rigidity, guarding, and rebound later. Rectal examination may reveal mass; guaiac positive with associated bleeding.

PATHOPHYSIOLOGY

The small bowel (intestine) extends from the pylorus to the ileocecal valve. The surface area is extensive, because its principle function is absorption of nutrients and peristalsis is constant. The duodenum begins at the pylorus where the common bile duct empties bile and pancreatic enzymes at its origin, and extends some 20 cm to the ligament of Treitz. The jejunum extends the next 100 to 110 cm, and is characterized by a larger lumen and thicker walls than the ileum, which is some 150 to 160 cm and terminates the small bowel at the cecum. With the exception of the proximal duodenum, all blood supply to the small bowel emanates from the superior mesenteric artery. The jejunum and ileum are tethered by only the mesentery and are freely mobile under normal circumstances.

Luminal obstruction may be intrinsically caused by Crohn's disease, foreign bodies, enterolith, Meckel's diverticula, or primary small bowel tumors. Extrinsic compression may be secondary to adhesions from prior surgery or radiation, other mass lesions in the abdomen, or strangulated bowel in a hernia (inguinal, femoral, Morgagni, or ventral). Vascular compromise, either from an embolic episode or underlying pathology, is a surgical emergency and must be recognized and treated early. Surgical consideration from a significant bleeding source within the small bowel is seen from arteriovenous malformations, Crohn's disease, ulcerations, or tumors. These are difficult to identify preoperatively and often are only found at the time of surgery or with intraoperative endoscopy.

DIAGNOSTIC STUDIES

Laboratory

CBC. Anemia may be present from chronc or acute blood loss. Elevated WBC is present in obstruction, perforation, and in the 20,000 to 30,000/mm^3 range with vascular compromise.

Chemistry Profile. Hypokalemia, hyponatremia, and hypochloremia occur in many cases. Acidosis is common in vascular compromise. Hypoproteinemia and hypoalbuminemia indicate chronic conditions.

Radiologic

Acute Abdominal Series. Including upright and flat film. Air–fluid level on an upright abdomen film is highly suggestive of small bowel obstruction. A left lateral decubitus view may show small amounts of air around the liver not seen on a routine chest x-ray. Dilated loops of small bowel are often present. Calcifications within the lumen may represent obstructive processes.

Chest X-ray. May show sympathetic pleural effusions and air beneath the diaphragm.

Upper GI Series. May show partial or complete obstruction. Gastrografin should be used when complete obstruction or perforation is suspected. Barium enema can be used to demonstrate terminal ileum lesions.

CT Scan of the Abdomen. Can often delineate location of obstruction or reveal bowel wall abnormalities, extrinsic masses, or abscess. Enteroclysis is sometimes helpful to identify intrinsic masses.

Other

Mesenteric Angiography. With significant active bleeding, can be helpful to define sources within the small bowel.

DIFFERENTIAL DIAGNOSIS

Traumatic. Not applicable.

Infectious

Gastroenteritis (Viral, Bacterial, or Parasitic). Usually with watery diarrhea and exposure history with personal contact or travel. Stool samples can document *Salmonella, Shigella, Clostridium difficile, Campylobacter,* and acid-fast bacilli.

Metabolic

Diabetic Ketoacidosis and Hyperthyroidism. Can cause abdominal pain and electrolyte imbalances. Both can be ruled out with blood glucose and appropriate thyroid panels.

Neoplastic

Paraneoplastic Syndromes. Caused by lung, prostate, or breast cancer; can cause electrolyte imbalances, leading to vomiting and abdominal pain. Appropriate history and x-ray studies can be helpful in excluding this entity.

Vascular

Portal Vein Thrombosis. Can cause abdominal pain; usually signs and symptoms of hepatic failure are present.

Vasculitis. Secondary to autoimmune disorders such as lupus, scleroderma, and Sjögren's syndrome, in rare cases, can mimic obstruction. A known history and negative abdominal series or CT are present.

Congenital. Not applicable.

Acquired

Colon Obstruction, Ileus, Cholecystitis/Cholelithiasis or Appendicitis. Ultrasound is effective in diagnosis of gallstones and noncompressible appendix. Flat plate with colon gas in absence of air–fluid levels suggests ileus.

TREATMENT

Medical. Nonacute small bowel obstruction can be treated with nasogastric suction, NPO, hydration, and IV antibiotics for a period of 3 to 14 days or longer, depending on the clinical situation. In some instances, decompression can be attained and surgery avoided. Monitoring with WBC, abdominal x-rays, fever curve, and physical examination for signs of deterioration are necessary. For patients who need prolonged decompression, nutritional status should be assessed and total parenteral nutrition instituted.

Surgical. The indications for surgical intervention are those patients in whom complete obstruction can be demonstrated despite cause. Patients with fever, elevation of WBC, peritoneal signs, or hemodynamic instability indicative of sepsis should be operated on early. Any suggestion of ischemic bowel is a surgical emergency, and prompt intervention is mandatory. Evidence of perforation or intraperitoneal free air is also a surgical emergency that demands early intervention. Those with incomplete obstruction secondary to demonstrated mass lesions (either intrinsic or extrinsic), Crohn's disease, or infectious origins deserve surgical consideration within hours to days, depending on their clinical situation. Postoperative obstruction within the first 6 weeks after abdominal surgery is a special consideration. An attempt at long-term (up to 30 days) trial of conservative management may be worthwhile. Because of the intense inflammatory changes of the small bowel during this time frame, the risk of small bowel enterotomies during surgery is extremely high, with fistula formation likely.

In elective cases or where time allows, bowel preparation, when possible, is suggested prior to surgery. Clear liquids for 48 hours before surgery, followed by bowel catharsis (Go-lytely, magnesium citrate) 24 hours prior. The bowel should be sterilized with 1 g each of neomycin and erythromycin base orally at 1200, 1400, and 2000 hours the day prior to surgery; the patient should be held NPO overnight.

Indications. Complete or incomplete (relative) obstruction, sepsis, ischemic bowel (a surgical emergency), perforation, or intraperitoneal free air.

Contraindications. Relative contraindications to surgery are poor patient health (cardiac, pulmonary, or renal failure), poor long-term prognosis, and personal preference.

TECHNIQUE OF SURGICAL ASSISTING

A midline incision is made from the umbilicus to the pubis and elongated as necessary. Care must be taken when entering the peritoneal cavity, because adhesions may be present or dilated small bowel may lie just under the surface. Once the abdominal cavity is entered, the small bowel must be held carefully, because it is often distended and friable. Enterotomies should be repaired as they are made (they are hard to find later). Apply only gentle countertraction as adhesions are lysed, and use only blunt-tipped instruments. If a segment of small bowel must be resected, normal proximal and distal bowel is identified and the mesentery between the two ends divided and tied. After resecting the bowel, the two ends are anastomosed either with stapling devices or by hand sewing in two layers. The mesentery is then approximated with chromic suture. Generous irrigation with body temperature saline is done before closure. If evidence of perforation or infection is present, drains and retention sutures may be placed or the wound skin left open to close secondarily.

PEDIATRIC CONSIDERATIONS

Small bowel atresia is evidenced within the first few days of life with bilious vomiting and bloating. Look for other developmental abnormalities in duodenal obstruction (30% have trisomy 21). The first few weeks of life, look for malrotation of the small bowel and midgut volvulus with typical symptoms. Intussusception is seen most commonly between 8 and 12 months. It is often preceded by viral gastroenteritis, so diagnosis is difficult, with paroxysms of crampy pain and vomiting. Bloody mucus (currant jelly stool) passed per rectum with vascular compromise. All should receive urgent surgical correction.

OBSTETRICAL CONSIDERATIONS

Increased risk for obstruction after 12 to 14 weeks of gestation with known associated factors, including pelvic inflammatory disease. Delay in diagnosis or intervention causes increased risk to fetus.

PEARLS FOR THE PA

In the patient with abdominal pain of small bowel disease, the clinical triad of elevated WBC ($>20,000/mm^3$), unexplained tachycardia, and acidosis is considered to be ischemic bowel until proven otherwise.

Splenic Rupture
James W. Becker, PA-C

DEFINITION

The spleen is a fist-sized, solid, vascular organ located in the left upper quadrant of the abdomen lateral to the stomach, under the diaphragm and above the colon. The spleen is normally not palpable, being tucked under the rib margin so that it is protected from blunt trauma. Certain physiological conditions (e.g., hematological or malignant) can cause splenomegaly and make the spleen more vulnerable. The spleen filters the blood and removes aging red blood cells and, during infancy, has a role in the development of new antibodies. Because a true surgical emergency is found with a ruptured spleen, it is discussed primarily.

HISTORY

Symptoms. The patient with a ruptured spleen may present in various ways, from obvious shock after a major trauma to the presentation of weakness and vague abdominal discomfort. The patient may experience anorexia, nausea, and possible emesis (nonbloody).

General. Most patients are able to give a history of some blunt abdominal trauma, although it may have been initially thought of as a trivial incident. Splenic preservation should be attempted in young and pediatric patients whenever possible.

Age. No correlation.

Onset. Symptoms usually appear shortly after the offending trauma. In about 5% of cases, the patient initially receives a splenic hematoma, which may slowly enlarge over several days. A delayed splenic rupture may occur 2 to 4 weeks after the traumatic event.

Intensity. Severity of symptoms usually increases with the passage of time, until the patient begins to lapse into shock from blood loss.

Aggravating Factors. Trendelenburg positioning usually makes the symptoms worse, although it may be necessary for maintaining blood pressure.

Alleviating Factors. The patient is usually more comfortable in a sitting position, allowing the pooling blood to drain away from the diaphragm.

Associated Factors. Enlarged spleen (more susceptible to trauma), other abdominal organ injuries, multisystem trauma.

PHYSICAL EXAMINATION

General. Depending on the circumstances of the extent of the trauma victim, the patient may exhibit dull abdominal pain, shoulder pain, or may be in shock. In the patient with splenomegaly, a gradual onset of early satiety, pressure in the upper abdomen, shortness of breath, and shoulder discomfort may be exhibited.

Cardiovascular. Tachycardia if significant blood loss or pain.

Gastrointestinal. Inspect for bruises, lacerations, or other deformities from trauma. The tympanic gastric air bubble may be in the midline or displaced into the right upper quadrant by an expanding splenic hematoma. Dullness in the left upper quadrant with tenderness indicates an enlarged spleen. Peritoneal signs exist if free blood from splenic disruption is present.

Pulmonary. Diminished breath sounds in the left base. Check for rib fractures.

PATHOPHYSIOLOGY

Splenomegaly itself is not a pathological process but rather a sign of an underlying problem. In cases of abdominal trauma, the spleen is the most commonly injured organ. The pediatric spleen serves as major site of new antibody formation, and splenic preservation should be attempted, especially if the patient is under the age of 2 years. In normal patients, the total amount of platelets contained in the spleen is about 30%, whereas the patient with splenomegaly may harbor up to 80% of the total platelet volume.

DIAGNOSTIC STUDIES

Laboratory
CBC. Rule out anemia from blood loss. Confirm adequate platelet count.

Chemical Profile. Preparation for general anesthetic. Review liver enzymes to rule out hepatic dysfunction or cirrhosis.

Amylase. Rule out associated pancreatitis from trauma.

Blood Bank. Obtain blood type and crossmatch for whole blood in the severe trauma patient, packed blood cells for the elective splenectomy patient, platelets for the thrombocytopenic patient, and fresh frozen plasma to correct any bleeding dyscrasia.

Serology. If history suggests, in the splenomegaly patient obtain a malaria smear and perform monospot tests.

Radiology
Flat and Upright Abdominal Films. To rule out space occupying mass in the left upper quadrant consistent with splenic hematoma/splenomegaly. In the trauma patient, check for free air.

Chest X-ray. Look for free air or rib fractures in the trauma patient.

Abdominal CT Scan. Check for splenic hematoma, ruptured spleen or, in the case of splenomegaly, look for splenic vein thrombosis, gastric varices, or cirrhosis.

Nuclear Medicine. Splenic scan to rule out intrinsic lesions of the spleen.

DIFFERENTIAL DIAGNOSIS

Traumatic
Blunt Trauma Without Splenic Rupture. Patient may have similar symptoms, but radiographic studies are negative for splenic rupture.

Infectious
Infectious Mononucleosis, Tuberculosis, Malaria. Splenomegaly can occur.

Splenic Abscess. Can occur with bacterial infections.

Metabolic
Chronic Anemia, Felty's Syndrome, Gaucher's Disease and Amyloidosis. Splenomegaly may occur.

Neoplastic
Leukemia and Lymphoma. Splenomegaly can occur.

Metastatic Carcinoma. May affect the spleen.

Vascular
Splenic Vein Thrombosis. Splenomegaly may occur.

Congenital
Hereditary Spherocytosis, Thalassemia, and Elliptocytosis. Splenomegaly may occur.

Acquired
Cirrhosis. Splenomegaly may occur in patients with portal hypertension.

TREATMENT

Medical. Recent data show an increasing incidence of nonoperative management of splenic trauma by close clinical monitoring and CT scan observation of the injury.

Surgical. Splenectomy can be performed as an open procedure and also by laparoscopic approach by an experienced surgeon. In cases of trauma, the open procedure is indicated. In patients who are surgically explored, there is an increasing incidence of splenic preservation by the use of absorbable mesh to tamponade the bleeding organ, which is recommended in the pediatric population. In the elective splenectomy patient, coordination with the hematologist is recommended for availability of adequate blood products and, if necessary, preoperative steroid preparation. All patients should receive pneumococcal vaccination prior to splenectomy, and the trauma patient should receive the vaccination prior to discharge. At the time of surgery, the splenic artery should be ligated first and then any blood products, especially platelets in the thrombocytopenic patient, should be administered. With a severely traumatized spleen, quick mobilization and hemostasis must be attained. Injury to the greater curvature of the stomach or the pancreas can occur, and dissection of these organs is essential. Postoperatively, blood counts and platelet counts should be monitored closely, because thrombocytosis may occur.

Indications. Acute or subacute rupture.

Contraindications. For acute hemorrhage, this is a surgical emergency and there are essentially no contraindications. For minor hemorrhage, observation may be employed.

TECHNIQUE OF SURGICAL ASSISTING

The PA assists with opening, retraction, hemostasis, and protection of other organs during splenic removal.

PEDIATRIC CONSIDERATIONS

Splenic preservation procedures are used whenever possible because during infancy, the spleen plays a role in the development of new antibodies.

OBSTETRICAL CONSIDERATIONS

In blunt trauma associated with pregnancy, the spleen is the most commonly injured intra-abdominal organ. General concerns in operative intervention during pregnancy include avoidance of x-rays and teratogenic drugs; adequate oxygenation; fluid, electrolyte, and blood volume normalization; appropriate sedation (to minimize the risk of premature labor); gastric decompression; treatment of urinary retention; measures to reduce the risk of deep vein thrombosis (antiembolism stockings or pneumatic compression hose); rest; and avoidance of antibiotic prophylaxis as indicated.

PEARLS FOR THE PA

An increasing number of patients with splenic trauma are being treated by nonoperative management and splenic preservation.

Monitor the post-trauma patient for delayed rupture of a splenic hematoma, which can occur 2 to 4 weeks after the event.

Monitor platelet counts after splenectomy for thrombocytosis.

Immunize the splenectomy patient for pneumococcus.

Further Reading

Bates, B: A Guide to Physical Examination and History Taking, ed 4. Philadelphia, J. B. Lippincott, 1987.

Corman ML (ed): Hemorrhoids. In Colon and Rectal Surgery, ed 3. Philadelphia, J. B. Lippincott, 1993.

Hardy JD (ed): Hardy's Textbook of Surgery, ed 2. Philadelphia, J. B. Lippincott, 1988.

Haubrich WS: Gastroenterology, ed 5. Philadelphia, W. B. Saunders, 1995.

Keighley MRB, Williams NS (eds): Surgery of the Anus, Rectum and Colon, vol I. London, W. B. Saunders Ltd., 1993.

Kempe CH, Silver HK, O'Brien D: Current Pediatric Diagnosis and Treatment, ed 8. Los Altos, Calif, Lange Medical Publications, 1984.

Labus J (ed): The Physician Assistant Medical Handbook. Philadelphia, W. B. Saunders, 1995.

Levien DH: Hemorrhoids. In Cameron JL (ed): Current Surgical Therapy, ed 5. St. Louis, Mosby–Year Book, 1995.

Levien DH (ed): Anorectal surgery. Surg Clin North Am 74(6):1994.

Netter F: Atlas of Human Anatomy. Summit, NJ, CIBA-GEIGY Corp., 1989.

Physician's Compendium of Drug and Patient Information, 1995. Secaucus, NJ, Compendium Publications Group Inc.

Rosen P: Emergency Medicine: Concepts and Clinical Practice, ed 3. St. Louis, Mosby, 1992.

Sabiston DC: Textbook of Surgery, ed 14. Philadelphia, W. B. Saunders, 1991.

Schwartz SI, et al: Principles of Surgery, ed 5. New York, McGraw-Hill, 1994.

Way LW: Current Surgical Diagnosis and Treatment. ed 10. Los Altos, CA, Lange Medical Publications, 1994.

Wilson JD, et al: Harrison's Principles of Internal Medicine, ed 12. New York, McGraw-Hill, 1991.

Zollinger RM, et al: Atlas of Surgical Operations, ed 7. New York, McGraw-Hill, 1992.

Chapter **5**

Gynecologic Surgery
Bartholin's Cyst/Abscess
Deborah E. Murray, PA-C, BS

DEFINITION

Nodular mass of Bartholin's gland (gland that keeps the vestibular surface moist) located in the inferior portion of the labium majus.

HISTORY

Symptoms. The cyst is frequently asymptomatic. An abscess of Bartholin's gland presents as a painful, ovoid mass.

General. Bartholinitis can be chronic with occasional acute exacerbations.

Age. Most common in the reproductive years.

Onset. Cyst may be present for years with occasional inflammation or infection.

Intensity. Asymptomatic to significant pain in presence of abscess.

Aggravating Factors. Infection.

Alleviating Factors. Medical and/or surgical treatment.

Associated Factors. None.

PHYSICAL EXAMINATION

General. Patient may appear in moderate to no distress.

Gynecologic. A complete pelvic examination should be performed. Evaluate for signs of infection such as vaginal discharge or purulent discharge from Bartholin's duct. Normally, Bartholin's glands are not palpable unless involved in a cyst or an abscess. A cyst is palpable as a small, nodular, usually nontender swelling. An abscess presents as a turgid, swollen, painful ovoid mass of the inferior labium majus.

PATHOPHYSIOLOGY

An abscess forms secondary to infection, often of gonococcal origin, but also commonly with coliform or polymicrobial organisms. *Bacteroides fragilis* is recovered in 15% of the cases. An abscess may subside to form a cyst when the main duct or one of its subdivisions are occluded.

DIAGNOSTIC STUDIES

Laboratory

Cervical Gonococcal Culture. Performed if discharge is present.

Complete Blood Count (CBC). If abscess is suspected; may show elevated WBC.

Radiology. Not applicable.
Other. Not applicable.

DIFFERENTIAL DIAGNOSIS

Traumatic
Hematoma. History of trauma, painful mass without evidence of infection.
Infectious. Not otherwise applicable.
Metabolic. Not applicable.
Neoplastic
Adenocarcinoma of Bartholin's Gland. Is extremely rare, occurring in approximately 1% of vulvar malignancies. An enlargement of Bartholin's gland in postmenopausal women should be considered malignant until proven otherwise through biopsy.
Vascular. Not applicable.
Congenital. Not applicable.
Acquired. Not applicable.

TREATMENT

Medical. Warm sitz bathes, analgesics, and appropriate antibiotics. No treatment is necessary if the patient is asymptomatic.
Surgical. If patient does not respond to medical treatment, surgery may be performed through excision of the cyst or, more commonly, marsupialization (drainage of the cyst followed by suturing the edges to those of the external excision).
Indications. If medical treatment fails.
Contraindications. Marsupialization should not be attempted until infection clears, because induration and edema make the procedure more difficult to perform.

TECHNIQUE OF SURGICAL ASSISTING

This is a relatively simple procedure, requiring no assistance. The PA is involved with diagnosis and management.

PEDIATRIC CONSIDERATIONS

Rare in children. (Rule out gonococcal infection and sexual abuse.)

OBSTETRICAL CONSIDERATIONS

Treat conservatively with rest, analgesics, and sitz baths. If infection is present, treat. Should the problem persist, reserve surgery for after delivery.

PEARLS FOR THE PA

Bartholin's cyst is frequently of gonococcal origin.

If the patient is asymptomatic, no treatment other than sitz baths, analgesics, and antibiotics is required.

A Bartholin's cyst is palpable, small, nodular, and usually non-tender, whereas an abscess is a turgid, swollen, painful ovoid mass.

Ectopic Pregnancy
Paul Taylor, PA-C, BS

DEFINITION

Ectopic pregnancy occurs when a zygote implants and grows outside the uterine cavity.

HISTORY

Symptoms. The classic triad of lower abdominal pain, amenorrhea, and vaginal bleeding is not commonly encountered.

General. Ectopic pregnancy is the great masquerader. The clinical presentation can vary from spotting to vasomotor shock with hemoperitoneum. Patients who present because of acute symptoms are usually at a more advanced gestational age compared with asymptomatic infertility patients who are being followed closely due to the risk of ectopic pregnancy.

The number of ectopic pregnancies continues to rise in the United States annually. Suggested reasons for the increase include the higher prevalence of risk factors, improvements in diagnostic methods, and the postponement of childbearing. The mortality rate is low, and when deaths occur, they are usually secondary to exsanguination following the rupture of the fallopian tube of an undiagnosed ectopic pregnancy. A diagnostic delay of 7 to 10 days is common in fatal cases.

Age. Women of childbearing age.

Onset. Generally 2 to 8 weeks. With rupture, symptoms are immediate.

Duration. Progressively worsening bleeding and lower abdominal pain.

Intensity. Worse as pregnancy progresses. Severe with rupture, with rebound tenderness and hypotension.

Aggravating Factors.   Abdominal pressure; delay in diagnosis and treatment.

Alleviating Factors.   None.

Associated Factors.   Minority race, advanced maternal age, low socioeconomic status, history of salpingitis, previous tubal surgery, progesterone-only contraceptives, progesterone-containing intrauterine devices (IUDs), ovarian hyperstimulation, prior *in vitro* fertilization and embryo transfer, and previous ectopic pregnancy (12% to 15% increase).

PHYSICAL EXAMINATION

General.   The patient usually appears in acute distress, bending over and holding the abdomen.

Gynecologic.   A full pelvic examination should be performed because symptoms tend to be nonspecific and can represent a myriad of pathologies. Specific findings in ectopic pregnancy include adnexa fullness (without rupture) and cervical motion and rebound tenderness (with rupture).

PATHOPHYSIOLOGY

Most patients presenting with an ectopic pregnancy do not have a recognized risk factor, suggesting dysfunctional problems in tubal transport or impaired implantation due to some abnormality in the conceptus. Sites of ectopic implantation are listed in Table 5–1.

DIAGNOSTIC STUDIES

Laboratory

Urine Pregnancy Test.   Can rule out ectopic pregnancy if the test is negative, because the urine test results are valid at the time that the ectopic

Table 5–1. Sites of Ectopic Implantation

Fallopian tube	
Ampullary segment	80%
Isthmic segment	12%
Fimbrial end	5%
Cornual and interstitial	2%
Abdominal	1.4%
Ovarian	0.2%
Cervical	0.2%

From Speroff L, Glass RH, Kase NG (eds): Clinical Gynecologic Endocrinology and Infertility, ed 5. Baltimore, Williams & Wilkins, 1994.

pregnancy becomes symptomatic. Serologic testing should be performed if further confirmation is required.

Serologic Measurements of Human Chorionic Gonadotropin (hCG). The hCG level increases at different rates in normal and ectopic pregnancies. In a normal pregnancy, the hCG approximately doubles every 2 days; an hCG greater than 6000 mIU/mL is usually associated with an intrauterine pregnancy (IUP). When the hCG titer is below 6000 mIU/mL and a transvaginal ultrasound fails to identify an IUP, the patient may be followed with serial hCG titers. If the titer does not double in 2 days, a laparoscopy is indicated. Laparoscopy is also indicated when the hCG titer is above 6000 mIU/mL and ultrasound shows no evidence of an IUP. In clinical practice, these guidelines are not always clear and definitive. It is important to note that the higher the hCG, the longer it may take for the titer to double.

CBC. Performed if hemorrhage is present (or suspected) to determine hemodynamic status. Serial hematocrits may be performed to identify a bleed.

Radiology

Ultrasound Imaging. Using a 5-MHz vaginal probe allows for visualization of the gestational sac at the time of the missed period. More importantly, the yolk sac becomes visible at 5 weeks, confirming the presence of embryonic tissue within the uterine cavity. Thus, the location of the pregnancy can be confirmed. Other important findings include a complex cystic mass in the adnexa or cul-de-sac, free fluid in the peritoneal cavity, or the lack of a gestational sac in the uterus that would normally be visualized using transvaginal ultrasound.

Other

Culdocentesis. Should only be performed when ultrasound is unavailable or in cases of emergency. Although the diagnosis of a hemoperitoneum is highly predictive of an ectopic pregnancy, a positive tap does not always correlate with tubal rupture and may be present in 1% to 2% of patients with an IUP.

Laparoscopy. Has the highest positive predictive value for diagnosing ectopic pregnancy as a single test and provides a correct diagnosis in over 90% of cases. Aggressive and liberal use of the laparoscope has resulted in a decrease in the delay of diagnosis, with immediate intervention following visualization.

DIFFERENTIAL DIAGNOSIS

Traumatic. Not applicable.

Infectious

Salpingitis. Negative pregnancy test; pain on bimanual examination; may have elevated WBC.

Infection of the Round Ligament with Normal IUP. Positive pregnancy test, associated with pain; pregnancy localized to the uterus.

Appendicitis. Possible occurrence with an IUP. Pregnancy localized to the uterus.

Metabolic

Ruptured Corpus Luteum. Usually presents later (8 to 12 weeks). Ultrasound may identify an IUP with fluid in the cul-de-sac; laparoscopy may be necessary to differentiate.

Endometriosis. Negative pregnancy test; pain usually associated with menstrual cycle.

Neoplastic

Ruptured Ovarian Cyst. Negative pregnancy test.

Vascular. Not applicable.

Congenital. Not applicable.

Acquired. Not applicable.

Other

Spontaneous Abortion. Os open to ring forceps, unlike ectopic bleeding with a closed os.

Adnexal Torsion. Seen on visual inspection of the tubes; must be reduced surgically.

TREATMENT

Medical. Improved detection expedites the delivery of care and allows for a greater degree of treatment options, ranging from traditional surgical approach to the more recent nonsurgical remedies. For those patients in need of acute care, serial examinations may not be possible. In such emergencies, a rapid urine test followed by transvaginal ultrasound establishes the diagnosis. The traditionally catastrophic presentation of a ruptured ectopic gestation and hemoperitoneum is no longer common. The diagnosis of the ectopic pregnancy is usually made prior to a rupture, while the patient is hemodynamically stable. Accordingly, treatment has shifted from immediate, life-threatening intervention to conservative methods, directed at preserving fertility and reducing morbidity. Repeat ectopic rates are similar comparing radical and conservative management. However, IUP rates seem to be higher after conservative tubal surgery. Thus, the patient's desire for future fertility should play a major role in management decisions. For women not desiring future fertility, a salpingectomy is performed. The goal of conservative management is removal of the products of conception while inflicting as little damage as possible to the involved tube. This can be attempted surgically or nonsurgically.

Methotrexate, a folic acid antagonist that interferes with DNA synthesis, has a long history of effectiveness in the treatment of trophoblastic disease. Considerable experience with its use in the treatment of tubal gestation now exists and the value of using methotrexate in the early treatment of persistent ectopic pregnancy is being realized. Methotrexate is a promising modality in properly identified patients. After administration, there should be a 15% decrease in the quantitative βhCG from day 4 to day 7. In the event of no such decrease, treatment may be repeated. Approximately one third of patients require a second cycle. Presently, there are no available studies where methotrexate has been used beyond a second cycle. If properly administered, methotrexate is 95% successful.

Multidose or single-dose methotrexate in most commonly used intramuscularly at a dose of 50 mg/m^2. Side effects include dermatitis, stomatitis, gastritis, liver enzyme elevations, bone marrow suppression, and pleuritis. Contraindications include active liver or renal disease, tubal rupture, positive fetal cardiac activity per ultrasound, or if the βhCG is greater than 5000 mIU/mL.

Surgical. Surgery remains the treatment method of choice and surgical technique is determined by various considerations:
- Condition of the tube (ruptured or unruptured)
- Location of the gestation within the tube (interstitium, isthmus, ampulla)
- Size of gestation
- Accessibility (presence of adhesions)
- Complications (e.g., bleeding)

Orthostatic blood pressure and pulse (to evaluate volume status) should be documented prior to surgery. Blood typing and cross match is performed for ruptured ectopic pregnancies (fluid in the abdomen on ultrasound). For those who have not ruptured, typing and screening is sufficient. It is important to follow the quantitative βhCG to zero postoperatively to confirm removal of all trophoblastic tissue.

The surgeon can choose to perform one of the following procedures using the laparotomy or laparoscopy approach.

Linear Salpingostomy. The procedure of choice for treatment on unruptured isthmic or ampullary gestation in patients who desire future fertility. Subsequent conception rate is about 60%, versus 40% after salpingectomy. Recurrent ectopic rate is about 13%.

Segmental Resection. Recommended for treatment of ruptured isthmic or ampullary gestation, especially when the contralateral tube is irreversibly damaged or absent. Reanastomosis of the proximal and distal segments can be performed when the tissues are less edematous.

Salpingectomy. Should only be performed if future fertility is not desired or the tube cannot be salvaged.

Another conservative surgical method, fimbrial expression or milking, consists of evacuation of a distal ampullary or fimbrial gestation by either digital expression or suction through the infundibular end of the tube. This technique has been associated with continued bleeding from the implantation site and high rates of recurrent ectopic gestation. Whenever a patient is treated with conservative surgery, she should be monitored postoperatively with serial hCG titers every 3 days until the levels are below the sensitivity of the assay to ensure the absence of trophoblastic tissue. An increase in serum hCG after an initial decline is highly suggestive of a persistent ectopic pregnancy. Management of this condition should be based on hCG levels, patient symptoms, and the surgeon's experience.

TECHNIQUE OF SURGICAL ASSISTING

One or two assistants may be required. Usually a camera port is placed at the umbilicus and two to three other ports for operating. A uterine manipulator is placed through the cervix to "drive" the uterus. Assistants may be used for "driving" the uterus, holding the tubes through an operating port, aiming the camera, and for irrigation, etc. Closing the ports with appropriate material is also a role of the assistant.

PEDIATRIC CONSIDERATIONS

Not applicable.

OBSTETRICAL CONSIDERATIONS

Not otherwise applicable.

PEARLS FOR THE PA

Ectopic pregnancy is the great masquerader, so always test hCG.

A rapid urine test followed by transvaginal ultrasound establishes the diagnosis.

Methotrexate is effective in the treatment of trophoblastic disease.

Endometriosis
Deborah E. Murray, PA-C, BS

DEFINITION

Endometrial tissue that occurs outside of the normal intrauterine location.

HISTORY

Symptoms.   Dysmenorrhea, acute and chronic pelvic pain, abnormal uterine bleeding, and dyspareunia.

General.   Dyspareunia may result from involvement of the uterosacral ligaments, cul-de-sac, and fornices.

Age. Most common in nulliparous women between the ages of 25 and 45 years. Not found in the prepubescent or postmenopausal periods.

Onset. Gradual.

Duration. Until treatment intervenes or menopause occurs.

Intensity. Dysmenorrhea can be severe. Symptoms are worse in nulliparous, older individuals.

Aggravating Factors. Menses, nulliparity, or delaying pregnancy until later in reproductive life.

Alleviating Factors. Pregnancy, hormonal or surgical intervention, and menopause.

Associated Factors. The combination of ovarian dysfunction and adhesions may cause infertility.

PHYSICAL EXAMINATION

General. Patient may appear in moderate distress secondary to pelvic pain.

Gynecologic. Rectovaginal examination is essential. Findings include nodules in the cul-de-sac, posterior fornix, and uterosacral ligament, and fixed retroversion of the uterus.

PATHOPHYSIOLOGY

Endometriosis is comprised of both gland and stroma. Lesions may grossly represent powder burns on the serosal or peritoneal surfaces. Endometriosis forms secondary to retrograde menstruation, causing implantation of endometrial tissue on the ovaries and perineum. A retrograde uterus may predispose to retrograde menses. The endometriotic tissue is responsive to the hormones of the menstrual cycle, thereby causing bleeding and increased symptoms during menstruation.

DIAGNOSTIC STUDIES

Laboratory data are not diagnostic for endometriosis.

Laboratory

WBC and Erythrocyte Sedimentation Rate. Normal values suggest endometriosis rather than PID.

Radiology

Barium Enema. As indicated to rule out a gastrointestinal source.

Intravenous Pyelogram. As indicated to rule out a renal source.

Other

Laparoscopy/Laparotomy. To provide definitive diagnosis.

Cystoscopy. Is performed if symptoms warrant.

DIFFERENTIAL DIAGNOSIS

Traumatic. Not applicable.
Infectious
Pelvic Inflammatory Disease. Elevated WBC and sedimentation rate distinguish from endometriosis.
Pelvic TB. Obtain TB skin test and thorough history of exposure.
Metabolic. Not applicable.
Neoplastic
Ovarian, Rectal or Sigmoid Neoplasms. Ovarian cancer is usually painless. Sigmoidoscopy rules out rectosigmoid cancer.
Vascular. Not applicable.
Congenital. Not applicable.
Acquired
Pelvic Congestion Syndrome. Pelvic examination under anesthesia helps differentiate. In endometriosis, the thickening and nodularity of the uterosacral ligaments and fornices do not decrease or disappear.

TREATMENT

Medical. Treatment is influenced by the patient's age and parity. The three methods of treatment include conservative, hormonal, and surgical. Conservative treatment includes reassurance and analgesics. Pregnancy can be curative. Hormonal treatment alone should be reserved for patients in whom a histological diagnosis of endometriosis has been confirmed or who refuse operations. The mainstay of therapy is oral contraceptives (the progesterones cause a pseudopregnancy, thereby causing atrophy of the endometrial glands and decreasing the symptomatology). Danazol and gonadotrophic-releasing hormone agonists are also effective. These do not cause a pseudopregnancy like the progestins; instead, they produce a pseudomenopause.

Surgical. Surgery may be conservative, in the form of laparoscopy and laser ablation of the implants, or more aggressive, with laparotomy and sharp dissection that may be indicated for those with larger implants. Postoperatively, the patient can be treated medically with oral contraceptives or may opt to become pregnant. If the patient has completed her family, bilateral tubal ligation may halt progression of the disease in that it prevents retrograde flow of menstrual fluid through the fallopian tubes into the pelvic cavity. Total abdominal hysterectomy and bilateral salpingo-oophorectomy should be an option only in those who fail all other treatment and have completed their family.

Indications. For ablation of implants. More aggressive management is reserved for those who have failed medical management, infertility (or desire infertility), or have an ovarian mass greater than 5 cm.

Contraindications. None.

TECHNIQUE FOR SURGICAL ASSISTING

Assist in opening and closing, hemostasis, adequate exposure with retraction, and pre- and postoperative care.

PEDIATRIC CONSIDERATIONS

Not present in the prepubertal age group. Endometriosis in the teen years should be treated conservatively unless complications arise.

OBSTETRICAL CONSIDERATIONS

Pregnancy regresses the endometriosis. Patients with adhesions from endometriosis are more prone to develop tubal pregnancies.

PEARLS FOR THE PA

Endometriosis presents with dysmenorrhea, which is progressive until treated.

It is most common in the nulliparous woman between the ages of 30 and 40 years.

Ovarian Cancer
Deborah E. Murray, PA-C, BS

DEFINITION

Malignant neoplasm of the ovary, most commonly epithelial in origin. Has highest mortality rate of all female genital tract cancers.

HISTORY

Symptoms. Vague abdominal discomfort, dyspepsia, urinary frequency, or asymptomatic.

General. The diagnosis is frequently not made until the patient presents with symptoms of advanced disease (increased abdominal girth, palpable pelvic and abdominal masses, ascites, and thrombophlebitis).

Age. All groups, but most common after age 50 years. A high index of suspension is warranted in premenarchal girls or postmenopausal women with pelvic mass.

Onset.   Can grow quickly and painlessly.

Intensity.   Normally mild. All ovarian tumors can cause severe pain secondary to torsion, infarction, or incarceration.

Aggravating Factors.   Nulliparity, infertility, and low parity may increase risk of developing epithelial tumors.

Alleviating Factors.   Early parity and oral contraceptives use reduce the risk of ovarian cancer.

Associated Factors.   Patients with two or more first-degree relatives with ovarian cancer are at higher risk. Twenty percent of ovarian tumors are metastatic, with primary sites being the breast, large intestine, and endometrium.

PHYSICAL EXAMINATION

General.   The patient may appear to be in no distress.

Breast.   Palpate for mass.

Gastrointestinal.   Measure abdominal girth. Palpate and percuss for omental mass and ascites.

Gynecologic.   Perform bimanual and rectovaginal examination for adnexal mass. If present, note whether mass is cystic, solid, unilateral, or bilateral (a solid mass suggests ovarian cancer). Note the size of the mass in centimeters.

Lymphatic.   Palpate for lymphadenopathy.

Pulmonary.   Auscultate for pleural effusion.

PATHOPHYSIOLOGY

Ovarian cancers are most commonly epithelial (80% to 90%), which is separated into serous, mucinous, endometrioid, undifferentiated, and clear cell types. The remainder arise from germ or stromal cells. Ovarian cancer grows locally, exfoliates, and then spreads, most frequently to the peritoneum, omentum, bowel surfaces, and retroperitoneal lymph nodes. Other more distant organs at risk are the breast, large intestine, endometrium, liver, lungs, pleura, kidney, bone, adrenals, bladder, and spleen.

DIAGNOSTIC STUDIES

Laboratory

CBC.   To evaluate for infection (elevated WBC) or anemia.

Chemistry Profile.   With emphasis on liver function tests that, if abnormal, suggest liver metastases.

Ca-125.   Is a surface protein found on ovarian cancer cells. The Food and Drug Administration (FDA) has limited its use to monitoring second-look surgery (surgery after a patient has undergone first-line de-bulking and chemotherapy and appears clinically free of disease) or as an aid to detect residual disease in those who have undergone first-line treatment. A normal value should not give a false sense of security. Ca-125 can be elevated in pregnancy, pelvic inflammatory disease (PID), and endometriosis.

Serologic Measurements of hCG. Performed as indicated to rule out intrauterine or ectopic pregnancy.

Radiology

Chest X-ray. To rule out pulmonary metastases.

CT—Abdomen, Pelvis, and Chest. As metastatic screening.

Intravenous Pyelogram. To rule out ureter and kidney involvement.

Lymphangiography. Positive in 30% of patients with ovarian cancer.

Proctoscopy—Upper/Lower GI Series. May be indicated, depending on the patient's symptoms.

Other

Laparoscopy. Used for definitive diagnosis, staging, and tumor de-bulking.

DIFFERENTIAL DIAGNOSIS

Traumatic. Not applicable.

Infectious

Tubo-ovarian Abscess. Presents with fever and bilateral low abdominal pain, whereas ovarian cancer is usually painless or with vague complaints.

Pelvic Inflammatory Disease. Presents with fever and bilateral low abdominal pain, whereas ovarian cancer is usually painless or with vague complaints.

Pelvic Tuberculosis (TB). Perform TB skin test and obtain a thorough history of exposure.

Metabolic

Functional Ovarian Cyst. Perform ultrasound, pelvic examination, and recheck after next menstrual cycle to make certain that the cyst has resolved.

Diverticulosis. Perform pelvic examination and ultrasound to rule out adnexal mass.

Endometriosis. Pain usually associated with menstrual cycle.

Ovarian Cancer. Usually asymptomatic.

Neoplastic

Rectal or Sigmoid Cancer. Differentiated with proctosigmoidoscopy and biopsy.

Uterine Myoma. The lesion most commonly confused with solid tumors of the ovary. After the pelvic mass reaches 12-week gestational size, the tumor has risen above the pelvic brim and the ovaries can no longer be palpated. At this point, ultrasound may be helpful for differentiation.

Vascular

Hemorrhagic Corpus Luteum Cyst. Presents with moderate to severe pelvic pain and pain on cervical motion. Ovarian cancer symptoms are usually mild or absent.

Congenital

Pelvic Kidney. Pelvic examination and ultrasound differentiate from ovarian cancer.

Acquired

Pregnancy or Ectopic Pregnancy. Positive serum pregnancy test and physical signs of pregnancy.

TREATMENT

Medical. Chemotherapeutic alkylating agents have been used most often in treating ovarian cancer. Other drugs include carboplatin, cisplatin, doxorubicin, hexamethylmelamine, and paclitaxel (Taxol). Single-agent and combination chemotherapy may be used. Intraperitoneal chemotherapy provides a high volume of agent to the confines of the ovaries and provides a better response rate for those with minimal disease, rather than those with more diffuse disease. Radiotherapy is usually reserved as an adjunct to surgery, for inoperable tumors, in patients unresponsive to chemotherapy, for persistent disease after primary treatment, or for palliative treatment.

Surgical. Surgery is an integral part of managing patients with ovarian cancer; therefore one should refer to a gynecologic oncologist who has extensive training in cytoreductive surgery. Maximum surgical effort should be performed during the operative procedure for staging ovarian cancer. Through maximum surgical effort, the patient is provided the best survival rate.

Upon opening the abdominal/pelvic cavity, ascites is identified, removed, and sent for cytologic evaluation. If no peritoneal fluid is present, 100 to 125 mL of normal saline is injected into the pelvic cavity, admixed in the pelvis, withdrawn with a syringe, and sent for cytology. Transabdominal hysterectomy and bilateral oophorectomy (TAH-BSO) is then performed, followed by examination of the pelvic peritoneum, paracolic gutters, omentum, both diaphragms, the spleen, and the liver. All abnormal tissue is removed as completely as possible. The large and small bowel are inspected and all lesions are removed or biopsied. The pelvic and para-aortic lymph nodes are sampled. For stage II and higher disease, surgery is followed by chemotherapy. If the patient is clinically free of disease at the end of chemotherapy, a second-look laparotomy is performed. The same procedures are followed in the second-look procedure, as well as lysing all adhesions and sending portions for pathology analysis.

Indications. Surgical exploration is indicated for all solid and bilateral adnexal masses and all masses greater than 5 cm in diameter. Also, the postmenopausal woman and premenarchal girl with adnexal mass should undergo surgery.

Contraindications. Chemotherapy and radiotherapy are given to patients unable to undergo surgery (e.g., poor medical condition and coagulopathy).

TECHNIQUE OF SURGICAL ASSISTING

Assist in opening and closing, hemostasis, adequate exposure through retraction, and pre- and postoperative care.

PEDIATRIC CONSIDERATIONS

Most ovarian neoplasms in children are of germ cell origin, the most common being the benign teratoma. Malignant ovarian tumors occurring in children include malignant teratomas, mixed germinal tumors, stromal cell tumors (Sertoli-Leydig type), embryonal carcinoma, polyembryoma, and choriocarcinoma. Treatment consists of surgery and chemotherapy.

OBSTETRICAL CONSIDERATIONS

Ovarian cancer is most common after age 50 years; therefore, it is quite rare in pregnancy. If there is a high index of suspicion, the patient should undergo laparotomy (early in the second trimester if possible). If a malignancy is found, the surgeon must properly stage the patient's disease. In younger patients, one would expect to find germ cell tumors, which are usually benign. As the patient approaches age 40 years, epithelial cancers are more common. Dysgerminoma and cystadenoma are the most common ovarian neoplasms observed in pregnancy.

PEARLS FOR THE PA

Ovarian cancer is frequently asymptomatic in the early stages of disease.

A solid, adnexal mass suggests ovarian cancer.

Distant organs at risk for metastases are the breast, large intestine, endometrium, liver, lungs, pleura, kidney, bone, adrenals, bladder, and spleen.

Pelvic Organ Prolapse
Paul Taylor, PA-C, BS

DEFINITION

Defective pelvic support, allowing the vagina, uterus, and adjacent organs to descend below normal positions (Fig. 5–1). Historically, prolapse has been named according to the organ lying next to that part of the vagina which has prolapsed. This terminology may incorrectly imply that there is an anomaly of the adjacent organ. Prolapse is actually a problem of vaginal and uterine support.

Urethrocele, Cystocele, Cystourethrocele. The urethra is approximately 4 cm long and fused to the lower 4 cm of the anterior vaginal wall. Descent of this portion of the vaginal is termed urethrocele. The bladder lies adjacent to the remaining portion of the anterior vaginal wall above the ureterovesical junction. Loss of support in this region is termed cystocele. A

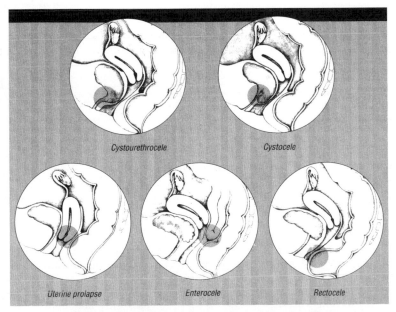

Cystourethrocele *Cystocele*

Uterine prolapse *Enterocele* *Rectocele*

Figure 5–1. Anatomy of pelvic organ prolapse. (From American College of Obstetricians and Gynecologists: Pelvic Support Problems. Patient Education Pamphlet No. APO 12. Washington, DC, © ACOG, April 1995.)

cystourethrocele occurs when support in the anterior vaginal wall is defective in both areas. Isolated urethroceles are rare.

Uterine Prolapse. Usually classified by describing the degree of descent of the uterine cervix when the patient strains.

Enterocele. The peritoneal fold (cul-de-sac or pouch of Douglas) extends approximately 3 cm below the junction of the posterior vaginal wall and the uterine cervix. This is the area in which an enterocele develops. A true enterocele is often referred to as a pulsion enterocele because it is filled with bowel and is distended by abdominal pressure.

Rectocele. This develops when the rectovaginal fascia (posterior vaginal wall) can no longer restrain the rectum in the normal position.

Procidentia. When the vagina and uterine cervix extend completely outside the body.

HISTORY

Symptoms. Anterior wall prolapse can lead to both stress incontinence and voiding difficulties. Stress incontinence is due to the lack of support at the bladder base, which results in a funnel effect on the urethra. Symptoms of incomplete bladder emptying are probably most common in patients who void by straining, which increases abdominal pressure to order force urine out of the bladder. This increasing abdominal pressure distends the cystocele, which becomes larger, and results in functional outlet obstruction as the urethra is compressed, resulting in prolonged voiding and an intermittent stream. In addition to these symptoms, many patients complain of urinary urgency and frequency.

The cardinal symptom of rectocele is difficulty in emptying the rectum. With a rectocele, straining leads to stool being pushed into the rectocele, and the harder the strain, the larger the rectocele becomes. Constipation is common in older women and may be due to a variety of causes, most of which have nothing to do with prolapse.

There are few symptoms related specifically to prolapse of the uterus, the vaginal apex, or to the formation of an enterocele. These patients usually complain of an uncomfortable bulge and/or urinary urgency and frequency and low back pain.

General. Most patients describe an underlying sense of pelvis insecurity that is difficult to describe.

Age. Women of childbearing age.

Duration. Symptoms usually worsen throughout the day as the prolapse is reduced from the previous night's bedrest. Ligaments and fascia stretch with gravitational pull on the structures above the vagina.

Intensity. Varies with the degree of prolapse.

Onset. Gradual.

Aggravating Factors. Anything that increases intra-abdominal pressure (e.g., coughing, straining, and lifting). Activities that may apply direct pressure to the supporting structures of the vagina (e.g., jogging, jumping on a trampoline).

Alleviating Factors. Lying down or sitting in a reclined position.

Associated Factors. The number of vaginal deliveries, obesity, prior hysterectomy, aging, chronic cough, obstructive pulmonary disease. Caucasian women are affected more than African-American women for unknown reasons.

PHYSICAL EXAMINATION

General. The patient may present in a very ordinary fashion. Patients with severe prolapse may sit down slowly in order to avoid compressing the prolapse.

Gynecologic. A number of clinical classification systems have been developed to describe the severity of prolapse. Until a formal system for the classification of prolapse has been agreed upon and comes into general use, the clearest method is probably descriptive (Table 5–2). The prolapse may be described simply by noting the position of the cervix (or bulge) in relation to the plane of the hymenal ring. The position that the bulge reaches during maximal straining can be estimated in centimeters above or below this point of reference (hymenal ring).

For example, a uterine prolapse could be described by noting that the cervix is descended 2 cm below the hymenal ring during straining. A similar assessment of a cystocele could be made by noting the location of the urethrovesical junction and the relative positions of the bladder and urethra.

The diagnosis of genital prolapse is made on physical examination. There are two fundamental points that must be made regarding the examination of patients with prolapse: the examination must be made with the patient straining forcefully enough to demonstrate the prolapse as its largest extent, and the clinician must examine each element of support independently.

Assessment is greatly aided by the routine use of a Sims vaginal speculum or by the posterior blade of an ordinary Graves speculum. This can be used to retract either the anterior or posterior wall while the other wall is being inspected. Having the patient cough or bear down while the speculum is positioned in the posterior vagina aids in the observation of bladder neck mobility and may facilitate the demonstration of stress incontinence. The importance of examining patients in the upright as well as the dorsal lithotomy position should also be emphasized. The right foot should be placed on a small stool or the footstep of the examining table

Table 5–2. Grading of Urogenital Prolapse

Above the hymenal ring: Probably not significant
At the hymenal ring: Borderline clinical significance
Below the hymenal ring: Clinically significant

and a vaginal examination should be carried out with the patient standing. A cystocele, rectocele, or uterine descent is often much more pronounced in this position than when the patient is lying down. The use of a thumb in the vagina with a forefinger in the rectum also allows a much better examination for the presence of an enterocele. Only those patients who complain of urinary incontinence should be examined with a full bladder and stress leaks noted.

Q-tip Test. Used to assess bladder neck mobility. The angle of the Q-tip in relationship to the horizontal can be measured using an orthopedic goniometer. A sterile, lubricated Q-tip is placed in the urethra and the resting and straining measurements are made. An upward movement of more than 30 degrees may be considered hypermobile.

PATHOPHYSIOLOGY

Vaginal birth is probably the most significant factor in the development of pelvic organ prolapse. Tissue trauma from the passage of the large human head through the female pelvis is presumably the common pathway linking prolapse and urinary incontinence. Avulsion of connective tissue from its normal attachments, neuromuscular damage, and alterations in the geometry of the pelvis are probably all important in the genesis of these problems.

Once the vagina has prolapsed below the introitus, it is the only structural layer separating the high pressure inside the abdomen from the much lower atmospheric pressure. Downward force created by this pressure differential puts immense tension on the supporting ligaments and fascia. This results in a dragging feeling noticed where the tissues connect to the pelvis sidewall (described as pressure in the groin) and a sacral backache caused by traction on the uterosacral ligaments. Exposure of the moist vaginal walls may lead to a sensation of wetness that the patient may confuse with urinary incontinence. This may also lead to ulceration of the vaginal wall.

DIAGNOSTIC STUDIES

The diagnosis of pelvic organ prolapse is made on physical examination.

Laboratory

Urinalysis and Culture and Sensitivity (C&S). To rule out concurrent UTI.

Radiology

CT Scan or Ultrasound. If there is a suspicion of a large pelvic or abdominal tumor.

DIFFERENTIAL DIAGNOSIS

Traumatic. Not applicable.
Infectious. Not applicable.
Metabolic. Not applicable.

Neoplastic

Pelvic or Abdominal Neoplasm.   Differentiated on physical examination and/or CT and ultrasound.

Vascular.   Not applicable.

Congenital

Pelvic Musculature Abnormalities.   May cause prolapse.

Acquired.   Not applicable.

TREATMENT

Medical.   Pelvic organ prolapse often exacerbates incontinence in elderly women. If the pelvic relaxation is symptomatic, a pessary may relieve symptoms without resorting to surgery. The pessary should be chosen so that it does not compromise bowel or bladder emptying. Some trial and error may be necessary to find the appropriate pessary. Cube pessaries are attractive because they tend not to compress the bowel or bladder. However, because these are held in place by suction effect, the cube may erode the vaginal mucosa if it is not removed daily. Gellhorn and ring or "doughnut" pessaries may compress bowel or bladder, but once fitted properly may be left in place for up to 3 months without removal. Only those women who do not suffer from atrophic vaginitis are candidates for pessary use. Estrogen vaginal cream is used concurrently with pessaries.

Surgical.   Age alone should not be the major reason for rejecting any given mode of therapy. Discussion of the quality of life with the patient and family, expected level of activity, and priority of symptoms will help individualize the management of prolapse. Furthermore, the associated factors that led to the prolapse will be contributory to recurrence (e.g., delay treatment until childbearing is completed prior to surgical repair of a cystocele or rectocele). Weight loss not only reduces the recurrence rate but improves surgical outcomes prior to surgery. Types of surgery performed for prolapse depend on the surgeon's skill and preference. The presence of stress incontinence also influences the type of procedure performed. If the prolapse operation is to be done vaginally, the needle suspension (e.g., Pereyra, Stamey) often provides additional urethral support. The simple anterior or posterior colporrhaphy may be all that is necessary for cystocele or rectocele repairs without incontinence.

Hysterectomy is the treatment of choice for symptomatic uterine prolapse. If a patient who wishes future childbearing decides to proceed with surgery, uterine support must be addressed. Imperfect uterine support may be improved by shortening the uterosacral ligaments and reattaching them to the back of the cervix. The Moschcowitz culdoplasty and the Halban culdoplasty obliterate the cul-de-sac, which prevents the formation of an enterocele. It is possible that hysterectomy can damage some elements important to pelvic support and that, over time, this may lead to the development of incontinence and prolapse. What is more likely, however, is that some patients who have had a hysterectomy for symptomatic pelvis relaxation without stress incontinence have gradually developed symptoms as a manifestation of the underlying problem for which they had their original surgery.

Indications. Symptomatic pelvic organ prolapse, failure of conservative treatment.

Contraindications. Desire for fertility (with certain procedures), inability to tolerate anesthesia.

TECHNIQUE OF SURGICAL ASSISTING

The assistant is used depending on the procedure and approach (abdominal or vaginal). A patient with a cystocele may be obese, which can make the procedure very technically difficult; therefore, exposure is crucial. Suction and countertraction are important. If the PA is tying the suspension sutures, be careful not to tie too tightly because it subsequently may cause postoperative urinary retention. A suprapubic tube may be left in place postoperatively to rest the bladder. The patient may require teaching for self-catheterization until she can void completely on her own. Self-catheterization is usually performed after attempting to void (with post-void residual measured) and is done three to five times a day.

PEDIATRIC CONSIDERATIONS

Not applicable.

OBSTETRICAL CONSIDERATIONS

Controlled deliveries and immediate repair of tears lessen the chance of developing significant pelvic organ prolapse.

PEARLS FOR THE PA

Regardless of the nomenclature, prolapse is a disorder of vaginal and uterine support.

Prolapse may be associated with voiding difficulties.

Vaginal birth is probably the most significant factor in the development of pelvic organ prolapse.

Urinary Incontinence
Paul Taylor, PA-C, BS

DEFINITION

The involuntary loss of urine, which may be due to increased abdominal pressure in the absence of detrusor activity (genuine stress incontinence [GSI]), the urge to void without a rise in abdominal pressure (detrusor instability [DI]), the continuous leakage of urine (bypass incontinence), or the result of incomplete voiding with overflow occurring from bladder distention (overflow incontinence). Accurate diagnosis of each of these conditions is crucial, because treatment for each is different.

HISTORY

Symptoms.   Clinical symptoms of GSI are usually consistent with leakage related to an increase in intra-abdominal pressure (e.g., cough, sneeze, lifting, or exercising). DI, bypass, and overflow incontinence may present with clinical symptoms of continued leakage, frequent nocturia, incomplete emptying, and a strong desire to void that cannot be suppressed.

General.   Histories in patients complaining of incontinence tend to be very misleading. Bladder diaries have been proven to be useful in documenting leakage episodes, frequency, nocturia, urgency, and 24-hour urine volumes.

PHYSICAL EXAMINATION

General.   The patient may be in no acute distress. There may be an odor of urine present; the patient may wear protective undergarments or dark clothing if leakage is a recurrent problem.

Gynecologic.   A Sims speculum can be used to examine the vaginal walls and to visualize a cystocele or urethrocele. Anterior wall defects can be a major clinical finding in evaluating a patient whose chief complaint is GSI. Additionally, atrophy and decreased muscle strength (levator ani muscle) and a hypermobile urethra contribute to the suspicion of GSI. Levator ani strength is tested by placing one or two fingers into the vagina and asking the patient to squeeze. The strength of the squeeze is graded at 1 (weak) to 5 (strong).

Neurologic.   Evaluate S2–S4 (lower micturition center), because urinary incontinence may be secondary to central nervous system lesions. The sensation of the inner thighs, perirectal, and vulvar areas should be tested. Testing the bulbocavernosus reflex (a gentle tap to the clitoris) should result in refectory contractions of the perirectal muscles. This represents the motor component of S2–S4.

PATHOPHYSIOLOGY

Up to 30% of older women are affected by urinary incontinence to some extent. Even a moderate degree of incontinence can interfere considerably with normal daily activities. Urinary incontinence is caused by lowered urethral resistance, inappropriate elevation in bladder pressure, or when urethral resistance is anatomically bypassed.

Urinary tract infections (UTIs) can simulate any lower urinary tract pathology. Diagnosis of incontinence established at the time of an undiagnosed UTI is inaccurate in 50% of patients. *Chlamydia* urethritis and interstitial cystitis may also contribute.

DIAGNOSTIC STUDIES

Laboratory
Urinalysis with Culture and Sensitivity.   The initial evaluation of all incontinence should begin with this study to rule out UTIs. If RBCs are present, urine should be sent for cytology.

CBC.   If a urinary tract infection is suspected.

BUN/Creatinine.   To rule out primary renal pathology.

Radiology
Intravenous Pyelography (IVP).   May be performed for recurrent UTIs and to evaluate for urinary tract pathology.

Other
Cystourethroscopy.   This procedure is performed under topical anesthesia, despite the potential effects on normal urethral function. The bladder and trigone are examined for gross pathology. The urethrovesical junction (UVJ) is examined while the patient is asked to hold urine, at which time the UVJ should be closed. If the patient has GSI, the UVJ funnels open. The urethroscope is slowly withdrawn, allowing a thorough examination for diverticula (which can simulate GSI) or exudate, and to evaluate urethral coaptation. Urethritis may simulate detrusor instability.

Q-tip Test.   A sterile Q-tip lubricated with K-Y jelly is introduced into the urethra and advanced to the UVJ. The resting and straining angles of the Q-tip to the horizontal are measured with a goniometer. A change of more than 35% is consistent with poor support of the UVJ. A negative test should rule out the diagnosis of poor UVJ support or hypermobility of the bladder neck.

Cotton Ball Test.   Cotton balls or a large tampon are inserted into the vagina. A Foley catheter is then placed and the bladder is filled to capacity with sterile water to which methylene blue dye has been added. The patient then ambulates, walks up and down stairs, sits, squats, coughs, and voids after 30 minutes. Special care is taken upon the removal of the vaginal pack to identify the location of any leakage (fistula). Vesicovaginal, urethrovaginal, and ureterovaginal fistulas may be diagnosed based on the location (upper, middle, or lower vagina) of the stain.

Multichannel Cystometrics/Urodynamics. Used to record concomitant pressures in the bladder, urethra, and abdomen (established by either vaginal or rectal pressure line) while filling the bladder. Additionally, a urethral pressure profile (UPP) measures the functional length and closure pressure at the UVJ. The patient may then void with pressure lines in place to determine the presence of a voiding dysfunction.

DIFFERENTIAL DIAGNOSIS

Traumatic. Not applicable.
Infectious
Urinary Tract Infection. Positive urinalysis and culture and sensitivity.
Chlamydial Urethritis. Presents with a urethral discharge; positive chlamydial culture.
Metabolic. Not applicable.
Neoplastic
Bladder Tumor. Positive urine cytology and imaging studies (e.g., IVP).
Vascular. Not applicable.
Congenital. Not applicable.
Acquired. Not applicable.

TREATMENT

Medical
GSI. The effectiveness is dependent on the presence of minimal GSI with high degrees of stress. Direct application of estrogen vaginal cream in addition to oral replacement has been proven to be effective. The use of estrogen for the atrophic urethra causes thickening of the mucosa and engorgement of the blood vessels beneath. This results in an increase of urethral pressure.

Kegel exercises promote hypertrophy and thickening of the striated periurethral muscle wall. The patient should tighten the pubococcygeal muscle 20 to 30 times a day. After 3 to 4 months of exercise, many patients report a 50% decrease in leakage.

Vaginal pessaries support the bladder base and restore the urethra to a normal anatomic position. Several types of pessaries are available to ensure the best fit. Care must be taken to ensure that the vagina is estrogenized; frequent examinations for lacerations or evidence of ulceration are necessary.

Periurethral collagen injections are a good option for nonsurgical candidates or surgical failures. This procedure is relatively simple, has a low morbidity, and can be performed on an outpatient basis. It can also be repeated as needed. Patients must have a immobile bladder neck in order for collagen to be successful.

DI. The combination of two therapies resolves more than 90% of the urge incontinence symptoms associated with DI. These include anticholinergic drugs, such as oxybutynin chloride (Ditropan) and imipramine, for up to 6 months and behavior modification techniques (e.g., bladder drills and biofeedback) to regain inhibitory control over the bladder.

Bypass Incontinence. Treatment is surgical.

Overflow Incontinence. May be due to a hypotonic bladder or scarred urethra. Hypotonicity may be treated medically with flavoxate HCl (Urispas) or bethanechol chloride (Urecholine) to achieve more complete emptying.

Surgical

GSI. The primary treatment should be surgical, either abdominally or vaginally, to correct the anatomic defect. The goal of surgery is to relocate the proximal urethra, support the bladder base, and increase the tension of the periurethral striated muscle. Although the majority of women who suffer from urinary incontinence are beyond their fertile years, a small portion may desire future fertility. The success rate of the first surgery for GSI is the highest. Subsequent pregnancy potentially will destroy the repaired anatomy. This does not mean that the desire for future fertility would prevent surgical repair. However, a conservative approach may be more appropriate in this instance.

Marshall-Marchetti-Krantz. Is performed retropubically using sutures placed between the periurethral tissue and periosteum of the symphysis pubis. Long-term results range from 85% to 89%.

Burch Colposuspension. Is also a retropubic approach; the full thickness of the perivesical vaginal wall is sutured to Cooper's ligaments. This procedure offers one of the highest degrees of patient satisfaction after 5 years (89% to 93%).

Transvaginal Needle Suspension. Has the advantage of requiring a shorter hospital stay and allowing simultaneous correction of the cystocele, enterocele, and rectocele. There are many modifications to the transvaginal needle suspension. These procedures have a success range of 61% to 94%.

Sling Cystourethropexy. Is the procedure to treat incontinence due to pure intrinsic sphincter deficiency (ISD). The urethra is open at rest and in normal anatomic position. The sling may be created with the use of synthetic material, round ligament, or rectus fascia muscle. The goal is to compress the urethra while enjoying a high degree of continence. Complications may include erosion into the urethra and a sling so tight that self-catheterization may be necessary in order for the patient to void.

DI. Treatment is primarily nonsurgical.

Bypass Incontinence. The fistula is identified with the cotton ball test (see diagnostic studies) and closed.

Overflow Incontinence. Urethral dilatation is necessary to relieve scarring.

Indications. Continued symptoms despite conservative treatment; anatomical defect.

Contraindications. Inability to tolerate anesthesia.

TECHNIQUE OF SURGICAL ASSISTING

Depending upon the type of surgery performed, the PA assists with hemostasis, closure of the defect, retraction, and support of the structures to be repaired.

PEDIATRIC CONSIDERATIONS

Enuresis in children may indicate a psychiatric disorder, developmental delay, or regression. The family history may be positive for similar problems. Support, counseling, and avoidance of punishment for the behavior may be of benefit. If enuresis continues, psychiatric referral may be required.

OBSTETRICAL CONSIDERATIONS

There is no correlation to underlying stress postpartum. There is a high incidence of fistulas (bypass incontinence) in third world countries due to uncontrolled deliveries.

PEARLS FOR THE PA

For DI, Ditropan and Imipramine may be used in open-angle glaucoma patients (open is OK). Normally, anticholinergics are not recommended for glaucoma patients with increased intraocular pressure.

A pessary is used preoperatively to reduce cystocele and urethrocele.

Ask the patient to stand and cough; if there is no leakage despite a history of incontinence, no work-up is necessary.

Uterine Cancer
Deborah E. Murray, PA-C, BS

DEFINITION

The most common cancer of the female pelvis. The most common cancer of the uterus is endometrial adenocarcinoma, of which early diagnosis of stage I (well-differentiated disease) provides an excellent prognosis. Uterine sarcomas account for 1% to 6% of uterine cancers and have a poor prognosis. Gestational trophoblastic disease, which is the most curable of all gynecologic malignancies, is discussed in the "Obstetrical Considerations" section.

HISTORY

Symptoms. The main symptoms are metrorrhagia (or postmenopausal bleeding in the older woman) and vaginal discharge.

General. Lesions in younger women tend to be less invasive and better differentiated, offering a better prognosis than lesions in older women.

Age. Primarily menopausal and postmenopausal women. Peak age is 55 years.

Onset. Endometrial adenocarcinoma remains localized in the endometrium for a prolonged period, and then may spread via the vascular route. Uterine sarcoma may cause rapid enlargement of the uterus.

Duration. Until diagnosis and appropriate treatment is instituted.

Intensity. Usually painless, unless advanced disease and metastasis is present.

Aggravating Factors. Unopposed estrogen, nulliparity, obesity, late menopause, polycystic ovary disease, and tamoxifen use.

Alleviating Factors. Addition of progesterone to regimen of hormone replacement therapy decreases the risk of uterine cancer.

Associated Factors. Hypertension, diabetes mellitus, arthritis, and hypothyroidism are common findings. Familial association does not appear to be strong.

PHYSICAL EXAMINATION

General. Patient may appear in no acute distress.

Breast. Palpate for sites of metastasis.

Gastrointestinal. Usually unremarkable. Palpate for masses.

Gynecologic. Observe for vaginal bleeding or masses extending through a dilated cervix (if present, suspect sarcoma). Bimanual examination may reveal enlarged uterus. Evaluate uterus for mobility, adnexa for masses, the parametrium for induration, and the cul-de-sac for nodularity. An endometrial aspiration biopsy may be performed in the office.

Lymphatic. Palpate all nodes with attention to the inguinal nodes.

Pulmonary. Auscultate for pleural effusion.

PATHOPHYSIOLOGY

Overall death rate is low due to early diagnosis and confinement to the uterus. Basically, the deeper the myometrial invasion and poorer the differentiation, the more adverse the prognosis. Endometrial adenocarcinoma is the most common uterine tumor, accounting for 80% of uterine cancers. It resembles normal endometrial glands. As the tissue becomes less differentiated, it becomes less vascular and has more atypia. Other less common types of endometrial carcinoma include mucinous, papillary serous, clear cell, squamous, undifferentiated, and mixed carcinoma.

Sarcoma of the corpus is much less common than endometrial carcinoma. Leiomyosarcoma is the most common of the sarcomas and arises from the uterine muscle. Endometrial sarcomas arise from the endometrial glands and stroma.

DIAGNOSTIC STUDIES

Laboratory
CBC.   To evaluate for infection (elevated WBC) or anemia.
Chemistry Profile.   With emphasis on liver function tests which, if abnormal, suggest liver metastases.
Radiology
Chest X-ray.   To rule out pulmonary metastases.
CT—Abdomen, Brain, Liver, and Bone Scans.   Performed as part of a full metastatic screen.
Intravenous Pyelogram (Optional).   If renal involvement is suspected.
Transvaginal Ultrasound.   May be helpful to evaluate for extrauterine involvement.
Other
Fractional Dilatation and Curettage (D&C).   Is the diagnostic procedure of choice for diagnosis.
Endometrial Aspiration Biopsy.   May be performed as indicated in the office setting.
Sigmoidoscopy and Barium Enema.   Performed if disease is palpated outside of the uterus.

DIFFERENTIAL DIAGNOSIS

Traumatic.   Not applicable.
Infectious.   Not applicable.
Metabolic
Benign Endometrial Hyperplasia.   Is usually caused by unopposed estrogen; diagnosed with endometrial biopsy.
Neoplastic
Carcinoma of the Cervix.   Differentiated through pelvic examination and biopsy. Usually presents with intermenstrual bleeding and postcoital bleeding.
Endometrial Polyps (Benign).   Are also common in postmenopausal women and present with vaginal bleeding; differentiated through fractional D&C.

Uterine Myomas. Tumors of the reproductive years, whereas uterine cancer is most common in postmenopausal years.

Vascular. Not applicable.

Congenital. Not applicable.

Acquired. Not applicable.

TREATMENT

Medical. Radiotherapy is used in high-risk, early-stage disease and in advanced disease. In patients with early, well-differentiated disease who wish to preserve fertility, irradiation has been used as a primary treatment. Intracavitary irradiation is used 4 to 6 weeks prior to hysterectomy to destroy superficial tumor and decrease the chance of metastasis. The most common systemic treatments for endometrial cancer are the progestogens (hydroxyprogesterone, medroxyprogesterone, and megestrol acetate). In stage III and IV disease, progestins have been used for palliation.

Surgical. Diagnosis is made by fractional D&C. This should be done before sounding the uterus to avoid contamination of the cervical sample. Total abdominal hysterectomy and bilateral salpingo-oophorectomy (TAH-BSO) is the treatment of choice for uterine cancer. Peritoneal fluid sampling should be obtained upon opening the peritoneal cavity. The para-aortic and pelvic lymph nodes should be sampled. Any large lymph nodes are removed and sent for histologic evaluation. Some authorities recommend frozen section for the depth of myometrial invasion and nodal sampling for grade I tumors with invasion over 50% or with cervical involvement.

Indications. TAH-BSO is indicated for most patients with uterine cancer unless preservation of fertility is desired in patients with early, well-differentiated disease.

Contraindications. Medically unsuitable patients with early disease may be treated with radiation therapy.

TECHNIQUE OF SURGICAL ASSISTING

Assist in opening and closing, hemostasis, adequate exposure with retraction, and pre- and postoperative care.

PEDIATRIC CONSIDERATIONS

None.

OBSTETRICAL CONSIDERATIONS

Endometrial carcinoma is extremely rare in pregnancy. It is usually focal and well-differentiated, with minimal or no invasion. TAH-BSO is the recommended therapy with adjunctive irradiation if indicated.

Gestational trophoblastic disease (GTN) is the most curable of all gynecologic malignancies and is preceded by molar pregnancy in 50% of cases. Diagnosis is made through an extremely high serum hCG titer and trophoblastic cells obtained on D&C sampling. Some patients have no localized disease in the uterus, only metastatic disease. Treatment involves close monitoring of the βhCG titer. Methotrexate is the chemotherapy of choice. If negative titers are not reached, the patient is switched to actinomycin D. The patient is considered in remission after three consecutive normal weekly βhCG titers. The βhCG titer should then be repeated bimonthly for at least 1 year. The patient must avoid pregnancy during this time, because a subsequent normal pregnancy cannot be differentiated from GTN by the βhCG determination. In those not desiring future fertility, hysterectomy may also be performed. Patients receiving both chemotherapy and hysterectomy go into remission sooner, receiving fewer doses of chemotherapy than those receiving chemotherapy alone.

PEARLS FOR THE PA

The overall mortality for endometrial cancer is low, because diagnosis is usually made early due to the warning symptoms of metrorrhagia or postmenopausal bleeding.

Further Readings

Berek JS: Novak's Gynecology, ed 12. Baltimore, Williams & Wilkins, 1996.

Devita VT, Hellman S, Rosenberg SA: Cancer: Principles and Practice of Oncology, ed 4. Philadelphia, J. B. Lippincott, 1993.

Hurt WG (ed): Urogynecologic Surgery. New York, Raven, 1992.

Speroff L, Glass RH, Kase NG (eds): Clinical Gynecologic Endocrinology and Infertility, ed 5. Baltimore, Williams & Wilkins, 1994.

Thompson JD, Rock JA. (eds): Tclinde's Operative Gynecology, ed 7. Philadelphia, J. B. Lippincott, 1992.

Wall LL, Norton PA, DeLancey JOL (eds): Practical Urogynecology. Baltimore, Williams & Wilkins, 1993.

Chapter 6

Head and Neck Surgery
Epistaxis
Carroll F. Poppen, PA-C

DEFINITION

Acute nasal hemorrhage.

HISTORY

Symptoms. Acute nasal hemorrhage can occur either spontaneously or after forceful nose blowing or trauma (e.g., nose picking or acute blunt trauma.)

General. Almost everyone has experienced a nose bleed at some time and most nose bleeds resolve without requiring medical attention. However, a nose bleed may be life threatening to those individuals with a bleeding disorder or who are old and debilitated.

Age. Any.

Onset. Usually spontaneous but may occur after trauma, Valsalva maneuver, or forceful nose blowing.

Duration. Usually resolves spontaneously within a few minutes.

Intensity. Can be severe and require nasal packing or transfusion.

Aggravating Factors. Atrophic nasal mucosa, systemic diseases that cause coagulopathies, foreign bodies, illicit drug use, or diseases involving the nasal tissue.

Alleviating Factors. Nasal constricting nose drops, local compression, and nasal packing.

Associated Factors. Bleeding disorders and medications that may affect the bleeding and clotting time.

PHYSICAL EXAMINATION

General. Patients usually have a normal general physical examination. May have evidence of easy bruising or findings of purpura, prominent and fragile vessels, and telangiectasia present on the tongue and fingers.

Head, Eyes, Ears, Nose, and Throat (HEENT). Patients may be actively bleeding from one or both nostrils, which may include anterior bleeding, posterior bleeding, or both. Crusts of blood and nasal clots may be present within the nasal cavity.

PATHOPHYSIOLOGY

The most common cause is a rupture of an anterior septal vessel, which accounts for approximately 90% of all nose bleeds; 10% of all nose bleeds occur from the posterior portion of the nose.

DIAGNOSTIC STUDIES

None may be required, depending on the history and physical findings.

Laboratory
PT/PTT, Bleeding/Clotting Time and Special Coagulopathy Studies.   May be required for recurrent or unremitting nose bleeds and in those in whom a coagulopathy is suspected.

Radiology
Computed Tomography (CT) or Magnetic Resonance Imaging (MRI) of the Base of the Skull.   Usually not required unless a nasal mass is suspected.

Other.   Not applicable.

DIFFERENTIAL DIAGNOSIS

Traumatic
Blunt Nasal Trauma.   Seen with behaviors such as nose picking. History reveals the cause.

Illicit Drug Use.   May be present on history or require a drug screen to expose.

Excessive Nasal Mucosal Dryness and Atrophy.   Excoriation of septum seen on physical examination.

Nasal Septal Perforation.   Seen on physical examination.

Traumatic Nasogastric or Nasal Tracheal Intubation.   History of recent intubation or attempted intubation.

Nasal Trauma.   History of trauma.

Infectious
Acute Upper Respiratory Infections.   Common symptoms of infection present. May be associated with prolonged nose blowing.

Tuberculosis (TB).   Positive TB test or chest x-ray.

Syphilis.   Positive Venereal Disease Research Laboratory (VDRL) test. Latent syphilis may initially cause a lesion followed by saddle deformity of the nasal septum.

Sarcoidosis.   Glistening or fish-scale appearance of the intranasal mucosa.

Acquired Immunodeficiency Syndrome (AIDS).   Human immunodeficiency virus (HIV) positive; more prone to epistaxis.

Wegener's Granulomatosis.   Physical findings of dry crusts of bloody mucus identified.

Metabolic
Bleeding Dyscrasia.   Multiple causes such as hemophilia, von Willebrand disease, clotting factor deficiencies, leukemia, thrombocytopenia, multiple myeloma, hereditary hemorrhagic telangiectasis, diabetes, hypertension, benign and malignant tumors, anticoagulant medications (e.g., aspirin, heparin, warfarin), alcoholism, liver disease, and chronic renal failure.

Neoplastic

Benign Tumors. Such as angiofibroma or inverting papilloma may present with or be associated with nosebleeds. CT/MRI should identify the lesion.

Malignant Tumors. Such as adenocarcinoma, esthesioneuroblastoma, lymphoma, melanoma, squamous cell carcinoma may present with or be associated with nosebleeds. CT/MRI should identify the lesion.

Vascular

Juvenile Angiofibroma. Is common in the adolescent male with nasal obstruction and epistaxis.

Congenital

Hereditary Hemorrhagic Telangiectasis (Osler-Weber-Rendu Disease). Associated with telangiectasia of the nasal septum and bleeding disorders.

Deviated Nasal Septum. Seen on physical examination.

Acquired

Foreign Body. Seen on physical examination.

TREATMENT

Medical. Approximately 80% to 90% of all nosebleeds can be controlled by direct application of pressure over the external nares. Vasoconstricting nose drops such as 1% Neo-Synephrine, Tyzine, oxymetazoline (Afrin), or cocaine solutions may be required in refractory cases.

Application of lubricating agents to the lining of the nose (e.g., saline nasal gel, K-Y jelly, Vaseline) may be beneficial.

Surgical. Several surgical options exist, depending on the severity and location of the bleeding. Often the use of an anesthetic agent and a vasoconstrictor (e.g., cocaine solutions) for control of hemorrhage with application of silver nitrate to the offending vessel will suffice. Electrocautery may be necessary, followed by nasal packing.

Indications. Uncontrolled bleeding despite usual medical treatment may include embolization, surgical reconstruction, or arterial ligation.

Contraindications. The patient's general health and extenuating medical conditions (i.e., pulmonary, cardiovascular, or liver disease).

Technique for Surgical Assisting. Proper visualization is a must. Nasal packing is usually required if oozing persists.

PEDIATRIC CONSIDERATIONS

Special attention to the amount of blood lost. Be suspicious of juvenile angiofibroma in teenage boys.

OBSTETRICAL CONSIDERATIONS

During pregnancy, thrombocytopenia may occur, especially if folic acid deficiency is present.

Facial/Sinus Fractures

William C. Perry, PA-C

DEFINITION

Fracture of the bones of the face, usually due to blunt trauma from a variety of causes (e.g., motor vehicle accident or assault).

HISTORY

Symptoms. Pain, tenderness, and swelling of the nose or face, external facial deformity with possible depressions or "step-offs," internal swelling of the nose with possible obstruction, septal hematoma, epistaxis, subcutaneous emphysema following nose blowing, subconjunctival hemorrhage, or paresthesias of the cheek.

General. The patient is usually able to give a history of the causative trauma. Suspicion should be raised when there is sufficient facial trauma in a unresponsive patient. Ask the patient if any clear, colorless drainage from the nose has been present, which could signify a cerebrospinal fluid (CSF) leak.

Age. All ages may be affected, but very young children have underdeveloped sinuses. A higher incidence of males than females, presumably due to the nature of the causative activity.

Onset. Acute, although symptoms may be initially unrecognized.

Duration. Facial/sinus fractures will heal if nondisplaced after 8 to 12 weeks. Symptoms resulting from the trauma (e.g., sinusitis) may be chronic.

Intensity. The patient may experience mild to intense pain, or the fracture may cause facial deformity and swelling. Significant fracture may be present that involves the skull base.

Aggravating Factors. Compromised airway, hemorrhage, open or contaminated wound, mechanism of injury, loss of consciousness, presence of intoxicants.

Alleviating Factors. Early recognition and evaluation, local measures such as ice and controlling bleeding.

Associated Factors. Other injuries (e.g., cervical spine, skull, neck, chest).

PHYSICAL EXAMINATION

General. Patients may present with obvious signs of facial trauma or have only slight bruising or swelling of the nose. A full and complete physical examination is performed on any trauma patient to evaluate for coexisting injury.

Nose. Visible deformity, bruising, edema, and epistaxis are common findings. Nasal obstruction may occur. Palpate for nasal depression and looseness of the nose and examine for septal hematoma (aspirate). Thin, watery rhinorrhea raises the possibility of a CSF leak from fracture through the skull base. The use of nasogastric tubes should be approached cautiously in patients with possible basilar skull fractures.

Midface. Evaluate symmetry (compare to photos if available; e.g., driver's license), palpate for bony step-offs and orbital rim defects. The maxilla is examined for correct dental occlusion and palpated for looseness by attempting to move the upper alveolar ridge/teeth.

Eyes. Enophthalmos, diplopia (from entrapment of the inferior extraocular muscles) should suggest a blow-out fracture of the inferior orbital floor. This can be demonstrated on radiographic studies. Examine for anterior chamber bleeding. If present, an ophthalmologic consult is necessary. Blindness may occur with severe trauma and significant ocular injury.

PATHOPHYSIOLOGY

The maxilla contains the upper teeth and maxillary antrum. The nasal bones attach medially to the maxilla.

The zygoma provides lateral support.

LeFort fractures are classified as

LeFort I: A transverse fracture across the apices of the upper teeth.

LeFort II: A pyramidal shaped fracture from the zygoma through the orbital floor and transversing the nasal bones.

LeFort III: Fracture separates the midface from the skull.

DIAGNOSTIC STUDIES

Laboratory

Full Chemistry Profile, CBC, PT, PTT, Platelets. Performed as a preoperative or trauma screen.

Radiology

CT Scan of the Facial Bones. Preferred for extensive or severe trauma after the patient is stabilized to evaluate the presence, extent, and structures involved.

Facial/Skull X-rays. In mild to moderate trauma, fractures of the nose, orbital rims, or zygoma may be demonstrated.

MRI Scan of the Facial Bones/Brain. The study of choice for brain and soft tissue evaluation. Is performed to evaluate the extent or presence of intracerebral injury. Three-dimensional scans may be available to further delineate the extent of the fracture.

DIFFERENTIAL DIAGNOSIS

Traumatic.   Not otherwise applicable.
Infectious
Sinusitis.   May be premorbid condition to the trauma. Fracture not seen on plain films or CT. CT may show fluid within the sinuses. Sinuses may be tender to palpation.
Metabolic.   Not applicable.
Neoplastic
Sinus and Skull Base Tumors.   May be a premorbid condition to the trauma. Bony erosion may be seen on radiographic imaging.
Vascular
Vascular Malformation.   May be noted on contrast studies.
Vascular Tear.   Causing bleeding; can be identified for repair.
Congenital
Absent or Hypoplastic Sinuses.   May be apparent on plain films.
Acquired.   Not applicable.

TREATMENT

Medical.   Generally, facial fractures are of a lower urgency in the severely injured patient. However, airway control and hemorrhage from fracture sites may necessitate more urgent treatment.

The primary goal with any trauma is to ensure a patent airway. Blunt trauma can result in significant tissue injury that compromises the airway. All efforts at fracture reduction or repair are worthless if the patient's airway is lost. Attention to the potential of cervical spine injury and the use of appropriate suctioning, oral airway management, intubation, and tracheotomy are important. Controlling of bleeding, fluid resuscitation, and treatment for shock follow.

Following initial evaluation and stabilization of the patient, attention can be given to facial fractures.

Definitive repair should be done within 7 to 10 days of injury, all other conditions permitting.

Surgical
Nasal Fractures.   Septal hematomas should be aspirated and drained. Closed reduction under local anesthetic (topical cocaine and infiltrated lidocaine [Xylocaine]) is the treatment of choice once swelling has subsided. Fractures should be supported with intranasal packing and external bridge of nose splints for protection. Open reduction and fixation may be required.

Facial and Midface Fractures.   Open reduction and fixation with miniplating is performed to restore proper alignment, stabilization, and restoration of function. More often necessary for displaced fractures. The goal of fracture treatment is to prevent complications, including loss of nasal support, nasal deformity, nasal synechiae or stenosis, recurrent of chronic sinusitis, mucocele or pyocele formation, non-union or malunion of fracture, malocclusion or limitation of motion, enophthalmos, ocular limitation of motion, blindness, persistent CSF leak, or meningitis.

PA Role in Surgery. The PA may be involved in the full aspects of care, including emergency room evaluation, assisting in the operating room, and postoperative follow-up. An assistant is frequently used in reconstructive procedures to help with hemostasis, maintain alignment, and to prepare bone grafts or mini-plates.

PEDIATRIC CONSIDERATIONS

With facial fractures, children should not be considered miniature adults, because developmental differences based on age exist. Sinuses may be small or undeveloped. Softer bony structures may mask significant soft tissue or intracranial injury. Early consultation with a pediatric otolaryngologist can augment the evaluation of the young trauma victim.

OBSTETRICAL CONSIDERATIONS

The need for anesthetic agents and surgical treatment necessitate the involvement of the obstetrician. Marginal airways and significant hemorrhage may be detrimental to the fetus.

PEARLS FOR THE PA

Do not delay treatment of life-threatening injuries while treating facial fractures.

Always rule out CSF leak in the patient with a suspected basilar skull fracture.

There are significant developmental differences in the facial and sinus structures between an adult and a child.

Laryngeal Trauma
William C. Perry, PA-C

DEFINITION

Any injury to the anterior neck that causes trauma to the exposed larynx and trachea. These exposed structures can become penetrated, crushed, or dislocated.

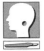

HISTORY

Symptoms. Hoarseness or any alteration to voice, dyspnea, pain, dysphagia.

General. The mechanical disruption, in addition to edema, may significantly threaten the airway. Causes include, but are not limited to, any patient with history of anterior neck trauma (e.g., sports injury ["clothes line" type injury], assault [strangulation], motor vehicle accident [steering wheel], or penetrating injury). There frequently is a witnessed trauma that can assist in diagnosis; however, patients can present with airway distress.

Age. All ages may be involved. Laryngeal fractures are less common in children due to cartilage softness, but soft tissue edema and bruising effects still threaten the airway.

Onset. Symptoms may be immediate (e.g., hemorrhage) or delayed due to local edema.

Duration. Local edema in mild trauma may resolve within 24 hours, but airway symptoms should be treated cautiously because urgent and catastrophic changes may occur.

Intensity. From mild discomfort or minimal bruising to stridor and obstruction.

Aggravating Factors. Prompt recognition and treatment of airway dysfunction.

Alleviating Factors. Maintaining airway patency.

Associated Factors. Associated neck trauma or cervical spine injury.

PHYSICAL EXAMINATION

General. The patient may appear relatively normal or may be in acute respiratory distress. Swelling or ecchymosis of the neck, stridor, hemoptysis, tenderness at trauma site, or symptoms of shock may be present. The neck and chest are palpated for subcutaneous emphysema.

A full and complete physical examination is performed on any trauma patient to evaluate for coexisting injury.

HEENT. Flexible fiberoptic examination of the larynx can be accomplished early in the uncompromised patient. Motion of the vocal cords, hematoma, or compromise of arytenoid function is readily determined.

Pulmonary. Percuss and auscultate for signs of pneumothorax or pneumomediastinum.

PATHOPHYSIOLOGY

The larynx is a structure consisting of the thyroid, cricoid, arytenoid, corniculate, and cuneiform cartilages, as well as the epiglottis. It is supported by internal and external muscles and held in place anterior to the fourth, fifth, and sixth cervical vertebrae. Its functions involve breathing, swallowing, and speech. Because of its anterior location in the neck, it can be involved in many forms of trauma.

DIAGNOSTIC STUDIES

Laboratory
Chemistry Profile, CBC, PT, PTT. Performed as part of the routine preoperative or trauma survey.
Arterial Blood Gases. Obtained in any patient with signs of respiratory compromise.
Radiology
CT Scan of the Larynx. The examination of choice; however, patients with significant, obvious trauma may not have the time necessary to wait for any special studies. In uncompromised patients, CT assists in the planning of repairs and may augment the endoscopic examination.
Arteriography. Indicated for penetrating wounds to rule out vascular injury.
Contrast Swallowing Studies. Performed to assess esophageal integrity.
Chest X-ray. May show pneumothorax or pneumomediastinum.
Cervical Spine Films. Utilized to rule out possible fracture. Free air may be noted.

DIFFERENTIAL DIAGNOSIS

Traumatic. Not otherwise applicable.
Infectious
Branchial Cleft Cyst. With infection, exhibits elevated white blood count (WBC), fever, warmth at the site. No history of trauma.
Parapharyngeal Infection. Elevated WBC, fever, warmth at the site. No history of trauma.
Metabolic
Goiter. May result in tracheal compression due to mass effect.
Neoplastic
Laryngeal Cancer. No history of trauma; seen on fiberoptic examination.
Vascular
Vascular Injury. Significant laryngeal trauma should raise the suspicion of vascular trauma.
Congenital. Not applicable.
Acquired. Not applicable.

TREATMENT

Medical. Protection of the airway is the immediate goal. Cricothyroidotomy may be used in the urgent phase and converted to a tracheostomy when the patient is stable. Attempts at intubation may further compromise an already marginal airway.

Surgical. Definitive treatment is aimed at fracture reduction, assurance of a stable airway, and restoration of the laryngeal functions of speech and swallowing. This most likely requires surgery, placement of an endolaryngeal stent or keel to maintain patency, and close follow-up after surgery to prevent complications of granulation tissue or stenosis. In surgery, exploration of the neck is performed to examine vascular and neural structures, because carotid artery and laryngeal nerve injury are possible.

Indications. To obtain or maintain airway patency and speech or swallowing functions.

Contraindications. Due to the acute nature, essentially none, but patients with severe coagulation defects or systemic disease that would prohibit anesthesia may have elective procedures deferred.

PA Role in Surgery. The PA assists with opening, closing, and exposure during surgery. Wound care and tracheostomy site follow-up are important postoperative considerations.

PEDIATRIC CONSIDERATIONS

Softer bony structures may mask significant soft tissue or intracranial injury. Early consultation with a pediatric otolaryngologist can augment the evaluation of the young trauma victim.

OBSTETRICAL CONSIDERATIONS

The need for anesthetic agents and surgical treatment necessitate the involvement of the obstetrician. Marginal airways and significant hemorrhage may be detrimental to the fetus.

PEARLS FOR THE PA

Prompt recognition and treatment of airway dysfunction are of primary importance.

Airway compromise may be immediate, due to the trauma, or delayed, due to edema.

Always rule out associated cervical spine and vascular injuries.

Nasal Polyps
Deborah Entrekin Whitehair, PA-C, MS

DEFINITION

Benign, pale or translucent tumors found in the nasal fossae, originating in the maxillary or ethmoid sinuses.

HISTORY

Symptoms. Nasal obstruction and pressure, rhinorrhea, anosmia, mouth breathing.

General. Usually the result of chronic inflammation in the nose and sinus or from allergies. Also can be part of a triad involving nasal polyps, aspirin sensitivity, and asthma.

Age. Children to adults.

Onset. Gradual, months to years.

Duration. Slow, will continue to grow and may recur if removed.

Intensity. Initially asymptomatic, but later cause nasal obstruction pressure.

Aggravating Factors. Vasomotor or allergic rhinitis.

Alleviating Factors. Surgical removal.

Associated Factors. Aspirin sensitivity, nonallergic asthma, chronic sinusitis, and cystic fibrosis.

PHYSICAL EXAMINATION

General. The patient may appear normal or may sound congested, with hyponasal phonation.

HEENT. Smooth, pale pear-shaped tumors that appear singular or in clusters in the nasal fossae, easily movable, nontender. May be unilateral or bilateral.

Excessive mucus may be present. The endoscopic nasal examination usually identifies the polyps in the middle meatus originating from the ethmoid sinus. Occasionally, they appear within the maxillary antrum and extend to the nasopharynx. The polyps may erode adjacent osseous structures in the nose.

PATHOPHYSIOLOGY

Edema of the sinus submucosa can form irregular folds within the sinus and result in polyp formation. The exact etiology of the polyp development is poorly understood.

DIAGNOSTIC STUDIES

Laboratory.   Usually not necessary, but increased eosinophils are commonly seen on nasal smear.

Radiology
Sinus Radiographs.   Soft tissue density that may totally opacify a sinus. Will not erode or destroy the sinus wall, as would be seen with a malignancy. If nasal obstruction is present for a long period of time, there may be changes with the nasal bones spreading and the bridge becoming wider.

Other.   Not applicable.

DIFFERENTIAL DIAGNOSIS

Traumatic
Facial Trauma.   May cause an obstruction of sinus secretions and lead to chronic inflammation of the nasal and sinus mucosa and polyp formation.

Infectious
Chronic Sinusitis of the Paranasal Sinuses.   Usually associated with headaches and facial pain.

Metabolic
Hypothyroidism.   Vasomotor rhinitis may be the result of endocrine disturbances and eventually lead to polyp formation.

Neoplastic
Malignant Tumors of the Paranasal Sinuses, Nasal Fossa or Septum.   Uncommon.

Squamous Cell Carcinoma.   The most common malignancy and is associated with nasal mass, facial swelling and pain, epistaxis, and palate swelling. The patient may present with a nonhealing lesion in the nasal vestibule or anterior portion of the septum.

Inverted Papilloma.   Unilateral tumor arising from the lateral wall of the nose that may intermittently bleed; may occur with nasal polyps or malignant nasal tumors. Patients present with nasal obstruction, epistaxis, or rhinorrhea.

Squamous Papilloma.   Benign wartlike tumor that occurs on the anterior nasal septum or lateral wall of the nose and may cause nasal obstruction or hemorrhage. May also involve the sinuses.

Vascular
Juvenile Angiofibroma.   Benign tumor found in teenage boys that can cause massive bleeding; may also arise from the lateral wall of the nose. Present with epistaxis, nasal obstruction and, occasionally, deformity of the cheek.

Congenital
Cystic Fibrosis.   Children with cystic fibrosis may have recurrent nasal polyps that can deform the nasal bones.

Acquired.   Not applicable.

TREATMENT

Medical.   Local or systemic decongestants or nasal corticosteroids are usually not effective in shrinking the polyp.

If allergies are the primary cause of polyp formation, desensitization, decongestants, and antihistamines help decrease the incidence of recurrence once they are removed.

Surgical. Surgical removal is the treatment of choice, especially in patients with complete obstruction, uncontrolled rhinorrhea, or nasal deformity. Postoperatively, topical nasal corticosteroids may decrease the incidence of recurrence and must be used indefinitely.

Indications. Nasal obstruction, uncontrolled rhinorrhea, nasal deformity.

Contraindications. Patients with major risk factors for general anesthesia.

PEDIATRIC CONSIDERATIONS

Nasal polyps develop in 25% of children with cystic fibrosis. Every child with nasal polyps, even in the absence of typical respiratory and digestive symptoms, should be tested for cystic fibrosis.

Nasal polyps in children are also associated with chronic allergic rhinitis, chronic sinusitis, and asthma. Children may often present with the complaint of persistent mouth breathing or hyponasal phonation.

OBSTETRICAL CONSIDERATIONS

No specific indications.

PEARLS FOR THE PA

Diagnosis is usually made by history and physical examination.

If epistaxis is present, along with nasal obstruction, the cause is probably not nasal polyps.

Treat all correctable underlying causes of polyp formation.

Nasopharyngeal Carcinoma
Joseph Roy Durio, PA-C, MA

DEFINITION

Nasopharyngeal carcinoma is, in general, a silent tumor that causes few symptoms. In approximately half the cases, the presenting symptom is lymph node metastases in the neck.

Tumors that are implicated include squamous cell cancer (71%), lymphoma (18%), miscellaneous (11%)—adenocarcinoma, melanoma, plasma cell myeloma, fibrosarcoma.

HISTORY

Symptoms

Nasal.   Purulent or bloody rhinorrhea (unilateral), posterior epistaxis, nasal voice, nasal obstruction.

Otologic.   Eustachian tube obstruction by edema or tumor, fullness to ear, conductive hearing loss.

Ophthalmologic.   Eye symptoms related to neurologic compromise (CN V, VI most frequent).

Neck.   Head, facial, and neck pain and neck mass.

General.   Fifty percent present with metastatic cervical nodes as the chief complaint. Carcinoma of the nasopharynx represents approximately 2% to 3% of all malignancies in Caucasians. Nasopharyngeal carcinomas (NPC) reveal a much higher genetic predisposition in the Chinese population, reaching 18%. NPC ranks 33rd in the United States among malignant tumors in males (first in Singapore).

Age.   Most patients in the United States are 50 to 70 years of age. Male : female ratio, 3 : 1.

Onset.   Slow growing, indolent.

Duration.   Progressive.

Intensity.   Asymptomatic to intense ear, face, or nasal pain.

Aggravating Factors.   Progressive growth leads to symptoms.

Alleviating Factors.   Radiation therapy.

Associated Factors.   Research shows that environmental and viral factors play a significant role in certain histologic types of NPC. High titers of the Epstein-Barr virus (EBV) are well established (increased in 70% of patients); polycyclic hydrocarbons, salted fish, sawdust, poor hygiene.

PHYSICAL EXAMINATION

General.   The patient may appear normal or in distress secondary to pain.

HEENT.   Lymph nodes are palpated in the neck for evidence of enlargement or tenderness. In the adult, the nasopharynx can be examined by gently pulling the tongue anteriorly and, with a heated mirror, inspecting behind the soft palate. The flexible fiberoptic scope is an extremely accurate and reliable tool in examining the nasopharynx. Evaluation with the fiberoptic scope reveals mass effect to the eustachian tube orifice or the area in the region of the fossa of Rosenmüller. A unilateral mass can also often be visualized with indirect laryngoscopy.

Neurologic.   May reveal cranial nerve abnormalities with CN V (trigeminal) and VI (abducens) most frequently involved.

PATHOPHYSIOLOGY

For unknown reasons, carcinomas of the nasopharynx arise immediately above the eustachian tube cartilage, in the depression known as the fossa of Rosenmüller. Cervical metastatic disease is common because the surface epithelium of the nasopharynx networks with lymphatic channels. Consequently, many patients first present with a neck mass in the posterior triangle.

DIAGNOSTIC STUDIES

Laboratory
Viral Capsid Antigen (VCA). May exhibit IgG and IgA antibodies.
Radiology
CT Scan. With contrast enhancement of the head and nasopharynx with soft tissue and bone; the study of choice.

DIFFERENTIAL DIAGNOSIS

Traumatic
Hematoma. Patient has a history of trauma. CT differentiates hemorrhage from neoplasm.
Infectious
Recurrent or Chronic Sinusitis. CT reveals fluid level in sinuses with no bony erosion.
Metabolic. Not applicable.
Neoplastic
Adenoid Cystic Carcinoma. Differentiated histologically with biopsy.
Melanoma. Differentiated histologically with biopsy.
Lymphoma. Differentiated histologically with biopsy.
Vascular
Juvenile Angiofibroma. Is common in the adolescent male with nasal obstruction and epistaxis.
Carotid Body Tumors. Differentiated on carotid arteriogram or MRI scan of the head/neck with gadolinium.
Congenital
Encephalocele/Choanal Atresia. May be associated with other anomalies. Differentiated on physical examination or MRI of the head.
Acquired. Not applicable.
Other
Nasal Polyps. Seen on examination of the nares. Growth or suspicious appearance may warrant removal.

TREATMENT

Medical. External beam radiation is used as the primary management of NPC with intracavity brachytherapy used as a supplement. Chemotherapy has no proven benefit.

Complications of radiation therapy may include xerostomia, dental caries, myelitis, fluctuating hearing loss, fibrosis of neck and pharynx, and pituitary dysfunction.

Pain control is essential and narcotics are prescribed based on the condition, level of discomfort, and the patient's prognosis.

Surgical. Surgical treatments play a limited role in excising NPC. Biopsy may be required to confirm the diagnosis and to rule out other causes.

Indications. To obtain tissue for definitive diagnosis.

Contraindications. Inability of the patient to undergo anesthesia; coagulopathy.

PA Role in Surgery. Depending on his or her experience level, the PA may assist with the diagnostic procedures and perform postoperative care, including co-ordination of ancillary services such as radiation therapy, oncology, social services, etc.

PEDIATRIC CONSIDERATIONS

Juvenile angiofibroma is a differential condition for NPC. It is common in the adolescent male with nasal obstruction and epistaxis.

OBSTETRICAL CONSIDERATIONS

Unilateral serous otitis media may be present.

PEARLS FOR THE PA

Unilateral serous otitis media is nasopharyngeal cancer until proven otherwise.

Five-year overall survival rate is 30% to 48%.

Otitis Media
Deborah Entrekin Whitehair, PA-C, MS

DEFINITION

Inflammation of the middle ear caused by pathogens from the nose or throat.

HISTORY

Symptoms. Ear pain, fever, enlarged tender cervical lymph nodes, and hearing loss.

General. Patient may have a history of persistent middle-ear fluid or recurrent ear infections. Children are usually irritable, have difficulty sleeping, and pull at their ears.

Age. Any, but most common in children younger than 5 years old.

Onset. Acute.

Duration. Becomes a chronic problem if not treated; may also recur after symptoms of upper respiratory infection.

Intensity. Mild to severe pain.

Aggravating Factors. Infections of the nose and throat.

Alleviating Factors. Antibiotic treatment.

Associated Factors. Serous otitis media, upper respiratory infections including viral infections.

PHYSICAL EXAMINATION

General. Patients generally present with fever; children may be crying and pulling at their ears.

HEENT. Normal external canal unless tympanic membrane has been perforated and purulent drainage is present. Nasal congestion with swollen turbinates. Throat inspection may be normal or postnasal drainage may be evident.

Tympanic Membrane. Erythematous, bulging, and unresponsive to pneumatic testing.

Neck. Enlarged, tender cervical nodes may be present.

PATHOPHYSIOLOGY

Streptococcus pneumoniae and *Haemophilus influenzae* are most common in children under the age of 5. In adults, *Staphylococcus aureus* and *Streptococcus* are more common. Other responsible pathogens include anaerobes, *Mycoplasma*, beta-hemolytic group A streptococcus, *Moraxella catarrhalis*, and *Pseudomonas*.

DIAGNOSTIC STUDIES

Laboratory

Culture and Sensitivity. If purulent drainage is present for appropriate antibiotic treatment.

Radiology. Not applicable.

Other

Audiologic Testing. Mild conductive hearing loss with a negative pressure in the middle ear noted on tympanometry.

DIFFERENTIAL DIAGNOSIS

Traumatic
Rupture of the Tympanic Membrane.   Can give infectious organisms an entrance into the middle ear. Positive traumatic history.

Infectious
Viral Otitis Media.   Slight thickening of tympanic membrane without marked hyperemia.

Bullous Myringitis.   Bleb or vesicle present on tympanic membrane; associated with a viral infection, but may have a secondary bacterial infection.

Chronic Otitis Media.   Persistent middle-ear effusion or painless drainage out the ear canal from the middle ear. Cholesteatoma may be present.

Metabolic.   Not applicable.

Neoplastic
Malignancies Involving the Middle Ear.   Rare, and when present, are associated with intense pain due to invasion of the bone and bleeding from the auditory canal.

Vascular.   Not applicable.

Congenital
Acute Otitis Media.   May be associated with sepsis, pneumonia, and meningitis in the newborn.

Acquired
Serous Otitis Media.   Sterile fluid in the middle ear with air fluid level or bubbles often noted; caused by eustachian tube dysfunction. May have history of allergic rhinitis.

TREATMENT

Medical.   Ten-day course of antibiotics.

In adults, amoxicillin 500 mg three times a day (use erythromycin if allergic to penicillin).

In children, amoxicillin 20 mg/kg/day, divided into three doses. If children are allergic to penicillin, use sulfisoxazole 150 mg/kg/day divided into four doses or trimethoprim/sulfamethoxazole 8 and 40 mg/kg/day. It may be useful to use long-acting decongestants twice a day for 10 days to relieve eustachian tube dysfunction and nasal congestion.

Persistent or recurrent otitis media needs to be treated with amoxicillin-clavulanate 40 mg/kg/day or cefaclor 40 mg/kg/day in three divided doses, or zithromax 10 mg/kg once daily for the first day, then 5 mg/kg once daily for 4 days.

Oral pain medicine as needed.

Auralgan otic drops may be used every 1 to 2 hours if no perforation is present to relieve pain.

If drainage is present, keep water out of ear canal.

Referral to ENT if the patient has persistent or recurrent infections.

Prophylactic treatment with antibiotic given once a day for 3 to 6 months is sometimes necessary in patients with recurrent infections.

Surgical. If the patient has severe ear pain, myringotomy and tympanocentesis may be necessary to drain the middle ear and provide immediate relief of pain. After adequate antimicrobial therapy, the tympanic membrane is re-evaluated for otoscopic evidence of the resolution of the otitis media.

For the patient with recurrent or persistent otitis media with effusion, a bilateral myringotomy with ventilation tube insertion is indicated. There are several types of ventilation tubes available. Some require a second surgery for removal, whereas others will fall out on their own. Most tubes should not remain within the tympanic membrane for more than 2 years because of the increased risk of scarring and permanent perforation. Once the tubes are out, the tympanic membrane must be evaluated to ensure that the myringotomy sites have closed.

Indications. This procedure is indicated if a significant hearing loss is present or if there is atelectasis of the tympanic membrane with pain, hearing loss, vertigo, or tinnitus.

Contraindications. Any patient considered to be a major surgical risk would continue antimicrobial therapy or have the myringotomy and ventilation tubes inserted under local anesthesia.

Role of the PA. The PA evaluates the ventilation tubes postoperatively to ensure that they remain patent and properly placed and that there is no evidence of infection.

PEDIATRIC CONSIDERATION

Otitis media is the most prevalent disease of childhood after respiratory tract infections. Infants and young children (4 months to 2 years) are at highest risk. Children who develop otitis media in the first year of life have an increased risk of chronic disease. Incidence is higher in males than in females. The high-risk populations include children with cleft palate and other craniofacial anomalies, children with Down syndrome, Alaskan natives, and native Americans. Incidence of otitis media is highest in the winter months. Some children may benefit from an adenoidectomy.

OBSTETRICAL CONSIDERATIONS

Sulfonamides, erythromycin, and ciprofloxacin should be used with caution. Tetracycline is contraindicated.

PEARLS FOR THE PA

Pain should resolve soon after antibiotic therapy begins.

Nose and nasopharynx should be carefully evaluated for causative factors such as adenoid hypertrophy or throat infection.

Follow-up evaluation of hearing is necessary.

Ventilation tubes should not remain in the tympanic membrane for more than 2 years.

Otoscopic examination is needed postoperatively to evaluate tube patency, placement, and persistent perforation once the tube is out.

Sinusitis

Carroll F. Poppen, PA-C

DEFINITION

An inflammation of the mucosal lining of the paranasal sinuses that leads to obstruction of the sinus ostia. May be due to infection, allergy, neoplasm, virus, or foreign body.

HISTORY

Symptoms.   Usually acute headache and face pain following an acute upper respiratory infection. Pain may radiate to the upper teeth and forehead. Presence of mucopurulent nasal discharge that may be blood tinged. Fever may or may not be present.

General.   Inquire as to recent sinus or dental surgery, history of pollen or environmental allergies, distant or acute trauma, presence of nasal polyps, known tumors, and symptoms of an upper respiratory infection (e.g., coryza, cough, sore throat, rhinorrhea).

Sinusitis is classified by the duration of symptoms. Acute suppurative sinusitis is an acute inflammatory process present for up to 3 weeks. Subacute sinusitis is an inflammatory process present from 3 weeks to 3 months. Chronic sinusitis is an inflammatory process lasting greater than 3 months.

Age.   Infant to elderly.

Onset.   Usually acute following an upper respiratory infection. May also be associated with acute allergic rhinitis or exacerbation of vasomotor rhinitis.

Duration. Several days to weeks.

Intensity. Headache, facial and dental pain. May require narcotic pain medication.

Aggravating Factors. Sneezing, nose blowing, Valsalva maneuver, and bending forward.

Alleviating Factors. Bedrest, analgesics, antibiotics, and possible hospitalization with intravenous hydration support.

Associated Factors. Allergic or vasomotor rhinitis, acute upper respiratory infection, nasal polyps, benign and malignant nasal tumors, adenoid hypertrophy, deviated nasal septum, choanal atresia, and dental abscesses (posterior upper molars).

PHYSICAL EXAMINATION

General. Fatigue, malaise, fever, nasal obstruction, and purulent nasal discharge usually are present.

HEENT

Nose. Acute mucosal inflammation with terminating engorgement and presence of purulent discharge.

Neck. Cervical adenopathy is usually absent.

Oral Pharynx. Presence of a purulent discharge in the posterior pharyngeal wall.

Sinuses. Acute tenderness may be present to palpation and percussion over the affected sinuses. Transillumination of the sinuses should be performed to evaluate for the presence of opacification.

PATHOPHYSIOLOGY

Any condition that causes blockage of drainage through the sinus ostium may cause sinusitis. The blockage may be direct (from a neoplasm or foreign body) or indirect due to inflammation (secondary to bacterial infection, allergy, or virus).

The most common bacterial causes are *Haemophilus influenzae, Streptococcus pneumoniae, Staphylococcus aureus,* and *Moraxella.* Anaerobes may be present in chronic sinusitis. Untreated, bacteria associated with the sinusitis may erode the bone and spread into the brain, causing an abscess.

DIAGNOSTIC STUDIES

Laboratory

Culture and Sensitivity. Endoscopically guided cultures from the middle meatus or aspirate from a maxillary sinus puncture are used to determine the causative agent and direct treatment.

CBC. Indicated if there is a suspicion of significant or systemic infection.

Radiology
Plain Films of the Paranasal Sinuses (Including Waters, Caldwell, and Lateral Views). Used to evaluate for air fluid levels within the sinuses.

Coronal CT Scanning of the Paranasal Sinuses. Will identify sinus inflammation, mucosal thickening, and fluid levels. Obstructive or erosive lesions may be identified.

CT/MRI of the Brain. Indicated if there is a suspicion of bacterial spread to the brain.

DIFFERENTIAL DIAGNOSIS

Traumatic
Acute Nasal Injuries. With blunt trauma to the nose, may cause congestion or symptoms of sinusitis. X-ray may reveal a fracture.

Barometric Trauma. Associated with scuba diving or air travel; may cause sinus congestion or exacerbate an existing sinusitis.

Multiple Facial Fractures. Secondary to motor vehicle accidents or other causes; may cause edema leading to sinusitis.

Infectious
Fungal Sinusitis. Acute fungal inflammatory process (usually *Aspergillus*) of the paranasal sinuses.

Neoplastic
Benign and Malignant Tumors. May be identified on CT/MRI of the sinuses. Common presenting symptoms include (in order) nasal blockage, bleeding, pain, and deformity.

Inverting Papilloma. Although not malignant, is very aggressive. Seen on physical examination. Requires biopsy for diagnosis.

Malignant. Lesions include squamous cell carcinoma, esthesioneuroblastoma, and adenoid cystic carcinomas (Cylindroma). Seen on CT/MRI.

Vascular
Juvenile Angiofibroma and Hemangiopericytoma. Occur in the maxillary sinus. Appear as an opacified sinus. May be difficult to differentiate from sinusitis.

Congenital
Choanal Atresia. Congenital anomaly of the posterior portion of the nose manifested by bony or membranous overgrowth.

Other
Nasal Polyps. Seen on physical examination.

Acquired
Apical Dental Infections. May be seen on oral examination. Root of tooth infection leads to sinusitis.

Foreign Bodies or Nasal Packing. Seen on nasal examination.

TREATMENT

Medical. Antibiotics are the keystone to medical management for acute and subacute sinusitis. The most common cause for treatment failure is inadequate antibiotic treatment. Patients with acute sinusitis should be treated for 7 to 10 days after resolution of nasal symptoms. Patients with subacute sinusitis should be treated for a period of 3 to 4 weeks. Patients with chronic sinusitis should be treated for 3 to 6 weeks. Antibiotic selection should include those medications that are effective in treating *Haemophilus influenzae, Streptococcus pneumoniae, Staphylococcus aureus,* and *Branhamella catarrhalis.* Consider a trial of anaerobe-sensitive antibiotics in those individuals with suspicion of an anaerobic infection. Analgesics, decongestants, and mucolytics should be considered. The use of antihistamines is reserved for those individuals with suspicion of allergic rhinitis as a predominating cause.

Surgical. Surgical management may be broken down into minor surgical procedures and major surgical procedures.

Minor Surgical Procedures

Maxillary Sinus Irrigation. The maxillary sinus position and shape lends itself to relative ease in irrigation. Irrigation can be accomplished by canalization of the middle meatal ostia, inferior meatal puncture, or anterior maxillary sinus wall puncture above the canine fossa. This procedure can be accomplished after adequate analgesia and vasoconstriction with the use of topical lidocaine (Xylocaine) or cocaine solution and 1% Neo-Synephrine. The main benefit of maxillary sinus irrigation is the removal of mucopurulent material from within the sinus cavity with production of material for general bacteriologic study.

Major Surgical Procedures. A major sinus procedure should be considered when an inadequate response from medical treatment is evident or impending complications are imminent. This procedure requires general anesthesia and hospitalization. Major sinus surgery is performed intranasally. After adequate general anesthesia and vasoconstriction of the nasal mucosa, an anterior ethmoidectomy is performed, followed by a middle meatal antrostomy (surgical enlargement of the maxillary sinus ostia) with evacuation of mucopurulent material from the maxillary sinus cavity. Postoperative packing with Vaseline-impregnated gauze and a nasal drip pad completes the procedure. Occasionally, an external ethmoidectomy or trephination of the frontal sinus may be acquired. The patient should remain hospitalized with adequate intravenous antibiotic coverage until symptoms have resolved. Nasal packing is removed in approximately 1 to 3 days postoperatively.

Indications. Surgical management of sinusitis should be considered to alleviate severe pain when it needs to be alleviated, when complications are impending, or when response to appropriate antibiotic/medical management is inadequate.

Contraindications. Inadequate initial antibiotic trial; inability of the patient to undergo anesthesia; bleeding disorders.

Role of the PA. The PA may assist with office procedures such as maxillary sinus drainage or irrigation and with the general medical or pre- and postoperative care of the patient.

PEDIATRIC CONSIDERATIONS

Children are treated aggressively with antibiotics in a similar manner as adults. Orbital involvement occurs more frequently in children due to the thin membrane (laminal paparicium) that exists between the globe and sinus. Evaluate closely for proptosis, deviation of the eyes, and central nervous system changes.

OBSTETRICAL CONSIDERATIONS

Teratogenicity of antibiotics must be evaluated prior to being prescribed.

PEARLS FOR THE PA

Any condition that blocks drainage from the sinus ostia may lead to sinusitis.

The most common cause of sinusitis is upper respiratory infection.

Always perform a complete and thorough examination to rule out other causes.

Tonsillitis

Joseph Roy Durio, PA-C, MA

DEFINITION

An acute infection of the lymphoepithelial tissues involving the palatine tonsils and surrounding area, including the tonsillar pillars and posterior pharyngeal wall.

HISTORY

Symptoms. The patient may present with dysphagia, fever, odynophagia, and tender cervical adenopathy. The tonsils may appear exudative, edematous, and enlarged. Additional symptoms may include myalgia, arthralgia, headache, or vomiting.

General. In the young patient, historical data may need to be augmented by a parent or caregiver.

Age. Any.

Onset.   Tonsillitis may present with sudden onset of sore throat, malaise, fever, anorexia, halitosis, muffled voice.

Duration.   The temperature may rise to 102 to 104°F in the first 24 to 48 hours. Often, the temperature is 104 to 105°F in children.

Intensity.   Discomfort and malaise with symptoms to upper airway obstruction, sleep disorders, or cardiopulmonary complications.

Aggravating Factors.   Hypertrophy of pre-existing tonsils, dehydration.

Alleviating Factors.   Warm saline gargles, acetaminophen.

Associated Factors.   Associated symptoms may include myalgia, arthralgia, headache, or vomiting.

PHYSICAL EXAMINATION

General.   Patient appears ill.

Neurologic.   Examination of the throat reveals pharyngeal edema (sometimes deeply purple), hypertrophy of tonsillar forms, edema and petechiae of the soft palate, and patchy white exudate that is easily wiped away.

Tender cervical adenopathy may also be present.

Bacterial pharyngitis may or may not present with exudative changes.

Presence or absence of exudate does not establish nor rule out a specific cause.

PATHOPHYSIOLOGY

The palatine tonsils are the largest accumulation of lymphoid tissue in Waldeyer's ring. The other components of this structure are the lingual tonsils, nasopharyngeal tonsils (adenoids), lateral pharyngeal bands, tubal tonsils of Gerlach (in Rosenmüller's fossa), and the nodules of subepithelial layer of the posterior pharyngeal wall.

The palatine tonsils, in conjunction with the previously mentioned tissues, have four functions: lymphocyte formation, antibody production, assisting in the acquisition of immunity, and localization of infection.

Common causative organisms of tonsillitis include beta-hemolytic streptococci, *Staphylococcus pyogenes*, *Haemophilus influenzae*, *Haemophilus parainfluenzae*, *Corynebacterium diphtheriae*, *Streptococcus pneumoniae*, and viruses (adenovirus and mononucleosis).

DIAGNOSTIC STUDIES

Laboratory

Throat Culture.   Performed to identify the causative organism and direct treatment.

Mono Spot.   If mononucleosis is suspected.

Radiology.   Not applicable.

DIFFERENTIAL DIAGNOSIS

Traumatic. Not applicable.
Infectious
Mononucleosis. Positive mono spot test.
Peritonsillar Abscess. Positive aspirant.
Tuberculosis. Recovery of acid-fast bacilli from the tissue.
Syphilis. Positive rapid plasma reagin (RPR) test performed as indicated.
Viral. Positive viral cultures.
Gonorrheal Pharyngitis. Positive culture; performed as indicated.
Diphtheria. Diagnosis is made clinically and confirmed on culture.
Lingual Tonsillitis. Seen on indirect examination.
Metabolic. Not applicable.
Neoplastic
Leukemia/Lymphoma/Cancer. Diagnosis made on biopsy; performed as indicated.
Vascular. Not applicable.
Congenital. Not applicable.
Acquired. Not applicable.

TREATMENT

Medical. Bedrest with hydration and antipyretics (e.g., acetaminophen). Antibiotics are instituted based on the results of the throat culture. Therapy may be started initially before the culture results are known, with penicillin still the first drug of choice, although erythromycin is useful in case of penicillin allergy. Antibiotics are given intramuscularly or orally based on the individual patient and chance of compliance.

Surgical. It is important to reserve surgery for those who have met the criteria or indications for surgery.

Indications. The tonsils are excised if there are four or more infections in a year despite adequate therapy, hypertrophy affecting orofacial growth or dental malocclusion, upper airway obstruction, dysphagia, sleep disorders, cardiopulmonary complications, peritonsillar abscess, failure of medical management, persistent foul taste or breath due to tonsillitis not responding to medical management, streptococcal carrier state unresponsive to appropriate antibiotic therapy, or unilateral tonsillar hypertrophy.

Complications of tonsillitis include peritonsillar abscess, cervical adenitis and abscess, post-streptococcal glomerulonephritis, rheumatic fever, neck abscess, and airway compromise.

Contraindications. History of bleeding abnormalities.

PA Role in Surgery. The PA may initially evaluate the patient and try conservative measures. Assisting with the removal of the tonsils and providing follow-up care are also assigned duties.

PEDIATRIC CONSIDERATIONS

Pediatric patients must meet the criteria (indications) to undergo tonsillectomy.

OBSTETRICAL CONSIDERATIONS

Internal tonsillectomy may be reserved for the postdelivery period. Always evaluate the efficacy versus risk to the fetus with any antibiotic therapy instituted.

PEARLS FOR THE PA

Patients should meet the criteria or indications before having the tonsils removed.

Asymmetric tonsils suggest the presence of lymphoma.

Further Reading

Ballenger JJ: Diseases of the Nose, Throat, Ear, Head, and Neck, 14th ed. Philadelphia, Lea and Febiger, 1991.

Paparella MM, Mrick SH, Gluckman JL, Meyerhoff WL (eds): Otolaryngology, 3rd ed. Philadelphia, W.B. Saunders, 1991.

Chapter **7**
Neurosurgery
Epidural Hematoma
Judy Nunes, PA-C, BS

DEFINITION

A collection of blood (hematoma) that occurs between the calvarium (skull) and dura mater that is usually due to head trauma.

HISTORY

Symptoms. Varies from a neurologically intact to a deeply comatose state. The classic presentation is a "triphasic story," which consists of a mild closed head injury (concussion), followed by a transient loss of consciousness. This is followed by a lucid interval, during which a patient is relatively asymptomatic (while the clot is accumulating). The patient then develops a rapid neurologic deterioration associated with a loss of consciousness and uncal herniation (once the clot has expanded farther).

Patients with epidural hematoma also may present with headache, subtle personality changes, speech disturbance, visual complaint, or focal weakness (depending on the cortical, anatomical location of the blood clot).

General. Epidural hematoma occurs in approximately 8% to 10% of patients who sustain severe head trauma. The most common cause is trauma due to motor vehicle accidents, falls, and sports-related injuries. Eighty-five percent of epidural hematomas are associated with a skull fracture.

Age. Most commonly seen in the second through the fourth decades of life. They are rarely seen in children less than 2 years of age, or in adults greater than 60 years of age, because of the adherence of the dura in these two patient populations. The male-to-female ratio is 4:1.

Onset. Variable, as neurologic signs and symptoms may occur within minutes to 48 hours after injury. Early recognition is key. The patient with a large epidural hematoma with neurologic compromise is a true neurosurgical emergency.

Intensity. Once an epidural hematoma has reached sufficient size, there is risk of uncal herniation and death.

Duration. If the cause of the hemorrhage is arterial (85%), signs and symptoms ensue rapidly and emergent treatment is necessary. If the cause is venous, the signs and symptoms are more likely to be delayed.

Aggravating Factors. Hypertension, any maneuvers that may increase intracranial pressure (e.g., suctioning, positioning).

Alleviating Factors. Surgical evacuation and hemostasis.

Associated Factors. Coagulopathy.

PHYSICAL EXAMINATION

General. Concomitant in the patient with an epidural hematoma, there may be a scalp contusion, skull fracture, subgaleal hematoma, brain contusion, subdural hematoma, or spinal cord injury. Therefore, a careful assessment of the head and neck with regard to obvious bony deformity (palpable step-off, etc.) and soft tissue swelling should be performed.

Neurologic. Level of consciousness is the single most important component of the examination. The pupils should be assessed for anisocoria; dilation (CN III—oculomotor), which should be ipsilateral to the epidura; and hemiparesis (often contralateral). Meningismus may also occur (check for nuchal rigidity, Kernig and Brudzinski signs), but only after the cervical spine has been cleared by x-ray.

PATHOPHYSIOLOGY

The initial head trauma is usually a low-velocity force that bends the skull inward, causing the dura to be stripped away from the skull and subsequently tearing meningeal blood vessels. The dura becomes separated from the bone and produces a tear in a blood vessel that normally lies against or within the bone. Blood then extravasates under arterial pressure and dissects the dura inward, away from the bone, allowing a hematoma to form and the brain gets displaced inward. The source of bleeding is arterial 85% of the time (usually the middle meningeal artery or its branches). It may also occur as a result of injury to the middle meningeal vein or sinus (draining veins of the brain). The mortality rate of patients with epidural hematomas is 20% to 50%.

The most common locations for epidurals to occur are

1. Temporal (middle meningeal artery) with associated temporal bone skull fracture. The expanding clot compresses the temporal lobe medially, which in turn causes downward herniation of the uncus through the tentorial notch. This may be apparent clinically by uncal herniation syndrome, which is manifested by decreased level of consciousness, dilation of the ipsilateral pupil (due to compression on the oculomotor nerve), and contralateral hemiparesis (due to the decussation of the descending pyramidal tracts).
2. Subfrontal, particularly in the very young and elderly, usually due to venous sinus or middle meningeal injury.
3. Occipital, with a fracture across the transverse sinus (at risk for Cushing's triad—elevated blood pressure, decreased respirations, and bradycardia).

DIAGNOSTIC STUDIES

Laboratory

PT/PTT/Bleeding Time. To rule out coagulopathy as a contributing factor in hematoma formation.

Chemistry Profile/Complete Blood Count (CBC). In anticipation of surgical intervention. Used as a baseline and to identify any coexisting metabolic abnormalities.

Radiology
Computed Tomography (CT) of the Brain (Noncontrast). The study of choice. An epidural hematoma appears as a lens-shaped lesion of high density adjacent to the skull and sharply demarcated by the dura, which is adherent to the inner table of the skull. Concurrent cerebral contusions or subdural hematomas may be identified.

Magnetic Resonance Imaging (MRI) of the Brain. Not as useful in the acute setting due to the time it takes to perform the study. Findings same as CT; concurrent intracerebral injury may be more clearly identified.

Other
Electroencephalogram (EEG). May be used postoperatively to screen for potential seizure activity.

DIFFERENTIAL DIAGNOSIS

Traumatic
Cerebral Contusion/Subdural Hematoma. May occur concomitantly with an epidural hematoma. May cause similar neurologic symptoms but without the triphasic history.

Metabolic
Hypoxemia. May cause decreased level of consciousness/neurologic deficit. Arterial blood gases/pulse oximetry reveal low O_2. CT of the brain is negative.

Hypoglycemia. May cause decreased level of consciousness/neurologic deficit. CT of the brain is negative. Serum glucose is diagnostic.

Neoplastic
Intracranial Lesion or Leptomeningeal Spread of Neoplasm. Contrasted CT scan of the brain or MRI differentiates neoplasm from blood.

Vascular
Venous Anomalies/Occult Vascular Lesions/Dural Fistulae. May rupture and cause signs/symptoms of epidural hematoma. May require surgical treatment, where the anomaly is detected. CT/MRI of the brain may reveal the vascular aberration.

Congenital. Not applicable.

Acquired
Drug Effect. May cause decreased level of consciousness/neurologic deficit. CT of the brain is negative. Toxicology screen is positive.

TREATMENT

An epidural hematoma is a potentially life-threatening lesion due to mass effect of the hemorrhage, which causes a rise in intracranial pressure. Approximately 30% of patients are surgically treated within 12 hours of injury and 75% within 48 hours after injury.

Medical. This approach may be taken if the patient is relatively asymptomatic (mild headache) and the epidural hematoma is small in size. Frontal and subfrontal lesions tend to be treated conservatively. Maneuvers to decrease intracranial pressure may be initiated (e.g., elevating the head of the bed, fluid restriction, hyperventilation). The patient is kept under close neurologic observation in the hospital.

Surgical. The goal of treatment is to preserve or restore neurologic function. Early treatment prevents extension of the dural tear to the inner table of the skull, thus extending over a large area, which may add to the arterial, venous, or dural sinus bleeding and result in a larger epidural collection.

A craniotomy is performed as rapidly as possible. A horseshoe or question-mark incision may be used. The scalp is incised sharply from the zygomatic arch within a fingerbreadth of the ear (to avoid the facial nerve) and hemostatic clips are applied to the skin to control bleeding. The temporalis fascia and muscle are divided, cauterized, and retracted. A burr (entry) hole is made in the temporal bone, and a high-speed drill is used to cut a bone flap. The dura is stripped from the inner table of the skull, and the epidural hematoma is then encountered. It may be suctioned or may present itself, depending on the pressure. The culprit artery is identified and coagulated with bipolar cautery. Control of the middle meningeal artery may require coagulation at the point of a dural tear or where the artery enters the skull (foramen spinosum). Once the clot is evacuated (specimen should be sent to pathology) and the vessel coagulated, hemostasis is obtained and the dura is irrigated. Tacking sutures may be used at the bone edges and center of the bone flap during closing in order to obliterate the epidural space. An intracranial pressure monitor or drain may then be placed, and the flap closed in layers.

Indications. Neurologic deficit with radiographic evidence of epidural hematoma with compression/mass effect. If CT is not available and patient is comatose with a dilated pupil, an exploratory burr hole ipsilateral to the dilated pupil may be performed emergently at the bedside.

Contraindications. Severe coagulopathy, clinical brain death.

PEDIATRIC CONSIDERATIONS

Infants and young children (younger than 2 years of age) have dura that is more adherent and are therefore less likely to have epidural hemorrhage. They are, however, more at risk for a delayed epidural hematoma due to a tear in the superior sagittal or transverse sinus. Epidurals in pediatric patients are more likely to be venous in origin.

OBSTETRICAL CONSIDERATIONS

Due to the potential life-threatening aspect of epidural hematoma, surgery should not be delayed. Special anesthetic considerations should be undertaken and an obstetrical consultation obtained.

PEARLS FOR THE PA

Classic triphasic presentation consists of mild head trauma followed by loss of consciousness, lucid interval, and rapid neurologic deterioration with loss of consciousness and uncal herniation.

Source of hemorrhage is usually the middle meningeal artery.

CT scan of the brain is the study of choice.

Most epidural hematomas are treated as a surgical emergency.

Glioma

Mary Loggins, PA-C, MS, MMSc

DEFINITION

Gliomas are one class of infiltrative, intrinsic brain tumors. They arise from those cells of neuroectodermal origin that ultimately become the supportive tissue of the brain. This supportive tissue evolves from four distinct neuroglial cells: astrocytes, oligodendroglia, ependymal cells, and neuroglial precursors (choroid plexus). One or more of these cell types may be found in any given glioma. When more than one cell type is present, the tumor is referred to as a mixed glioma. Gliomas are classified largely by their cytological and/or biological malignancy.

HISTORY

Symptoms. Patients are usually asymptomatic until the tumor grows to a point that it causes acute decompensation, either directly or indirectly. Direct effects reflect location and manifest as focal neurologic signs such as limb paresis (50%), visual field defects, dysphasia, seizures, pseudopsychiatric symptoms, and disruptions of long or short memory. These changes occur due to the physical bulk of the tumor and by the effects of the edema surrounding such tumors.

Indirect effects are manifested as increased intracranial pressure. Frequently gliomas cause a disturbance of cerebrospinal fluid (CSF) circulation, resulting in hydrocephalus. Under these circumstances, symptoms may include headache, nausea, vomiting, and altered mental status (drowsiness).

Ependymomas frequently cause ataxia. So-called butterfly gliomas (bifrontal) are known to cause mood disorders.

Seizure is a presenting symptom in approximately 50% to 75% of astrocytomas and 80% of oligodendrogliomas. Headache is a presenting symptom in approximately 50% of gliomas and is characteristically bitemporal and diffuse, present on awakening, and often associated with nausea and vomiting.

General. Intrinsic brain tumors such as gliomas rarely metastasize. Their characterization as malignant, therefore, comes not from metastatic potential, but from their aggressive biological characteristics and poor prognosis.

Age. Primary malignant brain tumors are the second most common cause of cancer death among those aged 0 to 34 years and the third most common cause of cancer death among men aged 35 to 50 years. The second most common brain tumors among adults are glioblastoma multiforme, anaplastic astrocytoma, and metastases. Oligodendrogliomas occur in greatest numbers among adults during the fifth decade; these are rare in children. The most common brain tumors among children are astrocytomas, medulloblastomas, and ependymomas. Ependymomas tend to be infratentorial among children, adolescents, and young adults, and supratentorial among adults.

Onset. Onset of symptoms can be gradual if the tumor is slow growing and less invasive, or acute if fast growing and highly invasive.

Duration. Survival rates of glioma patients reflect the malignancy of the underlying tumor. Patients with oligodendroglioma, a more slowly growing tumor, have a 30% to 50% five-year survival rate. Patients with ependymomas have a 15% to 50% five-year survival rate. Patients with high-grade gliomas have a 17-week life expectancy if treated with surgery alone, and a 37-week life expectancy if treated with surgery and radiation therapy.

Intensity. Intensity varies from subtle and slowly progressive to catastrophic and acute.

Aggravating Factors. Symptoms may be increased by factors that increase intracranial pressure (e.g., valsalva, overexertion, alcohol intoxication).

Alleviating Factors. Dexamethasone decreases cerebral edema and may initially reduce symptoms.

Associated Factors. There is an increased incidence of gliomas among patients with von Recklinghausen disease, especially gliomas of the optic nerve. Patients with tuberous sclerosis have a high incidence (50%) of subependymal giant cell astrocytoma, most commonly located at the foramen of Munro. There appears to be no association between the incidence of gliomas and immunosuppression or exposure to environmental carcinogens or viral infections. There is current controversy regarding the association between exposure to electromagnetic radiation (power lines, cellular phones) and development of brain tumors. To date, this association has not been adequately explored and there are no compelling data to support the association.

PHYSICAL EXAMINATION

General. The patient may appear normal, appear acutely ill, or exhibit overt neurologic abnormalities (e.g., hemiparesis, unusual personality, etc.).

Neurologic. Acute decompensation attributable to gliomas usually presents as altered mental status. There may be an alteration in the level of consciousness or more subtle manifestations such as disorientation or memory impairment. A complete neurologic examination is essential. Abnormalities noted generally reflect the location of the lesion. Motor strip lesions cause contralateral upper or lower extremity weakness. Sensory changes may follow the same pattern. Ataxia may be present. Lower extremity deep tendon reflexes may be pathologic and toes may be upgoing. Coordination of upper or lower extremities may be compromised. Cranial nerve function is impaired, depending on lesion location. Extraocular movements, pupil size, reactivity, and accommodation must be documented. Funduscopic examination may or may not initially reveal papilledema. Diminished visual acuity, visual field cuts, and third, fourth, and sixth cranial nerve palsies are often noted.

PATHOPHYSIOLOGY

The malignancy of gliomas is determined pathologically by
1. Increased numbers of mitotic figures
2. Increased vascularity
3. Lack of distinct tumor margins.

Low-grade tumors are generally avascular and, in 15% of cases, contain calcium deposits. High-grade tumors usually have vascular margins (which enhance in sectional imaging studies) with a necrotic (nonenhancing) center. Gliomas have no capsule or clear tumor margin. They invade the brain diffusely, depositing microscopic nests of tumor cells beyond what appears to be the periphery of the lesion. In adults, gliomas generally occur in the cerebral hemispheres; in children, the cerebellum is the more common site.

Astrocytomas have been classified in two different systems. In the first (Kernohan), the most benign tumor cytologically (but not necessarily biologically) is identified as Grade I, and the most malignant is Grade IV. Grade I tumors are composed almost completely of astrocytes and show increased cellularity. Grade II tumors have mild to moderate pleomorphism, but no mitotic figures. Grade III tumors have increased vascularity, necrosis, and frequent mitotic figures. Fifty to seventy-five percent of the astrocytes appear normal. Grade IV tumors are like grade III tumors, except few of the astrocytes appear normal.

The Ringertz classification condenses the four grades into three tiers. In the order of progressive malignancy, these are

1. Astrocytoma (well differentiated)
2. Anaplastic astrocytoma
3. Glioblastoma multiforme (GBM).

Glioblastoma multiforme is the most common adult cerebral tumor. It constitutes approximately 30% of all primary brain tumors and 50% of all gliomas.

Ependymomas are predominantly interventricular. These may, however, invade the cerebellum, brain stem, or cerebral hemispheres. These constitute 5% of all intracranial tumors and 9% of all gliomas.

Oligodendrogliomas constitute 4% of all primary brain tumors.

Included among low-grade astrocytomas are juvenile pilocytic astrocytomas and subependymal giant cell astrocytomas. Mid- and high-grade astrocytomas include gemistocytic astrocytomas, anaplastic astrocytomas, malignant astrocytomas, glioblastoma multiforme, and gliosarcoma.

DIAGNOSTIC STUDIES

Laboratory
CBC. WBCs may be elevated in cases of cerebral abscess or in patients taking corticosteroids.

Chemistry Profile/PT/PTT. Performed as part of the preoperative screen.

Radiology
CT Scan of the Brain. Performed with and without contrast. Low-grade astrocytomas do not enhance with contrast. They have reduced radiographic density compared to surrounding parenchyma. There is little or no edema and no mass effect. Often these lesions are calcified. Ependymomas are usually heavily calcified. High-grade astrocytomas tend to be large, ring-enhancing lesions with low-density centers. There usually is surrounding edema and mass effect. Fifty percent of oligodendrogliomas enhance and 90% of these are calcified.

MRI of the Brain. With and without gadolinium provides improved visualization of these lesions, once identified, and is especially helpful in defining low-grade astrocytomas.

Angiography. Is used on rare occasions to delineate blood supply to the lesion.

Other
Metastatic Work-up. Instituted if brain metastases are suspected with no known primary malignancy. Work-up includes CT of the chest, abdomen, and pelvis, and any serologic tests including acute reactants such as ESR, CEA antigen, serum electrolyte levels (hyponatremia, hypercalcemia, hypermagnesemia may be present). Liver function tests are performed, especially LDH and alkaline phosphatase, which may be elevated in metastatic disease.

Infectious Disease Work-up. Performed if the patient's history is highly suggestive of acute or chronic disease exposure or of immunocompromise. Brain abscesses usually are seeded in multiple lesions.

DIFFERENTIAL DIAGNOSIS

Traumatic
Subdural or Epidural Hematomas. Can cause acute altered mental status or seizure, symptoms that often herald the presence of gliomas. These lesions are easily differentiated by CT or MRI of the brain.

Infectious
Brain Abscess (Solitary). Is often difficult to differentiate by sectional imaging studies from gliomas. Most historical data relative to immune status and infectious disease exposure can be very suggestive clinically. Serologic diagnostic studies (e.g., acid-fast bacilli, toxoplasmosis titers, etc.), are also suggestive. However, differentiation between a single brain abscess and a glioma can only be achieved with certainty by biopsy.

Metabolic
Metabolic Derangement. May cause altered mental status (e.g., diabetic coma, hyponatremia, etc.). CT/MRI of the brain is negative and further investigation reveals the source.

Neoplastic
Metastatic Tumors. Those that most frequently metastasize to brain originate in lung, breast, kidney, gastrointestinal tract. Metastatic deposits are usually multiple, but when they are not, can be ruled out only by biopsy.

Meningiomas. Have a predictable radiographic appearance and typical location (in association with the meninges), which makes diagnosis by sectional imaging studies more comfortable. Generally, biopsy is performed at the same time as craniotomy for excision of the meningioma.

Vascular
Ruptured Aneurysm/Ruptured Arteriovenous Malformation. May present clinically in the same way as a glioma, although symptoms usually appear acutely. Cerebral angiography (digital substraction angiography) demonstrates the vascular anatomy of aneurysms and arteriovenous malformations, and differentiates them from gliomas.

Intracerebral Hemorrhage. Has a distinct CT or MRI appearance. Symptoms appear acutely rather than progressively. Occasionally, a glioma may be the source of the hemorrhage and, if suspected, follow-up CT or MRI with contrast is indicated.

Stroke. May present with focal neurologic symptoms. CT/MRI with contrast differentiates ischemic areas from neoplastic areas.

Congenital. Not applicable.

Acquired
Drug/Alcohol Intoxication. May present with altered mental status. CT/MRI negative; toxicology screen positive.

TREATMENT

Medical. Perioperative medical treatments for gliomas include steroid therapy (dexamethasone) to decrease cerebral edema before and after surgery. A typical postoperative steroid regimen includes dexamethasone

10 mg IV or PO q6h for 24 hours following surgery, then 6 mg IV or PO q6h for 4 additional postoperative days. Thereafter, the steroid dose is gradually tapered.

Usually, an H_2 blocker also is given to protect the gastrointestinal tract while steroid therapy is in effect. Anticonvulsants are given pre- and postoperatively and must be continued for a period of at least 2 years, possibly for life. Phenytoin (Dilantin) is the usual first choice because it can be administered intravenously as well as orally. The loading dose is 15 mg/kg, and the usual maintenance dose is 300 mg daily. The target therapeutic serum level of phenytoin is 10 to 20 μg/mL. Carbamazepine (Tegretol) is given when phenytoin is not tolerated. It is administered orally only. The usual dose for carbamazepine is 200 mg b.i.d with a target serum level of 4 to 12 μg/mL. A third choice is phenobarbital at 30 mg t.i.d. All patients on anticonvulsants should be monitored every 2 to 4 months for serum levels, liver function abnormalities, and pancytopenia.

Radiation therapy is used as an adjunct to surgery and has been shown to double the median survival rate for high-grade gliomas to 37 weeks. Radiation may be used in the absence of surgical treatment where the tumor location renders it inoperable. Intracavitary radiation occasionally is used for cystic tumors. The total radiation dose for gliomas varies with type, location, and size, but generally falls between 4500 and 6000 rads.

Oncological consultation can be obtained to consider chemotherapy, although definite benefit has not been established.

Experimental immunotherapy has not yet been found effective.

Surgical. Surgery is almost always required for diagnosing, grading, and treating gliomas. CT-guided stereotactic needle biopsy to establish diagnosis is preferred (when possible) over craniotomy with open biopsy in order to minimize morbidity. However, when a lesion is suspected of being highly vascular or when it is located in an area not safely approached stereotactically, an open craniotomy may be required for biopsy. In treating gliomas as opposed to diagnosing them, craniotomy is employed to debulk the tumor, and thereby reduce intracranial pressure, and to optimize subsequent adjuvant therapy.

Adjuvant therapy (radiation therapy) may be chosen without initial craniotomy and debulking when, on diagnosis, the tumor is found to be highly infiltrative and edematous. Subsequent to radiation therapy, the tumor quite often becomes necrotic. Surgery may then be elected to remove the necrotic tissue and thereby reduce the intracranial pressure.

Surgical exposure varies from a single burr hole for stereotactic needle biopsy access to excision of bone flap for open craniotomy. When a bone flap is removed, it is frequently reattached with titanium plates and screws. Because these are not affected by electromagnetic fields, the patient may undergo MRI postoperatively.

Typical tools used in craniotomies for glioma include stereotactic apparatus, ultrasound imaging, ultrasonic aspirator, microscope, somatosensory-evoked potentials, and laser ablation.

Disturbance of CSF circulation dynamics may result from gliomas and other brain lesions, resulting in acute hydrocephalus. Surgical intervention in the form of ventriculo-peritoneal or ventriculo-atrial shunting may be required.

Follow-up MRI scanning is required to determine the extent of excision and to evaluate for recurrence (continued growth).

Indications. For tumor diagnosis, grading, debulking, and reducing intracranial pressure.

Contraindications. Significant coagulopathy, brain death, inability to tolerate anesthesia.

PA Role in Surgery. The PA assists with the opening and closing of the craniotomy. Brain retraction and assistance with hemostasis may be required intraoperatively. One of the key roles of the PA is to coordinate ancillary services (e.g., radiation therapy, oncology, social services) and to provide education about the condition to the patient and family.

PEDIATRIC CONSIDERATIONS

Primary malignant brain tumors are the second most common cause of cancer death in children under the age of 15 years.

Oligodendrogliomas are rare in children.

Astrocytomas in children usually occur in the cerebellum.

Most optic nerve gliomas occur in children under the age of 10 years. These are usually benign juvenile pilocytic astrocytomas.

Brainstem gliomas occur more often in children than in adults.

OBSTETRICAL CONSIDERATIONS

Chemotherapeutic agents may seriously endanger a fetus and should be administered during pregnancy only if absolutely necessary.

PEARLS FOR THE PA

Particular care should be given to the explanation of the terms "benign" and "malignant" in any discussion of gliomas. Patients and their families need to understand that tumors can be malignant in terms of their aggressive characteristics and poor prognosis.

Because of the infiltrative nature of gliomas, complete surgical resection of these lesions is not possible.

Gliomas, even those that are low grade, usually recur. When they do recur, they frequently convert to a higher grade of malignancy. Therefore, close monitoring with follow-up sectional imaging studies is indicated.

Head Injury

James B. Labus, PA-C

DEFINITION

An injury to the brain sufficient to cause a transient loss of consciousness (concussion).

HISTORY

Symptoms. Memory loss, both retrograde (before the trauma) and antegrade (after the trauma), signs of increased intracranial pressure (headache, nausea, vomiting), or focal neurologic deficit.

General. The patient has a history of trauma, although he or she may not be able to recall the events surrounding the injury. It is important to obtain the mechanism and force of injury, if possible, from family, friends, witnesses, or from the ambulance personnel. Determine the last item the patient remembers prior to the event, as well as the most recent recollection (e.g., awakening in the ambulance). As with any trauma patient, obtain a full past medical history of concurrent illness. If the patient has had a period when he or she awoke after the trauma, then became lethargic, suspect epidural hematoma.

Age. Any, but more common in the second and third decades, when trauma is more prevalent.

Onset. Acute, although cerebral edema may not be manifested for 1 to 2 days.

Duration. Residual deficits may be permanent or resolve.

Intensity. Mild to life threatening.

Aggravating Factors. Alcohol use/abuse, underlying systemic conditions, hypotension, hypoxia.

Alleviating Factors. For mild concussion, rest and nonsedating analgesics may improve symptoms.

Associated Factors. Injuries to other organ systems, cervical spine injury, facial lacerations/fractures, development of subdural, epidural, or intracerebral hemorrhage.

PHYSICAL EXAMINATION

General. The patient may appear relatively normal or may have significant multiple trauma. The ABCs (airway, breathing, circulation) take precedence on the initial evaluation of any trauma patient. A full-body survey is performed to check for life-threatening or multisystem injury. Respirations may be regular, Cheyne-Stokes (intermittent pauses—

diencephalon), hyperventilatory (central neurogenic hyperventilation—midbrain), or irregular (ataxic—brainstem).

HEENT. The cervical spine must be cleared by x-ray (which includes C7) owing to a correlation between head injury and cervical spine injury. The tympanic membranes are viewed to rule out a hemotympanum. The mastoid area is observed for Battle's sign (bruising). Periorbital ecchymosis (raccoon eyes) may be present. Battle's sign and raccoon eyes are suggestive of a basilar skull fracture and the possibility of CSF leak (otorhinorrhea). If any nasal drainage is noted, it is checked for the presence of glucose (bloody nasal drainage is glucose positive because serum contains glucose).

Neurologic. Special attention is given to the mental status to obtain a baseline. Orientation, memory, and level of consciousness are documented. The Glasgow Coma Scale (Table 7–1) may be used or the specific findings documented. Avoid terms such as lethargic or obtunded and state in plain terms what the patient is able to perform. Mental status is repeatedly checked as an inpatient or, if the patient is discharged, by a family member or friend. A complete neurologic examination is performed. Cranial nerves (CN) are examined for abnormalities. Subfrontal injuries (CN I) may cause anosmia. CN III should be assessed for evidence of direct injury or palsy due to brain herniation. One of the more frequent findings in head

---

Table 7–1. Glasgow Coma Scale

The Glasgow Coma Scale is a practical means of monitoring changes in the level of consciousness based on eye opening and verbal and motor responses. The responsiveness of the patient can be expressed by summation of the figures. The lowest score is 3, the highest is 15.

Eyes	Spontaneously (eyes open, does not imply awareness)	4
Open	To speech (any speech, not necessarily a command)	3
	To pain (should not use supraorbital pressure for pain stimulus)	2
	Never	1
Best	Oriented (to time, person, place)	5
Verbal	Confused speech (disoriented)	4
Response	Inappropriate (swearing, yelling)	3
	Incomprehensible sounds (moaning, groaning)	2
	None	1
Best	Obeys commands	6
Motor	Localizes pain (deliberate or purposeful movement)	5
Response	Withdrawal (moves away from stimulus)	4
	Abnormal flexion (decortication)	3
	Extension (decerebration)	2
	None (flaccidity)	1
	Total Score _____	

From Youmans JR: Neurological Surgery, 4th ed. Philadelphia, W. B. Saunders, 1996, p. 65.

injury is that of CN VI palsy (abducens). Facial paralysis (CN VII) may be incurred from skull base fractures. Nystagmus or hearing loss may be present owing to an injury of CN VIII (acoustic/vestibular). For the comatose patient, cranial nerve testing should include corneal reflex, doll's eyes (if the eyes move with the head as if they were "painted on" and do not remain fixed on a distant point, it means the oculocephalic reflex is impaired), cold water calorics, and gag. Motor examination includes the presence of focal or unilateral weakness. Posturing, if present, is noted to be flexor or extensor. Sensory testing should include all dermatomes because concurrent spine and nerve root injuries may not be apparent on a quick screen. Sensation may be tested in the unresponsive patient by applying a painful stimuli on both sides of the body. Reflexes, cerebellum, and gait (if possible) are also examined for localizing signs.

Ophthalmologic. The eyes are evaluated for deviation and pupillary size is documented. Pupils fixed in mid-position suggest midbrain injury; pinpoint pupils imply pontine injury. An ipsilateral "blown" pupil is the cardinal sign of herniation. Papilledema is not initially seen, but funduscopic findings are documented and used as a baseline.

PATHOPHYSIOLOGY

The brain is protected from injury by surrounding CSF, which creates a cushion, and the skull. The facial bones with the associated sinuses absorb much of the impact of direct trauma and also protect the brain (although the injury can be disfiguring). When an injury occurs with enough force, the brain, which is mobile in the skull, can sustain damage. Contusion or shearing forces that involve the brain are termed diffuse axonal injury.

Contrecoup injuries occur when the mobile brain within the skull is contused opposite the site of trauma by an acceleration or deceleration type of injury (e.g., frontal contusion after occipital trauma).

Shearing of the axons and myelin sheath occurs as the brain undergoes rotation, acceleration, or deceleration at different speeds and is associated with petechial hemorrhages seen on CT scan.

Cerebral edema can occur in a specific area and be associated with a contusion, or occur diffusely throughout the brain. If the edema is significant, herniation and death can ensue.

Hemorrhage into the brain will *not* cause a drop in the hemoglobin and hematocrit, although associated scalp or facial lacerations may do so.

CSF leaks, usually due to a basilar skull fracture, may present acutely or in a delayed fashion. Cerebral edema initially may inhibit the leak. Conversely, delayed edema may cause an existing leak to cease.

DIAGNOSTIC STUDIES

Laboratory
Full Chemistry Profile, CBC, PT, PTT, Platelets. Are performed as a screening measure in trauma victims to rule out underlying abnormalities.

Drug Screen/Alcohol Levels.   Should be performed as a routine measure in trauma. Drug or alcohol intoxication may cause decreased responsiveness.

Radiology

CT of the Brain.   Should be performed as soon as possible. May show contusion, petechial hemorrhage, subdural or epidural hematomas, traumatic subarachnoid blood (subarachnoid hemorrhages can sometimes precede trauma). Bone windows must be obtained to look for skull fractures. Contrecoup findings are those of a cerebral contusion on the opposite side of the brain from where the trauma occurred. Special attention is given to the adequacy of the basilar cisterns, which are normally filled with CSF. A reduction in the size of this space is a significant finding, because it suggests diffuse cerebral edema. Hydrocephalus may be a delayed finding. Pneumocephalus (air within the intracranial compartment) is associated with basilar skull fractures.

MRI of the Brain.   Although more sensitive, is not commonly used for trauma screening owing to the time required in the scanner. May show sites of cerebral edema or coexisting pathology (e.g., neoplasm).

Skull X-ray.   Used to identify a skull fracture. Pneumocephalus (air in the cranial vault) or shift of calcified midline structures (e.g., pineal) may be identified. Obtaining skull x-rays must *not* delay brain imaging. More useful in the pediatric population.

Chest X-ray.   Pulmonary edema may result from head injury without primary pulmonary pathology.

Other

EEG.   Can be performed to evaluate the risk of seizure and the use of anticonvulsants following head injury. Also used to confirm brain death.

Cerebral Blood Flow.   Used to confirm brain death.

Isotope CSF Study.   Indicated to identify the location of a CSF leak from a basilar skull fracture.

DIFFERENTIAL DIAGNOSIS

Traumatic.   Not otherwise applicable.

Infectious

Meningitis.   May be a complication of head injury if a CSF leak is present.

Metabolic

Metabolic Coma.   Conditions such as diabetes may cause coma and lead to trauma. Serological evaluation should reveal the source.

Neoplastic

Brain Tumor.   Primary or metastatic; may be present in patients with a head injury. If a suspicious finding is evident on CT/MRI of the brain, contrast should be given.

Vascular

Intracerebral/Subarachnoid Hemorrhage.   May have occurred prior to the traumatic event (e.g., the hemorrhage occurred, which caused loss of consciousness and subsequent motor vehicle accident). Angiogram may be required as indicated to evaluate the source.

Congenital. Not applicable.

Acquired

Drug or Alcohol Use. Can cause altered mental status in the trauma patient. Drug testing and alcohol levels are positive.

TREATMENT

Medical. The initial physical findings should be documented and compared in subsequent examinations. If the patient is neurologically normal, there is no decreased level of consciousness, and no nausea/vomiting, there is capable support at home, the injury was of low velocity, and the CT/MRI are normal, the patient may be considered for discharge with follow-up in 1 day. If there is any uncertainty whatsoever, the patient should be hospitalized for observation. Intracerebral contusions, like bruises anywhere on the body, may not reach the maximal intensity for 1 to 2 days. The patient with a concussion may "talk and die" with the development of significant edema. Predictors of this phenomenon include reduced basilar cisterns on CT scan and clinical condition.

For mild concussion:

Vital signs and neurologic checks are performed every 1 to 2 hours.

NPO.

The head of the bed is kept elevated at 10 to 30 degrees.

Nonsedating analgesics (e.g., acetaminophen, codeine 30 mg) ordered.

Pulse oximetry may be applied and supplemental oxygen given to prevent hypoxia.

Fluid restriction to 75 mL/h D5 1/2 normal saline with 20 mEq KCl (fluid type may vary).

CT of the brain repeated for any change in neurologic status.

Acetaminophen or cooling blanket for fever, because hyperpyrexia may increase intracranial pressure.

For a severe head injury, the patient is hospitalized in the intensive care unit (ICU). The same measures listed above are applied, with the addition of the following:

Nutritional support is instituted via hyperalimentation or through a nasogastric (NG) tube (caution: *do not* place an NG tube in a patient with a known or suspected skull base fracture).

Electrolytes and CBC are performed daily to identify any metabolic abnormality (hyponatremia may result from injury to the brain) or infection in the early stages.

General care measures are undertaken (skin, urinary catheter, etc.) for those who are comatose or the patient who must remain at bedrest.

Prophylactic antibiotics are given for CSF leak. If the leak fails to resolve, surgical intervention may be necessary.

Anticonvulsants are used per the protocol of the physician. It is usually not necessary to treat the patient with anticonvulsants unless there is a suspicion of or a known seizure following the injury.

H_2 blockers are given due to the increased incidence of gastric ulceration following head injury.

Intracranial pressure (ICP) is of principal concern. If the patient has significant edema or contusion on CT, significant decreased level of consciousness, or impending herniation, he or she is intubated and hyperventilated to a pCO_2 of 25 to 30 (hypercapnia causes a rise in ICP). ICP monitoring devices may be placed, including ventriculostomy (which can also drain CSF), subarachnoid bolt, or ICP monitor. ICP may be normal in patients who have suffered a brain stem injury, although the patient may be comatose. Osmotic diuretics (e.g., mannitol) can be used to decrease ICP. Serum osmolalities should be followed and dosage adjusted to keep the osmolality from exceeding 320 mOsm/kg.

Steroids such as dexamethasone have little use in the acute setting of brain injury.

If the ICP fails to respond to these measures, sedation may be employed using barbiturates. At this point, neurologic examination is not possible. Treatment is based on the results of the ICP monitor. Prior to diagnosing brain death, the barbiturates must be reversed.

Post-traumatic rehabilitation is begun in the hospital and continued (as indicated) in the home or structured environment. The patient may have profound deficits that may improve or resolve over time. Physical, occupational, speech, and cognitive therapies may be implemented. Social services can assist with coordination of care.

Surgical. A craniotomy is performed to evacuate a significant hematoma. Careful attention to hemostasis is mandatory in order to prevent reaccumulation of blood. If the patient has acute herniation, a temporal lobectomy is sometimes used to decrease the intracranial volume. Depressed skull fractures can be débrided and elevated.

Ventriculostomies, subarachnoid bolts, or intracerebral monitors may be inserted through a burr hole at the time of surgery or in the ICU. For ventriculostomies, the ventricular catheter is inserted, through the cortical substance, into the ventricle. Strict sterile technique is required to prevent infection of the foreign body. CSF is obtained and sent for routine studies. The catheter is attached to an ICP monitor and drainage bag.

Persistent CSF leaks are repaired after adequate time for the resolution of cerebral edema has elapsed. Transposing pericranium or fascia lata into the site of the defect is performed.

Indications. If a post-traumatic hematoma is found to be causing significant shift of midline structures or if there is a depressed skull fracture. Persistent CSF leaks (timing and intervention are by surgeon preference).

ICP monitors are indicated when it is necessary to measure pressure to guide therapy.

Complications include infection, malfunction, intracerebral hemorrhage, inability to access the ventricle (with small ventricles).

Contraindications. Coagulopathy (hematoma will reaccumulate), minor hemorrhage or contusion that is not causing significant shift; brain death.

PA Role in Surgery. The PA assists with opening, closing, and hemostasis with the craniotomy. Assistance with harvesting fascia lata and pericranium is performed in procedures involving correction of CSF leaks. For ICP monitors, the PA may be assigned the task of maintaining patency, obtaining CSF for study, removing the device, and treating the patient based on the readings. When removing a ventricular catheter, it is important not to encounter any resistance. Resistance may signify that a blood clot has formed. Do not force removal, because the catheter may break. When closing the site, it is recommended to use a purse-string type of suture to prevent leakage of CSF from the site.

PEDIATRIC CONSIDERATIONS

The diagnosis and treatment for infant and pediatric trauma is basically the same; however, certain considerations must be taken into account. The infant's brain undergoes continued growth, and neural connections are forming. Therefore, head injury may disturb normal maturation and the child's ability to reach developmental milestones. The skull is not yet fused, the bones of the skull are soft, and myelination is not complete. With injury, the infant is more likely to suffer shearing-type injuries than contusions. Trauma may result in prolonged edema.

The history and physical examination pose some difficulty because transient loss of consciousness may not have been observed and cannot be communicated by the child. Orientation is difficult to assess. A period of amnesia may follow, with or without a definite loss of consciousness. The older child may have "traumatic automatism," which is a condition in which the patient continues with an activity but has no recollection of the activity (e.g., football injuries). Prolonged vomiting or focal finding, even by history (e.g., temporary loss of vision) suggest more severe injury; hospitalization is recommended.

Fontanelles are palpated to evaluate for increased ICP.

A history of seizure should be obtained. Seizures that occur immediately after the insult do not have a predictive value in the development of epilepsy. Seizures may occur as a delayed finding. There should be a low threshold of admission for the child with a head injury.

Additional diagnostic studies that are valuable in the pediatric population are skull x-rays and cerebral ultrasound. Fractures that are identified suggest an increased velocity of trauma. Ultrasonography can screen the intracranial contents for abnormalities without radiation (this does not supplant CT).

Children should be followed closely for electrolyte disturbances (e.g., sodium, potassium). Anticonvulsant use following head injury is controversial.

Child Abuse. Infants who present with subdural hematomas may have been victims of "shaken baby syndrome." This is associated with injury to the underlying brain. Child abuse should be suspected in infants and children who have intracerebral injury without surface injury (e.g., face, head, etc.), if there is conflicting or no history given for the injury, history is inconsistent with the child's developmental stage, there are multiple or recurrent injuries, delay in seeking treatment, abnormal parent–child interaction, or if the child is abnormally passive to medical care.

OBSTETRICAL CONSIDERATIONS

The risks versus benefits of diagnostic and therapeutic intervention need to be weighed based on the severity of the head injury. The fetus should be shielded if CT scanning is performed. The safety of MRI has not been established in pregnancy, but is not recommended during the first trimester. If the pregnant patient has suffered a severe head injury, fetal monitoring and obstetrical consultation are required.

PEARLS FOR THE PA

Cerebral edema may not be exhibited for 1 to 2 days after injury.

The reduction in the normal size of the basilar cisterns on CT suggests diffuse cerebral edema.

Serial evaluation of the patient is mandatory to assess for neurologic changes.

Hydrocephalus
James B. Labus, PA-C

DEFINITION

An expansion in the size of the ventricular system of the brain due to an accumulation of CSF. Hydrocephalus is classified as communicating due to reduced absorption of CSF or extraventricular obstruction, or noncommunicating (obstructive), due to a blockage of flow within the ventricular system. Another variant is normal-pressure hydrocephalus (NPH), which is a type of communicating hydrocephalus.

HISTORY

Symptoms. In adults, symptoms are usually related to signs of increased intracranial pressure (e.g., decreased level of consciousness, headache, nausea, vomiting). The patient may present with symptoms of focal neurologic deficit if the hydrocephalus is associated with a neoplasm. These symptoms may include personality change, hemiparesis, hemisensory loss, cranial nerve symptoms, balance difficulties, etc. The patient may have limited upgaze directly due to the hydrocephalus, or decreased visual acuity. NPH presents with a classic triad of dementia, urinary incontinence, and ataxia.

In infants and children, symptoms of hydrocephalus may be nonspecific (developmental delay, failure to thrive, lethargy, vomiting) or specific (increased head size, limited upward gaze, dilation of scalp veins). See pediatric considerations for presentations in infants.

General. For the infant or child, detailed data about the child's birth (e.g., premature), developmental delay, trauma, eating habits, academic achievement, memory, and activity must be obtained. In adolescents, precocious puberty or delayed endocrinological development may be encountered.

In the adult, inquire about focal neurologic signs or symptoms. In the elderly (data may be obtained from a family member or caretaker if the patient is demented) ask about mental function, gait stability, and urinary incontinence.

Age. Any, although aqueductal stenosis usually occurs at a younger age (including infants) and obstructive hydrocephalus more in older children and adults (depending on tumor pathogenesis). NPH in the elderly.

Onset. Acute or gradual, depending on the cause. Waxing and waning symptoms are sometimes encountered with intermittent CSF disruption (partial blockage is overcome when the CSF pressure behind the blockage is sufficient to allow returned flow).

Duration. May present acutely or with progressive symptoms.

Intensity. From mild, nonspecific symptoms to life-threatening increased ICP.

Aggravating Factors. Lumbar puncture, in the presence of increased ICP or mass lesion, may cause herniation of the brain and death.

Alleviating Factors. Identification and treatment.

Associated Factors. Intracerebral lesion, intracerebral hemorrhage (especially blood in the ventricular system), meningitis, or subarachnoid hemorrhage may cause inhibition of CSF flow.

PHYSICAL EXAMINATION

General. The patient may appear normal or may show overt signs of neurologic compromise.

Neurologic. A full and complete neurologic examination is performed to document the presence or absence of focal neurologic deficits due to mass lesions. The mental status should be ascertained to assess the degree of dementia present when evaluating for NPH. If a shunt is present for known hydrocephalus, it should be evaluated for function. Familiarity with shunt systems is essential when evaluating for patency. Usually, a bulb is palpable under the skin of the scalp. This bulb should compress and refill easily. In children, it is important to evaluate head circumference and compare it to established norms. Palpate the anterior fontanelle. A tense anterior fontanelle suggests increased ICP. Percussion of the skull may reveal a "cracked pot" sound. Observe for dilation of the veins of the scalp, which may suggest intracranial compromise. The cranium may also be transilluminated to evaluate intracranial contents.

Ophthalmologic. A full visual examination is performed with attention to acuity and extraocular muscle testing. Limitation of upgaze may be present owing to pressure from the third ventricle on the midbrain.

PATHOPHYSIOLOGY

The choroid plexi, which are located in the ventricular system of the brain, manufacture CSF at a rate of approximately 0.4 mL/minute. The CSF pathway begins at the lateral ventricle. CSF courses through the foramen of Monro into the third ventricle. It then goes through the aqueduct of Sylvius into the fourth ventricle, subarachnoid space of the brain and spinal cord, and basilar cisterns. From there it flows over the convexity of the brain, where it is reabsorbed by the arachnoid villi. The arachnoid villi arise from the dural sinuses, which allow absorbed CSF to enter the venous system.

Communicating hydrocephalus may be caused by obstructions of flow outside of the ventricular system (e.g., basilar cisterns) or from reduced uptake or failure of the arachnoid granulations to reabsorb CSF.

Noncommunicating hydrocephalus is caused by extrinsic compression of CSF flow within the ventricular system (e.g., neoplasm) or from aqueductal stenosis (primary, or secondary to extrinsic compression).

Any condition that interferes with the normal CSF flow may cause hydrocephalus. Conditions that cause adhesions include meningitis, hemorrhage, or tumor invasion of the meninges.

NPH is somewhat different in that the CSF is under normal pressure. Symptoms are thought to arise from flow of CSF into the cerebral substance through the ependymal cells that line the ventricles. NPH is one of the reversible causes of dementia.

DIAGNOSTIC STUDIES

Laboratory
Full Chemistry Profile, CBC, PT, PTT, Platelets, Bleeding Time. Performed as routine preoperative testing.

CSF Testing. Is performed after CT or MRI scanning rules out obstructive hydrocephalus or intracranial lesion. Evaluation may include glucose, protein, and cell count to rule out infectious processes, or special tests (e.g., cytology, acid-fast bacilli, India ink, cryptococcal antigen, etc.).

Radiology

CT Scan of the Brain. Used as a screening device to assess ventricular size and to determine which ventricles are affected. All of the ventricles are affected in communicating hydrocephalus. With obstructive hydrocephalus, the dilation may be unilateral, only affect the lateral ventricles, or affect the lateral and third ventricles. CT is used for postoperative follow-up to evaluate the patency of the shunt. CT should be performed with contrast if a mass lesion is suspected. If CT is negative and the index of suspicion is high for a lesion, MRI should be performed. CT can be used more efficaciously in the acute setting to evaluate for hemorrhage (subarachnoid, intracerebral, intraventricular).

MRI of the Brain. Performed with contrast if a mass lesion is suspected of causing obstructive hydrocephalus. CSF pathways can be visualized in detail on sagittal imaging. Aqueductal stenosis may be identified. More sensitive than CT in diagnosing small lesions.

Ultrasound. Can assess ventricular size in infants with an open fontanelle.

Isotope Cisternogram. Used to evaluate for NPH. Retention of isotope within the ventricles is considered positive.

Other

Shunt Tap. Performed only by experienced personnel. Used to measure CSF pressure and shunt patency. CSF can be sent for laboratory studies.

DIFFERENTIAL DIAGNOSIS

Traumatic

Intracranial Hemorrhage. May cause adhesions that inhibit CSF flow, especially if the hemorrhage has involved areas inhabited by CSF. Hydrocephalus may be a delayed finding.

Infectious

Meningitis. May cause adhesions that inhibit CSF flow; CSF positive. Hydrocephalus may be a delayed finding.

Metabolic

Cerebral Atrophy. May give the appearance of enlarged ventricles on CT scan. The perceived enlargement is due to loss of cerebral substance. The convexity of the brain appears atrophied compatible with the degree of ventricular "enlargement."

Neoplastic

Intracranial Lesion. May be responsible for obstructing CSF flow.

Vascular

Hemorrhage (e.g., Subarachnoid, Intraventricular, Intracerebral). May be responsible for obstruction or cause adhesions that inhibit CSF flow. Hydrocephalus may be a delayed finding.

Congenital

Aqueductal Stenosis.   Most frequently encountered congenital cause of hydrocephalus. Caused by a stenosis of the aqueduct of Sylvius. Congenital absence of the foramen of Luschka or Magendie is uncommon.

Arnold-Chiari Malformation.   A congenital anomaly in neurodevelopment; may give rise to hydrocephalus.

Acquired

Shunt Malfunction.   Shunt systems may become clogged with debris, infected, or become defective for mechanical reasons. Hydrocephalus may recur in this setting.

Other

Pseudotumor Cerebri.   May present with symptoms similar to hydrocephalus. CT reveals ventricles that may be smaller than normal. Papilledema is a hallmark feature. Shunting is sometimes required.

TREATMENT

Medical.   Not applicable.

Surgical.   Shunt procedures are performed to reduce the pressure of CSF on the brain and reduce cerebral damage. Shunting is performed by inserting a catheter into the lateral ventricle. This can be attached to an external drain (if shunting is thought to be temporary), or internalized with the CSF drained into the peritoneum (ventriculoperitoneal shunt), atrium (ventriculoatrial shunt) or, less commonly, to the pleura (ventriculopleural shunt). For communicating hydrocephalus, a lumboperitoneal (LP) shunt may be chosen. Although the LP shunt is noninvasive to the brain, it is less accessible and less reliable. Shunt system selection is a matter of preference. They are available as low-, medium-, and high-pressure systems, which are chosen depending on the condition and cause being treated.

The catheter is inserted into the ventricle through the cerebral substance via a burr hole. Pressure measurements and CSF for testing may be obtained. The distal catheter is tunneled under the skin to the insertion point. Insertion points include the peritoneum, the common facial vein of the neck to access the atrium, and the pleura. The catheters are attached and incisions closed.

In some instances, the surgeon may choose to remove a neoplasm that is obstructing flow without first placing a shunt catheter. This is a matter of preference and experience with these conditions.

Meticulous attention to sterile technique is mandatory as shunt infection can be a serious complication, especially in the shunt-dependent patient. Antibiotics routinely are given intra- and postoperatively. Other complications include shunt malfunction or hemorrhage (subdural or intracerebral).

Indications.   Acute or progressive hydrocephalus from any cause, preoperatively to reduce pressure from a lesion causing obstructive hydrocephalus; NPH.

Contraindications. Long-standing hydrocephalus with closed skull sutures, such as that seen in a patient with macrocephaly and extremely large ventricles. Shunting these individuals may shrink the brain, thereby causing traction on bridging veins, resulting in subdural hematoma.

PA Role in Surgery. When assisting with a shunt procedure, it is imperative to maintain meticulous sterile technique. Assisting is performed on both the ventricular and insertion site (peritoneum, atrium, or pleura). It is important after insertion of the ventricular catheter not to let copious amounts of drainage escape, which may decompress the ventricle and increase the risk of subdural hematoma formation. Care is also taken in closing the incision(s) not to incorporate the catheter into the sutures. Close attention to postoperative wound care is essential to prevent superficial infections that may result in a shunt infection.

PEDIATRIC CONSIDERATIONS

Hydrocephalus in the newborn or infant is usually due to congenital abnormalities, most often aqueductal stenosis. Intracerebral hemorrhage (more common in premature infants), especially associated with intraventricular blood, places the child at risk for development of hydrocephalus.

There is also a higher incidence of occurrence with spina bifida. Any child with symptoms of hydrocephalus should be examined for spina bifida. The converse is also true. Signs of spina bifida range from a dimple or hairy patch of the lower back to myelomeningocele, where the tethered spinal cord is seen exiting from the back. If spina bifida is present, a full neurologic evaluation is performed to assess the degree of neurologic compromise and determine treatment. Surgical treatments are available for significant disorders. Spina bifida may be associated with other nervous system, gastrointestinal, or urinary malformations.

Most children do quite well with the shunt procedure. Close follow-up is imperative to evaluate for potential shunt malfunctions or infections. As the child grows, lengthening procedures of the distal catheters may be required.

OBSTETRICAL CONSIDERATIONS

Prenatal amniotic α_1-fetoprotein (in high-risk individuals) should be performed to evaluate for spina bifida. Routine prenatal ultrasound can measure head circumference and note if there are any abnormalities that require further evaluation.

For the woman who becomes pregnant with a peritoneal catheter in place, it is imperative to assess the risks and benefits of converting to a ventriculoatrial system.

PEARLS FOR THE PA

Infants may present with nonspecific symptoms, such as failure to thrive or reach developmental milestones.

Hydrocephalus is frequently associated with spina bifida or intracerebral hemorrhage.

Limitation of upgaze is a pathognomonic finding.

NPH is one of the reversible causes of dementia.

Meningioma
James B. Labus, PA-C

DEFINITION

Meningioma is a neoplasm that arises from cells of the arachnoid layer of the meninges. Usually benign, this tumor is the most common intracranial neoplasm after glioma and accounts for approximately 15% of all intracranial tumors. Approximately 90% of meningiomas occur intracranially, with the remainder arising from the arachnoid of the spinal cord.

HISTORY

Symptoms. Are usually related to increased ICP. These symptoms include headache (which may be worse with Valsalva maneuver or with the head in the dependent position), nausea and vomiting, photophobia, or lethargy. Patients may also present with seizure, and a history of potential seizure must be obtained. Focal neurologic deficits such as hemiparesis, hemisensory loss, or cranial nerve abnormalities may be present. With tumors that affect the frontal lobe, progressive personality changes may be manifest, and it is important to obtain adjunct information from family members.

General. Meningiomas are usually slow growing and symptoms may be indolent as the intracranial vault accommodates for tumor growth. Symptoms may not be present during this growth phase. The patient develops symptoms when the intracranial compartment can no longer accommodate tumor growth. These symptoms may be slow and progressive or the patient may present with relatively acute findings.

Age. Incidence increases with advancing age; rare in childhood; women more often than men.

Onset. Slow and progressive as tumor growth progresses.

Duration. Tumor growth may be present for several years.

Intensity. The patient may be asymptomatic or present with seizure or signs and symptoms of increased ICP.

Aggravating Factors. Symptoms of increased ICP or the propensity to have a seizure may be worsened by maneuvers such as becoming overheated, Valsalva, or alcohol intoxication.

Alleviating Factors. Tumor removal; seizure prophylaxis.

Associated Factors. Patients with von Recklinghausen disease may have multiple intracranial neoplasms, including meningiomas. There is a correlation between breast carcinoma and meningioma. MRI of the brain is indicated when dealing with either of these conditions. Conditions that increase progesterone (pregnancy, medications) may increase the size of existing meningiomas.

PHYSICAL EXAMINATION

General. The patient may appear normal or have obvious neurologic deficit.

Neurologic. A full and complete neurologic examination is mandatory to evaluate for subtle abnormalities. The mental status examination may reveal changes in affect, reasoning, memory, or intelligence that may suggest frontal lobe involvement. Cranial nerves I to XII should be tested. Anosmia may be the only sign of an olfactory groove meningioma. Other skull base or posterior fossa meningiomas may exhibit cranial nerve anomalies. Motor and sensory evaluations may reveal a subtle hemiparesis or hemisensory loss. Cerebellar examination may herald the presence of a posterior fossa lesion.

Ophthalmologic. Proptosis may be present with certain locations of meningioma. Funduscopic examination may reveal papilledema, which signifies increased ICP. Visual field testing, either formally or to confrontation, should be performed to document any visual field deficits that may be present with occipital lobe lesions or lesions that affect the optic chiasm. Visual loss may be present with lesions that involve the optic nerve.

PATHOPHYSIOLOGY

Meningiomas are usually benign in that they do not invade brain tissue (although malignant meningiomas, which are uncommon, invade brain tissue). The cause of meningiomas is unknown. Sites of meningeal trauma have been implicated but not definitively proven.

Locations for the development of meningioma, in order of frequency, are parasagittal/falcine, convexity, sphenoid wing, olfactory groove, suprasellar, posterior fossa, ventricular, and optic sheath.

Treatment approach and prognosis are more related to tumor location than to histological type. Tumors of the skull base or those that involve the cavernous sinus may be unable to be completely resected.

Histological subtypes include syncytial (endotheliomatous), transitional, fibroblastic, angioblastic, and malignant. The angioblastic tumors are more vascular.

Meningiomas are usually well circumscribed and can be separated from surrounding brain. An exception to this is an *en plaque* meningioma, which occurs as a thin sheath.

There is a hormonal influence on meningiomas as well. Frequently, these tumors have progesterone receptors and, in the presence of endogenous or exogenous progesterone, become larger.

DIAGNOSTIC STUDIES

Laboratory
Full Chemistry Profile, CBC, PT, PTT, Bleeding Time. Are performed if surgery is being contemplated as routine preoperative screening. An elevated WBC may indicate the presence of an inflammatory lesion such as an abscess (the WBC may also be elevated if the patient has been placed on steroids for treatment of increased ICP).

ACTH, Prolactin, Growth Hormone, Thyroid Profile, LH/FSH. Are obtained if the tumor is believed to affect hypothalamic or pituitary function. A significant elevation of growth hormone or prolactin may indicate that the lesion is a pituitary adenoma with suprasellar extension, rather than a meningioma.

Radiology
CT Scan of the Brain. Performed with and without intravenous contrast, identifies most meningiomas. Meningiomas uniformly enhance with contrast. CT is limited in its ability to identify skull base or small meningiomas. Hyperostosis may be identified. Lesions of the posterior fossa may cause hydrocephalus, so documentation of ventricular appearance and size is necessary.

MRI of the Brain. Performed with and without gadolinium, MRI is the recommended study for evaluating the presence, extent of involvement and, in many cases, an indication of the vascular supply of meningiomas. Meningiomas uniformly enhance with gadolinium. Common sites of meningiomas are shown in Figure 7–1.

Skull X-ray. Rarely required due to the presence of CT and MRI, may reveal hyperostosis or shift of the calcified pineal or choroid plexus.

Magnetic Resonance Angiography (MRA) of the Brain. A noninvasive measure to identify feeding vessels and the extent of vascularization of a meningioma. This is usually done in anticipation of surgery for suspected vascular tumors.

MRI of the Spine. Performed with and without gadolinium, when indicated, if a spinal cord lesion is suspected.

Cerebral Angiography. Performed as indicated for suspected vascular tumors in anticipation of surgery. Meningiomas show a distinctive "tumor

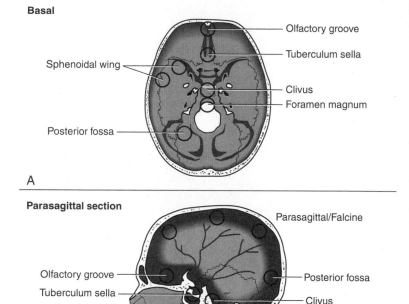

Figure 7–1. Common sites of meningiomas. (Redrawn from Kaye A (ed): Essential Neurosurgery. New York, Churchill Livingstone, 1991.)

blush." In some centers, feeding vessels to vascular lesions may be embolized to decrease intraoperative bleeding.

Other

EEG. Performed as indicated to determine the degree of cortical irritation, which may cause a seizure.

DIFFERENTIAL DIAGNOSIS

Traumatic

Cerebral Contusion. Blood is hyperdense on noncontrast CT. Hematomas are usually located within the parenchyma of the brain. A history of trauma accompanies the presentation. If an incidental tumor is suspected, contrast media should be given.

Infectious

Cerebral Abscess. Usually have a characteristic ring-enhancing appearance on CT/MRI. May have an elevated WBC and/or a history of recent dental procedure or other invasive procedures, which may introduce bacteria into the system.

Metabolic

Metabolic Disturbances. Those that cause neurologic changes. CT/MRI is negative for neoplasm.

Neoplastic

Glioma. No dural attachment is seen; less homogeneous enhancement; may be ring enhancing or surrounded by edema.

Cerebral Metastasis. May be multiple and small; no dural attachment; associated with surrounding edema; usually intraparenchymal.

Acoustic Neuroma. May be confused with a meningioma and the definitive diagnosis may be made intraoperatively. Acoustic neuromas usually have a characteristic appearance and occupy the internal auditory canal.

Pituitary Adenoma. Has an apparent point of origin in the pituitary fossa. If the tumor is large and extends into the suprasellar space, it may be confused with a meningioma. Hormonally active pituitary tumors can be differentiated with hormonal studies.

Other Primary Brain Neoplasms. Such as pinealomas, craniopharyngiomas, cysts, teratomas, etc. usually are differentiated by the lack of dural attachment, differences in contrast uptake, and radiographic appearance. Occasionally, it is necessary to make the diagnosis by biopsy or open craniotomy.

Vascular

Intracerebral Hemorrhage. Usually presents acutely. Blood is hyperdense on noncontrast CT. If an incidental tumor is suspected, contrast media should be given.

Congenital. Not applicable.

Acquired. Not applicable.

TREATMENT

Medical. One must always keep in mind the risks versus benefits of an operative procedure. In the elderly patient with an incidental small lesion consistent with a meningioma, it may be advisable to follow it with regular scanning. These tumors are slow growing and the time it takes to develop symptoms may be greater than the lifespan of the patient.

Seizure prophylaxis is given as indicated depending on presenting symptoms, tumor location, or EEG results.

For recurrent meningiomas in which the patient is not a candidate for further surgery, additional therapy may be required. Radiation therapy may be given using focused beam or a linear accelerator to arrest further growth of the tumor.

Studies are underway to evaluate the efficacy of mifepristone (RU 486), which blocks progesterone receptors, in the treatment of histologically proven, recurrent, or residual meningiomas that have demonstrated continued growth.

Surgical. In the preoperative phase, the patient may be placed on dexamethasone (2 to 10 mg q6h) to reduce cerebral edema. With vascular tumors, or tumors with an inaccessible vascular supply, preoperative embolization through an angiographic catheter may be performed by the surgeon or a skilled neuroradiologist.

A craniotomy is performed and the tumor and any accessible dural attachments excised. Dural grafting may be necessary. Some tumors involve the dural sinuses, which does not allow for total excision. Titanium plates may be used to reattach the skull flap. These plates tend to show less artifact on postoperative MRI scanning.

Postoperatively, measures to control intracranial pressure are ordered. These include head elevation at 30 to 45 degrees, dexamethasone in relatively high doses (10 mg q6h)*, and fluid restriction. Phenytoin, phenobarbital, or carbamazepine is given for seizure prophylaxis. Postoperative antibiotics are given at the surgeon's discretion.

With posterior fossa tumors, hydrocephalus may be present, which may require a shunting procedure prior to proceeding with tumor removal.

Risks of surgery include hemorrhage, stroke, infection, injury to the brain, or incomplete tumor removal.

It is important to follow the patient at regular intervals with MRI scanning because tumor recurrence is a possibility, even with tumors that were initially thought to be completely excised. This is especially true for tumors of the skull base, cavernous sinus, venous sinus, malignant tumors, or when it is known that complete tumor removal was not performed.

Indications. For symptomatic or larger tumors, surgery with attempted complete excision and eradication of the dural attachment is the treatment of choice. The major risk of not operating is that the tumor will continue to grow and may cause significant neurologic symptoms or become life threatening.

Contraindications. Significant coagulopathy, advanced age and absence of symptoms, inability of the patient to undergo anesthesia.

PA Role in Surgery. The PA assists in both the opening and closing of the craniotomy. During excision of the tumor, light traction of the brain or tumor may be necessary to remove the lesion and access feeding vessels.

PEDIATRIC CONSIDERATIONS

Meningiomas are rare in the younger age group, with only 1.5% of meningiomas occurring in children and adolescents. If a neoplasm is identified or suspected in a child, referral to a neurologist or neurosurgeon experienced in pediatrics is essential.

---

* Dexamethasone is usually continued at the higher dose for several days. After this, a slow taper is used (e.g., 6 mg q6h for 48 h, followed by 4 mg, 2 mg, 1 mg, on the same schedule). The slow taper is necessary because these tumors are slow growing and may take up significant intracranial volume; residual edema may persist for a prolonged period. In some cases, the dose may be reincreased if the patient's neurologic status deteriorates.

OBSTETRICAL CONSIDERATIONS

Because meningiomas tend to be sensitive to progesterone and increase in size during pregnancy, patients with a known meningioma should consider surgical excision prior to planning a pregnancy. If this is not possible, close observation of the tumor is necessary. Weighing the risks versus benefits of MRI scanning (not recommended during the first trimester and only performed during pregnancy if absolutely necessary) and surgical excision should be undertaken with the expectant mother. Much of this depends on the size of the tumor and danger to the mother during pregnancy and delivery.

PEARLS FOR THE PA

Meningiomas are almost always slow-growing, benign neoplasms.

Symptoms may be insidious as the brain accommodates for tumor growth.

Surgical excision is the preferred method of treatment.

Meningiomas may cause prolonged swelling in the postoperative phase.

Meningiomas are sensitive to progesterone, and avoidance of exogenous progesterone is recommended.

Obtain obstetrical, neurosurgical, and endocrinological consultation for the pregnant patient with a meningioma.

Metastatic Brain Lesion
James B. Labus, PA-C

DEFINITION

Spread of a tumor of extracerebral origin to the cerebral substance. The common sources are carcinomas of the lung, gastrointestinal tract, breast, liver/pancreas, prostate, female genital tract, kidney and urinary tract, and head and neck. Other conditions that may affect or metastasize to the brain are leukemia, lymphoma, melanoma, and sarcoma.

HISTORY

Symptoms. Usually referable to a focal neurologic finding (e.g., hemiparesis or hemisensory loss, dysphasia, etc.), symptoms of increased ICP (e.g., headache, nausea, vomiting, lethargy), or seizure.

General. Inquiry should be made as to a history of cancer. If this history is negative, investigate known risk factors for the development of tumors that metastasize to the brain. These questions would include occupational history, smoking, family history of cancer, change in bowel or bladder habits, or presence of bloody stools or melena.

Age. Increases with advancing age.

Onset. Usually relatively acute (days to weeks).

Duration. Progressive neurologic deficit.

Intensity. Mild to life threatening.

Aggravating Factors. Maneuvers that increase ICP such as alcohol abuse, becoming overheated, Valsalva.

Alleviating Factors. Recognition and treatment. Dexamethasone reduces cerebral edema and may lessen symptoms.

Associated Factors. Factors that are risks for developing the primary cancer. These include smoking, exposure to asbestos, industrial hazards (mining, volatile chemicals), tuberculosis, family history of cancer, close relative with breast cancer, or certain diets.

PHYSICAL EXAMINATION

General. The patient may appear normal or cachectic with signs of advanced cancer. A full physical examination is performed of all organ systems to attempt to identify the primary source or other regions of metastasis. Lymph nodes are palpated for enlargement. The lungs are auscultated and percussed for rales, rhonchi, or consolidation. A detailed abdominal examination is performed to check for masses, and kidneys are palpated for tenderness and masses. Breast examination is performed to evaluate for abnormal lumps. The skin is observed for lesions. A rectal examination is done to evaluate the prostate and to check for rectal lesions.

Neurologic. A full and complete neurologic examination is performed to evaluate for any subtle or overt focal findings. Ophthalmologic examination is done to evaluate for papilledema. If multiple metastases are present, the most obvious deficits may not be the sole findings.

PATHOPHYSIOLOGY

About 25% of patients with cancer have intracranial metastasis. Metastatic lesions may involve the dura, pituitary, leptomeninges, and the cerebral substance. Tumors tend to spread to the intracranial compartment in relation to their access to the blood supply. Primary tumors of the lung, and tumors that metastasize to the lung, tend to gain access to the vascular system and undergo hematogenous spread. Intracerebral lesions tend to be located in areas where the arteries narrow (gray–white matter junction).

DIAGNOSTIC STUDIES

Laboratory

Chemistry Profile, CBC, PT, PTT, Platelets. Are performed as routine preoperative evaluation and also to evaluate for any abnormalities. Electrolyte abnormalities may be present as a result of the disease process or from the cerebral lesion. Liver function or renal studies may be abnormal with tumor involvement. Bleeding dyscrasias may be encountered.

Carcinoembryonic Antigen (CEA). Elevated in gastrointestinal cancer.

Prostate-Specific Antigen. Elevated in prostate cancer.

Radiology

CT Scan of the Brain. With and without contrast is used as a screening measure for acute neurologic deficit. If a metastatic lesion is suspected, MRI should be performed. Lesions vary in size, enhance with contrast, and are classically associated with surrounding edema.

MRI Scan of the Brain. With and without gadolinium. Is done as an initial screen for acute neurologic deficit or performed if a metastatic lesion is suspected. Lesions vary in size, enhance with gadolinium, and are classically associated with surrounding edema. The increased sensitivity of MRI identifies multiple lesions that may be missed on CT.

Metastatic Work-up. Including chest x-ray, chest CT, abdominal CT, mammography, and bone scan as indicated is used to attempt to identify the primary lesion.

Other

EEG. May be used if the patient has experienced a seizure and the need for anticonvulsants requires assessment.

DIFFERENTIAL DIAGNOSIS

Traumatic

Intracerebral Hemorrhage/Contusion. Patients have a history of trauma. The hemorrhage/contusion resolves on follow-up CT/MRI.

Infectious

Intracerebral Abscess. May be encountered in patients with known cancer. Associated with fever, sepsis, elevated WBC, and possibly signs of meningitis (if the infection has involved the CSF). Lesions have surrounding edema and may be multiple. Biopsy may be required to differentiate.

Metabolic.   Not applicable.

Neoplastic

Meningioma.   Usually slow growing, not associated with significant edema, has dural attachment.

Glioma.   May cause significant edema and have the appearance of a metastatic lesion. Biopsy may be required to differentiate.

Lymphoma.   Associated with immunocompromised status. Biopsy may be required to differentiate.

Sarcoma.   Patient may have a history of radiation therapy with ports that involved the brain. Biopsy may be required to differentiate.

Vascular

Intracerebral Hemorrhage.   Blood appears as high density on CT and high signal on MRI without contrast. Associated with coagulopathy (e.g., disseminated intravascular coagulation, thrombocytopenia), which may accompany the cancer.

Stroke. May accompany cancer. CT/MRI reveal a low-density/low-signal image. This may be confused with edema. No enhancement with contrast.

Congenital. Not applicable.

Acquired. Not applicable.

TREATMENT

Medical. If cerebral lesions are multiple, and if a distant primary source is identified, radiation or chemotherapy is instituted per the protocol for the type of tumor diagnosed.

Anticonvulsants such as phenytoin, carbamazepine, or phenobarbital are given as a therapeutic measure in patients with a history of seizure, or as a prophylactic measure. Dexamethasone (2 to 10 mg q6h) is given to reduce cerebral edema. This should be given immediately after the presence of tumor with associated edema is recognized. Dexamethasone should be continued throughout radiation therapy owing to the risks of increased edema during therapy.

Surgical. Lesions are biopsied via needle through a burr hole or are excised or biopsied through a craniotomy. Radiation or chemotherapy is given postoperatively.

Indications. If a solitary tumor is causing significant deficit, has yet to be diagnosed, is in an accessible area, and the patient's lifespan (longer than 1 year) and clinical condition warrant, the lesion is excised. Surgical excision with adjunct radiation or chemotherapy is preferable to adjunct therapy alone. If a primary source is identified, it is often safer to biopsy the primary source rather than the cerebral lesion. Patients with multiple lesions without a known primary source may be candidates for needle biopsy for diagnostic purposes.

Contraindications. Multiple lesions are almost always a contraindication to surgery because every lesion is unable to be excised and there is no benefit to single lesion excision.

PA Role in Surgery. Assistance is performed with the opening and closing of the craniotomy. Brain or tumor retraction may be necessary for tumor removal. One of the most important roles of the PA in this instance is to provide education and support for the patient and family and coordinate consultants (e.g., oncology, radiation therapy, radiology, and other surgical services).

PEDIATRIC CONSIDERATIONS

If a cerebral lesion is identified in childhood, referral to a neurosurgeon with significant pediatric experience and access to specialized pediatric adjunct services (e.g., oncology, radiation therapy) is essential.

OBSTETRICAL CONSIDERATIONS

The risks versus benefits of diagnostic and therapeutic measures must be weighed when treating the pregnant patient.

PEARLS FOR THE PA

The diagnosis of metastatic lesion is based on histology because there are no specific symptoms or radiographic findings that can be used to definitively diagnose a metastatic lesion.

Patients with cancer can present with lesions other than those of the primary tumor.

Approximately 25% of patients with cancer have intracranial metastases.

Peripheral Nerve: Carpal Tunnel Syndrome
Carrie Gunn-Edel, PA-C

DEFINITION

A median nerve compressive neuropathy occurring at the wrist at the location where the median nerve enters the carpal tunnel and passes beneath the transverse carpal ligament.

HISTORY

Symptoms. Patients usually complain of numbness, tingling, and pain of the hand. Initially, the numbness is intermittent. Pain, numbness, and/or tingling of thumb, index, long finger, and medial aspect of the ring finger are the hallmarks of carpal tunnel syndrome, often with pain radiating up the arm into the shoulder (Cherington's sign). Patients often note nocturnal hand discomfort, decreased strength, and difficulty picking up fine articles. For obscure reasons, symptoms are often relieved by hanging the limb dependent.

General. It is important to obtain an occupational history to determine if there has been a repetitive use–type injury. The time of onset is characteristically in the early hours of the morning, induced by the acute wrist flexion of the "fetal" sleeping position, by altered fluid distribution in the lying position, and by increased blood flow to the limb for thermoregulation. Other contributing factors that should be obtained in the history include diabetes, pregnancy, use of birth control pills, thyroid disease, trauma, and rheumatoid arthritis.

Age. This syndrome occurs more frequently in adults 30 to 50 years of age, and is more common in women than men.

Onset. Gradual onset is usually the case, although it can be acute in nature, particularly when trauma is associated with an abrupt elevation of pressure in the carpal tunnel.

Duration. Chronic and progressive in the majority of cases.

Intensity. A preponderance of the time patients have a low-grade progressive pain that is initially mild. This is associated with tingling of fingers progressing to total numbness, thenar atrophy from abductor pollicis brevis muscle wasting, and an inability to pinch or abduct the thumb. Patients are often awoken at night because of the pain.

Aggravating Factors. Driving a car, reading a newspaper, talking on the telephone, and other sustained activities requiring wrist movement make the symptoms worse.

Alleviating Factors. Avoiding continuous wrist flexion, keeping the arms in dependent position, shaking out hands, nonsteroidal anti-inflammatory drugs (NSAIDs), and splinting the wrist help improve symptoms.

Associated Factors. Diabetes, pregnancy, thyroid disease, rheumatoid arthritis, and certain occupational activities are all associated with higher incidents of carpal tunnel syndrome, but the majority of cases are idiopathic.

PHYSICAL EXAMINATION

General. The patient may hold or splint the hand if the pain is severe. A wrist splint may be worn by the patient for prior carpal tunnel treatment.

Neurologic. Hand dominance is important when examining the wrist (the dominant hand is more frequently affected). Dryness of the skin may be noted over the thumb and radial two fingers. Decreased sensation can be detected with the Weinstein monofilament test and occasionally with two-point discrimination testing. Vibratory sensation is sometimes lost. A positive Phalen's test is demonstrated when finger tingling and numbness occurs after wrist flexion for 60 seconds. Tinel's sign (tapping over the median nerve) causes hypersensitivity, pain, or electrical-type sensation of the median nerve. A positive carpal tunnel test occurs when the reproduction of symptoms with direct compression over the median nerve can be demonstrated. Check for thenar atrophy and measure hand grip and strength, pinch strength (apposition and opposition), and wrist range of motion.

PATHOPHYSIOLOGY

A fibro-osseous canal on the ventral surface of the wrist, which the transverse ligament covers, forms the carpal tunnel. Passing through this tunnel are 10 structures, one of which is the median nerve. Owing to the nature of the carpal tunnel and its confining borders, a disparity between the size of the tunnel and an increase in volume of its contents causes an increase in intracarpal canal pressure and interference with median nerve conduction.

DIAGNOSTIC STUDIES

Laboratory
Serum Glucose.　To evaluate for diabetes mellitus as indicated.
CBC.　Elevated WBC in infectious process.
Thyroid Function Tests, Uric Acid, Pregnancy Test.　To evaluate for contributing conditions as indicated.
Radiology
Wrist X-ray.　Including anteroposterior (AP), lateral, and oblique views to define wrist anatomy or to rule out fractures.
Other
Electromyography (EMG).　The definitive test for carpal tunnel syndrome. Shows nerve entrapment over the wrist.

DIFFERENTIAL DIAGNOSIS

Traumatic
Colles Fracture.　Positive wrist x-ray.
Lacerations.　Signs of scar/laceration to wrist.
Injury to Carpal Bones.　Positive wrist x-ray.
Carpal-Metacarpal Dislocations.　May have a positive wrist x-ray or positive history or physical examination findings of a dislocation.
Extensive Hand Injuries.　Resulting in swelling (e.g., burns, contusions); positive history.
Infectious
Hand Infection.　Redness, swelling, tenderness, elevated WBC.
Foreign Body Reaction.　Foreign body may be seen on x-ray or on physical examination.
Tuberculosis (TB).　Positive history of; positive TB test.
Gonorrhea.　Positive history of; positive culture.
Metabolic
Diabetes Mellitus.　Positive history of; elevated serum glucose.
Thyroid Disease.　Abnormal thyroid function studies.
Gout/Pseudogout.　Positive history of; red, inflamed joints; may affect feet also; elevated uric acid (gout); responds to antigout therapy and/or NSAIDs.
Rheumatoid Arthritis.　Positive history of; joint deformities consistent with rheumatoid arthritis.
Scleroderma/Psoriasis.　May have associated rash.
Ectopic Calcifications.　May be palpated on examination or seen on x-ray.

Mucolipidoses. Systemic diseases in which there is thickening of the flexor mucopolysaccharidosis retinaculum.

Peripheral Neuropathy. Classically presents with stocking-glove, bilateral distribution symptoms. Feet usually involved.

Pregnancy. Positive pregnancy test and signs of pregnancy.

Neoplastic

Periosteal Chondroma or Bursae. May be palpated on examination or seen on x-ray.

Ganglion, Fibroma, Lipoma. May be palpated on examination or seen on x-ray.

Vascular

Raynaud Disease. May have cyanosis or erythema present.

Thoracic Outlet Syndrome (Neurovascular Compression Syndrome). EMG/NCV is normal. Adson manuever and hyperabduction test are often positive.

Aneurysm of the Median Artery. May be palpated on examination as a pulsatile mass.

Congenital

Systemic Disorders. With hypoplastic bone development may be noted on examination or seen on x-ray.

Weill-Marchesani Syndrome. Generalized connective tissue disorder.

Acquired

Cervical Disc Herniation/Cervical Spondylosis. Associated with pain, reflex change, or motor weakness in a dermatomal distribution. May have neck pain. MRI positive for lesion. Neck x-ray may reveal bone spurs in spondylosis.

TREATMENT

Medical. Night splinting with a wrist splint, NSAIDs, cortisone with lidocaine injection.

Surgical. Open carpal tunnel release is performed through a proximal, midpalmar incision over the wrist. This is extended down through the palmar fascia and through the transverse carpal ligament, which allows expansion of the carpal tunnel.

With endoscopic carpal tunnel release, a 5-mm incision is made at the distal wrist crease medial to the pisiform, and a 5-mm incision is made 4.5 cm distal in the palm. A scope is inserted, along with a probe to free up tissues from the transverse carpal ligament. The transverse ligament is incised without cutting the palmaris brevis muscle.

Indications. When conservative treatment fails with a minimum of 6 weeks trial or if symptoms recur following cortisone injections.

Contraindications. Pregnancy, acetylsalicylic acid (ASA)/antiinflammatory use (due to bleeding) within 7 days from surgery, contraindication to anesthesia, negative EMG results, and decreased wrist extension (which inhibits the use of the endoscope for carpal tunnel release).

TECHNIQUE OF SURGICAL ASSISTING

Providing adequate exposure for release of the median nerve. If open carpal tunnel release, the application of a plaster volar wrist splint in neutral position to 5 degrees extension is important for good results.

PEDIATRIC CONSIDERATIONS

Carpal tunnel syndrome can occur in children and adolescents but is not common.

OBSTETRICAL CONSIDERATIONS

Carpal tunnel syndrome may occur during pregnancy, but surgery is contra-indicated unless conservative treatment is not tolerated.

PEARLS FOR THE PA

Pain, numbness, and/or tingling of thumb, index, third finger, and medial aspect of ring finger are classic symptoms of carpal tunnel syndrome.

Peripheral Nerve Entrapment: Tardy Ulnar Nerve Palsy

James B. Labus, PA-C

DEFINITION

Entrapment of the ulnar nerve at the elbow, usually due to distant (tardy) trauma.

HISTORY

Symptoms. Numbness and tingling in the distribution of the ulnar nerve (fourth and fifth digits and the medial hand), atrophy of the hypothenar region, loss of strength. Discomfort may be present in the elbow region or forearm.

General. A history of elbow trauma should be ascertained and, although usually absent in most cases, will likely be the cause of the condition.

Other historical information should include the presence of other factors that may produce compression of the ulnar nerve. These include prolonged bedrest, extended pressure on the nerve (e.g., drivers who tend to rest their arm out an open window), primary joint disease (e.g., osteoarthritis), or ganglion cysts.

Age. Increases with advancing age; more prevalent with repeated, minor trauma in the working-age population.

Onset. Gradual.

Duration. Progressive.

Intensity. Muscle weakness may cause very little disability, even when severe. Paresthesias may be quite troublesome.

Aggravating Factors. Repeated elbow bending, activity that causes prolonged or repeated elbow pressure.

Alleviating Factors. Proper treatment of elbow fractures in the acute setting lessens the development of nerve entrapment later in life.

Associated Factors. Osteoarthritis, occupations that require multiple elbow bending and/or prolonged elbow pressure, protracted bedrest.

PHYSICAL EXAMINATION

General. The patient's hand may appear normal or have overt atrophy of the hypothenar area. In advanced cases, a "claw hand" may be observed.

Neurologic. Palpate the course of the ulnar nerve to rule out deformities or the presence of a ganglion cyst.

Interosseous muscle strength is tested by asking the patient to hold the fingers apart. Resistance is applied to push the fingers back together. Testing is then done with the patient attempting to hold the fingers together while the examiner tries to pull them apart. Adduction of the fingers is tested by asking the patient to hold a piece of paper between the fingers (fingers should be extended) while the examiner attempts to remove the paper. Flexor digitorum profundus testing is done by evaluating the flexion strength of the distal interphalangeal joint while holding the metacarpophalangeal and interphalangeal joints in extension. The strength of the contralateral hand should always be tested to evaluate for asymmetry.

Tinel's response is usually positive with entrapment of the nerve at the elbow. Using a reflex hammer, strike the area proximal and distal to the medial epicondyle. A positive Tinel's sign is elicited when the patient experiences paresthesias in the distribution of the ulnar nerve.

Reflex, motor, and sensory testing of the extremity is performed to assess for signs of nerve root compression.

Orthopedic. Palpation of the elbow and wrist should be performed to evaluate for any deformities that may cause nerve compression.

PATHOPHYSIOLOGY

The ulnar nerve course takes it medial to the medial epicondyle of the humerus. It travels distally through a fibrous opening that is composed of the attachment of the heads of the ulnar flexor muscle of the wrist. The cubital tunnel, which is formed by the attachments of this muscle, tightens during flexion of the elbow, which may cause nerve compression. Distant trauma that causes deformities to this area may lead to the development of nerve compromise. Other causes include repeated minor trauma, bone spurs due to arthritis, enlarged synovium, or enlarged head of the triceps muscle.

DIAGNOSTIC STUDIES

Laboratory
CBC, Chemistry Profile, PT, PTT, Bleeding Time. As routine preoperative studies if surgery is planned.
Radiology
Elbow X-ray. Used to assess anatomy if there is a history of trauma, clinical evidence of deformity, or osteoarthritis and surgery is contemplated.
Other
Nerve Conduction Studies. Diagnostic for tardy ulnar nerve palsy. Also localizes lesions of the nerve root, brachial plexus, or compression at the wrist.

DIFFERENTIAL DIAGNOSIS

Traumatic
Ulnar/Elbow Trauma. Due to any source (e.g., fracture, blunt trauma, gunshot wound), may cause acute injury to the ulnar nerve. Conservative therapy and observation for reinnervation is often used, but reanastomosis may be required for severed nerves.
Infectious
Osteomyelitis. Elevated WBC, fever; apparent on x-ray.
Metabolic
Diabetic Neuropathy. Usually affects both hands or the feet. The classic "stocking-glove" distribution of the numbness and EMG and nerve conduction velocity (NCV) will differentiate.
Neoplastic
Ganglion Cyst. Of the wrist may cause symptoms of ulnar nerve compression. EMG/NCV localizes the compression; cyst may be palpated.
Chest and Chest Wall Neoplasms. May cause compression of the brachial plexus. Chest x-ray is positive and EMG/NCV localizes the lesion. Other nerves may also be affected.
Vascular
Thoracic Outlet Syndrome. EMG/NCV is normal. Adson maneuver and hyperabduction test are often positive.
Congenital. Not applicable.

Acquired

Distal Ulnar Nerve Compression. Less common than compression at the elbow; usually due to traumatic or repetitive use injuries. NCV localizes the compression to the wrist.

Other

Cervical Radiculopathy. Most frequently is associated with pain in the neck, shoulder, and proximal arm. MRI of the cervical spine may reveal nerve root compression. EMG/NCV localizes the lesion to the nerve root.

TREATMENT

Medical. Conservative measures may be employed for symptoms that are minor and have no functional impairment. NSAIDs are used initially to help resolve the symptoms. Patient education, cessation of heavy lifting, and alleviation of repeated pressure on the nerve may also be of benefit.

Surgical. There are three major surgical procedures used in the treatment of tardy ulnar nerve palsy.

1. Decompression of the nerve may be performed by opening the cubital tunnel.
2. Decompression of the nerve and medial epicondylectomy.
3. Transposition of the nerve with medial epicondylectomy. This involves moving the nerve into a new location to prevent further compression.

The failure rate of the surgery (regardless of which procedure is selected) is approximately 15% with excellent results in approximately 60% of patients, and intermediate results in the remainder.

Indications. Surgery may be necessary if symptoms are severe or if there is atrophy or significant functional impairment.

Contraindications. Absence of severe symptoms, inadequate trial of conservative therapy for more minor lesions, and contraindications to anesthesia.

PA Role in Surgery. The PA assists in opening and closing of the incision. Protection of the nerve during medial epicondylectomy is also an important function. The nerve may be shielded with an instrument, pad, or sponge. Transposition of the nerve requires the nerve to be held in place and kept clear of any overlying sutures.

PEDIATRIC CONSIDERATIONS

Not applicable.

OBSTETRICAL CONSIDERATIONS

Transient paresthesias may be experienced by pregnant women. Most of these resolve postpartum. If the symptoms fail to resolve, additional investigations may be necessary.

PEARLS FOR THE PA

Numbness and tingling of the fourth and fifth digits and the medial hand, atrophy of the hypothenar region, and loss of strength are the hallmark symptoms of ulnar nerve palsy.

Tardy nerve palsy is usually due to remote elbow trauma.

NCV confirms the diagnosis.

Pituitary Adenoma
James B. Labus, PA-C

DEFINITION

Pituitary adenoma is a neoplasm arising from the anterior lobe (adenohypophysis) of the pituitary gland and accounts for 8% to 10% of all intracranial tumors. They are classified as prolactin secreting (40%), growth hormone (GH) secreting (20%), nonsecreting (20%), adrenocorticotropic hormone (ACTH) secreting (15%), prolactin and GH secreting (5%), follicle stimulating hormone (FSH) and luteinizing hormone (LH) secreting (1% to 2%), thyroid stimulating hormone (TSH) secreting (1%), and acidophil stem cell nonsecreting (1% to 2%).

HISTORY

Symptoms. Symptoms are due to active endocrine secretion by the tumor, endocrine dysfunction, or compression of adjacent neural structures. Non–tumor-specific symptoms include headache, diplopia (with involvement of cranial nerves III, IV, and VI), visual field cut (with optic nerve or chiasm compression), hypothalamic syndrome (abnormalities of thirst, appetite, sleep, temperature regulation, and occasionally diabetes insipidus or syndrome of inappropriate antidiuretic hormone [SIADH] secretion), facial pain (with cranial nerve V involvement), and CSF rhinorrhea. The patient may present with symptoms of hypopituitarism such as decreased energy level, muscle weakness, anorexia, and episodic confusion.
Prolactin
Hypersecretory. Females may present with breast growth, galactorrhea, and amenorrhea and males may be impotent.
Hyposecretory. Females may have failure of postpartum lactation.

GH

Hypersecretory. Patients present with acromegaly characterized by (after the growth plates have fused) increased size of the hands and feet, mandibular prominence (prognathism), skin changes, hoarseness, new onset or worsening of snoring, heat intolerance, carbohydrate intolerance, neuropathic symptoms, and cardiac symptoms (e.g., congestive heart failure [CHF]). Before the growth plates fuse, patients may present as pituitary giants.

ACTH

Hypersecretory. Patients present with Cushing's syndrome characterized by fat deposits in the face, trunk, and cervicothoracic area; skin changes; spontaneous bruising; new growth of facial hair; fatigue; and weakness.

Hyposecretory. Hypercortisolism (Addison's disease). Includes weakness, hyperpigmentation, nausea, vomiting, anorexia, loss of body hair, amenorrhea.

TSH

Hypersecretory. Patients present with thyrotoxicosis characterized by toxic nodular goiter or Graves' disease.

Hyposecretory. Hypothyroidism includes cold intolerance, lethargy, periorbital edema, and decreased sweating.

FSH/LH. Patients present with hypogonadism.

General. Nonsecreting tumors tend to grow to larger size owing to the relative endocrinologic silence; therefore, patients tend to present with symptoms of neural compression.

Patients may be reticent to discuss certain symptoms or the symptoms may be dismissed by the patient as normal. Inquiry should be made as to energy level, visual field disturbance (e.g., with driving or participating in sporting activities), thirst and urinary habits, presence of double vision in certain fields of gaze, positional clear colorless drainage from the nose, galactorrhea, menstrual history, impotence, changes in ring or shoe size, increase in snoring, new weight gain, and new or additional facial hair.

Age. Any, but GH tumors tend to present in the third and fourth decades; prolactin tumors tend to present with symptoms in the childbearing years with infertility.

Onset. Usually slow and insidious.

Duration. Progressive without treatment.

Intensity. Patients may be asymptomatic or present with severe endocrinologic disturbance. GH tumors may be life threatening owing to nasopharyngeal closure (resulting in sleep apnea) or cardiac disturbance.

Aggravating Factors. None.

Alleviating Factors. Appropriate therapy.

Associated Factors. Are due to endocrine dependent organs. Thyroid abnormalities, diabetes mellitus, and hyper/hypotension.

PHYSICAL EXAMINATION

General.   Observe the patient's general appearance. ACTH tumor patients have truncal obesity, moon facies, and a "buffalo hump." GH tumor patients have the appearance of acromegaly.

Vital signs should be evaluated for hypertension, postural hypotension, and pulse rate and rhythm. Patients with GH tumors and CHF may be dyspneic.

Cardiovascular.   Evaluate GH tumor patients for CHF by inspecting neck veins for distention; auscultate for S3 gallop (the hallmark finding).

Extremities.   Test strength to evaluate for generalized weakness and inspect for wasting, which may be present in patients with ACTH tumors.

HEENT.   Palpate for thyroid enlargement or goiter. Test for CSF rhinorrhea by asking the patient (while sitting) to lean over. Observe for clear colorless fluid coming from the nose. The fluid may test glucose positive on glucose stick if it is CSF (if any blood is present, the glucose test is void because blood contains glucose).

Neurologic.   A full neurologic examination needs to be performed in all patients with a suspected or known intracranial lesion. Test eye movements for paresis (cranial nerves III, IV, VI). Check the sensation of both sides of the face (cranial nerve V). Sensory examination should be performed in GH tumor patients if there is any symptom of peripheral neuropathy.

Ophthalmologic.   Fundoscopic examination may show optic atrophy with long-standing optic nerve or chiasm compression. Papilledema may be present with increased ICP. Visual fields are tested, initially to gross confrontation, then by formal means through an ophthalmologic consultation. Suprasellar tumor extension and compression of the optic chiasm classically causes a bitemporal hemianopsia.

Pulmonary.   Moist rales may be heard on auscultation or the chest may be dull to percussion in GH tumor patients with CHF.

Skin.   Evaluate skin for turgor, acne, sweat production, and greasy appearance (GH and ACTH). ACTH tumor patients may have purple striae and hirsutism.

PATHOPHYSIOLOGY

The pituitary is divided into two lobes. The anterior lobe (adenohypophysis, from which tumors arise) develops from Rathke's pouch, an ectodermal derivative. The posterior lobe (neurohypophysis) is formed from the infundibulum, which develops from the floor of the diencephalon. The pituitary gland is under control of the hypothalamus in the form of hypothalamic releasing hormones. The anterior pituitary normally secretes GH, TSH, ACTH, prolactin, FSH, and LH, whereas the posterior pituitary secretes antidiuretic hormone (ADH) and oxytocin. When tumors develop, they may oversecrete certain hormones or, if a local mass effect is present, inhibit release of normal circulating hormones, eventually culminating in what is known as a panhypopituitary state.

Tumors are classified as to size. Microadenomas are less than 10 mm in size. Macroadenomas can grow to a much larger size, extend superiorly, and compress the optic chiasm, hypothalamus, or third ventricle; extend laterally and involve the cavernous sinus; or extend inferiorly into the sphenoid sinus, potentially causing CSF rhinorrhea. Macroadenomas tend to erode the sella. The sella then enlarges and remodels itself to accommodate the mass. This accounts for the large sella seen on plain x-rays or CT images.

Only 10% of pituitary tumors are invasive and permeate the pituitary capsule, bone, and dural sinuses. Most of these tumors are either prolactin secreting or nonsecreting. Metastasis from pituitary carcinoma to distant extracranial sites or from seeding within the CSF pathways is rare.

DIAGNOSTIC STUDIES

Laboratory

Electrolytes.   May see hypokalemia with ACTH tumors.

Thyroid Function Studies.   It is likely that the hypothalamic-pituitary-thyroid axis is intact if serum thyroxine is normal. If the serum thyroxine is low, a thyrotrophin releasing hormone (TRH) study is performed. A baseline thyroid stimulating hormone (TSH) level is drawn, followed by an IV injection of 500 μg of TRH. TSH levels are obtained at 30 and 60 minutes after the injection. A normal test reveals an increase of twice the baseline level of TSH at 30 minutes. A low TSH response indicates a pituitary abnormality. A delayed TSH response (60 minutes) indicates a hypothalamic abnormality.

Hormone Assays by Radioimmunoassay (RIA)

Prolactin (females, 0–23; males, 0–20 ng/mL).   Levels greater than 200 almost always indicate a tumor, greater than 1000 suggest an invasive tumor.

GH (females < 10; males < 5 ng/mL).   Elevated with GH tumors.

ACTH.   Using dexamethasone suppression test. Urine and plasma free cortisol are normally suppressed with low-dose dexamethasone (0.5 mg q6h). Levels are also suppressed with high-dose dexamethasone (2 mg q6h) in pituitary-dependent Cushing's disease. There is no suppression of levels in nonpituitary Cushing's.

Radiology

Plain Skull X-rays (True Lateral).   Show an enlarged sella with macroadenomas. May see bony erosion.

High-resolution CT Scan with Contrast (Including Coronal Views of the Sella).   Visualizes micro- and macroadenomas. May see enlarged ventricles with a large tumor obstructing the third ventricle.

MRI Scan with Gadolinium (Including Coronal Views of the Sella).   The most sensitive test to identity micro- and macroadenomas. Suprasellar and lateral extension to the optic chiasm and cavernous sinuses, respectively, can be evaluated. May see hydrocephalus with large tumor obstructing the third ventricle.

Cerebral Angiogram.   To rule out giant aneurysm if the diagnosis of pituitary tumor is uncertain. Used less frequently since the advent of MRI.

Other

ECG.   To rule out arrhythmia.

Echocardiogram.   To rule out cardiomegaly in GH tumor patients.

Sleep Studies.   To rule out sleep apnea in GH tumor patients.

DIFFERENTIAL DIAGNOSIS

Traumatic

Basilar Skull Fracture.   With avulsion of the pituitary stalk. History of trauma. Raccoon eyes, Battle's sign, or hemotympanum may be present; may have CSF rhinorrhea; CT/MRI may show intracranial air in the acute phase.

Infectious

Pituitary Abscess.   Presence of tissue destruction. Histologically differentiated by the presence of cell necrosis and polymorphonuclear lymphocytes.

Metabolic

Sarcoidosis.   May involve the hypothalamus or pituitary gland. Well-circumscribed mass seen on CT/MRI. Requires histological confirmation.

Neoplastic

Adrenal Adenoma/Carcinoma.   May have elevated ACTH production from adrenal tumors, oat cell cancer of the lung, or other ectopic sources; 90% of patients with an elevated ACTH have a pituitary source.

Craniopharyngioma.   Cystic tumor, usually with flecks of calcium seen on CT/MRI. May enlarge the sella owing to pressure on the intrasellar contents.

Glioma.   Affecting the hypothalamus or optic nerve. MRI may identify an intramedullary tumor or enlargement of the optic nerve.

Meningioma.   May occur in the suprasellar region. May see dural enhancement with homogeneous enhancement of the tumor on MRI with gadolinium.

Granular Cell Tumors.   Such as chordomas, germinomas, teratoid tumors. May affect the pituitary. Requires histological confirmation.

Vascular

Giant Aneurysm.   May resemble an extrasellar pituitary tumor. Angiogram may be necessary to differentiate.

Congenital

Rathke's Cleft Cyst.   Likely a derivative of Rathke's pouch. May be confused with craniopharyngioma.

Acquired

Empty Sella Syndrome.   Can be seen congenitally, postoperatively, due to pseudotumor cerebri or postradiation therapy. There is herniation of the arachnoid into the sella. This can occur with elevated ICP or hydrocephalus. Patients may be asymptomatic, have nonspecific symptoms, or present with CSF rhinorrhea.

Postpartum Females. May have transient increased size of hands, feet, or nose due to circulating fetal GH.

TREATMENT

The type of treatment is dependent on the degree of endocrinological or neural compromise. There are no medically curative measures, only therapies directed at reducing the excessive hormone levels or size of the tumors.

Medical. Prolactin-secreting tumors can be treated with the dopamine agonist bromocriptine (Parlodel), which inhibits prolactin synthesis and release. A daily oral dose may reduce or normalize the prolactin level, reduce tumor size, improve galactorrhea, and allow for resumption of menses and fertility. Drug cessation results in a resumption of the hyperprolactinemic state and regrowth of the tumor. Side effects include nausea, vomiting, and postural hypotension.

GH and mixed GH and prolactin tumors may respond to bromocriptine, which can reduce GH levels up to 75%. Much larger doses are required to achieve this result.

ACTH tumor patients have been tried on a variety of medical therapies with variable results, including adrenal toxins, serotonin antagonists, and bromocriptine.

Panhypopituitary patients require repletion of deficient hormones by treatment with hydrocortisone, thyroxine, or DDAVP (if diabetes insipidus is present).

Radiation therapy is indicated for patients who have undergone subtotal excision of the tumor, patients in whom general anesthesia and surgery is contraindicated, or if postoperative endocrine levels remain elevated.

Surgical. Surgery may be performed through the transphenoidal approach if the tumor is confined to the sella. If there is suprasellar extension, the transphenoidal route can be used to diagnose the lesion and for an attempt remove the tumor through the sella. If this is unsuccessful, a craniotomy may be required. A craniotomy may be used for persistent suprasellar tumors in order to reduce neural compression (e.g., optic chiasm).

Complications include injury to the pituitary gland, causing transient or permanent endocrinopathies, CSF leak, bleeding, injury to the optic chiasm, and infection.

Postoperative attention to intake and output at hourly intervals is essential due to the possibility of transient or permanent diabetes insipidus. If the output is 300 mL or more for 2 consecutive hours, STAT electrolytes, serum, and urine osmolalities are drawn. Sodium and serum osmolalities are elevated and urine osmolality decreased with diabetes insipidus.

Parenteral hydrocortisone is given and weaned down to a maintenance dose (20 mg every morning and 10 mg in the late afternoon). Thyroxine or testosterone replacement may also be needed.

Indications. GH tumors causing acromegaly, ACTH secreting tumor, patients with Cushing's disease, failure of medical treatment (bromocriptine), and neural compression.

Contraindications. Coagulopathy, inability to undergo anesthesia.

Role of the PA. The PA may assist with the transphenoidal or craniotomy approach. Frequently, packing of the defect is required to prevent CSF leakage. For this, a fat or muscle graft is used. Care must be taken when obtaining these grafts not to devascularize the skin by removing fat directly under the dermis. Deeper fat can usually be excised. Nasal airways may be placed intraoperatively to assist with healing of the nasal mucosa. These are removed on about postoperative day two. Close attention to fluid status is mandatory.

PEDIATRIC CONSIDERATIONS

Pituitary tumors in children may result in retarded development of secondary sex characteristics or, in the case of GH, in pituitary gigantism.

OBSTETRICAL CONSIDERATIONS

Bromocriptine should not be used in the pregnant patient owing to the risk of congenital malformations and spontaneous abortion.

PEARLS FOR THE PA

Always consider pituitary adenoma in the differential diagnosis of endocrine abnormality or unexplained visual field deficit.

There is no medical cure for pituitary adenomas, only those that inhibit hormone secretion or shrink tumor size.

CSF leak and transient diabetes insipidus should be monitored for in the postoperative period.

Spinal Cord Injury
Judy Nunes, PA-C, BS

DEFINITION

Damage to the neuronal elements of the spinal cord, usually due to trauma, as a result of penetration, malalignment, angulation, or intrusion of bony parts or soft tissues of the spinal canal, or foreign body, that results in neurological deficit.

HISTORY

Symptoms. Quite variable. The patient usually has neck pain and may have weakness (incomplete injuries) or complete paralysis below the level of injury that includes the loss of sensation and deep tendon reflexes (in the acute phase) and is accompanied by bowel or bladder dysfunction. In a high cervical injury, respiratory distress or diaphragmatic breathing may occur, as well as spinal shock (hypotension with bradycardia).

General. Most spinal cord injuries occur in males and are related to motor vehicle accidents (MVA), falls, and water sports. Predisposing factors include a pre-existing canal stenosis or spondylosis. The most common site of injury is C5 to C6, where the greatest flexion/extension occurs ("fulcrum" of the cervical spine). The thoracolumbar junction is also a fulcrum for spinal motion, and injury to this area is usually due to motor vehicle accidents or falls.

Age. Most commonly seen in those 13 to 34 years old.

Onset. Most neuronal insult occurs at the time of injury, with resultant neurologic deficit.

Duration. Neuronal damage occurs owing to initial injury (mechanical compression), with potential delayed secondary injury of ischemia, hemorrhagic necrosis, infarct, and edema. The neurologic deficit is almost always permanent (approximately 98%).

Intensity. Variable, from mild paresthesias to complete paralysis.

Aggravating Factors. Hypotension, hypoxemia, inadequate immobilization causing secondary injury.

Alleviating Factors. Surgical decompression (although usually not performed until the patient has stabilized and cord edema has resolved), adequate oxygenation, and steroids (methylprednisolone) may improve function or prevent further cord insult to some degree.

Associated Factors. As with any trauma patient, multiple organ systems can be involved but symptoms may not be apparent owing to the cord injury. Additional spinal fractures (thoracic or lumbar) may occur distal to the site of cord injury.

PATHOPHYSIOLOGY

Traumatic spinal cord injury ranges in severity from soft tissue injury to fracture with resultant paralysis or possibly death. There are an estimated 200,000 injuries to the spinal column each year, with approximately 10,000 cases of severe spinal cord injury in the United States alone. The primary insult (trauma) to the spinal cord results in pericapillary hemorrhage and ischemia, with potential infarct occurring within 4 to 6 hours after injury. Secondary injury is thought to be due to central hemorrhagic necrosis, which generally extends two levels above and two levels below the level of injury. Once the hemorrhage has occurred, edema and ischemia ensue, with disruption of cellular membranes.

Mechanisms of injury include

Fracture/Dislocation: Which results in an acute reduction in canal diameter and distortion of cord tissue. Approximately 50% to 60% of these injuries occur in the cervical spine.

Flexion: Most vulnerable area of injury in the cervical spine is C5 to C6. If rotation occurs, may result in "locked facet."

Extension: Greatest risk at C4 to C5 and a common injury in patients involved in rear-end MVA collisions.

Compression/Axial Loading: Tends to occur with diving and falls; often, burst fractures are seen with sharp bony fragments violating the spinal canal.

Approximately 40% to 60% of cervical spine injuries result in a neurologic deficit, with a mortality rate of 40% for high cervical injuries (occiput to C4). The thoracolumbar junction is also a fulcrum for spinal motion, with 35% of patients sustaining a complete injury, 40% partial injury, and 25% neurologically intact.

PHYSICAL EXAMINATION

General.   Consider concomitant injuries and potential hemodynamic instability in trauma patient, particularly in the comatose patient. Consider the spine to be unstable until proven otherwise.

Neurologic.   Once spinal shock has abated, a careful, thorough assessment of neurologic function is essential to document the degree of initial injury and to provide a baseline against which neurologic change (both progression or regression) may be measured. Emphasis on signs relating to spinal cord function include a detailed motor examination, including all extremities with respect to major muscle groups is performed and rated on a scale of 0 to 5 (0 = paralysis, 1 = weak flicker, 2 = weak, but some active contraction, 3 = can hold against gravity, 4 = slight weakness, 5 = intact strength; Table 7–2). Tone of the extremities should also be documented.

A detailed sensory examination is performed involving all dermatomes, including pin prick and light touch. The patient is examined from caudad-cephalad, both anterior and posterior and bilaterally in order to document a "sensory level" (the lowest level of intact neurologic function). Proprioception and vibratory sensation should be evaluated.

A rectal examination is mandatory to assess tone and check for saddle anesthesia.

Deep tendon reflexes should be checked throughout all extremities, as well as abdominal wall and cremasteric reflexes where applicable. Evaluate for Babinski's sign, clonus, and hyperreflexia, although these may not be apparent on initial evaluation. The patient may present with flaccidity and areflexia in the acute setting.

Table 7–2. Cervical and Lumbar Myotomes

Upper Extremities		Lower Extremities	
Elbow flexor, Shoulder abductor	C5–6	Hip flexion	L1–3
Elbow extensor	C6,7,8	Hip adduction	L2–4
Wrist extension	C6,7	Hip adduction	L5
Hand intrinsics	C8, T1	Knee flexion	S1–2
		Knee extension	L3–4
		Plantar flexion	S1
		Plantar extension	L4–5

From Youmans JR: Neurological Surgery, 4th ed. Philadelphia, W. B. Saunders, 1996, p. 65.

There are several spinal cord syndromes that may be encountered, depending on the anatomic location and mechanism of injury:

- Transverse cord injury syndrome: Complete loss of motor and sensory function below the level of injury. Spinal shock must have abated in order to diagnose, and if there is any evidence of sacral sparing, the lesion is incomplete.
- Brown-Séquard syndrome: Occurs with a hemisection of the lateral half of the spinal cord, which results in damage to the descending motor fibers in the corticospinal tract and cell bodies in the ventral horn. Generally seen in penetrating injury to the spinal cord, such as gunshot or stab wounds. It is manifested clinically as ipsilateral weakness/paralysis, and loss of vibratory and position sense with contralateral loss of pain, temperature, and gross touch. The axons of the dorsal columns do not cross until the level of the medulla; therefore, one sees ipsilateral loss of vibratory and position sense. The fibers of the lateral spinothalamic tract that relate to pain and temperature cross within two segments above the level of entry into the spinal cord (i.e., contralateral loss of pain, temperature, and touch).
- Central cord syndrome: Usually seen with hyperextension injury. Generally a good prognosis for recovery. Clinically manifest as greater weakness in the arms than in the legs (arm and hand fibers are more centrally located in the corticospinal tract). Often accompanied by urinary retention and sacral sparing. Discrimination, vibratory, and position sense are usually intact (dosal column is preserved).
- Anterior cord syndrome: Seen with hyperflexion injuries (ventral cord injury). Clinically manifested as loss of pain, temperature, and light touch, and preservation of vibratory and position sense

(dorsal column functions). This is due to compromise of the anterior spinal artery, which supplies the anterior two thirds of the cord, and which may result in ischemia or infarct in the ventral horns, lateral spinothalamic tracts, and descending motor fibers, with sparing of the dorsal columns.

DIAGNOSTIC STUDIES

Laboratory
Full Chemistry Profile, CBC, PT, PTT. Performed as part of the trauma or preoperative screening process.
Radiology
Cervical Spine Films. Initial study should be cross-table lateral of cervical spine. Complete cervical spine series should include AP, lateral, odontoid, and swimmer's views. All seven cervical vertebrae must be visualized. Once the initial series is cleared, a complete study should include flexion/extension views. This is done to evaluate for malalignment or ligamentous injuries and should be performed with qualified assistance to prevent neurologic injury (or worsen an existing deficit).
Laminograms (Tomograms). May be helpful, particularly in patients with ankylosing spondylitis, or to visualize fractures in more detail.
CT Scan. Best to evaluate bony detail with fine-cut (2 mm) study; allows visualization of atlas-axis articulations; assess for fracture, subluxation, facet abnormalities; should include sagittal reconstruction views.
MRI. Best to visualize spinal cord and evaluate soft tissues (e.g., ligamentous integrity, evidence of traumatic disc herniation, hematoma).

DIFFERENTIAL DIAGNOSIS

Traumatic. Not otherwise applicable.
Infectious
Epidural Abscess. May be due to bacteria (staphylococcus), virus, tuberculosis (with IV drug abuse, immunocompromised host). Patients are usually febrile, with severe spine pain.
Metabolic
Subacute Combined Degeneration. Such as seen with vitamin B_{12} deficiency; may cause loss of posterior column function.
Demyelinating Disorders. Such as multiple sclerosis may cause paralysis. The patient may have a history of the condition, demyelinating lesions are seen on MRI, or the CSF is positive.
Neoplastic
Bony Metastases. Especially of the prostate and lung; may cause pathologic fractures and cord compression. Differentiated on MRI as lesion; appears as high signal, suspicious for lesion.
Lymphoma. May cause direct cord compression. Differentiated on MRI.

Intramedullary Mass. Such as meningioma, neurofibroma; may cause direct cord compression. Lesion seen on MRI.

Vascular

Infarction. Patients may have a history of microvascular disease. Infarction seen on MRI.

Spinal Cord Arteriovenous Malformation. May rupture or "steal" blood from the spinal cord tissue. Seen on MRI scan.

Occult Vascular Lesion. May cause hemorrhage; seen on MRI scan.

Congenital

Ankylosing Spondylitis. Tend to develop fractures across the disc space and develop epidural hematomas that may cause cord compression/injury.

Acquired

Vascular Surgery. Patients may have had an acute onset after a major vascular procedure that has caused hypoperfusion of the spinal cord.

TREATMENT

Medical. The goal of therapy is to preserve current neurologic function, prevent further compromise, and provide anatomical stability. Treatment begins at the scene of the injury with the basic trauma concept of airway, breathing, and circulation. The spine is immobilized with a cervical collar, backboard, and sandbags. Intubation, if necessary, is performed without neck extension prior to hospital transport.

A relatively recent development is the institution of high-dose steroids to improve neurologic functional outcome, both sensory and motor, when administered within 8 hours of injury.

Spinal Cord Injury Protocol. 30 mg/kg bolus of methylprednisolone over 15 minutes, then wait 45 minutes and begin 23 hours continuous infusion of 5.4 mg/kg/h.

Ganglioside GM$_1$. Gangliosides are complex acidic glycolipids that are found in high concentrations in the central nervous system and are thought to form a major component of cell membranes. Treatment is experimental, but promising, and thought to induce regeneration and restore neuronal function postinjury.

General Care. Measures are undertaken from the moment the patient enters the emergency room. Vital autoregulatory functions such as heart rate, blood pressure, peristalsis, and bowel and bladder control are all affected by the injury. The patient should be placed on cardiac monitoring because asystole in the early phases may occur. Vasopressors may be required to maintain blood pressure. A nasogastric tube is placed because ileus is a common initial problem. Meticulous skin care is mandatory because many patients have no sensation to warn of a developing decubitus ulcer. A urinary catheter is placed owing to urinary retention.

Treatment of Malalignment. Skeletal traction (e.g., Gardner-Wells tongs) may be useful to reduce a dislocation and restore anatomical alignment. The amount of weight depends on patient age, size, and level of injury, but generally is begun at or below 5 lbs per interspace (e.g., C5 injury would require 25 lbs of traction). The neurologic examination is closely monitored for change. Cervical spine x-rays are performed with the patient in traction to document alignment, particularly as additional weight is added. This is a temporizing measure.

Halo vest fixation may be used to provide immobilization of the cervical spine pre- or postoperatively while healing occurs. This is the most effective external immobilizer, and generally is worn for 3 months. The advantage to the halo orthosis is early mobility.

Surgical. Surgical intervention may be necessary, and timing of such is often quite controversial. The goal of surgical therapy is to decompress the neural elements, restore anatomical alignment, and provide stability so that functional rehabilitation is optimized. Surgery usually is postponed until spinal cord edema has abated.

The determination of spinal instability can be difficult and may be defined using a three-column concept. Instability is defined as disruption of greater than one column.

Anterior column = anterior longitudinal ligament, anterior body

Middle column = posterior longitudinal ligament, annulus, posterior body

Posterior column = facet joints, ligamentum flavum, lamina, posterior spinous process, interspinous ligaments

Treatment of Fractures—Cervical

Atlanto-Occipital Dislocation. There is potential for brain stem compression (often fatal), and segmental fixation may be used to provide stability with fusion from occiput to C4, autologous bone graft and stabilization with a Luque rod or Steinmann pin. These patients are at risk for vertebrobasilar insufficiency.

Jefferson Fracture. Burst fracture of the ring of C1 (atlas) due to axial loading, is often stable, and may be treated with immobilization in a Philadelphia collar. If there is significant ligamentous disruption, internal fixation may be necessary.

Odontoid Fractures. Three basic types (usually due to hyperflexion injury):

Type 1: Tip of odontoid process, generally a stable fracture

Type 2: Base of the ondontoid process, generally unstable, and most common type of odontoid fracture. There is a high rate of non-union with this type fracture.

Type 3: The base of the odontoid process and body of C2, which may be treated with halo vest fixation or with a surgical approach if there is a non-union. With a combination C1 to C2 fracture, internal fixation is usually performed with sublaminar wires or lateral mass plating.

Hangman's Fracture. Fracture of lamina and pedicle with dislocation of body of C2 over C3; is considered unstable, with halo vest fixation the treatment of choice.

Locked Facet. Must be reduced then immobilized, usually with a halo orthosis. May require surgical intervention to reduce.

Teardrop Fractures. Are generally stable injuries and are treated with a Philadelphia collar.

Vertebral Body Fracture. Burst fractures with instability. If there is neural compression greater than 50%, kyphotic angulation greater than 25%, or reduction of the anterior body height by 50%, it is considered unstable. If bony fragments are present in the canal, decompression and fusion with stabilization (e.g., pedicle screw fixation) may be performed. Corpectomy is sometimes necessary. If compression is less than 50%, a cervical collar may be adequate.

Treatment of Fractures—Thoracolumbar

Flexion-Compression. Anterior wedge compression fracture with disruption of the anterior column. It is considered a stable fracture and treated with bedrest and external orthosis.

Burst Fracture. Axial compression injury with disruption of the anterior and middle columns; considered unstable. Treatment is quite controversial and may include bedrest with a brace if neurologically intact, or pedicle screw fixation with corpectomy in the presence of neurologic deficit, loss of body height, angulation, or retropulsion of bony fragments into the canal.

Flexion-Distraction Injury (Chance). Disruption of the posterior ligaments; usually treated with internal fixation.

Indications. Increasing neurologic deficit, evidence of cord compression by disc or hematoma, bony injury to vertebrae with cord compromise, nonreducible fracture or dislocation despite traction, and instability after a trial of halo vest fixation.

Contraindications. Immediately postinjury because cord edema may be significant and surgical intervention may cause additional damage; inability to undergo anesthesia; any time when the risk of intervention is greater than the benefit.

PEDIATRIC CONSIDERATIONS

Pediatric patients are more likely to have injury between occiput and C2.

Pediatric patients have laxity of ligaments, incompletely ossified vertebrae, and shallow facets.

Relative weight of head to torso ratio is greater than in adults.

OBSTETRICAL CONSIDERATIONS

Meticulous detail must be given to all vital functions in the pregnant patient who has suffered a spinal cord injury in order to reduce the chance of secondary injury to the fetus. A serum pregnancy test is indicated for trauma patients of childbearing age.

PEARLS FOR THE PA

Factors affecting recovery include the force of injury, extent of neurologic deficit, ability to realign and decompress, presence of irreducible cord compression, persistent instability, time between injury and realignment, ability to treat hypoxemia and shock.

Complete cervical spine series visualizing all seven vertebrae is mandatory.

CT scan is the study of choice for bony detail.

MRI is used to assess cord injury, soft tissue, ligamentous disruption, and evaluate for hematoma and edema.

Subarachnoid Hemorrhage

David A. Adams, PA-C

DEFINITION

Subarachnoid hemorrhage (SAH) occurs when blood leaks into the subarachnoid space, either primarily when vessels that traverse the subarachnoid space rupture (as in the case of aneurysms of the circle of Willis) or secondarily when a hemorrhage into the parenchyma of the brain ruptures through to the subarachnoid space. Rupture of an intracranial saccular or berry aneurysm is the most common cause of spontaneous SAH in adults. The management of morbidity and mortality remains significant despite advances in diagnosis, perioperative care, and surgical treatment.

HISTORY

Symptoms. The majority of intracranial aneurysms rupture into the subarachnoid space. This event produces a dramatic and characteristic clinical syndrome. Typically, the patient experiences a sudden severe headache described as violent, bursting, or explosive, usually as the worst headache of the patient's life. It is often associated with nausea, vomiting, transient loss of consciousness, meningismus, and photophobia. A less severe hemorrhage may present with an acute headache of moderate intensity, sometimes associated with nausea and vomiting, followed within 24 to 48 hours by the development of low back pain. The back pain, which may be associated with radicular pain, is believed to be caused by irritation of the cauda equina by blood in the CSF settling in the dependent lumbar thecal sac. Focal deficits and a depressed level of consciousness are common findings. Focal neural damage occurs in approximately 50% of patients, causing symptoms that include weakness, paralysis, speech and sensory disorders, seizures, and visual alterations. Five to ten percent of patients have convulsions at the time of rupture.

General. SAH is one of the few afflictions capable of causing instantaneous death in an otherwise healthy individual. In as many as 40% of patients with SAH, there may be a history of minor rupture or warning leak or other symptoms referable to the aneurysm. The majority of patients with warning leaks have a major SAH within 4 weeks of their minor hemorrhage. Some clinical findings such as a unilateral third nerve palsy can help to localize the aneurysm; however, the majority of aneurysms cannot be localized on the basis of clinical findings alone.

Age. About two thirds of intracranial aneurysms become symptomatic between the ages of 40 and 65 years. There is a slight female predominance.

Onset. Usually acute, but warning hemorrhages may occur.

Duration. The subarachnoid blood and subsequent vasospasm resolve after approximately 10 to 14 days.

Intensity. The initial neurologic insult seen with SAH may result in immediate death, permanent or transient neurologic deficit, or minimal symptoms.

Aggravating Factors. None.

Alleviating Factors. Essentially none, but prompt diagnosis, control of ICP, and obliterating the source improve mortality.

Associated Factors. Patients with hypertension, atherosclerotic vascular disease, Ehlers-Danlos syndrome, polycystic kidney disease, and coarctation of the aorta are more prone to develop aneurysms. For those who have had SAH, vasospasm may occur.

PHYSICAL EXAMINATION

General. The patient often rests quietly in bed, resisting neck and extremity movement with eyes closed owing to photophobia and with back and legs flexed to reduce tension on the irritated nerves and meninges. Vomiting, sweating, and chills may be apparent. The patient may also present in a comatose state. Vital signs may reveal fever or alterations in heart rate due to autonomic disturbances.

HEENT. Nuchal rigidity is the most frequent sign of meningeal irritation. Visual disturbances, especially diplopia caused by extraocular nerve palsies, are common. A CN III palsy in an awake patient suggests a posterior communicating artery aneurysm; in a comatose patient, it heralds herniation. A fundoscopic examination may reveal papilledema caused by increased ICP, blood around the disc from hemorrhage into the optic nerve sheath, or optic atrophy as a result of pressure on the optic nerve from a large aneurysm.

Neurologic. A full and complete neurologic examination is performed. The level of consciousness must be assessed because approximately 50%

of patients show some alteration. The more common neurologic deficits referable to hemispheric dysfunction include hemiparesis, aphasia, anosognosia, memory loss, and abulia. The patient is assigned a grade based on the clinical presentation. A commonly used method is the Hunt and Hess system (Table 7–3).

PATHOPHYSIOLOGY

Intracranial aneurysms are found in 4% of adults at autopsy and are multiple in 20% of cases. Rupture is the mechanism of clinical presentation in over 90% of patients who are later found to have an aneurysm. Approximately 26,000 cases of SAH resulting from aneurysm rupture occur each year in the United States.

Aneurysms are caused by a combination of congenital and acquired factors and, rarely, may be caused by trauma, infection, or tumor. They are thought to arise from defects in the muscularis media, particularly at arterial bifurcations where the muscular coat is incomplete. From the time of diagnosis, unruptured aneurysms are thought to bleed at a cumulative rate of 3% per year. Approximately 85% of congenital aneurysms are located on the anterior portion of the circle of Willis, whereas 15% are located at the posterior portion. Most symptomatic aneurysms range in size from 0.5 to 1.5 cm in diameter. Unruptured aneurysms that are detected clinically or at autopsy are usually less than 6 to 7 mm in diameter. Rupture is not common in unruptured aneurysms of less than 5 mm in diameter. Aneurysms of 2.5 cm and larger begin to act as an intracranial mass, resulting in symptomatology related to pressure and mass effect. Because most aneurysms lie free in the larger subarachnoid cisterns under the brain, they commonly rupture into the subarachnoid space. However, in over half of patients, the aneurysm ruptures into the brain and ventricles as well. The two major potential complications of SAH are rebleeding and cerebral arterial vasospasm with subsequent infarction. Vasospasm is

Table 7–3. Hunt and Hess Grading System

Grade	Description
1	Asymptomatic, or minimal headache and slight nuchal rigidity.
2	Moderate to severe headache, nuchal rigidity, no neurologic deficit (except cranial nerve palsy).
3	Drowsiness, confusion, or mild focal deficit.
4	Stupor, moderate to severe hemiparesis, possible early decerebrate rigidity and vegetative disturbances.
5	Deep coma, decerebrate rigidity, moribund.

From Kaye A (ed). Essential Neurosurgery. New York, Churchill Livingstone, 1991.

defined as radiographically measurable constriction of cerebral arteries after SAH. About 30% of patients with angiographic spasm develop ischemic neurologic deficits. Although the exact cause of vasospasm is poorly understood, it is probably related to the irritant effect of a blood constituent or breakdown product on the external vessel wall in addition to mechanical changes.

The precise cause of SAH is not found in approximately 15% of cases.

DIAGNOSTIC STUDIES

Laboratory
Full Chemistry Profile, CBC, PT, PTT.   Performed as routine preoperative screen to identify any underlying metabolic or hematologic anomaly.
Type and Cross Match.   Used if surgery is imminent.
Radiology
CT Scan.   Without intravenous contrast to evaluate for the presence of subarachnoid, intracerebral, subdural or intraventricular blood, hydrocephalus, or mass effect. In 5% to 10% of cases, the CT scan is negative.
Four-vessel Cerebral Angiography.   Used to identify the cause of the SAH, location of an aneurysm(s), and the presence or absence of vasospasm. May also reveal an arteriovenous malformation.
MRI/MRA.   Used as screening for potential aneurysm or to differentiate aneurysm from neoplasm.
Other
Lumbar Puncture.   Used to confirm SAH if a CT scan is negative or is not available. Blood in the CSF (which does not diminish as CSF is withdrawn) or xanthochromia is positive for SAH.

DIFFERENTIAL DIAGNOSIS

Traumatic
Head Injury.   CT may reveal traumatic subarachnoid blood associated with cerebral contusion. Primary SAH may lead to an acute loss of consciousness, causing trauma.
Infectious
Meningitis.   CT negative for subarachnoid blood. Lumbar puncture reveals decreased glucose, elevated protein; culture positive.
Metabolic
Hypertensive Intracerebral Hemorrhage.   History of hypertension, no aneurysm seen on angiography; may have no subarachnoid component to hemorrhage.
Pituitary Apoplexy.   May cause subarachnoid hemorrhage (rare). Angiogram negative; true lateral skull film may reveal enlargement of pituitary fossa, associated with endocrinological disturbance.

Neoplastic
Brain Tumor. May cause hemorrhage; may have no subarachnoid component to hemorrhage: CT/MRI may show changes constant with neoplasm. CT/MRI with contrast may show lesion.

Vascular
Cerebral or Spinal Cord Arteriovenous Malformation. May present as SAH; differentiated on MRI/MRA or angiography.

Migraine. Negative CT/MRI angiography (performed as indicated). May have history of migraine or headache may follow a common pattern (approximately 99.6% of patients with new onset headache are eventually diagnosed with benign headaches).

Congenital
Coagulation Defects. May cause intracerebral hemorrhage; history of coagulation defect.

Acquired
Iatrogenic Anticoagulation. May cause intracerebral hemorrhage; may have no subarachnoid component to hemorrhage; elevated PT, PTT, or bleeding time; positive history of taking anticoagulants (e.g., warfarin, heparin), or history of a condition requiring anticoagulation (e.g., prosthetic heart valve).

TREATMENT

Medical. The goal of initial management in patients with SAH is to reduce increased ICP, prevent secondary neurologic damage from vasospasm, prevent rebleeding, and to diagnose and treat the causative factor.

For treatment of increased ICP, an ICP monitor (ventriculostomy, subarachnoid bolt, or intracerebral monitor) may be used to guide therapy. The ventriculostomy provides the added benefit of the ability to drain CSF. Additional methods may include elevating the head of the bed or, in more extreme cases, the use of mannitol. Treatment will be tempered by the need to prevent cerebral vasospasm. Sedatives and analgesics are given to help calm the patient. Factors that may increase ICP (overstimulation, cough) are avoided.

Cerebral vasospasm typically occurs on about the fourth day following the SAH and continues for 10 to 14 days. This process may lead to hypoperfusion of the brain with resultant infarct or death. Although not preventable, its effect can be moderated. Hypervolemia is instituted to keep the central venous pressure at 12 mm Hg. The increased fluid necessary also dilutes the blood to some degree, which makes it easier for the blood to pass through the spastic vessels. The calcium channel blocker nimodipine is given (60 mg q4h) to reduce spasm. This drug is thought to work on the microvasculature because angiographically apparent spasm persists. Significant hypertension is controlled to prevent rebleeding; however, adequate blood pressure is maintained (at or slightly above the patient's baseline) to maintain cerebral perfusion. It is important to identify and definitively treat the causative source to prevent rebleeding. Antifibrinolytic drugs have no benefit owing to the secondary risks of systemic thrombosis.

Anticonvulsants such as phenytoin, carbamazepine, or phenobarbitol may be given to prevent seizure.

Surgical. Timing of surgery is based on established norms and the surgeon's experience. If an aneurysm is identified, surgery can be performed early or late. Surgery is not performed during the time period when vasospasm exists (day 4 to day 10 to 14).

Early surgery has the benefit of obliterating the source of the bleed acutely and preventing rebleeding. This is generally selected for the patient who is of low grade (clinically stable). Delayed surgery may be elected if the patient is of a higher grade (unstable) in order to allow for healing of the brain from the initial insult or to allow for the clinical condition to stabilize. This may require a second angiogram to confirm the absence of vasospasm.

Microsurgery is performed through a craniotomy (pterional or temporal in most cases). The aneurysm is treated by placing a clip across the neck of the aneurysm, by wrapping or reinforcing the dome of the aneurysm (if the neck is not accessible or is not present) or, less commonly, by ligation of the parent vessel.

Another method that may be implemented is endovascular occlusion of the aneurysm through an angiographic catheter. This is performed by the surgeon or by a neuroradiologist specially trained in neurointerventional techniques.

Arteriovenous malformations are treated surgically, with or without preoperative endovascular occlusion of feeding vessels.

If the cause of the SAH is not found, the patient undergoes further evaluation after approximately 6 months because the aneurysm may have been initially thrombosed and recanalize.

Indications. Clinically stable patients in whom an aneurysm is identified. Higher grade patients would be surgical candidates if there is a significant intracerebral hematoma.

Contraindications. Clinically unstable; cerebral vasospasm; coagulopathy.

PA Role in Surgery. The PA assists with the opening and closing of the craniotomy. It is imperative to enlist assistance with aneurysm surgeries because rupture of the aneurysm may occur intraoperatively. If rupture occurs, the assistant uses the suction device to allow visualization and clipping to take place. It is important to keep the suction tip away from the aneurysm so as not to inadvertently tear the vessel or suction other important structures. This can be accomplished by placing a patty on the suction tip or by placing the suction tip on bone. Identify intracranial landmarks in anticipation of a rupture.

PEDIATRIC CONSIDERATIONS

SAH is uncommon in children and, if present, is usually due to a arteriovenous malformation.

OBSTETRICAL CONSIDERATIONS

Meticulous detail must be given to all vital functions in the pregnant patient who has suffered an SAH to reduce the chance of secondary injury to the fetus. A serum pregnancy test is indicated on all patients of childbearing age.

PEARLS FOR THE PA

Always rule out subarachnoid hemorrhage in patients with acute onset headache, because up to 40% of patients will have a minor rupture or warning leak and progress to rupture.

Surgery can be performed early or late, depending on the patient's clinical condition.

Cerebral vasospasm occurs from about day 4 to 14 after SAH and results in significant morbidity and mortality.

Subdural Hematoma

Judy Nunes, PA-C, BS

DEFINITION

A collection of blood that is located between the dura mater and calvarium (skull), which is often due to traumatic injury to bridging veins or brain laceration. Associated with a progressive neurologic deficit.

There are three major types of subdural hematoma (SDH): acute, subacute, and chronic.

HISTORY

Symptoms. Patients may present as comatose or asymptomatic, but commonly complain of persistent headache, with or without focal neurologic deficit (usually contralateral hemiparesis). The mental status may wax and wane (especially in patients with chronic subdurals). Seizures are possible.

General. Acute subdural hematoma (SDH) usually occurs after head trauma with a rapid progression of symptoms. Most patients have significant progressive neurologic deficit within 48 hours postinjury.

Subacute hematoma symptoms occur within 48 hours to 2 weeks postinjury.

Chronic subdural hematoma symptoms occur greater than 2 weeks post-injury. Often seen in the elderly, particularly in those with alcohol dependence with some degree of brain atrophy, or patients on anticoagulation therapy. Patients are generally amnestic for the traumatic event, which may have been quite trivial.

Age. May occur as a result of traumatic birth, but are more prevalent in the elderly.

Onset. Variable, depending on the extent of the bleed and setting (e.g., patients on ASA, Coumadin). From immediate (acute subdural hematoma) to weeks or even months before symptoms are apparent (chronic subdural hematoma).

Duration. Progressive if left untreated.

Intensity. Variable from asymptomatic to comatose.

Aggravating Factors. Coagulopathy, anticoagulation therapy (Coumadin, ASA).

Alleviating Factors. Surgical evacuation and decompression.

Associated Factors. Brain atrophy, alcohol use/abuse, anticoagulation therapy, coagulopathy.

PHYSICAL EXAMINATION

General. Consider potential associated neurologic injuries (e.g., skull fracture, epidural hematoma, contusion, spinal cord injury) or multitrauma. A full trauma survey is performed as indicated.

Neurologic. A full and complete neurologic examination is performed. Level of consciousness may be diminished in patient with a large subdural collection (usually acute). Patients often present with a progressive neurologic deficit, particularly a hemiparesis (check for pronator drift), Babinski's sign (contralateral to the subdural collection). Evaluate sensation, gait (if able), cerebellar functions, and reflexes to evaluate for any additional focal findings. A unilateral CN III palsy suggests herniation.

PATHOPHYSIOLOGY

Subdural hematoma occurs when bridging veins (cortical veins that "bridge" the cortex and dural sinuses) are disrupted or lacerated and the brain is contused, resulting in hemorrhage into the subdural space through thin, pia-arachnoid membranes. The blood spreads out over the convexity of the brain. If it reaches significant size, it may cause cortical compression, mass effect, and shift with progressive neurologic deficit and possible herniation and death. If the collection is relatively small, the clot may be eventually lysed by the fibrinolytic cascade (usually liquefies within 7 days) and become enveloped by a fibrous tissue membrane with friable capillaries. These membranes form after approximately 2 weeks and may be a potential source of repeat hemorrhage, resulting in an expanding lesion. As blood cells lyse, fluid osmotically flows into the hematoma. If the subdural fluid continues to accumulate, the bridging veins may be further stretched and there is potential for a mixed acute and chronic subdural process.

DIAGNOSTIC STUDIES

Laboratory
Full Chemistry Profile, CBC. Performed as routine trauma or preoperative screen to evaluate for underlying metabolic or hematologic anomalies.
PT/PTT/Bleeding Time. To evaluate for coagulopathy; mandatory in patients on Coumadin or heparin.

Radiology
CT Scan of the Brain. Is the study of choice with three densities: soft tissue, subdural, and bone windows. The appearance of the subdural hematoma is variable depending on the age of the hematoma. Acute subdural hematomas appear as hyperdense, biconcave extra-axial lesions (crescent shape). If large enough, they may cause shift of midline structures with mass effect. Subdural hematomas may also be bilateral or "balanced."

Subacute subdural hematomas appear isodense on CT scans and are therefore easy to miss. Subdural windows are most helpful in demonstrating this type.

Chronic subdural hematomas appear hypodense on CT and may have a blood–fluid level. Membranes tend to calcify over time and may be visualized more easily with a contrast enhanced study.
MRI of the Brain. May be helpful to gauge the "age" of the clot (e.g., presence of hemosiderin).

DIFFERENTIAL DIAGNOSIS

Traumatic
Epidural Hematoma. Acute presentation with lucid interval of an initial loss of consciousness followed by awakening and subsequent lapse in consciousness. Appears more local on CT than a subdural hematoma; frequently associated with a skull fracture.
Cerebral Contusion. Similar acute presentation; contusion seen on CT.

Infectious
Subdural Empyema. May have a history of ear/nose/throat (ENT) or sinus procedure; infected subdural collection; associated with elevated WBC, fever; surgical evacuation identifies it as an infection.

Metabolic
Hypoxemia, Hypoglycemia. May present as altered mental status. Serological evaluation should reveal the source; CT/MRI of the brain is negative.

Neoplastic
Carcinomatosis Meningitis. Diffuse arachnoidal involvement. Enhances with contrast on CT/MRI of the brain; CSF may be positive for tumor cells.
Vascular
Intracranial Aneurysm, Arteriovenous Malformation. May rupture and cause neurologic deficit. CT/MRI differentiates from subdural hematoma.
Congenital
Birth Trauma. May cause intracerebral hemorrhage or subdural hematoma. CT/MRI used for diagnosis.
Acquired
Subdural Hygroma. Caused by a tear in the pia-arachnoid that acts as a one-way valve with leakage of CSF into the subdural space.

TREATMENT

Varies with acuteness of the lesion, size, and ability of brain (elastance and compliance) to accommodate or compensate.
Medical. Conservative management can be employed if the lesion is less than or equal to 5 mm (thin-rim or skim subdural), with minimal neurologic deficit.
Anticonvulsants such as phenytoin, carbamazepine, or phenobarbital are given as indicated.
Surgical
Acute Subdural Hematoma. If large (often holo-hemispheric) and associated with neurologic deficit, it should be evacuated as early as possible. A craniotomy may be necessary to evacuate the hematoma (solid clot) and gain control of bleeding points (e.g., bridging veins or cortical arteries). If the dura appears tense (bluish hue), it is incised in a cruciate fashion to achieve a very rapid decompression. If the subdural is holo-hemispheric, a large flap is raised in order to rapidly decompress the temporal fossa and allow for visualization of the cortical veins, and to create a dural-traction flap. The subdural clot is irrigated with warm normal saline or lactated Ringer's solution to loosen and wash away the clot. It may be necessary to resect a portion of the frontal or temporal lobe if it does not appear viable as a result of the compression from the subdural clot. Hemostasis is obtained. A dural graft may be necessary (with pericranium, fascia lata, or commercial/cadaver type) and a drain may be left (Jackson-Pratt type) in the subdural space. Dural tenting sutures are placed to obliterate the epidural space and the craniotomy is closed in layers.
Chronic Subdural Hematomas. Are usually drained with two to three burr holes. The dura is coagulated beneath the burr hole, and a cruciate incision is made. The subdural space is irrigated until clear, and a Jackson-Pratt type drain is placed. If membranes are thought to be the source of recurrent hemorrhage, they may be preventing re-expansion of the hemisphere and a formal craniotomy may be necessary for extirpation.

Indications. Greater than 1 cm subdural collection with focal cortical distortion/shift of midline structures, with presence of neurologic deficit; impending herniation.

Contraindications. Significant coagulopathy must be corrected or any surgically evacuated hematoma will soon redevelop.

PEDIATRIC CONSIDERATIONS

In the newborn, subdural hematoma may result from traumatic delivery, underlying vitamin K deficiency, coagulopathy, or perinatal asphyxia.

In infants, subdurals tend to be bilateral and present with seizures, lethargy, and irritability. Low-grade fever and anemia are often present. The head may demonstrate biparietal enlargement. Consider child abuse. Look for associated fractures (skull or rib injuries consistent with shaken baby syndrome). Persistent subdurals may require shunting (subdural to peritoneal diversion), but in infants may often be managed with subdural taps via the anterior fontanelle using a 20-gauge spinal needle posterior to the coronal suture (never aspirate).

OBSTETRICAL CONSIDERATIONS

Meticulous detail must be given to all vital functions in the pregnant patient who has suffered a head injury to reduce the chance of secondary injury to the fetus. A serum pregnancy test is indicated on trauma patients of childbearing age.

PEARLS FOR THE PA

Subdurals are most commonly found in elderly patients on anticoagulation therapy, or in those with alcohol dependence.

Episode of trauma is often trivial and forgotten by the patient with a chronic SDH.

Three entities include: acute—within 48 hours; subacute—48 hours to 2 weeks; and chronic—greater than 2 weeks.

CT scan is the study of choice with three densities: brain, blood, or subdural windows, and bone windows.

Common signs and symptoms include a persistent headache and progressive neurologic deficit, especially a hemiparesis or pronator drift.

Further Reading
Allen MB Jr, Miller RH (eds): Essentials of Neurosurgery: A Guide to Clinical Practice. New York, McGraw-Hill, 1995.

Friedman AH, Wilkins RM (eds): Neurosurgical Management for the House Officer. Baltimore, Williams & Wilkins, 1984.

Kaye A (ed): Essential Neurosurgery. New York, Churchill Livingstone, 1991.

Kempe LG (ed): Operative Neurosurgery, Vol. 1. New York, Springer-Verlag, 1985.

Long DM (ed): Current Therapy in Neurological Surgery, ed 2. Philadelphia, BC Decker, 1989.

Netter FH, Jones HR Jr (eds): The CIBA Collection of Medical Illustrations, Vol. 1: Nervous System Part II—Neurologic and Neuromuscular Disorders. West Caldwell, NJ, CIBA Pharmaceutical Company, 1986.

Ropper AH, Kennedy SF (eds): Neurological and Neurosurgical Intensive Care, ed 2. Rockville, MD, Aspen Publishers, 1988.

Schwartz SI, et al: Principles of Surgery, ed 5. New York, McGraw-Hill, 1994.

Wilkins RH: Traumatic intracranial hematomas. In Rengachary SS, Wilkins RH (eds): Principles of Neurosurgery. New York, Mosby-Wolfe, 1994, pp. 19.2–19.3.

Youmans JR (ed): Neurological Surgery, ed 4. Philadelphia, W. B. Saunders, 1996.

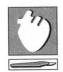

Chapter **8**

Organ Procurement

Michael G. Phillips, PA-C, BHS, CPTC, and
Demosthenes Y. Lalisan, I, BS, MBA, CPTC

HISTORY

The first long-term successful kidney transplant was performed by Dr. Joe Murray and his associates at the Peter Bent Brigham Hospital in Boston in 1954. During the years since this historical transplant procedure, the medical community has perfected techniques not only for improved survival of kidney transplants but also for heart, lungs, heart/lungs, liver, pancreas, small bowel, and abdominal organ cluster transplants. This tremendous growth in the success of organ transplantation comes from greatly improved surgical techniques, preservation solutions, and new immunosuppressive drugs, which have immensely enhanced graft survival.

As reported in the *United Network for Organ Sharing Update* in December of 1995, there are over 40,000 potential transplant recipients on the national waiting list. This list continues to grow due to the lack of organs for transplantation. Areas in which the practicing physician assistant (PA) can contribute include recognizing potential donor situations and working with hospital personnel to ensure that families are given the opportunity to consider donation.

The role of the PA in organ procurement, preservation, and distribution covers a multitude of jobs and responsibilities. These include professional education, public education, organ donor identification and management, surgical intervention (with the transplant surgeon and recovery teams), preservation of the organs postrecovery, as well as sharing organs among transplant centers on a nationwide basis. The PA's training and education is well suited for assisting the transplant surgeon in the preoperative stage and postoperative management of transplant recipients. In many cases, the PA, along with the transplant surgeon, follows organ recipients for long-term care.

The field of organ transplantation has developed into an accepted mode of treatment for those patients suffering end-stage organ disease. The organs transplanted have expanded to include almost all vital organs throughout the thoracic and abdominal cavities.

APPROACH TO THE DONOR FAMILY

The Uniform Anatomical Gift Act grants the legal right for any persons, prior to death, to donate any of their organs or tissues to medical research, education, or therapy. In instances where the wish to donate has not been disclosed prior to a person's death, consent for organ and tissue donation must be obtained from the legal next of kin in the following priority:

1. Spouse
2. Adult child
3. Parent

4. Adult sibling
5. Legal guardian
6. Any other person authorized to dispose of the body
Signed, written consent is preferred, but under extenuating circumstances, a witnessed verbal consent by phone is satisfactory.

Required request or routine inquiry policy has been initiated by many states. This policy states that designated personnel routinely approach the families of potential organ and tissue donors and provide them with information concerning organ and tissue donation. This policy is now law in many states and is being federally mandated for hospitals that accept Medicare and Medicaid reimbursement.

There is no set time frame for obtaining consent. However, it is best if families are given time to grieve. The revelation of the death of a loved one must be uncoupled from the request for organ and tissue donation. Ideally, the discussion should take place in a private room. The participants should include (but not be limited to) the legal next of kin and family decision maker, who may or may not be the same person. For this reason, an acute understanding of family dynamics and a full assessment of the social and medical information received from the physician and other hospital personnel is mandatory. Time should be allowed (and encouraged) for family discussion. If possible, the decision to donate should be by consensus. Informed consent is then obtained for organ and tissue donation. The consent informs the family regarding the need for transplant, the surgical procedure, the estimated time necessary for procurement, the tests necessary to ensure the quality of the donated organs and tissues and, in some cases, the need for an autopsy by a pathologist. The family should also be aware that there is no additional cost for donation.

The PA may assume an active role in any or all aspects of the approach to the donor family, including discussion about organ and tissue donation with a family and early contact with the hospital's designated organ procurement organization (OPO). Any assistance provided to the organ procurement coordinator optimizes the donation process.

PROTOCOL FOR ORGAN PROCUREMENT

The initial step in the donation process is the referral of a potential donor to the designated OPO by the physician, PA, nurse, or any personnel assigned by the hospital. Suitability of a potential organ and tissue donor is determined by the OPO and appropriate transplant surgeons. A potential organ and tissue donor must meet specific criteria concerning past medical and social history, current illness or injury, and age limits. These criteria, according to the organs or tissues evaluated for transplantation, are OPO specific. It is helpful to be familiar with the hospital chart and family dynamics before initiating a referral. Initial contact with an OPO should not be construed as a commitment to donation; rather, it is a first step in the evaluation of a terminal patient as a potential donor.

The first decision in donor triage is whether or not the potential donor's diagnosis is a terminal neurologic injury that will result in the declaration of brain death. Usually, only this type of diagnosis permits both vascular organ and tissue donation from the same donor. Unsuccessful resuscitation or cardiopulmonary cessation permits only tissue donation. Only after consent is obtained, brain death is declared, and the coroner's approval is obtained (when applicable), can the vascular organ and tissue donation proceed. In the case of cardiopulmonary cessation, cardiac death has to be documented in order for tissue donation to proceed.

After consultation with transplant surgeons, the organ procurement coordinator arrives at the hospital to perform a donor evaluation that includes a physical examination. It is at this point the PA and other medical personnel may be quite helpful in providing pertinent information concerning past medical and social history, current medical status, and prognosis. Applicable consents and declarations of death should also be verified at this time. If this has not been done, the coordinator works with the attending physician regarding proper protocols followed in the declaration of deaths, and obtains consents from the family and coroner (if applicable).

Donor management should be considered the beginning of organ preservation for transplantation. Medical management of the vascular organ donor is assumed by the OPO. Phillips' rule of hundreds is an excellent guideline for management of the adult donor: $BP \geq 100$ mm Hg, PaO_2 ~ 100 torr, and urine output ≥ 100 mL/h. General management goals include maintaining adequate organ oxygenation via the ventilator, restoring and maintaining circulatory volume, maintaining body temperature at $37°C$, balancing electrolyte levels, and avoiding infection. Laboratory tests and physician consult(s), when applicable, are ordered to assess each individual organ's function. Operating room time is scheduled based on the completion of these assessments and estimated time of arrival of the procurement team. The PA may be requested to assist in any of the management steps. Management suggestions are also welcomed by the OPO.

Organ allocation and assembly of procurement teams occur simultaneously and in synchrony with donor management. This function may be accomplished by another organ procurement coordinator at the OPO office or laboratory.

Anesthesia and respiratory personnel are needed to assist in transporting the donor to the operating room. With the assistance of the organ procurement coordinators, transplant surgeons recover all organs suitable for transplantation. It is paramount that the anesthesia team maintain adequate ventilation, monitor any hemodynamic changes, and administer any drugs when requested to do so. The recovery of organs optimal for transplantation requires a great amount of coordination and teamwork among all personnel involved.

TECHNIQUES IN ORGAN PROCUREMENT

The following is a general overview of the recovery procedures involved for each transplanted organ. Although the recovery techniques for each organ are discussed separately, they occur simultaneously during a multi-organ procurement.

DONOR CARDIECTOMY

A median sternotomy is performed. The pericardium is opened in a vertical direction and the incision is extended laterally at the level of the diaphragm. Pericardial sutures are then placed. The superior vena cava is dissected free and encircled with a suture placed at least 4 to 5 cm above the sinoatrial node. The aorta is dissected up to the level of the innominate artery. The aorta and main pulmonary artery are separated in order to allow placement of the aortic cross clamp. The inferior vena cava is also dissected free circumferentially and a pursestring suture is placed in the ascending aorta at the proposed cardioplegia site.

After administration of 300 U/kg of heparin, the cardioplegia needle is inserted into the ascending aorta and secured using the pursestring. The superior vena cava is divided between ties. The inferior vena cava is divided at the right atrial vena cava junction. The heart is allowed to beat until it is empty. The aortic cross clamp is applied and cardioplegia is administered. Cold topical saline is administered to the heart.

Once cardioplegia has been given, the needle is removed and the purse-string is secured. The inferior vena cava transection is completed, pulmonary veins are divided, and the aorta and pulmonary arteries are divided. The heart is lifted from the chest and the remaining attachments are divided. Care is taken to avoid the trachea and main stem bronchi posteriorly.

DONOR LUNG AND HEART/LUNG RECOVERY

Through a median sternotomy incision, the pericardial cavity is opened and the cut edges secured with stay sutures. The ascending aorta is dissected free from the main pulmonary artery and pursestring sutures are placed in these vessels, respectively. The trachea is dissected between the aorta and superior vena cava and then encircled by an umbilical tape. The superior vena cava is dissected superiorly from investing pericardium and a ligature is passed around this vessel.

After the donor is given heparin, the ascending aorta and main pulmonary artery are cannulated. The lungs are fully inflated to avoid perfusion with areas of atelectasis. Prostacyclin (500 μg) is then injected into the superior vena cava, followed by ligation of this vessel and transection of the inferior vena cava. When the heart is decompressed, the ascending aorta is cross clamped and preservation solutions are administered to the heart and lungs.

The tip of the left atrial appendage is amputated to vent the left side of the heart. The left atrial cuff is fashioned by making an incision in the left atrial wall midway between the confluence of the left pulmonary veins and the atrioventricular groove, and then continuing circumferentially around the orifices of the veins. A similar venous cuff is created on the right side. The superior vena cava is divided, the main pulmonary artery and ascending aorta transected, and the heart removed following division of the pericardial reflection.

The pericardium anterior to the hilum of each lung is then excised and pulmonary ligaments are divided. The lung block is excised by dividing mediastinal soft tissue and pleura anterior to the esophagus or stapling the esophagus and removing the entire mediastinal contents anterior to the vertebral column. The trachea is clamped and divided with the lungs fully inflated. On the back table, the lungs are separated by dividing the pulmonary artery bifurcation, mediastinal soft tissue, and by stapling the trachea and dividing the left main bronchus between the two staple lines.

DONOR NEPHRECTOMY

The en bloc nephrectomy is the usual technique by which both kidneys and segments of aorta and vena cava are included as a single specimen. A standard midline incision is adequate, although some surgeons use a chevron incision to provide maximal abdominal exposure. Mannitol (25 to 50 g IV) is given early to increase diuresis and to minimize renal cellular edema.

Beginning in the right lower quadrant, the mesocolon is freed along the line of Toldt, from the cecum to the hepatic flexure, and medially to the midline. The inferior edge of the small bowel mesentery is then divided. The right colon and small bowel are then eviscerated from the abdominal cavity. The third and fourth portion of the duodenum is elevated, exposing the left renal vein. Just superior to the left renal vein, the superior mesentery artery can be palpated. Next, the posterior edge of the mesentery of the left colon and sigmoid over the aorta is incised to the level of the inferior mesenteric artery, which is ligated and divided. The dissection is continued along the posterior peritoneum in a caudal direction into the pelvis. The ligament of Treitz is divided and the duodenum and other retroperitoneal structures are dissected free of the left renal vein. The abdominal contents are rotated to the left upper quadrant and eviscerated out of the abdominal cavity.

The abdominal aorta is isolated and ligated securely above the bifurcation, and a perfusion cannula is inserted proximally. The distal vena cava is now isolated. Both ureters are freed from deep within the pelvis to just below the lower pole of each respective kidney. Frequently, before mobilizing the kidneys, 100 mg IV of furosemide is given in an attempt to increase the renal vascular blood flow and to maximize diuresis. Isolation of the kidneys is now begun. The gonadal veins are ligated. The superior mesenteric artery and frequently the celiac artery are isolated, ligated, and cut. The proximal aorta and vena cava are isolated. Large vascular clamps are placed around the great vessels in an open position. Approximately 5 minutes after the addition of 300 U/kg of heparin and a vasodilator, the vena cava is vented distally and the aortic clamp is now applied above the celiac axis. Retrograde perfusion through the aortic cannula is immediately begun *in situ.* Usually 2 liters of preservation solution is flushed through the aorta. During the *in situ* flush the abdominal organs are bathed in iced saline. After lifting the distal vessel clamps, as well as both ureters and kidneys cephalad, the remaining dissection is completed.

DONOR HEPATECTOMY

A midline incision is extended from the suprasternal notch to the pubis. Initial mobilization begins with division of the falciform and the left triangular ligament. An aberrant left hepatic artery, when present, will travel in the gastrohepatic ligament. If none is encountered, a window is created in the gastrohepatic ligament. The porta hepatis should be palpated for pulsation of the common hepatic artery and for a potential aberrant hepatic artery. The common bile duct is dissected, ligated, and divided distally. The gallbladder is incised at the fundus and irrigated with saline in order to prevent autolysis.

Mobilization of the terminal ileum, right colon, and duodenum proceeds with the identification of the origins of the renal veins. Elevation and reflection of the transverse colon and small intestine to the right facilitates dissection and cannulation of the inferior mesenteric vein, in preparation for portal perfusion.

The distal aorta is dissected at the level of the iliac bifurcation and encircled with two umbilical tapes. An umbilical tape is passed around the supraceliac aorta in order to facilitate later cross clamping.

Heparin is administered intravenously. The umbilical tape is tied to occlude the distal aorta, and the flushed aortic cannula is inserted through an aortotomy. In rapid succession, the inferior vena cava is divided at the atriocaval junction, the supraceliac aorta is cross clamped, and the aortic and portal catheters opened wide to cold preservation solution. Iced saline is immediately placed in the abdominal cavity.

The initial flush (e.g., preservation flush) requires 5 to 10 minutes. Following the flush of the liver, the right hemidiaphragm is divided circumferentially, allowing the liver to be reflected superiorly toward the chest cavity. The arterial dissection is performed, beginning with identification and ligation of the gastroduodenal artery. The common hepatic artery is dissected proximally toward the celiac axis. Next, the splenic artery is identified and ligated. Once fully exposed, the aorta is transected below the clamp. The anterior portal vein, mesenteric vein, and splenic vein are identified and ligated, respectively. Then the aorta is transected between the origins of the celiac and the superior mesenteric artery. The remainder of the mesentery is divided to the spine between the transected aorta. The vena cava is transected above the origins of the renal veins. The liver can now be removed by dividing the remaining diaphragm and retroperitoneal attachments.

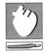

DONOR PANCREATECTOMY

Upon entering the abdomen, the arterial supply to the liver should be ascertained. The gastrocolic omentum should be divided. Dissection of the porta hepatis is then undertaken. The common bile duct is identified and divided. The gastroduodenal artery is then identified and ligated, and the common hepatic artery dissected back to the celiac where the origin of the splenic artery is identified. The portal vein should then be dissected in preparation for its division just prior to the *in situ* flush.

The right colon and small bowel should be mobilized to expose the retroperitoneum. The duodenum and head of the pancreas can then be mobilized to identify the inferior vena cava and aorta. At this point, the pancreas dissection is complete. The donor should be given heparin and a distal aortic cannula placed. The portal vein can now be cannulated for the portal flush.

DONOR HEART VALVE AND BONE TISSUE RECOVERY

Heart valves may be recovered from vascular donors whose hearts have been deemed unsuitable for transplant, as well as from cardiac death donors. Bone tissue may be recovered from vascular donors following organ recovery in addition to cardiac death donors.

The heart is surgically removed via a median sternotomy. The pericardium is opened and the heart is dissected free. Care should be taken in order to obtain adequate length on the aorta and pulmonary artery. Dissection of both great vessels should be taken beyond their bifurcations, respectively. Large sections of pericardium are also recovered at this time.

The long bones of the legs and iliac crests are recovered via bilateral incisions made from the superior aspect of the iliac crest and carried to the medial malleolus. Prior to the long bone recovery, fascia lata, patellar tendons, and Achilles tendons are recovered. Humeri are recovered via bilateral incisions made from the superior aspect of the deltoid to the medial aspect of the elbow.

DONOR CORNEAL RECOVERY

The corneal removal procedure may be performed in any controlled access space and an operating room is not required. The surgical procedure begins by rinsing the eye with sterile physiological saline followed by preparation of the corneal area and sterile draping. If an enucleation procedure is to be performed, the muscles of the eye are identified and clipped. This is followed by isolation and cutting of the optic nerve. If the cornea is to be removed *in situ*, the sclera is scraped with a sterile scalpel blade working from the limbus circumference outward to approximately 2 to 4 mm. Using a separate blade, a cut is made approximately 2 mm from the limbus and the tenotomy scissors are used to cut the cornea from the scleral rim. The excised cornea, with a surrounding rim of sclera, is placed in an antibiotic-containing preservation media.

POSTDONATION FOLLOW-UP

Following an organ or tissue donation, a personal letter is written to the donor family by the procurement coordinator. General information concerning the condition of the transplant recipient(s) is provided in a manner that does not compromise the confidentiality of the recipient(s), yet provides reassurance to the donor family of the value of their generosity. A similar letter is sent to the physicians and other hospital personnel who have assisted in the donation. If applicable, letters are also sent to the medical examiner, coroner, and funeral home.

An on-site visit is made to the donor hospital by the organ procurement coordinator following the recovery. During this visit questions that have arisen post-donation are answered. Suggestions to improve future working relationships between the hospital and procurement organizations concerning the donation process are addressed.

Donor family liaison programs have been adopted by some organ procurement organizations around the country. The purpose of these programs is to offer assistance to the donor families during their grief and bereavement process and to validate their decision to donate. This may allow for anonymous correspondence to occur between donor and recipient families via the family liaison coordinator.

SUMMARY

The growth of organ and tissue transplantation has been rapid during the last 40 years; more specfically, in the last 20 years. The role of the PA in this field of medicine has been exciting. As transplantation has grown, so has the acceptance of physician extenders in the practice of medicine, specifically in the field of transplantation. This chapter has attempted to highlight the multifaceted areas of organ and tissue transplantation.

Further Reading

Flye MW: Atlas of Organ Transplantation. Philadelphia, W.B. Saunders, 1995.

Phillips MG: Cadaver-donor nephrectomy. In Glenn JF (ed): Urologic Surgery. ed 3. Philadelphia, J.B. Lippincott, 1983, pp 329–335.

Phillips MG: Organ Procurement, Preservation and Distribution in Transplantation. Richmond, William Byrd Press, 1991.

Phillips MG, Mainous PD: UNOS Organ Procurement Coordinator's Handbook. Richmond, VA, UNOS, 1995.

Shumway SJ, Burdine J, Belman RM III: Combined harvest of heart and lungs: Techniques and results. Transplant Proc 1991;23:1236.

Sollinger HW, Vernon WB, D'Alessandro AM, Kalayoglu M, Stratta RJ, Belzer FO: Combined liver and pancreas procurement with Belzer-UW solution. Surgery 1989;106:685–691.

Starzl TE, Hakala TR, Shaw BW, et al: A flexible procedure for multiple cadaveric organ procurement. Surg Gynecol Obstet 1984;158:223.

Starzl TE, Hakala TR, Shaw BW, et al: An improved technique for multiple organ harvesting. Surg Gynecol Obstet 1987;165:343–348.

Sundaresan S, Trachiotis GD, Aoe M, Patterson GA, Cooper JD: Donor lung procurement: Assessment and operative technique. Ann Thorac Surg 1993;56:1409–1413.

Chapter 9

Orthopedics

Foot: Clubfoot (Talipes Deformity)

Richard E. Donnelly, PA-C, BS, BS

DEFINITION

Talipes, derived from the Latin words talus ("ankle bone") and pes ("foot"), is a term used to describe any congenital foot anomaly. Clubfoot is a hereditary foot deformity of unproved cause and is a rotational subluxation of the talocalcaneonavicular complex. Clinically, true clubfoot is a triad of midfoot and forefoot adductus, hindfoot varus, and heel equinus. There is controversy over whether soft-tissue or hard-tissue changes are actually the primary cause of this disorder. The term "intrinsic clubfoot" was coined to differentiate the malpositioned or malformed talus from the extrinsic clubfoot, which has normal anatomy, with the deformity secondary to uterine packing, or in utero positioning.

HISTORY

Symptoms. Infants are often evaluated shortly after birth, but it is often difficult to determine the degree of severity at that time. With involvement in multiple other joints including upper extremities, it is quite easy to classify this child in the severe teratogenic category. Conversely, a foot may appear to be quite stiff on initial examination but, after one or two castings, many of the components are already corrected.

General. The incidence in the general population is approximately 1 per 1000 births, and if one child in a family has the deformity, the incidence among siblings rises to 2.9 per 100. Nongenetic, extrinsic factors that may result in clubfoot deformity include arthrogryposis multiplex congenita, amniotic band (Streeter's) syndrome, and certain drugs taken during pregnancy (aminopterin). The initial evaluation of the child includes notation of the patient's age, prior treatment, and an estimate of the actual severity of the clubfoot.

Age. Present at birth; a 1 : 2 male-to-female ratio.

Onset. Intrauterine.

Duration. Residual deformity or effects last through life, even with correction; conservative or surgical treatment does not correct the entire deformity. Regardless of the form of treatment, the resultant foot is smaller, less mobile, and the calf relatively atrophic.

Intensity. May be disabling.

Aggravating Factors. Not applicable.

Alleviating Factors. Early recognition and treatment.

Associated Factors. Myelodysplasia, arthrogryposis, and congenital hip dysplasia, myelomeningocele.

PHYSICAL EXAMINATION

General. The patient may present with only the foot anomaly or with significant congenital defects.

Orthopedic. Inward rotation of the whole foot may be present, and the ankle joint appears in extreme equinus position. The Achilles tendon is also shortened and may be attached medially on the calcaneus; creases and dimpling over the sinus tarsi region may be seen. The neurovascular units are usually intact. Because the osseous structures of the infant foot are small, it is nearly impossible to ascertain their true anatomic relationship by simple clinical evaluation. The abundant heel fat pad can easily hide a great deal of hindfoot equinus. Likewise, the absence of soft-tissue definition can make a moderate amount of hindfoot varus clinically difficult to appreciate.

PATHOPHYSIOLOGY

Clubfoot has been presumed to be a myopathy or a neuropathy, but the evidence is inconclusive. Theories include the malformed talus, the malrotated talus, a growth arrest on the medial border of the foot secondary to contractile tissue, and an abnormality of the navicular position. The primary deformity seems to be present in the head and neck of the talus: the neck is foreshortened to absent with medial deviation, the articular surface of the head is inclined plantarward. Because of the plantarward declination of the talar neck, the talar body lies more anterior in the ankle mortise than in the normal foot. The hindfoot therefore declines into equinus and developmental contracture of both the ankle and subtalar joint capsules. Due to the medial and plantar-deviated head of the talus articulating with the anteromedial portion of the calcaneus, the posterior calcaneus is rotated laterally and held in close proximity of the lateral malleolus. The combination of rotation and varus of the calcaneus widens the sinus tarsi and brings the Achilles tendon insertion medial to the calcaneal midline. The midfoot likewise adapts to changes in the head and neck of the talus. The navicular is smaller than normal and medially displaced. The remainder of the midfoot seems to follow the talar neck and rotated calcaneus. The cuboid is displaced beneath the third cuneiform and rotated toward the medial side of its normal articulation with the calcaneus, whereas the forefoot follows the varus and adducted contour of the midfoot.

DIAGNOSTIC STUDIES

Laboratory. Not applicable.

Radiology

Feet and Hip X-ray. Anteroposterior (AP) and lateral x-rays are indicated for treatment and diagnosis on the initial evaluation. The AP view is obtained with the plantar surface flat on the film cassette in pseudostanding position. The lateral view likewise should be obtained in a pseudostanding position with the ankle as neutral as possible. These studies are also indicated during treatment to determine appropriate correction during casting and in the postoperative phase.

DIFFERENTIAL DIAGNOSIS

There are no differential conditions.

TREATMENT

Medical.   In general, the position in utero "extrinsic clubfoot" and mild intrinsic feet can be corrected with casting. Three-stage casting is used according to the Kite method. If a more severe true intrinsic clubfoot is present, the casting is preliminary to surgery, which is carried out when it is obvious that casting is not making progress. Casting stretches the skin and corrects many of the components of clubfoot, such as adductus of the forefoot, some supination or varus, and some malrotation, although often it does not relieve the equinus.

Surgical.   A single surgical procedure should be complete, with release or reconstruction of all the pathologic components that exist at the time. The surgical procedure is carried out according to the degree of deformity in regard to soft-tissue and bony abnormalities. Postoperatively, while in the operating room, the foot is placed essentially in the corrected position and covered with extensive soft dressings, including abdominal pads and extensive sheet cotton (Robert Jones–type dressing). A plaster or fiberglass shell is applied from the toes to above the knee, which allows the skin to heal without tension, swelling to be controlled to a minimum, avoids ischemia of the foot, and helps control postoperative pain. Casting is preferred over taping, manipulations, and various forms of bracing. Most clinicians agree that when casting is no longer effective, as extensive as possible a one-stage surgical procedure is preferable to multiple serial procedures.

Indications.   Failure of casting to relieve the deformity.

Contraindications.   Inability to tolerate anesthesia, inadequate trial of casting.

TECHNIQUE OF SURGICAL ASSISTING

The PA assists with maintaining traction on the tendons as they are resutured. Applying the cast and following the progress of the patient while being casted is an important duty of the PA.

PEDIATRIC CONSIDERATIONS

This is a pediatric condition.

OBSTETRICAL CONSIDERATIONS

Genetic counseling should be instituted when clubfoot has been identified in a relative. This is especially true for the woman who has had a previous affected child. Avoidance of known teratogenic factors is essential.

PEARLS FOR THE PA

This disorder is a lifelong condition, because treatment does not entirely correct the deformity.

Extrinsic and mild intrinsic clubfoot can be treated initially with casting.

Foot: Hallux Valgus

Richard E. Donnelly, PA-C, BS, BS

DEFINITION

Hallux valgus (bunions) occurs at the metatarsophalangeal (MTP) joint of the great toe and is defined as a MTP angle greater than 15 degrees or a first metatarsal to second metatarsal angle greater than 10 degrees.

HISTORY

Symptoms. Most patients complain of pain, swelling, and erythema over the medial aspect of the MTP joint with certain footwear. Numbness may be present with more severe lesions.

General. Modern footwear has made bunions more common than in the past. Only 10% of bunions are inherited; the other 90% are acquired through wearing improper shoes. Eighty percent of bunions occur in women, mainly due to fashionable footwear.

Age. The onset of bunions can occur as early as mid to late teens, but usually occurs in the fourth to sixth decades. Tends to worsen with age.

Onset. Chronic.

Duration. Bunions can last an entire lifetime and never need correction.

Aggravating Factors. Footwear is the main aggravating factor for this deformity. Narrow, high-heel type shoes are the greatest offenders. Heel height of 2 inches increases the forefoot pressure by 66%, and a 1-inch heel increases the pressure by 22%.

Alleviating Factors. Wider shoes and heel heights of less than 1 inch help to lessen symptoms, but may not be enough to alleviate symptoms entirely.

Associated Factors. Heredity plays a relatively small role in the formation of hallux valgus. Patients with rheumatoid arthritis have a higher incidence than the normal population. In some cases, osteoarthritis may occur more readily due to incongruity of the joint. Hammer-toe deformity of the second toe occurs more frequently in individuals with severe hallux valgus.

PHYSICAL EXAMINATION

Orthopedic. The hallmark of hallux valgus is the valgus deformity occurring at the MTP joint of the great toe. There is enlargement and thickening of the medial capsule of the joint with prominence of the medial eminence, enhancing the appearance of this deformity. Generally, there is erythema over the medial aspect of the joint and tenderness with palpation or movement. With the more severe deformities, paresthesia or numbness may occur distally into the great toe. This is due to compression by shoes over the dorsal medial branch of the medial plantar nerve, which passes superficially over the medial joint area.

PATHOPHYSIOLOGY

Through decades of wearing narrow shoes, hallux valgus deformity forms and progresses. The lateral deviating forces applied by narrow, pointed shoes tend to stretch the medial capsule and other ligamentous structures of the great toe at the metatarsal phalangeal joint. With time and force, the lateral structures, the flexor hallux brevis and longus, begin to bowstring, thus creating even greater force on the distal toe, deviating it laterally or into valgus. The constant irritation of the medial eminence and capsule by the shoe enlarges and thickens these structures. With rheumatoid arthritis, the laxity of joint tissues due to the disease process increases the likelihood of hallux valgus deformity, along with degeneration of the joint cartilage.

DIAGNOSTIC STUDIES

Laboratory
CBC, Erythrocyte Sedimentation Rate, Uric Acid, Rheumatoid Profile. Performed as indicated to rule out systemic conditions.

Radiology
Foot X-rays. Standing radiographs are necessary to assess properly the degree or severity of hallux valgus and to rule out any other pathology that may be present.

DIFFERENTIAL DIAGNOSIS

Traumatic. Not applicable.
Infectious
Joint Infection. Painful swollen joint, elevated WBC, erythema, warmth.
Metabolic
Gout, Pseudogout. Periodic, acute attacks of joint swelling and pain without history of a specific injury. Elevated serum uric acid levels with gout.
Rheumatoid Arthritis. Twenty percent of patients initially present with foot problems; positive rheumatoid factor.
Neoplastic. Not applicable.
Vascular. Not applicable.
Congenital. Not applicable.
Acquired. Not applicable.

TREATMENT

Medical. Conservative treatment consists of wider shoes, and sometimes a hallux valgus night or day splint. Shoe modification by stretching the shoe over the medial aspect of the foot may be of some benefit.

Surgical. The severity of the deformity, the patient's age, functional outcome required for the patient, the expected patient outcome, and underlying disease process influence which bunion procedure is indicated for a satisfactory results.

Resection arthroplasty is a resection of the base of the proximal phalanx, used mainly in older, inactive patients with severe deformities. The great toe is shortened, and the patient loses plantar flexion strength. Distal osteotomies are the most common procedure and are osteotomies of the distal metatarsal near the metatarsal head, used for mild to moderate deformities. The majority of cases are fixed to prevent slipping or malunion.

Distal realignment with proximal osteotomies/arthrodesis addresses the proximal first metatarsal and first metatarsal cuneiform joints with soft-tissue realignment at the distal end of the ray. These procedures are used for deformities that are moderate to severe. Greater correction is afforded with these procedures while retaining function of the MTP joint. Corrections generally are long lasting and allow better footwear and improved pain relief. Internal fixation is used.

MTP arthrodesis is a fusion of the first MTP joint, used as a salvage procedure. This procedure is indicated in patients with rheumatoid arthritis involving the MTP joint, those with failed MTP joint replacements, secondary complications of prior surgery (e.g., hallux varus), and severe osteoarthritis of the MTP joint. Women who wish to wear high heels may have difficulty because the toe will not bend to accommodate.

Indications. The criteria for correction are painful hallux valgus and difficulty fitting in shoes.

Contraindications. For cosmetic purposes alone. This is due to the relative risks of surgery: loss of or decreased range of motion that occurs with most procedures, scaring, and rate of recurrence of hallux valgus.

TECHNIQUE OF SURGICAL ASSISTING

The PA may assist with exposure and repair of the defect. Identification and counseling patients as to the options of treatment are primary responsibilities of the PA.

PEDIATRIC CONSIDERATIONS

Bunion surgery prior to bone maturity is a relative contraindication. Usually, conservative treatment and patient education allows individuals to get along until they reach an age of bone maturity.

OBSTETRICAL CONSIDERATIONS

Use caution performing x-rays and prescribing potentially teratogenic drugs. Surgery can be delayed until after delivery.

PEARLS FOR THE PA

Hallux valgus is caused by improper footwear in 90% of cases.

The mainstay of treatment is changing from a narrow-toed to wider footwear.

Surgery may be required if the deformity is severe.

Fractures

Richard E. Donnelly, PA-C, BS, BS

DEFINITION

A fracture is the loss of structural integrity or discontinuity of bone, ranging from stress reaction of the bone, compression, to frank disassociation of the cortex and cancellous structures. Fractures may occur secondary to metabolic disease (e.g., osteoporosis, osteopenia, osteomalacia), Charcot arthropathy (in peripheral neuropathy), and pathologic causes (e.g., tumors and metabolic diseases). Stress fractures occur because of increased repetitive force over time. Traumatic forces that produce frank fractures caused by blunt or twisting forces are the most common.

Union.   Union of a fracture has been achieved when a pain-free, functional status has returned, with no clinical mobility at the fracture site, and no pain is present on palpation or application of deforming stress across the fracture site.

Delayed Union.   When a fracture has failed to unite within an expected time frame.

Malunion.   Nonosteounion of a fracture, usually united by fibrous tissue.

Non-union.   Failure of the bone ends of a fracture to unite after 9 months of attempted healing.

Open Fracture.   When bone extrudes through a break in the skin and overlying soft tissue.

Transverse Fractures.   Usually occur by a bending force or direct blow to the bone; can occur in certain pathologic conditions.

Oblique Fracture.   Usually is produced by torsion and loading. It has rather short fracture ends and usually heals well.

Spiral Fracture.   Caused by a twisting or rotatory force that is loaded; tends to break with sharp ends.

Compressive Fractures.   Usually are not markedly displaced and can be of the greenstick type or torus buckling of the cortex; often seen in children. Adult fractures include compression of vertebrae. These are often seen in osteomalacia or osteoporosis and certain pathologic conditions such as myeloma or metastases.

Comminuted Fractures.   Are seen with associated soft-tissue injuries that are sometimes severe. Usually the result of direct, violent blows that produce multiple fragments.

Segmental Fractures.   Can result in devitalization of a segment of bone. Reduction is quite difficult and union is slow; should be treated by a consultant.

Impacted Fractures.   Are those that result from direct, violent blows that drive bone fragments firmly together. These quite often are seen in the shoulder.

Avulsion Fractures.   Are those in which indirect force against a muscle mass pulls off a fragment of bone. These often are seen around the rotator cuff of a shoulder, the patellar tendon, the hamstring, and in fractures in which the Achilles tendon pulls loose.

Fracture-dislocations.   Occur with dislocations of the joint. These are always complex injuries that require consultation.

HISTORY

Symptoms.   Patients usually have a sudden onset of pain, with progressive swelling or deformity in the area of fracture.

General.   Most fractures occur as result of trauma from a blunt or twisting force of a direct or indirect nature. Fractures without a history of trauma usually have a poorer prognosis. Stress fractures occur more frequently in weight-bearing bones, and usually are a benign condition brought on by excessive repetitive stress. The hallmark is pain over the area of fracture (point tenderness).

Age.   Traumatic fractures may occur at any age but occur more frequently in the second decade to the fifth decade of life in more active patients. Pathologic fractures or fractures due to metabolic causes usually occur later in life. Stress fractures can occur at any age but occur in more active patients.

Onset.   Sudden with trauma. Stress fractures usually are insidious in nature, whereas pathologic fractures may present with sudden onset of pain with a spontaneous fracture without history of trauma.

Duration.   Fractures usually heal within 6 weeks. Tibia fractures may take up to 12 weeks or longer. Charcot arthropathy–type fractures may take up to 6 months or longer.

Intensity.   Depends on type of injury or type of fracture and bone involved. Acute fractures may cause significant pain and deformity or cause neurovascular compromise. Early Charcot arthropathy may be painless, and warmth and deformity may occur before pain is noted.

Aggravating Factors.   Activity of the limb or area of fracture may cause greater displacement of the fracture or delayed mal- or non-union.

Alleviating Factors.   Immobilization of the fracture, elevation, and ice help with decreasing pain. Compression, if it is not restrictive, may help pain and swelling.

Associated Factors.   Metabolic disease, drug-induced osteoporosis or osteopenia, tumors or metastatic disease, osteoporosis, age, and activity at risk for trauma are factors that may place individuals at a higher risk.

PHYSICAL EXAMINATION

General.   The patient usually is in significant distress with an acute fracture. With stress fractures, the patient may be in relatively no distress or favoring the involved area.

Orthopedic. Observation and inspection for obvious deformity, open wounds, severity of edema, and discoloration is performed before the limb or area is touched. Palpation for pulses distal to the area of injury and testing for sensory and motors defects distal is essential. Bone fragments are sharp and can sever vessels and nerves easily, whereas swelling can compromise neurovascular structures. When the fracture is not obvious by inspection, palpation over the injured area or area of pain elicits point tenderness if a fracture is present. Crepitation can sometimes be felt as the bone ends move; the examiner must be cautious not to cause further displacement of the fracture or further damage to soft tissue. Joint stability should be evaluated with injuries near or around joints.

PATHOPHYSIOLOGY

Fractures occur when an injuring force exceeds the mechanical strength of the involved bone. These forces may be applied directly or indirectly. Biomechanically, failure of the bone leading to a fracture results from tension, compression, or shear forces acting on the bone.

Pathologic fractures are caused by weakening in the bone secondary to tumor invasion or other metabolic bone defects. This is due to either primary tumors of bone, metastatic tumors to bone, or weakening of bone due to metabolic abnormalities. As the tumor invades the bone, it decreases the bone's mineralization—usually of the cancellous bone first—because of its high metabolic state. As the tumor invades the cortical structure, the bone structurally becomes weak and is unable to support the body weight or force placed upon it, and thus the bone fractures.

Pathologic fractures may also occur in bones afflicted with generalized disease processes such osteoporosis and osteomalacia. Osteoporotic fractures can be grouped into at least two recognized groups: spine "crush-fractures" or compression fractures of the vertebrae, and long-bone fracture syndrome. Compression fractures of the vertebrae mainly occur in women 10 to 15 years after menopause. Long-bone fractures, especially those involving the proximal femur and humerus, occur in the elderly and more commonly in women than men. Osteomalacia may be suspected in patients who complain of chronic skeletal pain and tenderness, slowly healing bilateral fractures, or proximal muscle weakness.

In traumatic fractures it is obvious that the external force has overcome the ability of the bone to resist and it therefore fractures.

DIAGNOSTIC STUDIES

Laboratory
Full Chemistry Profile, CBC. As part of a full metabolic work-up. Indicated for pathologic fractures to assess the cause. Other tests are indicated by abnormal values of the basic tests (e.g., protein electrophoresis).

Radiology

X-ray. Is the study of choice. Minimum views are the AP, lateral, and oblique. Special views may be indicated for special situations, (e.g., sunrise view for patella fractures, or sesamoid view [foot]).

Tomograms. May help to visualize fractures through joints or difficult bones or assess joint involvement.

CT Scan. Is much better for evaluating fractures of the calcaneus, midfoot region, and intra-articular and wrist fractures.

Bone Scan. May be used for stress fractures and to assess the extent of bone tumors. With suspected stress fractures, the bone scan does not indicate increased uptake within the first 3 days following the fracture.

Other

Electromyelography (EMG)/Nerve Conduction Velocity (NCV). Is used to diagnose peripheral neuropathy with Charcot arthropathy.

Bone Density Studies. Used to confirm osteoporosis.

DIFFERENTIAL DIAGNOSIS

Traumatic

Ligament Injuries, Dislocations. Differentiated on x-ray.

Infectious

Osteomyelitis. Elevated WBC and ESR. Bony destruction may be present on x-ray.

Metabolic

Charcot Arthropathy. Presence of peripheral neuropathy, more common in those with diabetes mellitus.

Osteoporosis, Osteopenia, Osteomalacia. Differentiated on x-ray; bone density studies may be required.

Paget's Disease. Osteolytic lesions may be seen on x-ray. Usually affects the pelvis and skull.

Chronic Renal Disease. Elevated BUN and creatinine.

Neoplastic

Primary and Metastatic Tumors, Bone Cysts. Differentiated on radiographic studies.

Vascular

Avascular Necrosis. Most often associated with profound femoral head changes on x-ray. Commonly fractured just distal to the femoral head below the necrotic head. Comparison x-ray views often are helpful.

Congenital. Not applicable.

Acquired. Not applicable.

TREATMENT

Medical. Most stress, compression, and nondisplaced fractures can be treated conservatively with splint or cast immobilization. Some fractures lend themselves to closed reduction and cast immobilization. With current techniques and equipment, this is becoming less common and is not a standard of care.

Four interdependent variables—comminution, bone quality, energy of injury, and displacement—contribute to the ability of the fracture to remain in a stable position once it has been manipulated into an anatomical position.

Comminution: tends to increase directly with energy of injury and patient age. Comminution is important in predicting the intrinsic stability of fracture reduction.

Bone Quality: Due to osteopenia of bone, reflects a direct relationship to the fracture's tendency to shorten and the ability to achieve a strong interface with fixation materials; has a direct relationship with treatment options.

Energy of Injury: Low-energy injuries occur more often in older women with postmenopausal osteoporosis. High-energy injuries occur more often at a younger age and present more difficulties in management. With higher energy of injury come greater degrees of displacement, comminution, and higher risk of instability.

Displacement: The greater the extent of displacement, the more likely soft-tissue stripping and instability will occur. The extent of displacement is directly proportional to the associated swelling, neurovascular compromise, and risk of open fracture. The degree of displacement must be considered in contemplating treatment.

Surgical. Most fractures—especially displaced fractures of long bones, intra-articular, hand, and midfoot—require open reduction internal fixation (ORIF). Primary bone healing is not guaranteed by anatomical reduction; however, inadequate reduction contributes to delayed union or nonunion. Inadequate immobilization also has deleterious effects, but more so in some bones such as the tibia.

Severe open fractures are more prone to develop non-union, probably due to soft-tissue stripping and poor vascularity. Injuries most commonly associated with delayed union or non-union include open fractures, segmental or highly comminuted fractures, and fractures iatrogenically devitalized at the time of open reduction. A relative increase of non-union in fractures associated with multiple injuries has been reported.

Complications associated with fractures may arise from the initial injury or subsequent management. Systemic complications include shock, adult respiratory distress syndrome (ARDS), thromboembolic disease, fat emboli, and hypercalcemia. Local sequelae include delayed union, malunion, non-union, avascular necrosis, Sudeck's atrophy, post-traumatic arthritis, and hypertrophic ossification.

Successful fracture healing is dependent on a viable soft-tissue envelope. Local soft-tissue destruction following blunt trauma involves vascular and lymphatic destruction, increased local vasodilatation, and increased capillary permeability. The ensuing swelling, hemorrhage, and increased tissue pressure lead to local tissue hypoxia. The skin and soft tissue are particularly vulnerable to pressure necrosis from an overlying cast, occlusive bandage, or poorly applied traction device, especially in the lower extremity.

Vascular injury is an infrequent complication. Accurate diagnosis requires a high index of suspicion. Approximately 75% of all vascular injuries occur in the extremities.

The incidence of nerve injury in orthopedic trauma is relative low and is usually due to deep lacerations and penetrating wounds. Glenohumeral dislocations and humeral shaft fractures account for most of the nonpenetrating nerve injuries in the upper extremity and are as high as 33% in shoulder dislocations. Any fracture or dislocation of the elbow may damage a contiguous nerve. Posterior dislocations and fractures of the femoral head may be associated with sciatic nerve injury.

Increased tissue pressure is the key to the pathogenesis of compartment syndrome. Elevated local tissue pressure in a closed compartment of a limb decreases the local arteriovenous gradient. Local blood flow and oxygenation are diminished, compromising tissue function and viability. The pressure required to diminish microcirculation is usually less than that of aterial blood pressure; the larger arterial vessels that pass through the affected compartment remain patent and the distal blood flow is intact. As a result, distal pulses are almost invariably present.

TECHNIQUE OF SURGICAL ASSISTING

When assisting, it is critical that good exposure is maintained and adequate reduction of fracture parts is maintained while fixation is performed. It is up to the assistant to ensure these conditions are maintained while the surgeon performs the fixation. Keeping hands out of the surgical field allows a greater area for the surgeon to maneuver and facilitates a large exposure area for viewing the bone for fixation.

PEDIATRIC CONSIDERATIONS

When working with pediatric patients, comparison x-rays become necessary in order to differentiate or detect subtle fractures or fractures of growth plates. Some long-bone fractures with angulation will remodel and heal over time in line of force and become straight or physiologically normal (this usually occurs before puberty).

OBSTETRICAL CONSIDERATIONS

No surgical treatment is mandated during pregnancy. Use caution in performing x-rays and prescribing analgesics.

> ## PEARLS FOR THE PA
>
> *Comminution, bone quality, energy of injury, and displacement contribute to the ability of the fracture to remain stable once it has been manipulated into an anatomical position.*
>
> *Complications of fractures include inadequate healing, vascular or nerve injury, and compartment syndrome.*

Fractures: Ankle
Richard E. Donnelly, PA-C, BS, BS

DEFINITION

Any excessive force about the ankle joint can cause destruction of not only the bony architecture but often the ligamentous and soft-tissue components. Ankle fractures may be classified along anatomical lines, such as monomalleolar, bimalleolar, or trimalleolar, or by mechanism of injury, such as supination-eversion (supination-external rotation), supination-adduction, pronation-abduction, or pronation-eversion (pronation-external rotation).

HISTORY

Symptoms.   Pain and swelling are the prominent symptoms.

General.   A thorough history of the mechanism of injury and the force involved help in diagnosis and management. Most injuries occur with a twisting type of motion of the ankle; usually the foot remains fixed and the rest of the body rotates, creating a large, twisting force. Hiking, running, court sports, climbing, and jumping are the more common activities associated with ankle injuries. High-impact accidents such motor vehicle or motorcycle accidents are also causes of lower extremity injuries.

Age.   May occur at any age, but more often in the second through forth decades of life and in the later seventh and eighth decades of life.

Onset.   The onset of pain and swelling occurs suddenly with injury, although swelling can be insidious, whereas the pain is progressive.

Duration.   Fractures usually take 6 to 8 weeks to heal in a normal situation and if immediate treatment is initiated.

Intensity.   Usually the intensity of pain and swelling is directly related to the severity of injury and the amount of force involved.

Aggravating Factors.   Continued activity on a fractured ankle causes further pain and swelling, as well as progression of fracture displacement and possible widening of the mortise.

Alleviating Factors. Nonweight bearing (rest), elevation, ice, and compression lessen or alleviate pain and swelling to some degree. The most important factor is early diagnosis and treatment of ankle fractures.

Associated Factors. Distal lower extremity and foot fractures; tendon and ligamentous injuries.

PHYSICAL EXAMINATION

General. The patient may be in significant distress, limping and guarding the injured ankle. Neurovascular status must be evaluated early in the examination.

Orthopedic. Visual examination of the ankle usually reveals swelling over the affected areas. Ecchymosis may be present with acute injury but usually is manifested later in the course. Frank deformity can indicate obvious fracture or dislocation (swelling may be misleading). Point tenderness over the involved area is more indicative of a fracture, especially if it is over a bony prominence rather than a ligamentous structure. Ankle stability must be evaluated in all injuries to rule out unstable fractures, ligamentous disruptions, and mortise integrity. The use of the anterior drawer and talar tilt test before and after fixation may be helpful to evaluate ligamentous tears and stability. Palpation of the proximal fibula should be done to evaluate for a proximal fracture of the fibula, which is seen with medial ankle injuries in which the interosseous ligament is disrupted.

PATHOPHYSIOLOGY

The ankle joint consists of the articulation between the tibia and talus, the talus and fibula, and the tibia and fibula, with distal projections from the medial side of the tibia and from the distal fibula, which form malleoli. Along with the capsule and stabilizing ligaments, these structures form a geometric constraint to transverse movement of the talus. In the stance phase of gait, up to 20% of the upward force is absorbed by the lateral malleolus.

Supination-eversion injuries result in a spiral fracture of the distal fibula and a rupture of the deltoid ligament or fracture of the medial malleolus. Supination-adduction injuries result in a transverse fracture of the distal fibula and a relatively vertical fracture of the medial malleolus. Pronation-abduction injuries produce a transverse fracture of the medial malleolus and a short, oblique fracture of the fibula. Pronation-eversion injuries produce a tear of the deltoid ligament or fracture of the medial malleolus and a spiral fracture of the fibula relatively high above the level of the ankle. Trimalleolar fractures involve the medial malleolus, fibula, and the posterior lip of the articular surface of the tibia, allowing posterior and lateral displacement and external rotation with supination of the foot.

The medial malleolus may remain intact with a tear or avulsion of the deltoid ligament.

DIAGNOSTIC STUDIES

Laboratory.   Not applicable.
Radiology
Ankle X-ray.   Including AP, lateral, and mortise views. Evaluate the integrity or widening of the mortise. Stress views may be warranted to check talar tilt for ankle integrity and stability.

DIFFERENTIAL DIAGNOSIS

Traumatic
Tendon/Ligament Injuries.   To the Achilles, posterior tibial, or peroneal tendons; lateral, deltoid, interosseous ligament. May be present with or without ankle fracture. Differentiated on examination and radiographic studies.
Proximal Fibula Fracture.   High index of suspicion should be maintained. X-ray and examination will diagnose.
Infectious
Joint Infection.   Frank swelling and pain of a single joint without history of trauma. WBC may be elevated; joint may exhibit erythema or warmth.
Metabolic
Gout, Pseudogout.   Periodic, acute attacks of joint swelling and pain without history of a specific injury. Elevated serum uric acid levels with gout.
Reflex Sympathic Dystrophy.   Is manifested by swelling, pain, color changes, and temperature fluctuation of the skin.
Neoplastic.   Not applicable.
Vascular
Deep Vein Thrombosis.   Is usually manifested by calf or medial thigh tenderness, swelling above the ankle, and positive Homans sign.
Congenital.   Not applicable.
Acquired.   Not applicable.

TREATMENT

Medical.   The goal of treatment is to restore function to the same level as before insult. Restoring the original anatomy is the single best means of restoring normal function. Closed treatment of ankle fractures is not recommended except when the initial displacement is within acceptable limits. As a general rule, the mechanism of forces that produced the fracture is reversed by closed reduction manipulation. Monomalleolar fractures lend themselves to closed reduction more easily than do bimalleolar and trimalleolar fractures. Closed reduction of displaced ankle fractures usually does not exactly restore the anatomy and may require repeated reduction attempts in order to maintain alignment. Bimalleolar fractures treated by closed methods may develop a 10% non-union rate of the medial malleolus fragment, and up to 20% of bimalleolar fractures are intra-articular injuries to the talus and tibia and are left untreated when closed methods are attempted. Cast immobilization for closed, nondisplaced ankle fractures is the treatment of choice, usually nonweight bearing for a period of 3 to 4 weeks, then weight bearing for another 3 to 4 weeks.

Surgical. For most bimalleolar fractures, open reduction and internal fixation of both malleoli is recommended. Anatomical restoration of the distal tibiofibular syndesmosis is essential. In the majority of instances, the fibular fracture is fixed with a semitubular plate and screws and the medial malleolus is fixed with one or two screws; on occasion, screw fixation for the fibula may be adequate. Indications for open reduction of the posterior malleolus or posterior tibial fragment depend chiefly on size and displacement. If the fragment involves 25% to 30% of the weight-bearing surface, it should be anatomically reduced and held with internal fixation. The posterior fragment should be fixed before either the medial or lateral fragment is fixed. This requires direct exposure to allow anatomical reduction of the articular surface of the posterior tibia.

Indications. If frank deformity is present and neurovascular status is compromised, this is an indication for immediate reduction of the ankle, if only temporarily, to restore circulation and viability to the foot. Bimalleolar and trimalleolar fractures frequently require ORIF for anatomical restoration.

Contraindications. Closed, nondisplaced ankle fractures may be casted. Any contraindication to anesthesia.

TECHNIQUE OF SURGICAL ASSISTING

Good retraction of soft tissues is essential and distraction of the tibiotalar joint is necessary for good visualization for the reduction of a posterior fragment. The ability to maintain reduction while fixation is applied is very beneficial.

PEDIATRIC CONSIDERATIONS

If there is point tenderness over the distal malleoli and the growth plates are still present on x-ray, even though there is no obvious fracture or displaced bone fragment, an injury to the physis must be suspected until proven otherwise. Comparative x-ray views of the opposite ankle are helpful for pediatric injuries but are not conclusive. Salter I fractures of the growth plate are difficult to detected by x-ray because they are produced by a shear force across the epiphysis, causing separation. This type of fracture is diagnosed most often by clinical evaluation, but displacement can occur if the periosteum is torn. Salter II and III fractures are much easier to identify by x-ray than Salter I fractures.

OBSTETRICAL CONSIDERATIONS

No surgical treatment during pregnancy. Caution should be used in performing x-rays and prescribing analgesics.

PEARLS FOR THE PA

Most ankle injuries occur with a twisting type of motion.

Assess ankle stability with all injuries.

Rule out concurrent proximal fibular fracture.

Fractures: Distal Radial
Richard E. Donnelly, PA-C, BS, BS

DEFINITION

Classification of distal radial fractures is based on anatomy, mechanism of injury, and involvement of articular structures. Classifications include bending (metaphysis fails under tensile stress [Colles, Smith]), compression (fracture of the joint surface with involvement of the subchondral and metaphyseal bone ["die-punch"]), shearing (fractures of the joint surface [Barton, radial styloid]), avulsion (fracture of ligament attachments [ulna, radial styloid]), and combinations (with high-velocity injuries).

Extra-articular Fracture.   Those fractures that do not involve either the radiocarpal or distal radioulnar joint. If displaced, there must be an injury or disruption of the distal radioulnar joint, unless there is a fracture of the ulna proximal to the distal radioulnar joint.

Intra-articular Fracture.   Includes any fracture that extends into the radiocarpal or radioulnar joint and is displaced more than 2 mm.

HISTORY

Symptoms.   The most notable symptom is localized pain in the area of the distal radius. There is pain and swelling noted at the onset of the injury with notable deformity in some cases.

General. Usually due to low-energy trauma. This type of fracture usually occurs when the patient falls on an outstretched arm while trying to break a fall.

Age. The greatest frequency of distal radius fractures occur in two age groups: 6 to 10 and 60 to 69 years of age.

Onset. Occurs suddenly with falling on outstretched arm.

Duration. Fracture healing may take 6 to 8 weeks or longer, but early immobilization is encouraged.

Intensity. In the younger age group, the pain is intense and patients usually come in to be treated right away, whereas in the older age group, the patients may have a lower intensity of symptoms, attributed by the patient to a sprain or a flare up of arthritis, unless there is frank deformity.

Aggravating Factors. Continued use of the hand increases swelling and pain and may cause a stable fracture to become unstable.

Alleviating Factors. Immobilization, elevation. Ice initially helps pain and swelling.

Associated Factors. Metabolic disease (e.g., osteoporosis, osteomalacia, patients on high-dose or long-standing steroid use) that may cause osteopenia of the bone may predispose patients to higher risk of fracture with a fall.

PHYSICAL EXAMINATION

General. The patient may appear in acute distress or with mild symptoms of pain.

Orthopedic. Observe for obvious deformity, edema, ecchymosis, and loss of function. Palpation is performed to assess location of maximum point tenderness, amount and quality of edema, pulses, and neurological status. The active function of distal structures should also be assessed. If the median nerve (which may be contused) shows decreased function due to a swollen wrist, carpal canal pressures are measured and used to differentiate median nerve contusion from acute compressive neuropathy.

PATHOPHYSIOLOGY

Distal radial fractures fall into two groups, those of low impact or high impact. Low-impact injuries are those in which the patient falls on an outstretched hand (usually occurring in the older, aged patient who has osteoporosis or some other metabolic disease that causes osteopenia). High-impact fractures usually occur in the younger age group (due to contact sports, motor vehicle, or bicycle accidents).

Approximately 80% of axial loads are supported by the distal radius and 20% by the triangular fibrocartilage and distal ulna. Reversal of the normal palmar tilt of the distal radius can have deleterious effects, such as significant transfer of load onto the ulna with progressive angulation of the distal radius. Pain, decreased grip strength, and a midcarpal instability pattern seen on lateral radiographs are the hallmarks of this dynamic intercarpal instability.

Loss of dorsal tilt and shortening of the distal radius may result in dysfunction of the distal radioulnar joint with limitation of forearm rotation and ulnar impingement.

DIAGNOSTIC STUDIES

Laboratory. Osteopenia evaluation.
Radiology
X-ray. Including AP, lateral, and oblique views. The study of choice in diagnosing fractures.
Tomography. May be required in some instances to assess the degree of fracture and involvement of articular structures.
CT Scan. Can be used to view intra-articular fractures not adequately visualized on routine films.
Other
Examination Under Anesthesia. With radiographic control may be necessary (especially in pediatrics) to assess the fracture.

DIFFERENTIAL DIAGNOSIS

Traumatic
Sprain, Dislocation of the Wrist. Differentiated on physical examination and radiographic studies.
Infectious. Not applicable.
Metabolic
Osteoporosis, Osteomalacia, Arthritis. May predispose the patient to having a fracture. Diagnosed on physical examination and radiographic studies.
Neoplastic
Pathologic Fractures. Secondary to primary or metastatic tumors. Lesion seen on radiographic studies.
Vascular. Not applicable.
Congenital. Not applicable.
Acquired
Carpal Tunnel Syndrome. More insidious in nature; symptoms of pain, numbness, or weakness in the distribution of the median nerve. EMG positive.
Steroid Use. May predispose the patient to having a fracture. History of use.

TREATMENT

Medical. The goal of treatment is to restore a relatively normal, anatomical alignment of the displaced fracture. The general aspect of fracture management relates to the loading expectations of the hand and wrist. This represents a combination of age, occupation, handedness, and lifestyle, along with the patient's expectations, psychological outlook, associated medical conditions, and compliance. Functional result has a significant relationship to the quality of the anatomical restoration and function as reflected in grip strength and endurance.

Extra-articular. Most minimally displaced, noncomminuted fractures are managed with closed reduction and immobilization in mild flexion of 10 to 20 degrees and ulnar deviation of 15 degrees.

Because the hand is more functional in a neutral or slightly pronated position, this is the preferred position for immobilization. Smith fractures are more stable in supination. Reduction is performed by gentle traction to the hand manually, with countertraction on the humerus with the elbow flexed. The displacement is reduced gently after disimpaction of the fracture. Postreduction x-rays are taken to ensure good anatomical reduction. X-rays are taken at 1 or 2 weeks to ensure reduction is maintained. Redisplacement of fractures during cast immobilization is not uncommon, and remanipulation has been a common practice.

Intra-articular. Most require surgical correction.

Surgical

Extra-articular. Treatment includes percutaneous pinning of distal fragment, metal external skeletal fixation devices and, rarely, ORIF. Extra-articular fractures with extensive comminution but not associated with undue soft-tissue swelling are amenable to percutaneous pinning. When instability exists and maintenance of length and alignment is deemed important, application of external skeletal fixation is recommended. ORIF is indicated in those rare instances in which the preceding methods are unsuccessful.

Intra-articular. High-energy fractures and fracture dislocations require relocation of the articular anatomy to ensure hand and wrist function and to prevent post-traumatic arthritis. Most of these fractures require ORIF, especially those that demand high function or loading of the wrist and hand.

Indications. Patients in whom the maintenance of anatomy is important because of functional demands.

Contraindications. For extra-articular fractures, inadequate trial of conservative management. Relative in those with low-demand activities. Those who cannot undergo anesthesia.

TECHNIQUE OF
SURGICAL ASSISTING

When assisting, it is critical that good exposure is maintained and adequate reduction of fracture parts is maintained while fixation is performed. It is up to the assistant to ensure that these conditions are maintained while the surgeon performs the fixation. Keeping hands out of the surgical field allows a greater area for the surgeon to maneuver and facilitates a large exposure area for viewing the bone for fixation.

PEDIATRIC CONSIDERATIONS

When working with pediatric patients, comparison x-rays become necessary in order to differentiate or detect subtle fractures or fractures of growth plates. Some long-bone fractures with angulation remodel and heal over time in the line of force and become straight or physiologically normal (usually occurs before puberty).

OBSTETRICAL CONSIDERATIONS

No surgical treatment during pregnancy. Caution is used in performing x-rays and prescribing analgesics.

PEARLS FOR THE PA

Distal radial fractures are classified as extra-articular and intra-articular.

The median nerve may be contused.

Pain, decreased grip strength, and a midcarpal instability pattern seen on lateral radiographs are the hallmarks of this fracture.

Fractures and Dislocations of the Elbow

Edward D'Ettorre, PA-C, and
Richard E. Donnelly, PA-C, BS, BS

DEFINITION

Dislocation of the elbow is the displacement of the ulna and radius off the distal humerus. Fractures of the elbow can involve all three bones that make up the elbow joint (distal humerus, proximal radius, and ulna and olecranon process).

HISTORY

Symptoms. Patients relate sudden onset of pain, swelling, and an inability to move the elbow. They may complain of swelling with distal paresthesias or dysesthesias.

General. Fractures and dislocations of the elbow occur when the patient falls on an outstretched arm or experiences direct trauma to the elbow.

Age. Elbow dislocations occur equally in adults and children. Fractures of the olecranon, radial head, and proximal ulna are seen more commonly in adults.

Onset. Sudden with injury.

Duration. Dislocations and fractures of the elbow require approximately 6 to 8 weeks to heal, but require early mobilization to prevent contractures.

Intensity. Most elbow injuries are very painful.

Aggravating Factors. Movement of the elbow after initial injury intensifies the pain and swelling and potentiates further soft-tissue injury.

Alleviating Factors. Immobilization of the elbow lessens the pain; ice helps decrease the swelling. Immediate reduction of the fractures or dislocation helps the most in alleviating symptoms.

Associated Factors. Dislocations of the elbow may be associated with fractures.

PHYSICAL EXAMINATION

General. Most patients refuse to use the upper extremity and want to hold it as still as possible.

Orthopedic. Swelling and the patient's hesitation to move the elbow after injury makes it difficult to examine the extremity. Inspect and observe for deformity, discoloration, or pallor distally. Distal pulses should be palpated for and recorded. Neurological examination for sensory and motor function in the hand should be done as soon as possible after injury and followed closely throughout the course of the acute stages. Neurovascular status after reduction or immobilization should be followed closely as well.

PATHOPHYSIOLOGY

Dislocations of the elbow cause considerable soft-tissue damage and may involve neurovascular structures. Joint stiffness caused by intra-articular and peri-articular adhesions is a common complication. A less common but more serious cause of stiffness is post-traumatic ossification—a condition in which new bone forms in the hematoma beneath the damaged periosteum and joint capsule.

With fractures, injury to the brachial artery may occur, which may lead to impairment of the circulation to the forearm and hand and cause Volkmann's contractures, which occur when the flexor muscles of the forearm and sometimes peripheral nerve trunks suffer ischemic changes. The affected tissue is replaced with fibrous tissue, which contracts and draws the wrist and fingers into flexion.

Peripheral nerve trunks affected by ischemia may cause sensory and motor paralysis, paresthesias, or dysesthesias, which may be temporary or permanent.

DIAGNOSTIC STUDIES

Laboratory
Full Chemistry Profile, CBC, PT, PTT. As routine, preoperative screen.

Radiology
Elbow X-rays. AP, lateral, and oblique views are minimum. Precise interpretation may be difficult. Minimally displaced fractures may be poorly visualized. The presence of the fat pad sign (area of radiolucency posterior to the distal humerus on lateral view) should alert the clinician to the likelihood of an occult, usually intra-articular, fracture.

DIFFERENTIAL DIAGNOSIS

Traumatic
Epicondylitis. Tenderness to palpation over the humeral epicondyle and radiocapitellar ligament, aggravated by wrist extension or wrist flexion (see topic epicondylitis of the elbow).

Strain, Sprain. No dislocation or fracture found on examination or radiographic studies.

Olecranon Bursitis. Tenderness of the bursa. No dislocation or fracture found on examination or radiographic studies.

Infectious
Infection of Olecranon Bursa. Erythema, warmth, and tenderness of the bursa; WBC may be elevated. No dislocation or fracture found on examination or radiographic studies.

Metabolic
Gout, Pseudogout. Periodic, acute attacks of joint swelling and pain without history of a specific injury. Elevated serum uric acid levels with gout.

Rheumatoid Arthritis. Positive rheumatoid factor.

Neoplastic
Tumors. May be palpated on examination or seen on radiographic studies.

Vascular. Not applicable.
Congenital. Not applicable.
Acquired. Not applicable.

TREATMENT

Dislocation. Dislocations of the elbow should be reduced as soon as possible, usually under anesthesia. Reduction is performed by pulling with steady, gentle force on the forearm with the elbow semiflexed while direct pressure is applied behind the olecranon. Reduction should be confirmed by x-ray and clinical examination, as well as making sure there are no postreduction fractures. After reduction, it is recommended that the elbow be splinted at 90 degrees of flexion for 3 weeks, followed by early mobilization with range-of-motion (ROM) exercises. A sling also may be used to help support the arm and relax the muscles.

Complications include neurovascular injury (uncommon) and joint stiffness.

Fractures of the Condyles of the Humerus. Relatively uncommon. An undisplaced fracture requires 3 weeks of protection in a splint, followed by active ROM exercises. Displaced fractures are more serious due to the potential of permanent disability. If closed reductions are unsuccessful, ORIF is recommended. Condylar fractures are prone to non-union, deformity, and osteoarthritis.

Epicondylar Fractures. Nondisplaced fractures usually are uncomplicated and only symptomatic treatment is required. Displaced fractures are seldom severe and usually do not require reduction. The elbow should be immobilized with a posterior splint for 3 weeks to relieve pain. After splinting, active ROM exercises should be started. Complications include displaced fracture fragments into the joint that cause decreased motion of the joint and pain. Impingement of the ulnar nerve can occur.

Fractures of the Olecranon Process. Nondisplaced fractures are treated with protection with a posterior splint for 2 or 3 weeks, then ROM exercise is started. Surgery is advised for displaced fractures due to the difficulty of maintaining reduction with closed methods. If there is good reduction and a secure fixation, gentle ROM exercises may begin immediately postoperatively. With comminuted fractures, realignment of the fracture fragments rarely is possible. Fragments are excised and the triceps muscle is secured to the bone "stump" of the ulna. Immobilization is maintained for 3 weeks, then active ROM is begun.

Radial Head Fractures. If the radial head shows only minimal damage radiographically and the articular surface appears reasonably smooth, conservative treatment is recommended with posterior splinting with the elbow at 90 degrees and the forearm midway between pronation and supination for 3 weeks. This is followed by active ROM. With severely comminuted or displaced fractures, surgery is indicated. The entire radial head is excised. Postoperatively, the elbow is immobilized in a splint for 10 to 14 days and then active ROM exercises are begun. Complications are infrequent and function usually is restored to normal or almost normal. Occasionally some joint stiffness or osteoarthritis may occur.

Fracture of the Proximal End of the Ulna with Dislocation of the Radius. The ulna is angled forward and the radial head is dislocated forward. Accurate and perfect reduction is essential but rarely is possible with closed methods. ORIF is usually required with splinting or casting of the entire limb for 4 to 6 weeks or longer until the fracture shows healing.

Indications. Displaced fractures of the condyles of the humerus (potential for permanent disability), inability to maintain reduction with ole-cranon process, comminuted or displaced radial head, and proximal radial fractures.

Contraindications. Inadequate conservative therapy (closed reduction) when applicable. Patient intolerance of anesthesia.

TECHNIQUE OF SURGICAL ASSISTING

When assisting, it is critical that good exposure is maintained and adequate reduction of the fracture parts is maintained while fixation is performed. It is up to the assistant to ensure that these conditions are maintained while the surgeon performs the fixation. Keeping hands out of the surgical field allows a greater area for the surgeon to maneuver and facilitates a large exposure area for viewing the bone for fixation.

PEDIATRIC CONSIDERATIONS

Supracondylar and condylar epicondylar fractures of the humerus occur more commonly in children.

OBSTETRICAL CONSIDERATIONS

No surgical treatment during pregnancy. Caution is used in performing x-rays and prescribing analgesics.

PEARLS FOR THE PA

Neurovascular status must be assessed and followed acutely during and after treatment.

The presence of the fat pad sign on x-ray suggests fracture.

Fractures/dislocations should be reduced as soon as possible.

Fractures: Hip
Stephen M. Cohen, PA-C, MS, BS

DEFINITION

Classification of fractures of the hip is based on anatomical description and includes fractures of the acetabulum, femoral neck fractures (intracapsular fracture of the femoral neck), intertrochanteric fractures (most common in the elderly), and subtrochanteric fractures (rarest form; pathologic or high-energy trauma).

Fractures of the hip are defined as stable (stress and impacted fractures) or unstable (generally displaced or comminuted fractures).

HISTORY

Symptoms.   Patient may complain of local hip, groin, and often thigh or knee pain.

General.   The two major causes of hip fracture are low-energy trauma in the elderly with osteoporotic or pathologic deteriorating bone stock, and high-energy trauma that often causes open or displaced hip fractures due to motor vehicle accidents, falls, pedestrian mishaps, and which may occur at any age. One of four mechanisms is often present: (1) a fall producing a direct blow over the greater trochanter; (2) lateral rotation of the extremity while the head is fixed by the anterior capsule; (3) cyclical loading, producing microfractures that become complete with minor trauma; and (4) pathologic conditions (e.g., systemic conditions such as osteogenesis imperfecta or local conditions such as tumors or fibrous dysplasia).

Age.   Eighty percent occur in those over age 60 years. Females are affected more often than males. Femoral neck fractures occur mostly in those over age 50 years.

Onset.   Acute, although symptoms may be relatively nonspecific. Stable-appearing fractures may displace at a later time if not surgically stabilized.

Duration.   May take weeks to months before the patient is able to bear weight.

Intensity.   Mild or moderate pain to immobility.

Aggravating Factors.   Osteoporosis, metastatic and primary cancer, hyperparathyroidism.

Alleviating Factors.   Maximizing dietary calcium and physical activity during adolescent growth; discouraging smoking, steroid, and alcohol use; estrogen replacement therapy, fall prevention (e.g., walker, cane, rails, etc.).

Associated Factors.   Anticonvulsant drugs, senile dementia and other neurologic disease, psychotropic medication, renal disease.

PHYSICAL EXAMINATION

General.   In high-energy trauma, carefully evaluate for other subsystem injuries.

Neurologic.   Often is difficult or misleading due to pain and lack of cooperation by the patient. Nerve injuries are rare in closed fractures.

Orthopedic.   Note the attitude of the extremity in displaced fractures (flexed, abducted, shortened, externally rotated). Stable fractures have minimal shortening and deformity. Impacted fractures often present in the valgus position (angulated, apex medial). Fractures typically present with thigh swelling, gross deformity, and the inability to move the hip or knee.

The patient may be able to move the extremity actively or may experience groin or hip pain during ROM testing. With fracture of the femoral neck, motion of the hip causes pain. If fragments are stable, pain may only be present at the extremes of passive range of motion. Patients with stable fractures may be able to walk.

Vascular. Evaluation of pulses is critical in the evaluation of hip fracture. Ancillary tests such as Doppler pulse assessment or angiography may be necessary.

PATHOPHYSIOLOGY

Normal anatomy of the hip: Angle of inclination (femoral neck to shaft angle) is normally 125 to 130 degrees. Blood supply is from the retinacular and intramedullary vessels from the intertrochanteric region, which course from the intertrochanteric area to the femoral head through the neck. Nerve supply is via the obturator nerve, which also supplies a sensory branch to the medial thigh and motor to some hip adductors. This is responsible for referred pain to the inner thigh and knee if irritation occurs due to hip fracture.

Bone density rises to a peak at 35 to 40 years in both sexes, with men having a higher bone density at all times than women. There is a steady loss of bone density at a rate of 1% to 2% per year, with women having 10 years of accelerated loss after menopause. Exercise-induced amenorrhea may produce irreversible bone density losses.

Classification of fractures:

Femoral Neck Fractures (Garden System)
1. Garden I: Incomplete or impacted fracture.
2. Garden II: Complete nondisplaced fracture.
3. Garden III: Complete with partial displacement; posterior periosteum (retinaculum of Weilbrecht) intact.
4. Garden IV: Complete fracture with total displacement.

Subtrochanteric Fractures: Are rare and usually seen in pathologic conditions or high energy trauma.

DIAGNOSTIC STUDIES

Laboratory
Full Chemistry Profile, CBC, PT, PTT. Used in preoperative screening.

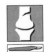

Radiology
Hip X-ray. Should include AP, "frog-leg," lateral, and full AP pelvic views to evaluate for the presence of fracture. Gentle traction and internal rotation may be needed to maximize AP quality. A 45-degree oblique pelvic view is performed for suspected acetabular fracture. Repeat x-rays in 10 to 14 days if no radiolucent fracture line is present and a stress fracture of the femoral neck is suspected, because deforming forces may displace fragments (muscle action, body weight, fascia).

Femur X-ray. Of the entire femur length to evaluate for distal femur or knee injury.

Tomogram/Bone Scan. Indicated for suspected occult and stress fractures.

CT of the Hip. The preferred test for acetabular and pelvic fracture evaluation.

Angiography. Used as indicated to evaluate vascular status.

Other
Doppler Pulse Assessment. Used as indicated to evaluate vascular status.

DIFFERENTIAL DIAGNOSIS

Traumatic
Greater/Lesser Trochanter, Sacral, Iliac, Pubic Ramus Fracture. May mimic hip fracture pain; identification made on x-ray with full AP pelvis view helpful.

Infectious
Pathologic Fracture. Through an area of occult infection. The infection may have no signs and symptoms and present as a fracture. Comparison x-ray views delineate unilateral bone architecture changes.

Metabolic
Osteomalacia, Calcium Depletion, Hyperparathyroidism. Low-energy trauma most often has an underlying metabolic bone process.

Neoplastic
Pathologic Fracture. Through an area of primary or secondary tumor. Index of suspicion should be high with a primary tumor history. Comparison x-ray views highlight subtle bone changes.

Vascular
Avascular Necrosis. Most often associated with profound femoral head changes on x-ray. Commonly fractured just distal to the femoral head below the necrotic head. Comparison x-ray views are often helpful.

Congenital
Congenital Hip Dysplasia, Osteogenic Imperfecta. Past medical history often details underlying process. Radiographic findings of long-term deformities.

Acquired
Osteoporosis. Increased frequency of association with increasing age of patient. May be difficult to differentiate from metabolic process. Often associated with low-energy trauma in the elderly.

TREATMENT

Medial

Primary Evaluation and Treatment. Minimize motion during initial phases of assessment. Distal neurovascular status is assessed before and after stabilization. Stabilization is performed with a gentle traction splint (e.g., Thomas) or Buck traction with 5 to 8 pounds of weight. The patient should be positioned for comfort and splinted "where it lays" for transport.

Intravenous fluids are given for IV access and hemodynamic treatment. The patient is kept NPO in case surgery is required. A cold pack may be applied to reduce swelling. IM or IV analgesia is provided after documentation of a fracture. Vital signs and electrocardiogram (ECG) are monitored, especially in the elderly. A full evaluation is undertaken in the event of a fall to determine a reason for the fall (e.g., neurologic, cardiovascular). Orthopedic and medicine consultations are obtained as needed. The patient is admitted for surgical evaluation.

Surgical. The goal of surgery is to provide stable fixation and early mobilization.

Neck Fractures. Requires hip prosthesis or pins. An impacted fracture is surgically treated because there is a high rate of displacement without surgery. For unstable neck fractures, reduction and internal fixation is the treatment of choice. Plans are made for internal fixation versus total arthroplasty.

Intertrochanteric. Nails or screws are used with side plates.

Subtrochanteric. Nonoperative measures may be used if the patient's medical condition does not allow for surgery or if bone quality is so poor that secure fixation would be difficult. Operative options include conventional medullary nails or screws (a Zickel nail is used for pathologic fracture), nails with a long sideplate, external fixation for open fractures, or delayed internal fixation.

Nondisplaced Stress Fractures of the Femoral Neck. Treatment is begun with crutch ambulation with minimal weight bearing and instructions not to use the leg for leverage or in stressful positions. Partial weight bearing may begin in 5 to 6 weeks. Full healing of the stress fracture may take 3 to 6 months.

Nondisplaced Fractures. Traction and spica casting are not advised in adults because immobilization of the hip region with casts is unreliable and may require prolonged bedrest with resulting complications. Skeletal traction has similar complications. These fractures are treated with skillful neglect and rehabilitation, pinning, or capsulectomy for hematoma evacuation (controversial).

Displaced Fractures. In the young patient, displaced fractures are treated with closed reduction, pinning with multiple screws, or a compression screw and sideplate. Muscle pedicle graft may be used with nonanatomic reduction. In the elderly patient, ORIF with a hip screw and sideplate versus hip replacement are used. Closed reduction is also an option.

Complications. Complications of hip fracture and surgery include deep vein thrombosis (preventive measures include pneumatic venous compression, compression stockings, anticoagulation, early ambulation), thrombophlebitis, pulmonary embolus, non-union (10% to 35%), avascular necrosis (adults, 40%; children, 50% to 100%), late segmental collapse, malunion, pseudoarthrosis, premature fusion of growth plate (more common in older children), post-traumatic arthritis, hardware loosening or implant failure, loss of fixation, compartment syndrome of the thigh, fat emboli, infection and sepsis, nerve injury or palsy, heterotopic bone formation, and bleeding.

Indications.   Internal fixation is recommended for all displaced and unstable fractures.

For hip replacement, the relative indications are age greater than 70 years, Pauwels type III fracture, femoral head fracture mostly on the weight-bearing surface, fracture/dislocation or osteoporosis of the femoral head, or low-demand patients to facilitate care. Absolute indications for hip replacement are unreduceable fractures, femoral neck fracture with fixation loss postoperatively, pre-existing hip lesions, malignancy, uncontrolled seizures, old femoral neck fracture, Garden type IV fracture, patient cannot tolerate more than two operations, mentally retarded/psychotic patients.

Contraindications.   Medical conditions that delay surgery; complications of multiple system trauma.

TECHNIQUE OF SURGICAL ASSISTING

The PA plays an active role in surgical preparation and postoperative care. Intraoperatively, first assisting is provided and includes duties such as positioning of the patient, helping with exposure, application of hardware, and closing.

PEDIATRIC CONSIDERATIONS

Hip dislocations are much more common than fractures in children because the cartilaginous structure of the hip requires less force to dislocate. The capsule usually tears off the pelvis. Hip fractures are extremely rare and follow high-energy trauma (automobile bumpers are about the same height as a child's greater trochanter). Vascular studies explain the high rate of avascular necrosis following hip fracture. Most traumatic hip fractures in neonates are transepiphyseal (high avascular necrosis risk).

Pediatric Femoral Neck Fractures and Avascular Necrosis Prediction

Type I: Transepiphyseal fractures are often associated with dislocation. Avascular necrosis almost 100%.

Type II: Transcervical is the most common type in pediatrics (50%). Avascular necrosis related to displacement in 35% to 78%.

Type III: Cervicotrochanteric accounts for 37% of all pediatric hip fractures. Avascular necrosis risk of 20% to 25% with high risk in varus deformity.

Type IV: Intertrochanteric is the least common and avascular necrosis is rare.

OBSTETRICAL CONSIDERATIONS

A hip fracture in a pregnant patient may necessitate a Cesarean delivery. Coccyx fracture occurring during vaginal delivery may mimic the pain of a hip fracture. Placenta previa and abruptio are not uncommon with high-velocity trauma of the hip. Fracture immobilization that requires the patient to remain in a right lateral position may require manual manipulation of the fetus to the left side of the abdomen to prevent aortic compression. Intracapsular bleeding in hip fractures may be more extensive in the pregnant patient. Normal hormone changes in pregnancy make the hip more resistant to trauma.

PEARLS FOR THE PA

Early ambulation and physical therapy reduces morbidity and mortality: 15% mortality in the hospital; 33% mortality by 1 year; of survivors, only two thirds return to their own home.

Stable-appearing fractures may displace if not surgically stabilized due to forces of weight bearing and using the leg for leverage.

It is important to protect body pressure points (e.g., sacrum, heels, malleoli) from decubitus ulcers.

Fractures: Stress

Richard E. Donnelly, PA-C, BS, BS

DEFINITION

A stress fracture is the bony expression exhibited by hypertrophy of normal bone that results from a summation of stress brought about by overuse. It is most commonly seen in the metatarsals of the foot.

HISTORY

Symptoms. Pain usually occurs after some extended activity, and is described as an ache, stiffness, or tiredness in the foot.

General.   Patients relate no specific injury, but have a vague and insidious onset of pain, usually with exertion.

Age.   May occur in all age groups but more often in those over the age of 30 years, with increasing frequency with age.

Onset.   Insidious onset of a vague ache.

Duration.   May last for an extended period of time due to the insidious onset and vague symptoms, but is usually progressive in nature. If treatment is initiated soon after onset of symptoms, the usual course is 6 to 8 weeks of protection in a cast or protective shoe. Callus formation around the fracture site may appear at 4 to 6 weeks.

Intensity.   Progressive symptoms with continued activity and insidious onset.

Aggravating Factors.   Activity continues to aggravate symptoms.

Alleviating Factors.   Rest, elevation, and immobilization.

Associated Factors.   Congenital shortening of the first metatarsal has been implicated as a relative factor predisposing to stress fractures of the second metatarsal.

PHYSICAL EXAMINATION

General.   Neurovascular status must be assessed. A history of diabetes mellitus or of other disease processes that may cause peripheral neuropathy may exist; such states predispose patients to develop Charcot arthropathy, which appears as stress fractures of the metatarsal-cuneiform region of the foot.

Orthopedic.   There is point tenderness over the involved area. A fullness may be palpated over the area if the fracture is forming callus. Mild to moderate swelling is usually present, and ecchymosis around the involved area may be visible. Pain is accentuated with dorsiflexion or percussion of the involved metatarsal shaft.

PATHOPHYSIOLOGY

Stress fractures are recurrent microfractures of the bone that occur secondary to repetitive loading, increased frequency, and magnitude of stress forces. Microscopically, there are increased levels of osteoclastic and osteoblastic activity. Initially, vascular congestion occurs with osteoclastic-mediated bone resorption in the haversian canals and interstitial lamellae. Small cracks appear at the cement lines of the haversian systems, which propagate into microfractures. Simultaneously, new bone formation occurs as a result of increased periosteal osteoblastic activity (Wolff's law). Stress fractures appear to develop when normal bone remodeling is disrupted and osteoblastic activity is outpaced by osteoclastic resorption.

DIAGNOSTIC STUDIES

Laboratory
CBC. As indicated to rule out infection (elevated WBC).
Radiology
X-ray. Of the involved area, taken with 10 to 14 days of onset of symptoms, usually do not demonstrate a fracture. Two to three weeks following the development of pain, a fine line may appear on x-rays.
Other
Technetium-99 Bone Scan. Shows increased activity in the area of fracture and is usually positive at or shortly after the onset of pain.

DIFFERENTIAL DIAGNOSIS

Traumatic
Lisfranc Injury. A strain, sprain, or dislocation of the first through third metatarsals and medial cuneiform and middle cuneiform (foot).
Infection
Osteomyelitis. Seen on x-ray; elevated WBC.
Metabolic
Charcot Arthropathy, Osteopenia. Secondary to other metabolic or drug-induced processes such as rheumatoid arthritis, chronic corticosteroid use.
Neoplastic
Pathologic Fractures. Differentiated on x-ray, physical examination.
Vascular. Not applicable.
Congenital. Not applicable.
Acquired. Not applicable.

TREATMENT

Medical. Stress fractures of the foot usually respond to avoidance of impact loading for 4 to 8 weeks. The use of a short-leg walking cast is suggested for those patients who have severe symptoms or who are required to be active for their jobs. Activity is limited until pain subsides. Ridged-sole shoes with a well-supported arch are recommended for 4 to 6 weeks for those who are relatively inactive or not casted. Patients are rehabilitated with progressive activity within the limits of pain.

Surgical. If indicated by symptoms or x-ray pathology, stress fractures may be fixed with Steinmann pins; this is rarely indicated.
Indications. Rarely indicated.
Contraindications. Inadequate conservative trial, patient inactive (relative), or inability of the patient to tolerate anesthesia.

TECHNIQUE OF SURGICAL ASSISTING

When assisting, it is critical that good exposure and adequate reduction of fracture parts are maintained while fixation is performed. It is up to the assistant to ensure that these conditions are maintained while the surgeon performs the fixation. Keeping hands out of the surgical field allows greater area for the surgeon to maneuver and facilitates a large exposure area for viewing the bone for fixation.

PEDIATRIC CONSIDERATIONS

Uncommon in pediatrics and adolescence.

OBSTETRICAL CONSIDERATIONS

No surgical treatment during pregnancy. Use caution in performing x-rays and prescribing analgesics.

PEARLS FOR THE PA

Stress fractures are most common in the metatarsals of the foot.

It is important to obtain a history of concurrent illness that may predispose the patient to developing stress fractures.

Conservative treatment is the mainstay of therapy.

Fractures: Supracondylar Humerus

John W. Bullock, PA-C, BA, BS

DEFINITION

A fracture that occurs through the distal metaphysis of the humerus just proximal to the level of the epicondyles in children.

HISTORY

Symptoms. Patient presents with a history of trauma and unwillingness to move the elbow. Deformity may be noted. Numbness or weakness may be present with associated nerve injury.

The views expressed in this material are those of the author and do not reflect the official policy or position of the United States Government, the Department of Defense, or the Department of the Air Force.

General. Ninety-eight percent are fractured with the elbow in extension.

Age. Eighty-five percent are in children younger than 10 years of age, with incidence peaking at 5 to 8 years of age. Rare after age 15 years. 2:1 predominance in boys.

Onset. Sudden, after a fall on the outstretched arm.

Duration. Until appropriate treatment is instituted.

Intensity. Pain may be severe.

Aggravating Factors. Ischemia, secondary injury to the brachial artery.

Alleviating Factors. Immobilization, analgesics.

Associated Factors. Nerve injuries occur in about 7% of the fractures, usually the radial or median nerve in extension-type fractures and the ulnar nerve in flexion-type fractures.

PHYSICAL EXAMINATION

General. The neurovascular status is assessed because the brachial artery can be stretched and lacerated against the sharp end of the proximal fragment. The circulation must be checked carefully and recorded with special attention to the "5 Ps": pain, pallor, pulselessness, paresthesias, and paralysis. The skin may be cool and there may be loss of passive finger extension due to swelling in the flexor compartment.

Orthopedic. Inspection may show an S-shaped deformity of the elbow caused by the flexion of the distal fragment, the anterior spike of the proximal fragment, and the posterior prominence of the olecranon. Supracondylar fractures present with tenderness in the supracondylar area over both the medial and lateral supracondylar ridges.

Evaluation for compartment syndrome is imperative because the median nerve and the radial artery both can be compressed by swelling in the anterior compartment of the forearm. Volkmann's ischemic contracture is the end result of muscle necrosis caused by the occlusion of the microcirculation. The fingers are pulled into flexion and the wrist is pulled into flexion and pronation by the mats of fibrous tissue that form in the necrotic muscle. It is the most feared sequela of a supracondylar fracture.

PATHOPHYSIOLOGY

During the ages when supracondylar fractures are prevalent, there is a relative laxity of the elbow ligaments that allows increased motion, particularly hyperextension. At the moment of greatest displacement the distal fragment and the forearm are pushed backward, pulling the brachial artery and median nerve against the sharp, distal end of the proximal fragment.

DIAGNOSTIC STUDIES

Laboratory

CBC, Full Chemistry Profile, PT, PTT. As routine preoperative screen.

Radiology

Anteroposterior and True Lateral X-rays. Essential for diagnosis. The lateral view should be taken with the film between the body and the elbow, with the arm at the side and the elbow bent 90 degrees. This shows fat pad signs (relative soft-tissue lucencies) indicative of intra-articular effusion and posterior displacement of the ossification center of the capitellum in relation to a line drawn along the anterior cortex of the humerus. This "anterior humeral line" normally should pass through the center of the ossification center of the capitellum. This relationship of the anterior humeral line to the capitellum will be disrupted in up to 95% of minimally displaced supracondylar fractures.

Other

Doppler Evaluation or Arteriogram. Evaluation of distal circulation may be required.

DIFFERENTIAL DIAGNOSIS

Traumatic

Lateral Condylar Physis Fracture, Avulsion of the Medial Epicondyle, Radial Neck Fractures. May present with effusion. These are distinguished through palpation for the site of maximum tenderness.

Posterior Elbow Dislocation. In a dislocation, the olecranon is more prominent because it is posterior to the epicondyle; in a supracondylar fracture, the relationship between the epicondyles and olecranon is maintained.

Infectious. Not applicable.
Metabolic. Not applicable.
Neoplastic. Not applicable.
Vascular. Not applicable.
Congenital. Not applicable.
Acquired. Not applicable.

TREATMENT

Medical. Treatment is surgical.

Surgical. A successful closed reduction can be held by casting with the elbow flexed (less popular due to possible circulatory compromise) or via various traction methods (also less popular due to inconvenience and long hospital stays). Except for undisplaced fractures, the most popular way to manage supracondylar fractures is via closed reduction and percutaneous pinning. Reduction and fixation should be accomplished as soon as possible because the humeral metaphysis heals rapidly and the fragments usually are immobile after about 1 week. Secondly, if open reduction is needed, delay of more than 96 hours carries with it a significant risk of stimulating myositis ossificans.

Closed reduction is performed under general anesthesia (to obtain relaxation not possible with regional anesthesia). After adequate reduction (demonstrated via x-ray and by the ability to fully flex the arm) the position is held by percutaneous pins. If the fracture is unreducible, closed, or if there is vascular compromise, an open reduction is performed and held with pins. The pins are removed after approximately 3 weeks, and active range of motion is started at the child's own pace.

Indications. Mandatory exploration if there is vascular compromise. All except the most minimally displaced fractures must be reduced and held until healed. Surgery allows early motion.

Contraindications. The risks of doing nothing outweigh the risk of surgery in this age group.

Complications. Vascular damage, compartment syndrome, Volkmann's ischemic contracture, median nerve damage, malunion, myositis ossificans.

TECHNIQUE OF SURGICAL ASSISTING

The assistant stabilizes the proximal fragment during the closed reduction and ensures the stability of the reduction while it is being fixed by the pins.

PEDIATRIC CONSIDERATIONS

This is a pediatric fracture.

OBSTETRICAL COMPLICATIONS

This is a pediatric fracture. In the rare case of a fracture in an obstetrical patient, reduction must be attained under regional anesthesia. Use caution in performing x-rays and prescribing analgesics.

PEARLS FOR THE PA

Don't accept inadequate or low quality x-ray views.

Delayed forearm pain may indicate muscle ischemia.

Always evaluate the neurovascular status with attention to the "5 Ps": pain, pallor, pulselessness, paresthesias, and paralysis.

Musculoskeletal Tumors

Franklin A. Trejos, PA-C

DEFINITION

Neoplastic process of bone or soft tissue that may be benign, malignant, infectious, or inflammatory in nature. The tumor nomenclature describes the tissue, or type of cells from which the tumor arose, and how the tumor behaves. Tumors vary according to their histological aggressiveness or tumor grade. The higher the grade, the more aggressive the tumor. There are benign tumors that are very aggressive, quite destructive, difficult to control, and behave in a malignant fashion. Malignant tumors are treated most effectively using a multispecialty approach.

HISTORY

Symptoms. Swelling, pain, and dysfunction. Some patients complain of night pain that is relieved by aspirin. Other patients who have no mass may point specifically to an area of pain in the soft tissue. Other presentations include a gradual, insidious, enlarging mass or progressive deformity without pain.

General. A careful, meticulous history must be taken to elicit accurate clinical information. A high index of suspicion is essential in order to recognize the organic basis of swelling, pain, and dysfunction without a history of trauma (e.g., a teenager with atraumatic knee pain lasting longer than expected, or an older patient in a high-risk group for metastatic disease). Location of lesions may occur wherever there is bone, muscle, soft tissue, or neurovascular structures. Common injuries or musculoskeletal complaints that do not behave or resolve as expected must be investigated.

Age. All ages. Tumors can be developmental abnormalities and are appreciated as the skeleton matures.

Onset. The onset of symptoms is largely variable. Musculoskeletal tumors can present from a large, fungating mass to a subtle, incidental radiographic finding. Other tumors present only in adulthood and are picked up by accident on routine x-ray.

Duration. Highly variable; tumor origin, grade, size, and location affect the prognosis. Patients with a soft-tissue osteosarcoma of an extremity can be treated very effectively and with very good cure rates. Tumor is usually found earlier, leading to earlier treatment and better prognosis. Pelvic osteosarcoma tends to be larger before it becomes symptomatic or is found as a mass. The size, location, and relationship to vital structures, along with grade and tumor origin, determines prognosis of pelvic malignancies.

Intensity. Variable levels of complaints. Some patients have asymptomatic masses; others have injury pain that does not improve and is difficult to control. Musculoskeletal complaints that do not improve as expected need to be investigated. Glomus tumors can be exquisitely tender when palpated but have no mass present.

Aggravating Factors. Activity, weight bearing, and position.

Alleviating Factors. Pain medicines, aspirin, nonsteroidal anti-inflammatory drugs (NSAIDs), positional, rest.

Associated Factors. Deformities, lesions, or bowel and bladder changes may be present that lead to suspicion of a tumor. Distal neuropathy or vascular changes secondary to direct tumor invasion on neurovascular compression from tumor growth may also occur. Joint effusion may occur if a lesion is in or near a joint or joint capsule.

PHYSICAL EXAMINATION

General. Observe for deformity and asymmetry of contralateral parts. Examine the patient sitting, standing, and walking, looking for asymmetry of musculoskeletal systems, gait, as well as limp or loss of use of any limb. Palpation of localized painful area and comparing to the contralateral side for subtle differences may be helpful. Evaluate range of motion of the nearest joints, including rotational motion and force. Benign-appearing symptoms that persist must be investigated. Any painless subfascial tissue mass must be considered malignant until proven otherwise.

Neurologic. Neurologic examination is performed to note subtle differences in sensory and motor function.

Vascular. Changes must be evaluated for distal compromise to the limbs.

Gastrointestinal, Genitourinary, Gynecologic. Functions must be evaluated for suspected pelvic or spinal tumors.

PATHOPHYSIOLOGY

Primary tumors of the musculoskeletal system are derived from nonepithelial elements of the soft tissue that supports and contributes to the function of the musculoskeletal system and those tumors that arise *de novo* in bone. Secondary malignant tumors usually arise in the epithelial elements and metastasize to bone.

Staging. There are several systems of staging, but only the two major systems are reviewed here. The first is the American Joint Commission of Cancer (AJCC) system. This is used mostly by general surgeons when dealing with soft-tissue sarcomas. It has a four-point grading scale based on the tumor's histologic appearance (Table 9–1).

The second system is the American Musculoskeletal Tumor Society (Enneking) system. This system addresses the unique problems related to sarcomas of the extremities and soft tissue. This applies to tumors of the

Table 9–1. American Joint Commission on Staging (AJCS)

Stage	Grade	Size	Nodal Metastasis	Distant Metastasis
IA	1	<5 cm	No	No
IB	1	≧5 cm	No	No
IIA	2	<5 cm	No	No
IIB	2	≧5 cm	No	No
IIIA	3	<5 cm	No	No
IIIB	3	≧5 cm	No	No
IVA	Any	Any	Yes	No
IVB	Any	Any	Any	Yes

bone and soft tissue and is generally preferred by orthopedic oncologists. The Enneking staging system uses a three-point system based on the histopathological grade and the anatomical site, intracompartmental (A) or extracompartmental (B) (Table 9–2).

Malignant tumors resemble their cell type of origin and can be primary in tissue other than the original tissue cell of origin. The tumor cell origin has specific characteristics in and of itself that differentiate the tumor type cytologically as well as clinically, including aggressiveness, the preferred tissues most often invaded, appearance on x-ray, and age of patient affected. Tumors can be separated into large groups such as hemopoietic, chondrogenic osteogenic, lipogenic, neurogenic, vascular in origin, or unknown.

DIAGNOSTIC STUDIES

Laboratory
CBC, Full Chemistry Profile, PT, PTT. As routine preoperative screen.

Immunoglobulin Electrophoresis, Alkaline Phosphatase, Acid Phosphatase. If indicated, to rule out multiple myeloma or lymphoma.

Table 9–2. Enneking Staging System

Stage	Grade	Compartment	Metastasis
IA	Low	Intra	No
IB	Low	Extra	No
IIA	High	Intra	No
IIB	High	Extra	No
IIIA	Any	Intra	Yes
IIIB	Any	Extra	Yes

Radiologic

Plain Radiographs. Of the affected area are the single most important diagnostic study for bone neoplasm. It is helpful for the investigation of soft-tissue lesions that are mineralized, as well as lytic lesions.

MRI. To determine the extent of any tumor involvement, the size of the tumor, and the presence or extent of tissue invasion. Vital in the management of bone and soft-tissue sarcomas. This study can provide crucial information, increasing the ability to safely excise lesions that where formerly thought to be inoperable. MRI is very sensitive to reactive edema and easily affected by biopsy procedures.

Bone Scans. Total-body technetium-99 scan is very site specific and provides useful information about the lesion. It can detect multiple lesions as well as bone reactions to overlying soft-tissue tumor. In metastatic disease, the bone scan is very helpful in detecting or identifying all bone areas involved. It is used in follow-up evaluations for spread, recurrence, and metastases.

CT Scan. To determine the extent of any tumor involvement, the size of the tumor, and the presence or extent of tissue invasion. An essential part in staging and necessary for planning treatment, particularly when planning surgical procedures. CT is particularly helpful with bone lesions and soft-tissue lesion of high contrast. It is essential that it be performed prior to an invasive procedure such as biopsy or even fine-needle aspiration (FNA).

Metastatic Work-up. Should be performed on clinically suspicious masses to rule out metastases.

Chest Tomography. Provides helpful information about certain bone tumors that have the propensity to metastasize to the lung.

Angiography. Helpful for evaluating bone and soft-tissue sarcomas. It is particularly helpful for planning limb salvage procedures, to outline the tumor, and to show blood supply to the tumor.

Ultrasound. Very limited application. Can confirm cystic versus solid lesion. If done, it should be followed by CT or MRI.

Other

Biopsy. Includes FNA, Tru-Cut needle biopsy, and open procedures. Invasive procedures such as biopsies must not preceed imaging studies, because they may interfere with interpretation of the results.

DIFFERENTIAL DIAGNOSIS

Traumatic. Any pathologic fracture needs to be worked up to rule out a tumor.

Infectious

Osteomyelitis. Can appear similar to a tumor and must be ruled out by history (prior infection/sepsis) and laboratory studies (elevated CBC, ESR).

Neoplastic

Metastatic Tumor.   May have evidence of primary tumor elsewhere.

Bone Cysts.   Include solitary bone cyst (simple or unicameral bone cyst), juxta-articular bone cyst (intraosseous ganglion), metaphyseal fibrous defect (nonossifying fibroma), eosinophilic granuloma, fibrous dysplasia and ossifying fibroma, myositis ossificans, and parathyroid adenoma (brown tumor). Differentiated on physical examination, radiographic studies, or biopsy.

Metabolic

Inflammatory Arthritis.   May have elevated ESR; differentiated from neoplasm on x-ray.

Vascular

Aneurysmal Bone Cyst.   Differentiated on x-ray; Doppler evidence of an erosive aneurysm.

Congenital

Ollier's Disease.   Multiple enchondroma is a rare, nonfamiliar dysplasia that is usually seen on one half of the body.

Maffucci Syndrome.   Multiple enchondromas, multiple soft-tissue hemangiomas.

Acquired

Stress Fracture.   Due to repetitive stress; differentiated from neoplasm on x-ray (see topic stress fractures).

Other

Herniated Disc.   Causes radicular symptoms (pain, numbness, weakness) in a dermatomal distribution (see topic cervical and lumbar intervertebral disc disease).

TREATMENT

Evaluation of musculoskeletal masses is best performed by a sarcoma team that consists of an orthopedic oncologist, radiologist, radiation oncologist, medical oncologist, and pathologist. All masses must be considered malignant until proven otherwise by physical examination or staging investigations.

All investigations must be completed before considering any invasive procedure. No biopsy of any kind should be performed until all staging procedures are complete. Deviating from these recommendations can change the course of treatment and the final outcome.

Biopsy.   Proper technique of biopsy may mean the difference between the patient undergoing a limb-sparing procedure versus an amputation. A culture of soft tissue should always be performed on bone lesions. Techniques include open incisional biopsy (advised in most instances) and FNA. The biopsy incision should always be carefully considered in relation to the possible definitive surgery later. All biopsy incisions and drain sites need to be resected if the lesion is proven to be malignant. FNA applications include confirmation of metastases from a known cancer, biopsy of a lesion that is not easily accessible by open biopsy, staging of certain lesions by bone marrow aspiration, and for confirming suspected local recurrence when an experienced pathologist is available.

Medical. The three major modalities in treatment of malignant musculoskeletal tumors are surgery, chemotherapy, and radiotherapy. Treatment depends on a number of factors, including type and extent of the tumor. In most instances, a combination of two or more modalities is required for the best outcome. In tumors of high-grade malignancy, such as osteosarcoma, the immediate concern is with complete removal of the primary tumor. A high percentage of patients have micrometastases present at the time of first evaluation. Adjuvant chemotherapy therefore becomes an integral part of the treatment plan.

Metastatic lesions to bone can be very destructive to the integrity of bone structure involved. The primary disease, pathologic fracture, or potential pathologic fracture must be treated. The goal is for ambulatory activity, particularly when the lower extremity is involved; hence the popularity of rigid internal fixation of pathologic fractures of long bones. The effectiveness of the treatment and likely prognosis is essential before the lesion and fracture are interfered with surgically.

Chemotherapy. Essential in the treatment of small round cell tumors such as Ewing's sarcoma; plays an important role in the treatment of osteosarcoma. It has a promising role in soft-tissue sarcomas and is helpful in selected cases of metastatic disease. The chemotherapeutic approach remains controversial and is a frequently changing area of treatment. Palliative chemotherapy is given only in the setting of symptomatic metastases or unresectable primary tumors.

Curative Chemotherapy Plus Radiotherapy. In a group of tumors referred to as "round cell" or "blue cell" (Ewing's sarcoma, primitive neuroectodermal tumor, Askin's tumor), it is recommended that a combination of radiotherapy and chemotherapy be used.

Curative Chemotherapy Plus Surgical Excision. Used in osteosarcoma. Adjuvant chemotherapy has been established as an essential part of the management of osteogenic sarcomas. For soft-tissue sarcomas, the role for routine adjuvant chemotherapy has not been proven, but it has been used for primitive tumors in young patients, after marginal local excision where radiation cannot be delivered, and in some patients with very advanced disease who are undergoing preoperative radiation for debulking of the disease.

Radiotherapy. Important in the role of management of sarcomas arising in bone or soft tissue. Used for both curative and palliative treatment. It may be used alone or in conjunction with surgery or chemotherapy. Radical (curative) radiotherapy may be used alone to ablate local disease in sites where surgical resection is impossible (e.g., vertebral column). Local control rates are good for Ewing's sarcoma using only radiotherapy and chemotherapy. Complex planning procedures are required to spare normal tissue from the high-dose radiation. Thoughtless placement of biopsy scars and unnecessary exploration at the time of surgery compromise radiotherapy. Tumors disseminate into wider tissue planes, which make it impossible to treat tumors radically without severe late damage to normal tissue. Palliative radiotherapy can be used to palliate symptoms from incurable sarcoma.

Surgical. The guiding principle in surgical intervention is complete removal of the primary tumor with maximum retention of function and minimum possibility of local recurrence. In extremity tumors, this was typically accomplished by amputation. Currently, limb salvage or preservation procedures have become possible because of the effectiveness of adjuvant chemotherapy and radiotherapy in limiting the extent of surgical resection required.

Intralesional Excision. This procedure is equivalent to an incisional biopsy, often referred to as debulking or curetted, where the tumor is removed in piecemeal fashion. Macroscopic disease remains and local recurrence is guaranteed.

Marginal Excision. Essentially an excisional biopsy or "shell-out" procedure that transgresses the pseudocapsule (reactive zone) and leaves behind microscopic tumor. All tissue planes encountered during the excision are contaminated. In high-grade tumors, 100% local recurrence is expected; in low-grade lesions, a high likelihood of local recurrence is expected. A marginal excision is inadequate for high-grade tumors without adjuvant therapy.

Wide Excision. The mass is removed intracompartmentally with adequate but viable normal surrounding tissue. A wide margin is thought to be adequate in most cases.

Radical Excision. This is an extracompartmental excision whereby the tumor and surrounding tissues are removed by dissecting along planes that are separated from the tumor and its tissue of origin. At least one anatomical structure surrounding the tumor in both longitudinal and transverse planes should be removed.

Surgery and Adjuvant Radiotherapy. Surgery combined with radiotherapy has improved local tumor control so that less radical and mutilating surgery can be performed. Limb salvage and preservation procedures commonly use this modality.

Preoperative Radiotherapy. Has the advantages of a small treatment volume, the presence of normal blood vessels *in situ* and thus fewer hypoxic cells present, and surgery is facilitated by fibrosis of the reactive zone and avoidance of delays due to surgical complications. The disadvantages are poor wound healing, postsurgical pathology is difficult to interpret, and the patient may decide to refuse surgery after radiotherapy is completed.

Postoperative/Radiotherapy. Has the advantages of the full pathology report being available, avoids surgical delay due to complications from radiotherapy, and provides better wound healing. The disadvantages are that larger radiation treatment volume is required (if there is wide surgical disruption of tissues, the radiotherapy treatment will be severely compromised) and inappropriately placed biopsy or drain sites can make postoperative radiotherapy impossible.

Patient Follow-up. Routine follow-up of the patient at appropriate intervals remains the best clinical evaluation to detect recurrence or metastatic disease. In most sarcomas, the concern for pulmonary metastases is evaluated with periodic chest x-rays. For superficial and distal tumors, clinical examination is most reliable. For deeper, proximal, and axial tumors, CT scans are preferable. Bone scans may remain hot for 2 to 3 years when bone is involved and are unreliable indicators of local recurrence during that time. In general, patients are seen every 3 months for the first 2 years, then every 6 months for a three-year period, and yearly thereafter.

Treatment of Metastatic Disease. The detection of metastatic pulmonary disease is not the signal to cease all curative efforts. These lesions may respond to additional chemotherapy and may be surgically resectable. Aggressive approach to metastectomy is recommended. A patient should be considered for resection of skeletal or pulmonary metastases if the primary disease is or can be controlled or a complete metastectomy can be performed. A 20% to 25% salvage rate can be expected in well-selected cases.

World Health Organization Modified Classification of Bone Tumors

Bone-forming Tumors

  Benign: Osteoma, osteoid osteoma, osteoblastoma (benign osteoblastoma)

  Indeterminate: Aggressive osteoblastoma

  Malignant: Osteosarcoma (osteogenic sarcoma), juxtacortical osteosarcoma (periosteal, parosteal osteosarcomas), periosteal osteosarcoma

Cartilage-forming Tumors

  Benign: Chondroma (enchondroma), osteochondroma (osteocartilaginous exostosis), periosteal chondroma, chondroblastoma (benign chondroblastoma, epiphyseal chondroblastoma), chondromyxoid fibroma

  Malignant: Chondrosarcoma, mesenchymal chondrosarcoma, dedifferentiated chondrosarcoma

Giant Cell Tumor (Osteoclastoma)

Marrow Tumors

  Ewing's sarcoma, malignant lymphoma, myeloma

Vascular Tumors

  Benign: Hemangioma, lymphangioma, glomus tumor (glomangioma)

  Intermediate or Indeterminate: Hemangioendothelioma, hemangiopericytoma

  Malignant: Angiosarcoma

Other Connective Tissue Tumors

  Benign: Desmoplastic fibroma, lipoma

  Malignant: Fibrosarcoma, malignant fibrous histiocytoma (MFH), liposarcoma, malignant mesenchymoma, undifferentiated sarcoma

Other Tumors

  Chordoma, adamantinoma of long bones, neurilemoma (schwannoma, neurinoma), neurofibroma

Tumor-like Lesions

Solitary bone cyst (simple or unicameral bone cyst), aneurysmal bone cyst, juxta-articular bone cyst (intraosseous ganglion), metaphyseal fibrous defect (nonossifying fibroma), eosinophilic granuloma, fibrous dysplasia and ossifying fibroma, myositis ossificans, parathyroid adenoma (brown tumor)

Indications. For diagnosing, staging, and debulking the lesion.

Contraindications. Essentially none, because the risk of the lesion outweighs other considerations. Adjunct therapy may be given to those patients who cannot tolerate anesthesia.

TECHNIQUE OF SURGICAL ASSISTING

Caution is practiced in any surgical procedure dealing with neoplasms in order to prevent cellular spread. If drains are required, the drain site should be brought out in line with the incision, and close to the incision.

PEDIATRIC CONSIDERATIONS

Tumors can be developmental abnormalities and are appreciated as the skeleton matures. A high index of suspicion for musculoskeletal tumors needs to be maintained in pediatric patients who present with swelling, pain, dysfunction, or a mass.

PEARLS FOR THE PA

A multidisciplinary approach (sarcoma team) is imperative to provide the best possible outcome for the patient.

Swelling, pain, dysfunction, or a mass in the absence of trauma is suggestive of a musculoskeletal tumor.

Musculoskeletal complaints that do not improve as expected require investigation.

Invasive procedures such as biopsies must not preceed imaging studies, because they may interfere with interpretation of the results.

Amputations are no longer the required therapy for limb tumors due to adjunct treatment measures.

The detection of metastatic pulmonary disease does not preclude treatment.

OBSTETRICAL CONSIDERATIONS

The risk versus benefit to the mother and fetus must be assessed when ordering radiographic or invasive studies to be performed on a pregnant patient.

Adult Reconstructive Surgery

Richard E. Donnelly, PA-C, BS, BS, and
Edward C. D'Ettorre, PA-C

DEFINITION

The replacement of joints with artificial parts. This can be a partial or total joint replacement with metal, ceramic, or plastic parts.

HISTORY

Symptoms. Patients usually complain of gradual onset of pain over several years with gradual loss or decrease in activity of the involved limb or joint.

General. Most joint replacements are done for degenerative joint disease due to osteoarthritis, rheumatoid arthritis, and avascular necrosis, or due to fractures, mainly in the shoulder and hip.

Age. The average age for joint replacement is 65 to 70 years of age, but may occur as early as the fourth decade of life and as late as the tenth decade.

Onset. The onset of pain may be acute if the joint has been damaged due to trauma, but is usually insidious with progressive pain and limited activity.

Duration. Total joint replacement has a 90% to 95% satisfaction rate for up to 15 to 20 years for the hip and knee joints, and 90% satisfaction at 10 years for shoulders. Other joints are less satisfactory (e.g., elbows, ankles, and digits).

Aggravating Factors. Artificial joints are mechanical devices; wear with time is accelerated in those activities that tend to add additional stress (e.g., running or jogging, lifting over 50 lbs [greater than 10 to 20 lbs for the upper extremity]).

Associated Factors. There is a 1% risk for infection for the lifetime of the prosthesis. The artificial part may become loose between the bone–prosthesis interface (approximately 5% to 10% at 20 years). Total hip replacements have a 3% incidence of dislocation; the risk is greatest during the first 6 months. Total shoulder replacements have a greater risk of dislocation.

PHYSICAL EXAMINATION

General. The patient is noted to have decreased function in the involved joint (e.g., limping to the examination room, limited unilateral arm swing, etc.).

Orthopedic. The range of motion is the greatest concern with total joint replacement. The preoperative range of motion should be recorded, then followed postoperatively at 6 weeks, 1 year, 2 years, etc., up to 5 years, then at 5-year intervals. The vascular and neurologic status should be evaluated and recorded preoperatively, and followed closely postoperatively for the first 6 weeks. Extremity strength is also important and should be evaluated; if weakness is present, an attempt to strengthen the extremity before surgery is recommended, if feasible.

PATHOPHYSIOLOGY

There are two classes of artificial joint prosthesis—cemented and pressfit (bone ingrowth). Bone ingrowth prostheses are used more frequently in the younger age group, with hybrid knee and hip prostheses and the humeral component of the shoulder, in the hope that bone ingrowth will give longer life to the prosthesis. The cemented prosthesis is used in older persons, mainly with elbows and the glenoid component of the shoulder, due to improved results with this technique.

DIAGNOSTIC STUDIES

Laboratory
CBC, Full Chemistry Profile, PT, PTT. As routine preoperative evaluation.

Type and Screen. Most larger joints (e.g., knee and hip) require blood transfusions. Autologous donations are recommended.

Radiology
AP and Lateral X-rays. Of the involved joint are minimum. With total knee arthroplasty, full-length standing AP views are helpful for varus valgus alignment. Hip x-rays with 100 mm markers to judge magnification for prosthesis templating is also helpful.

DIFFERENTIAL DIAGNOSIS

There are no differential conditions.

TREATMENT

Medical. Because this is a procedure, the concept of conservative management does not apply.

Surgical. At the present time, the most satisfactory joint replacement outcomes have been with the knee and hip. The shoulder also has good outcomes, but is not as predictable. Elbow replacement is improving and is satisfactory in limited cases. Total ankle replacement has not proven to be very satisfactory, with early failure rates. Joint replacement in digits (toes, fingers) has not proven to be long lasting and has a high degree of failure in a short period of time. Salvage procedures for the latter joints following failure of total joint replacement are also difficult and have a high degree of dissatisfaction, mainly due to bone loss and shortening of the involved bones.

Most orthopedists use prophylactic antibiotics in total joint arthroplasty and recommend antibiotic coverage for patients undergoing dental work, gastrointestinal or genitourinary procedures, and for bronchoscopy.

There is an approximately 50% incidence of deep venous thrombosis and a 10% incidence of pulmonary embolism in patients undergoing lower extremity total joint arthroplasty who are not prophylactically anticoagulated. Therefore, high-risk patients (severe lower limb varicosities, history of previous thrombosis or thrombophlebitis of the lower extremity, cardiac arrhythmias, or other conditions related to thrombosis formation) should be anticoagulated. Anticoagulants are most effective when continued from the day of surgery until the patient is fully ambulatory. Compression stockings are also used to help prevent embolic formation in the lower extremities postoperatively. Even with these precautions, there is a risk of an embolic episode for 6 months.

Warfarin (Coumadin) has been the main anticoagulant agent used for prophylaxis. Low molecular weight heparin sodium (Lovenox) may also be used. Aspirin, in small doses, once or twice daily, may be used as a preventive agent for thrombosis.

Indications. Patients who have pain sufficient to interfere with quality of life or limit their activity are considered for joint replacement.

Contraindications. Inactivity (relative), inability to tolerate anesthesia.

TECHNIQUE OF SURGICAL ASSISTING

Familiarity with prosthesis material is important. Traction and exposure during the procedure are the primary roles of the PA.

PEDIATRIC CONSIDERATIONS

Rarely required in children unless significant congenital defects exist.

OBSTETRICAL CONSIDERATIONS

No surgical treatment during pregnancy. Use caution in performing x-rays and prescribing analgesics.

Spine: Cervical and Lumbar Intervertebral Disc Disease

Susan Lemens, PA-C, and
James B. Labus, PA-C

DEFINITION

Herniation or extrusion of the nucleus propulsus (HNP) of an intervertebral disc, which compromises a neural structure, causing neurologic symptoms (radiculopathy). Radiculopathy refers to a dysfunction of a specific nerve root (pain, sensory deficit, muscle weakness, or abnormal reflex).

Cervical. Most herniated discs occur in areas with increased mobility, C6–C7, followed by C5–C6. May cause myelopathy, which refers to a disorder (compression) of the spinal cord with accompanying symptoms of painless weakness, sensory anomalies, or bowel and bladder dysfunction.

Lumbar. Most herniated discs occur in areas with increased axial load (lumbar, L4–L5, and L5–S1). Sciatica describes pain and neurologic dysfunction specifically localized to the L4, L5, and S1 roots that supply the sciatic nerve.

HISTORY

Symptoms. Usually severe and unilateral pain, numbness, or weakness radiating to an extremity in a specific dermatomal pattern. Worse with activity and better with rest.

General. Inquire as to the distribution and character of the pain, presence of bowel or bladder dysfunction, activities (e.g., flexion or extension) that exacerbate or relieve symptoms, any worsening with Valsalva maneuvers, mechanism of injury (if applicable), prior spinal injury or surgeries, onset of symptoms, and any subjective evidence of numbness or weakness. Careful documentation needs to be performed on work-related injuries.

Cervical. Neck pain (discogenic neck pain) may be the only complaint with an HNP. Obtain a history of any painless weakness, gait difficulty, generalized sensory deficit (numbness, temperature, proprioception), bowel or bladder dysfunction, and subjective evidence of Lhermitte's sign (electrical shock radiating down the spine with neck flexion).

Age. 25 to 45 years of age. Infrequent after the age of 65 years unless associated with degenerative conditions of the spine such as spinal stenosis (spondylosis).

Onset. Usually acute. There is not always a precipitating event (more common with cervical HNP). Symptoms may be intermittent, with acute flares.

Duration. Usually requires intervention, conservative or surgical, to improve symptoms. May take weeks to months of conservative therapy.

Intensity. Varies. Pain is often described as sharp, shooting, or electric shock–like; radiating down the extremity; associated with activity; or may be a dull, persistent ache.

Aggravating Factors. Pain increases with walking/activity. Occasionally coughing, sneezing, or straining (Valsalva maneuvers) elicit symptoms.

Alleviating Factors. Appropriate intervention may improve symptoms.

Cervical. Guarding of neck movement or splinting the arm may be used by some patients.

Lumbar. Lying down with hip and knee slightly flexed, or leaning forward and slightly flexing the lumbar spine.

Associated Factors. May be, but not always, associated with low back or neck pain. Paraspinous muscle spasm can be associated with HNP. Risk factors include smoking, obesity, prolonged daily driving, or repetitive heavy lifting, twisting, or bending.

Cervical. HNP may compromise the spinal cord.

Lumbar. May cause symptoms of cauda equina syndrome (see lumbar spinal stenosis).

PHYSICAL EXAMINATION

General

Cervical. The patient may be in significant distress, holding the neck in a neutral position. Palpate the neck for any lesion that may contribute to the symptoms.

Lumbar. The patient may be in significant distress and walk with a stooped posture. He or she may prefer to perform the history while standing. Careful examination is performed to rule out other causes such as palpation of the abdomen to rule out abdominal and pelvic tumors and aortic aneurysms. Peripheral pulses must be tested when vascular claudication is suspected. Inguinal hernia must also be ruled out if the presenting symptom is groin pain.

Neurologic/Orthopedic. Range of motion of the spine (including flexion, extension, lateral bending and rotation) is often limited due to spasm of the paraspinous muscles. Palpate the spine for step-offs, spasm, or obvious deficits. A sensory examination is performed, noting the distribution of numbness. Always compare proximal to distal (may signify peripheral neuropathy) and all dermatomes. Motor examination should include all major muscle groups of the extremity, checking for weakness or atrophy. Reflexes are often diminished or absent on the affected side. Evaluate Babinski's sign to rule out upper motor neuron disease.

Cervical. Spurling's cervical compression test is performed and is positive if arm pain is reproduced. Hoffman's response is elicited by holding the third finger extended and flicking the nail. It is positive if the hand flexes in response (signifies possible upper motor neuron disease).

Lumbar. Observe gait and posture while the patient is traveling to the examination room. Repeat the examination in the room and compare the findings. The patient often limps, favoring the affected leg. There is sometimes an acute scoliosis, an involuntary attempt to reduce nerve root tension by bending to the affected side. The sciatic notch is palpated for the reproduction of pain in the leg. On motor examination, the examiner is not able to overcome gastrocnemius; therefore, ask the patient to walk on the heels and toes, noting any asymmetry.

The straight-leg raising test and femoral stretch (nerve tension tests) are performed. The straight-leg raising test is performed with the patient supine. The leg is passively raised and, if positive, the patient experiences radicular pain. The crossed straight-leg raising test is performed on the nonpainful leg and is positive when the patient experiences the same pain in the opposite leg as the one being raised. This test is highly suggestive of an HNP. The femoral stretch is performed with the patient on his or her side, facing away from the examiner. The leg is dorsally flexed and a positive test occurs when the patient experiences pain in the involved leg (indicative of upper lumbar nerve root compression). Range of motion of the hip is assessed to rule out a primary hip disorder. A rectal examination must also be performed, testing sphincter tone and sensation, when cauda equina syndrome is suspected. Specific nerve roots and their correlated examination findings are listed in Table 9–3.

PATHOPHYSIOLOGY

The intervertebral disc is made up of a strong outer capsule, called the annulus fibrosis, which is made up of crossing collagen fibers; and the softer, inner nucleus pulposus, made up of linear collagen fibers. When the fibers of the annulus are disrupted (as in degenerative changes or with trauma), extrusion of the nucleus material occurs. The herniated nucleus compresses the nerve root as it exits the foramen, causing a radiculopathy.

Disc ruptures may be subcapsular, where the nucleus migrates from the central region of the disc into the annulus, causing a bulging of the capsule; or the nuclear material may extrude through the annulus, protruding into the spinal canal, sometimes breaking off and becoming a free fragment, compromising the nerve root above.

Table 9–3. Specific Nerve Roots and Examination Findings

Nerve Root	Muscle	Reflex	Sensory
C5	Deltoid, biceps	Biceps	Lateral arm
C6	Biceps, wrist extensor	Brachioradialis	Radial forearm, 1st and 2nd digits
C7	Wrist flexor, digit extensor, triceps	Triceps	3rd digit
C8	Intrinsic hand muscles		Ulnar forearm, 4th and 5th digits
T1	Intrinsic hand muscles		Ulnar forearm
L4	Tibialis anterior	Knee jerk	Anterior thigh, medial leg
L5	Extensor hallucis longus		Posterolateral leg, dorsal foot
S1	Gastrocnemius soleus	Ankle jerk	Posterior leg often to the ankle

Cervical. The nerve root lies rostral to the corresponding vertebral body number (e.g., the C5 nerve root exits between C4–C5). The disc may rupture centrally and if large enough capacity may compress the spinal cord.

Lumbar. The nerve root lies caudal to the corresponding vertebral body number (e.g., the L5 nerve root exits between L5–S1).

DIAGNOSTIC STUDIES

Laboratory

CBC with Differential, Sedimentation Rate, Full Chemistry Profile. Are needed to rule out metabolic and infectious causes.

Radiology

Cervical X-rays. May show degenerative disease, bone spurs, fracture, disc space narrowing, or prior fusion. The size of the spinal canal can be deduced. Flexion and extension views should be obtained in the setting of neck pain following trauma to rule out spinal instability.

Lumbosacral X-rays. May show fracture, narrowed disc space, end-plate erosion, degeneration, spondylolisthesis, prior surgical defects, spina bifida (occulta), or bone spurs.

MRI. Is probably the best imaging study for evaluating patients suspected of having disc disease. T2-weighted images best identify the herniated or extruded disc and associated neural compromise. MRI is also helpful in identifying far lateral disc herniations that would not be seen on myelogram/CT. Tumors or other intraspinal pathology may be identified. The presence of increased signal in the cervical spine at the level of an HNP suggests edema and cord injury.

Myelography Followed by CT.   Is an invasive procedure that should be reserved for special indications: when MRI cannot be performed due to metallic implants or severe claustrophobia, equivocal MRI findings, or more detailed surgical planning. HNP and some intraspinal lesions can be identified. Bony encroachment on the neural foramen can be more easily seen on this study.

Other

EMG/NCV.   Is useful in ruling out peripheral neuropathies and to identify the specific nerve root involved.

Vascular Studies.   May be needed when symptoms suggest vascular claudication.

DIFFERENTIAL DIAGNOSIS

Traumatic

Cervical Strain.   Pain usually localized to the neck and intrascapular region. Examination is normal.

Lumbosacral Strain.   Causing minor symptoms of radiculopathy. Examination is usually normal except for muscle spasm. Straight-leg raising testing negative. Pain may involve the posterior thigh to the knee.

Fractures.   With retropulsion of vertebral body fragment into the canal.

Thoracic HNP.   May cause myelopathic symptoms. MRI of the thoracic area will rule out.

Spine Fracture.   Usually seen on x-ray. CT may be required to identify subtle fractures. In the cervical spine, C7 needs to be viewed.

Infectious

Discitis.   Usually associated with severe back pain with movement. Back pain greater than leg pain. Seen in IV drug abusers, postsurgery, immunosuppressed (e.g., diabetic) patients, or after gastrointestinal or genitourinary procedures.

Epidural Abscess or Hematoma.   May be seen after spinal anesthesia placement. Meningeal irritation signs may be present (nuchal rigidity, Kernig's, Brudzinski); seen on MRI.

Tuberculosis and Lyme Disease.   Can also cause back pain associated with a mild radiculopathy. Positive titers.

Herpes Zoster (Shingles).   Usually associated with a rash in the distribution of the pain.

Metabolic

Peripheral Neuropathies.   Diabetic neuropathy the most common. Stocking-glove distribution numbness; hyperesthesia.

Rheumatoid Arthritis.   Positive rheumatoid factor.

Osteoporosis.   May cause spine pain without radicular findings. Hypodense bone seen on x-ray; bone density measurements may be required.

Ankylosing Spondylitis.   Fusion seen on cervical x-rays.

Neoplastic

Tumors.   Intradural (e.g., meningioma), extradural (e.g., metastasis), peripheral nerve (e.g., neurofibroma), intra-abdominal, pelvic, and brachial plexus (e.g., Pancoast) tumors can all compromise neural structures, presenting with symptoms similar to HNP.

Vascular

Vascular Claudication. A careful vascular examination must be done to rule out peripheral vascular or abdominal aortic aneurysmal disease.

Thoracic Outlet Syndrome. Entrapment of the brachial plexus and vascular structures (see Thoracic Outlet Syndrome, Chapter 13).

Congenital

Perineural/Meningeal Cysts. Seen on myelogram/CT or MRI.

Conjoined Nerve Roots. Seen on myelogram/CT or MRI.

Tethered Cord. May have findings of spina bifida (e.g., dimple or hairy patch in the lumbar area); seen on myelogram/CT or MRI.

Scoliosis. Significant scoliosis is apparent on examination. May cause foraminal compromise. MRI may be inadequate if the scoliosis is severe.

Spondylolisthesis. Due to a defect of the pars interarticularis. A palpable step-off may be present. Seen on x-ray. Back pain with activity is more common.

Acquired

Spinal Stenosis (Spondylosis). Usually seen in the older population. Narrow spinal canal, facet hypertrophy, and bone encroachment on the foramen seen on myelogram/CT or MRI.

Facet Joint Synovial Cysts. Seen on myelogram/CT or MRI.

Peripheral Neuropathies. Such as a femoral neuropathy, carpal tunnel syndrome, or tardy ulnar nerve palsy may be mistaken for radiculopathy. EMG/NCV positive.

Other

Malingering. More common with secondary gain. Examination and radiographic studies differentiate.

TREATMENT

Medical. Initial treatment should include a brief episode of bedrest (only 2 to 3 days is recommended), analgesics, NSAIDs, muscle relaxants, physical therapy (which helps to strengthen supporting muscles), traction (better for cervical than lumbar disease), and epidural steroid injections.

Cervical. Splinting with a soft cervical collar may be of some benefit. Epidural steroid injections should only be administered by someone with significant experience.

Lumbar. Over 50% of patients with a radiculopathy due to HNP notice improvement in their symptoms with medical treatment alone.

Surgical. The goal of any surgery is to relieve the pressure on the nerve root by removing the offending disc fragment. It is important to maintain spinal stability.

Cervical. The most common procedure is the anterior discectomy and fusion using the patient's own iliac crest or cadaver bone. This removes the fragment, and the addition of the fusion maintains the integrity of the disc space height. Occasionally, especially with multilevel discectomies, a titanium plate is used to further stabilize the fusion. A posterior approach is sometimes used to open the foramen or attempt to remove the extruded disc fragment (used more for far lateral herniations). X-rays are obtained at intervals postoperatively to assess healing and position of the bone graft.

Lumbar. The most common procedure performed for HNP is a standard open hemilaminectomy, discectomy, and foraminotomy. Other procedures include microdiscectomy (similar to an open discectomy with the addition of a surgical microscope), which has the advantage of a smaller incision, less anatomical disruption, possibly a shortened hospital stay, and less blood loss. Percutaneous endoscopic discectomy and laser-assisted procedures are relatively new and controversial, with limited results in studies and are contraindicated in spinal stenosis and with free disc fragments. Chemonucleolysis using chymopapain has a high complication and failure rate and is not recommended.

Indications

Cervical. Failure of medical treatment with persistent severe pain and positive neurologic examination findings; myelopathy.

Lumbar. Failure of medical treatment with persistent severe pain and positive neurologic examination findings. Recurrent episodes of radiculopathy. Urgent indications for surgery include cauda equina syndrome or acute progressive motor deficit (foot drop).

Contraindications. Poor surgical candidate because of severe medical illness. Inadequate conservative trial.

Cervical. Prior multilevel fusions (relative).

Lumbar. Predominant symptoms of low back pain and absence of confirmation of HNP by imaging studies.

TECHNIQUE OF SURGICAL ASSISTING

As in any procedure, it is of utmost importance to protect the neural structures at all times. Many times one is working in very small areas of exposure such as during a microdiscectomy, so fine, calculated movements are necessary. Previous experience with working under a microscope is helpful.

Cervical. The PA frequently assists with harvesting of the bone graft. Caution is taken to prevent injury to the lateral femorocutaneous nerve or to not perforate the peritoneum.

Lumbar. The PA often retracts the nerve root so that the disc can be removed. Light traction is usually all that is required, because firm or overzealous retraction may injure the nerve root or tear the dura.

PEDIATRIC CONSIDERATIONS

Radiculopathy secondary to disc disease is very uncommon in children. Children often have few neurologic findings and the disc material is very firm, fibrous, and strongly attached to the endplate.

OBSTETRICAL CONSIDERATIONS

Pregnancy is often associated with low back pain and sciatica. Often the strain of labor precipitates a herniated disk. Treatment during pregnancy is conservative.

PEARLS FOR THE PA

Radiculopathy refers to a disorder of the nerve root that causes pain, numbness, or weakness in a dermatomal pattern.

Many symptomatic disc herniations respond well to conservative treatment, and surgery should only be considered after failure of medical management.

Urgent indications for surgery include symptoms of myelopathy and cauda equina syndrome or acute progressive neurologic deficit.

Spine: Lumbar Spinal Stenosis
Susan Lemens, PA-C

DEFINITION

Lumbar spinal stenosis refers to the decrease in the anterior-posterior dimension of the spinal canal, which causes direct neural compression or compromise of the blood supply to the cauda equina or nerve roots, resulting in neurogenic claudication or radiculopathy. It is a degenerative condition of the spine that can be acquired or caused by a congenitally narrowed spinal canal. Most common location is at L3–L4–L5. May cause central compression of the lumbar or lumbosacral nerves in the thecal sac or lateral recess, compromising the nerve roots in the neural foramen.

Cauda equina syndrome is defined as central spinal canal stenosis that produces specific symptoms of cauda equina compression, including sphincter disturbance (urinary retention/fecal or urinary incontinence, decreased anal tone), saddle anesthesia (perianal, buttock, and posterior-superior thigh numbness), muscle weakness, severe pain, and sexual dysfunction.

HISTORY

Symptoms. The major symptom is that of neurogenic claudication (pseudoclaudication). Defined as unilateral or bilateral hip, buttock, thigh, or leg pain along the compromised nerve root distribution. May occur with prolonged activity. Pain is described as a rubbery feeling or dull ache in the legs, sometimes associated with subjective weakness or numbness. Usually not well localized to a specific dermatome, often because several nerve roots are affected.

General.   A careful history for any associated trauma, malignancy, or systemic illness (e.g., peripheral vascular disease) must be taken to rule out other causes of back pain radiating to the legs.

Age.   Usually occurs in the later decades of life (greater than 50 years of age). Stenosis is more likely the cause of neurogenic claudication or radiculopathy than disc disease in patients greater than 55 years of age.

Onset.   Insidious. Gradual, progressive onset, usually over years.

Duration.   Slow rate of progression with symptoms that may be intermittent. The distance that patients may walk prior to developing claudicatory symptoms may vary from day to day in mild to moderate cases. Exercise tolerance is usually well defined and consistent in very severe cases of spinal stenosis.

Intensity.   Moderate to severe pain, described as a dull ache that increases with activity.

Aggravating Factors.   Pain made worse with standing, walking, straining such as coughing or lifting, and/or sitting.

Alleviating Factors.   Pain slowly resolves with rest. Relieved by changing posture and "opening" the spinal canal. Positions such as forward flexion (e.g., bending over a shopping cart), squatting, lying down, and/or sitting.

Associated Factors.   Back pain, paresthesias, weakness, sensory loss, bowel or bladder changes such as incontinence or urinary retention, due to involvement of the cauda equina. Previous minor to moderate trauma to the lumbar spine can contribute to degenerative changes of the spine several years later.

PHYSICAL EXAMINATION

General.   The patient may be in no acute distress or may walk with a stooped posture and guarding of the spine.

Vascular.   It is important to differentiate between neurogenic and vascular claudication. Vascular examination, including palpation of the peripheral pulses and abdominal aorta for aneurysmal disease and tenderness, is required.

Orthopedic.   Careful examination of the hip, including various stress maneuvers, is necessary to rule out hip disease. FABER test refers to an acronym for **f**lexion, **ab**duction, and **e**xternal **r**otation of the hip. This test stresses the hip joint without necessarily exacerbating nerve root compression symptoms.

Neurologic.   Neurologic examination is sometimes normal. Straight-leg raising test (Lasèque's sign) is very useful to differentiate sciatica from hip pain. With the patient supine, lift the straightened leg by the ankle until the point of pain. Positive results occur when pain is elicited at less than 60 degrees. Primarily stretches the L5 and S1 nerve roots. May be more useful in patients with disc disease.

Rectal examination is performed (testing anal tone and sensation) when cauda equina syndrome is suspected. The examination should include careful testing of gait, lumbar spine palpation and range of motion, muscle strength, sensation, and reflexes. Gait may be antalgic and slightly stooped forward. Range of motion is often decreased, with pain reproduced with extension. Motor examination may reveal a weakness in the affected nerve root distribution (see Table 9–3). Reflexes are often normal.

PATHOPHYSIOLOGY

Lumbar spinal stenosis is usually the result of degenerative changes in the spine, including spondylosis, facet hypertrophy, ligamentum flavum hypertrophy or thickening, foraminal stenosis, and disc degeneration, which compromises the thecal sac and nerve roots. Symptoms result from ischemia and nutritional compromise of the lumbosacral nerve roots due to an increased metabolic demand caused by exercise.

DIAGNOSTIC STUDIES

Laboratory

CBC with Differential and Sedimentation Rate. To rule out disc space infection.

Full Chemistry Profile. To rule out other systemic illnesses (e.g., diabetes mellitus).

Radiology

Lumbosacral X-rays. Should include AP, lateral, flexion-extension, and oblique views. Useful to identify bony anatomy and degenerative changes such as bone spurs and decreased disc space height. Also useful to evaluate spondylolisthesis and the diameter of the spinal canal.

CT Scan. With sagittal and axial views is used for identifying bony abnormalities in more detail, but does not evaluate the neural structures with great detail.

Water Soluble Myelography Followed by CT. Better defines the neural structures and degree of narrowing of the spinal canal and compression of the thecal sac, but is invasive. Metallic implants (e.g., from prior fusion) may cause significant artifact.

MRI. Is less optimal than CT for visualizing bony structures; however, clearly defines the neural structures and disc space, especially on T2-weighted axial and sagittal images.

Other

EMG. Is used to exclude peripheral neuropathies and identify specific nerve root pathology.

Vascular Studies. Transcutaneous oximetry, ankle/brachial indices, and Doppler flow studies are performed to rule out vascular claudication if suspected.

DIFFERENTIAL DIAGNOSIS

Traumatic
Lumbar Fracture. Usually acute presentation. May have associated radicular or neuropathic signs and symptoms. Seen on spine x-ray or CT scan.

Infectious
Disc Space Infection, Epidural Abscess. Can cause similar symptoms. With discitis, back pain is more severe than leg pain. May occur after such procedures as epidural pain blocks or placement of epidural catheter or, more rarely, some gastrointestinal or genitourinary procedures.

Osteomyelitis. Can produce similar symptoms; back pain is the usual presenting symptom.

Metabolic
Diabetic Peripheral Neuropathies, Paget's Disease, Pott's Disease, Osteoporosis, and Fluorosis. Can contribute to spinal stenosis or present with similar symptoms. Differentiated on serologic, physical examination, and radiographic studies.

Vascular
Vascular Claudication. Is due to ischemia of an exercised muscle and is often described as pain in the distribution of the specific muscle group. Sensory loss is in the stocking distribution versus a dermatomal distribution. Pain is precipitated by walking a specific distance. Relief is immediate with rest, and patient does not need to sit or change positions. Peripheral pulses are almost always diminished or absent.

Expanding Abdominal Aortic Aneurysms. Can also cause back pain with associated symptoms of vascular claudication.

Intraspinal Vascular Lesions. Spinal–dural arteriovenous malformations and fistulas can cause similar symptoms but usually produce a myelopathy rather than a radiculopathy.

Neoplastic
Bone and Intraspinal Tumors. Bony metastases may occur from lymphoma, lung, breast, or prostate cancer. Primary spinal tumors include chordomas, neurofibromas, meningiomas, lipomas, astrocytomas, and ependymomas, although these are very rare. Differentiated on CT, myelography, or MRI.

Congenital
Scoliosis, Spondylolysis (Defect in the Pars Interarticularis) Causing Spondylolisthesis, Achondroplasia. Developmental causes of stenosis. Seen on physical examination or radiographic studies.

Acquired
Iatrogenic Radiculopathy. (e.g., postlaminectomy failed back syndrome, post fusion, arachnoiditis.) History of surgery. May require radiographic evaluation to diagnose.

Other

Spondylolisthesis. Slippage of one vertebrae on another, which may cause radicular symptoms with activity. Palpable step-off on palpation of the spine; seen on spine x-ray.

TREATMENT

Medical. The degenerative process of spinal stenosis is irreversible, so medical treatment is usually palliative. Conservative treatment does not slow the progression of spinal stenosis, but may control symptoms and enable the patient to delay or avoid surgery in selected cases.

Conservative treatment includes:

Bedrest (because symptoms are insidious, this is usually reserved for acute, severe flares of back pain and is only recommended for no more than 2 to 3 days)

Physical therapy, which helps to strengthen the paravertebral and abdominal muscles that support the spine

Drug therapy, including NSAIDs, analgesics, or muscle relaxants

Lumbar epidural steroid injections, which involve local injection of a steroid and anesthetic agent such as methylprednisolone and bupivacaine into the epidural space or at various trigger points; risks include CSF leak ("wet tap"), epidural abscess, or hematoma formation

Lumbosacral orthoses such as corsets or braces for patients with low-grade spondylolisthesis and back pain

Surgical. The procedure most commonly performed for severe lumbar stenosis is a decompressive lumbar laminectomy. Stabilization procedures (fusion) may be required in high-grade spondylolisthesis. Through a vertical midline incision, the spinous processes and lamina are removed. A foraminotomy is used to decompress the exiting nerve roots. If a fusion is necessary, it is performed by placing iliac crest autograft between and over the transverse process and supplementing the autograft with instrumented fixation such as pedicle screws and rods or plates, creating a solid construct.

Indications. Urgent surgical intervention is necessary when acute severe neurologic deficits present, such as a foot drop or cauda equina syndrome (mentioned above). Indications for elective decompression include intolerable pain despite conservative measures or slowly progressing neurologic deficit.

Contraindications. Poor surgical candidate because of severe medical illness. Low back pain as the predominant symptom. Imaging studies that show only mild to moderate stenosis.

TECHNIQUE OF SURGICAL ASSISTING

As in any neurosurgical procedure, it is of the utmost importance to protect the neural structures at all times. Exposure and keeping the area clear of debris is one of the important tasks of the assistant. Many times one is working in very small areas of exposure, so fine, calculated movements are necessary.

PEDIATRIC CONSIDERATIONS

Not applicable.

OBSTETRICAL CONSIDERATIONS

No surgical treatment during pregnancy. Use caution in performing x-rays and prescribing analgesics.

PEARLS FOR THE PA

Degenerative lumbar spinal stenosis refers to an age-related narrowing of the lumbosacral spinal canal, causing symptoms of neurogenic claudication.

The mainstay of successful elective surgical treatment is proper patient selection. Best results occur in patients with symptoms of true neurogenic claudication (pain), positive neurologic examination findings, and solid imaging findings to support the diagnosis.

Strains, Sprains, and Tendon Injuries
Richard E. Donnelly, PA-C, BS, BS

DEFINITION

Strain. Minimal injury of acute stress to a ligament, muscle, or tendon.

Sprain. Micro tear, partial tear, or complete tear of one or more ligaments around a joint. Classified as grades I through III. Grade I is a micro tear of a ligament without instability; grade II is a partial tear of a ligament that may or may not have some degree of joint instability or widening; and grade III is a complete tear of ligaments about a joint with resultant instability or widening of the joint.

Tendon Dysfunction. The inability of the tendon muscle complex to function. This is due to elongation or rupture of the tendon, decreasing its ability to pull on the bone attachment.

HISTORY

Symptoms. Ordinarily, there is a complaint of pain, swelling, and bruising localized to the involved tissue.

General. Many joints are affected by sprains and strains with relative frequency. These include the ankle, fingers, wrist, elbow, shoulder, and knee. Defining the mechanism of injury should allow prediction of the location and nature of the injury. Usually, the patient is involved with some sort of physical activity. The mechanism of injury is most often a twisting-type action about the joint involved. The symptoms are consistent with the severity of injury and should be graded as best possible. Chronic tendon dysfunction has an insidious onset with progressive symptoms.

Age. Occur at a greater frequency in the ages between the second and forth decade, but may occur at any age. Chronic tendon dysfunction occurs in the older age groups, usually beginning in the fifth decade.

Duration. Duration of injury varies according to severity of injury. Mild injuries of strains improve over a 1- to 2-week period, whereas complete tears may take 6 to 8 weeks to heal.

Intensity. The intensity varies from mild to severe, depending on the severity of injury and area of injury.

Aggravating Factors. Continued activity or use of the injured part increases pain and swelling of acute injuries. Weight-bearing activity on lower extremities increases injury and symptoms.

Alleviating Factors. Conservative treatment improves symptoms. Immobilization may be necessary to alleviate symptoms.

Associated Factors. Certain metabolic diseases and medications may predispose or place individuals at a greater risk of ligament or tendon injury. Patients with rheumatoid arthritis and other connective tissue diseases are at higher risk than the normal population. Fluoroquinolones and the corticosteroid class of drugs also put patients at risk.

PHYSICAL EXAMINATION

General. Early, careful observation and documentation of distal neurovascular function are vital. Circulatory function should be assessed by examining capillary fill and peripheral pulses. Both sensory and motor function of the major peripheral nerves should be tested.

Orthopedic. Observation of the injured limb is important in order to note any obvious deformity, edema, or discoloration. The injured limb is compared to the contralateral limb in order to note subtle differences that may exist. Palpation of regional anatomy should be performed and individual structures tested, with attention to local tenderness, crepitation, deformity, or swelling. Point tenderness localizes the area of injury. Stability of the joint can be tested with a drawer test or stress test of the ligament involved. The drawer sign is the subluxation of a joint with anterior and posterior stress applied to the bones that make up the joint. The stress test is medial or lateral stress applied to the joint, looking for joint opening or widening. These tests may need to be compared with the opposite limb to check for reliability.

PATHOPHYSIOLOGY

Soft-tissue injury about a joint occurs from a sudden increase in force, long-standing receptive load, degenerative changes of tissue, or a combination of these factors. A sudden increase in force across a joint that is beyond the ability of tissue to adjust to or stress that causes the tissue to give way, producing a fracture, ligament tear, or tendon injury. A long-standing reparative force over time will cause fatigue of the tissue, causing micro tears which, with continued force and time, progress to complete tears or stress fractures, as seen in endurance sports. Degenerative changes that develop with age and certain conditions such as connective tissue diseases predispose tendons and ligaments to become weak and tear.

DIAGNOSTIC STUDIES

Laboratory
ESR, Rheumatoid Factor. As evaluation for connective tissue disease, as indicated.
Radiology
X-ray. Plain AP, lateral, and oblique views are minimum and help rule out avulsion or stress fractures. Joint widening or irregularities may be seen as well. Stress views of the involved joint also may show instability and joint widening, which indicates complete tear and disruption of the joint ligaments.
MRI. May be helpful if plain films are nonspecific and partial or tendon and ligament tears are suspected.

DIFFERENTIAL DIAGNOSIS

Traumatic
Fractures. Including avulsion or stress fractures or osteochondral injuries of the joints. Ruled out on x-ray.
Infectious
Infection. Any chronic soft-tissue swelling inflammation should raise the suspicion of infection. WBC, ESR may be elevated.
Metabolic
Connective Tissue Disease. History of chronic inflammation, early morning joint stiffness, pain, and swelling. May have elevated ESR or positive antinuclear antibody or rheumatoid factor.
Gout, Pseudogout. Periodic, acute attacks of joint swelling and pain without history of a specific injury. Elevated serum uric acid levels with gout.

Neoplastic
Tumors. Soft-tissue tumors, nodules, or lumps (e.g., edema) without history of trauma or injury should be suspicious of neoplastic disease. Confirmed on radiographic studies.

Acquired
Ganglion Cyst, Joint Effusion. May be due to degenerative joint disease. Differentiated on physical examination.

TREATMENT

Medical. Proper initial management includes protection or immobilization of any significant ligament injury. Acutely, RICE (**R**est, **I**ce, **C**ompression, **E**levation) for the initial 1 to 2 days in mild injury may be all that is required. In more severe injuries, immobilization or nonweight bearing for 2 to 3 weeks may be necessary, with up to 6 weeks of treatment required. Early mobilization is indicated with some injuries and in conditioned athletes. For chronic conditions, stabilizing braces or orthoses may be necessary to stabilize and provide functional use.

Surgical. Most injuries do not require surgical intervention. Those injuries or conditions that leave the joint unstable may require surgical repair. Ligament reattachment, ligament reinforcement, and tendon repair or transfer are all procedures used for treatment.

Indications. Joint instability in the patient in whom there are high demands for the joint (e.g., competitive athletes).

Contraindications. Inadequate conservative therapy, inability to undergo anesthesia, and relative in those patients in whom there is not a high demand for the joint.

TECHNIQUE OF SURGICAL ASSISTING

Maintaining tension on ligaments and tendons during repair and providing adequate exposure are the primary roles of the PA.

PEDIATRIC CONSIDERATIONS

Always rule out growth plate injuries by using comparison x-rays. Treatment is the same as in adults.

OBSTETRICAL CONSIDERATIONS

No surgical treatment during pregnancy. Use caution in performing x-rays and prescribing analgesics.

PEARLS FOR THE PA

Rest, ice, compression, and elevation (RICE) is the mainstay of therapy.

It is best to refrain from using injectable steroids due to the weakening effect on the ligaments and tendons.

Sprains: Achilles Tendon Rupture

Richard E. Donnelly, PA-C, BS, BS

DEFINITION

Tear in the Achilles tendon, an overuse syndrome, which may be partial or complete. It is believed to be the result of both tendon degeneration and mechanical overload.

HISTORY

Symptoms. Acute onset of pain and inability to step off is the hallmark. May be accompanied by an audible snap. Swelling and ecchymosis may occur in the distal aspect of the leg and posterior aspect of the ankle over the next 1 to 2 hours. There is difficulty with ambulation, inability to ascend stairs or stand on tip-toes, with complaints of weakness.

General. Achilles tendon rupture, a common overuse injury in athletes (especially weekend athletes), is more often associated with the left heel cord. It is usually the result of an indirect trauma that occurred while performing some sort of sports activity, with no pre-existing symptoms. A typical history is a middle-aged man employed in a white-collar profession who reports that he felt sudden pain in his calf while playing a sport.

Age. Men in their third through fifth decades of life are more often affected.

Onset. Most often acute. Some patients may have prerupture symptoms of progressive pain (peritendinitis), especially in athletes who have overtrained (overuse injury). The early symptoms of local tenderness or burning pain are experienced after strenuous sports activities. Later, symptoms start when exercise commences. As the condition becomes more chronic, the local tenderness increases and the pain is caused by increasingly less activity. In advanced stages, the pain occurs with activities of daily living or at rest.

Duration. Most ruptures will take up to 6 to 8 weeks to heal. Chronic rupture, if left untreated, may require reconstructive surgery and Achilles tendon lengthening, and takes longer to heal.

Aggravating Factors. Continued activity, going up stairs or inclines.

Alleviating Factors. Rest, elevation, and no ambulation combined with early treatment.

Associated Factors. Systemic diseases, such as rheumatoid arthritis, systemic lupus erythematous, primary and secondary hyperparathyroidism, hyperlipidemia, gout, and diabetes mellitus. Long-term oral corticosteroid use in an older population predisposes patients to a relative increased risk of nontraumatic rupture. Fluoroquinolone therapy (pefloxacin, ofloxacin, ciprofloxacin, enoxacin) has been associated with peritendinitis of the Achilles tendon. A history of local corticosteroid injection of the Achilles tendon may have a deleterious effect on the tendon and may predispose it to rupture.

PHYSICAL EXAMINATION

General. The patient may present in significant distress with an acute rupture. The neurovascular status of the foot is evaluated by checking the posterior nerve and artery, as well as the peroneal nerve. Rupture of the gastrocnemius soleus complex and tibialis posterior tendon must be evaluated.

Orthopedic. The patient is examined lying in a prone position with the feet extended off the examination table. A visual defect may be seen in the distal aspect of the Achilles tendon if edema has not concealed it. A palpable defect also is noted approximately 2 to 6 cm proximal to the insertion of the tendon on the posterior calcaneus. Partial Achilles tendon ruptures may be seen with pain, weakness, swelling, and bruising but without a palpable defect. With a complete rupture, patients are unable to perform a single heel rise test. This test is done by having the patient stand on the affected foot while holding the opposite foot off the ground and trying to rise up on the tip toes of the affected foot. The Thompson-Doherty squeeze test is positive. This test is performed while the patient is still on the examination table. The examiner squeezes the patient's calf muscles of the affected leg while observing the foot; if the foot does not plantar flex or move, this indicates a positive test, because if the tendon is intact the foot will plantar flex with this maneuver. To confirm a questionable squeeze test, results are compared with the opposite leg.

PATHOPHYSIOLOGY

The mechanism of Achilles tendon injury results when the patient pushes off with the weight-bearing forefoot while extending the knee (e.g., at the start of a sprint); experiences sudden, unexpected dorsiflexion of the ankle (such as when slipping on a stair or ladder); or suffers violent dorsiflexion of the plantar-flexed foot (such as when falling from a height). No true synovial sheath surrounds the tendon, but there is an outer covering of areolar connective tissue in which elastic fibers are interposed, known as the peritenon. Peritenon surrounds the tendon, which is continuous proximally with the fascial envelope of the muscle and blends with the periosteum of the calcaneus. The proximal muscle and the distal insertion are well supplied with vessels, which decrease in number toward the tendon segment that is more prone to rupture.

Two theories are suggested to explain the cause of Achilles tendon rupture, one of tendon degeneration and another of mechanical overload. In the clinical setting of rupture, both sets of factors usually are involved. In some patients with complete rupture, preceding symptoms of pain, swelling, and warmth of a variable period suggest a role for inflammation.

DIAGNOSTIC STUDIES

Laboratory
CBC, Full Chemistry Profile, PT, PTT. As routine preoperative screen.
Radiology
Ankle X-ray. Are rarely necessary to establish the diagnosis of ruptured Achilles tendon.
MRI. Distinguishes inflammation, degeneration, and incomplete or complete tendon ruptures. Because of the high water content, the normal Achilles tendon is seen as a dark band, easily differentiated from surrounding tissue. With tendon rupture a visible discontinuity of the tendon is seen, with thickening of more than 6 mm at the ends in the anteroposterior plane. Incomplete rupture shows thickening of the tendon with structural changes longitudinally and horizontally within the tendon.
Ultrasonography. Readily depicts pathologic changes in tendons that clearly differ from healthy, asymptomatic tendons or central tendon degeneration.

DIFFERENTIAL DIAGNOSIS

Traumatic
Other Tendon or Ligament Injury. Such as severe ankle sprain, tibialis posterior tendon dysfunction or rupture, and medial gastrocnemius tear. Negative examination findings for Achilles tendon rupture.
Infectious. Not applicable.
Metabolic. Not applicable.
Neoplastic. Not applicable.
Vascular. Not applicable.
Congenital. Not applicable.
Acquired. Not applicable.

TREATMENT

Medical. Achilles tendon ruptures can be treated nonsurgically in the nonathletic or low-end recreational athletic patient, particularly those over 50 years of age. Nonoperative treatment usually involves a long-leg cast for a period of 4 weeks, then a short-leg cast for a period of 8 weeks. The foot is placed in a plantar-flexed position to allow good approximation of the tendon ends, and the foot is progressively dorsiflexed over a period of time with cast changes of 2-week intervals. Following cast immobilization, a supervised physical therapy program with progressive dorsiflexion and strengthening of the muscle groups involved is recommended for several months.

Surgical. Surgical repair can be technically difficult because the tendon usually does not rupture in a clean fashion, but more often shows multiple shredded ends. For this reason, there is no single accepted technique. Percutaneous repair or open primary repair may be used with or without augmented tendon or fascia reinforcement. A thorough understanding of the anatomy of the surgical approach is necessary in order to avoid problems with skin, neurovascular structures, and so that the ends of the tendon have adequate apposition. Complications of surgical treatment include skin and tendon necrosis, wound infection, and nerve damage. Rehabilitation occurs over a period of several months. With use of a TheraBand (elastic band), early progressive strengthening and stretching exercise activities are begun. Active and passive range-of-motion exercises of the ankle are taught to the patient. The patient is progressively advanced to weights and may also use a Cybex machine for testing strength, power, and endurance of the calf muscles. Completely ruptured tendons that have been surgically repaired have significantly more muscle power than those treated nonsurgically.

It is recommended that the foot be placed in the neutral position within 1 week to 10 days after surgery to achieve the positive results of tension.

Indications. Surgical repair is the treatment of choice for those patients who are young and athletic, providing the treating physician does not delay diagnosis and treatment (less than 1 week, and preferably less than 48 hours).

Contraindications. Inactive patients (relative), inability to tolerate anesthesia.

TECHNIQUE OF SURGICAL ASSISTING

Traction is maintained on the ruptured tendon ends during repair. Handling of the tissues is done with gentle pressure as to the placement of forceps and retractors to avoid further tissue trauma. Care is taken with skin closure, to allow good approximation of the skin edges without excessive tension on the wound edges and to prevent skin necrosis.

PEDIATRIC CONSIDERATIONS

Always rule out growth plate injuries by using comparison x-rays. Treatment is the same as in adults.

OBSTETRICAL CONSIDERATIONS

No surgical treatment during pregnancy. Use caution in performing x-rays and prescribing analgesics.

PEARLS FOR THE PA

The hallmark of Achilles tendon rupture is acute pain and the inability to perform a single heel raise test (step-off).

Conservative therapy may be used for the inactive patient.

Sprains: Acromioclavicular Injuries
John W. Bullock, PA-C, BA, BS

DEFINITION

Traumatic injury to the acromioclavicular joint of the shoulder.

HISTORY

Symptoms. Pain and decreased range of motion of the shoulder.

General. Most commonly caused by a direct fall on the point of the shoulder with the arm adducted at the side. History should be directed to determining the mechanism of injury and level of postinjury performance.

Age. Any, but most frequent in second decade of life. Male : female ratio, 5 : 1.

Onset. Acute, traumatic.

Duration. Varies, based on severity. Type I: generally recover full

---

The views expressed in this material are those of the author and do not reflect the official policy or position of the United States Government, the Department of Defense, or the Department of the Air Force.

range of motion and have no pain within 2 weeks; type II: most recover fully, with some having residual pain and stiffness for up to 5 years.

Intensity. Varies.

Aggravating Factors. Occupational demands on shoulder. Low-demand patient (e.g., an office worker) has a better long-term prognosis than a heavy laborer.

Alleviating Factors. None.

Associated Factors. None.

PHYSICAL EXAMINATION

General. Observation of the contour of the shoulders with patient seated. Look both anteriorly and from above so that anteroposterior displacement can be assessed.

Orthopedic. Palpate the entire clavicle for areas of tenderness or soft-tissue deficiency. If there is obvious subluxation or dislocation, carefully assess motion in the anteroposterior plane. Support the arm to see if there is spontaneous reduction of the acromioclavicular joint.

Assess the neurovascular status of the arm by palpating distal pulses and evaluating motor and sensory function (Table 9–4).

PATHOPHYSIOLOGY

This injury usually occurs when the patient falls with arm adducted, striking the shoulder against the ground or a wall, causing a displacement of the scapula in relation to the clavicle. The clavicle remains in its normal anatomic position, whereas the scapula and shoulder girdle are driven inferiorly.

Acromioclavicular injuries are actually a continuum of ligament injuries, beginning with injury to only the acromioclavicular ligaments (type I). As the force is increased, the injury extends to the coracoclavicular ligaments (type II), followed by the deltoid and trapezius musculature (type III), until, ultimately, the overlying fascia or even the skin over the acromioclavicular joint can be torn (see Table 9–4).

DIAGNOSTIC STUDIES

Laboratory

CBC, Full Chemistry Profile, PT, PTT. As routine preoperative screen.

Radiology

Acromioclavicular X-ray. Two views are routine: (1) AP view with 10 to 15 degrees cephalic tilt (Zanca view), if possible both shoulders should be imaged simultaneously on one large (14 × 17) cassette; (2) axillary lateral. Stress views are optional and should be used only for patients with suspected type III injuries so that they can be differentiated from the lesser type II injuries. These views are not necessary to diagnose types IV, V, or VI (see Table 9–4).

AP stress view: same as aforementioned AP view, except that weights (10 to 15 lbs) are suspended from each arm with wrist straps. The weights should not be held by the patient.

Lateral stress view (Alexander or shoulder forward view): Patient set up as for scapular lateral (Y) view, except both shoulders are thrust forward.

DIFFERENTIAL DIAGNOSIS

Traumatic
Glenohumeral Dislocation. Rule out with axillary, lateral x-ray.
Rotator Cuff Injury. Positive drop arm test (see topic rotator cuff).
Infectious. Not applicable.
Metabolic
Bursitis. X-ray negative for fracture. Bursa tenderness.
Neoplastic
Tumor. Affecting the shoulder joint or brachial plexus may cause reduction in shoulder motion.
Vascular. Not applicable.
Congenital. Not applicable.
Acquired. Not applicable.

TREATMENT

The optimum treatment is controversial and varies greatly between different authors and different communities. The classification system, based on underlying pathoanatomy, is crucial to determining appropriate treatment (see Table 9–4).

Medical. None.
Surgical. There are two major approaches for acute injuries—acromioclavicular joint fixation and coracoclavicular fixation.

Acromioclavicular Joint Fixation. Is accomplished using some type of pin fixation that crosses the joint. Various techniques are used. The advantages are easy exposure, fixation can be used if coracoid fracture is present, and anteroposterior displacement can be controlled. The disadvantage is that of pin breakage or migration (if the pin breaks, it usually does so at the level of the joint, thereby necessitating redisruption of the joint surface for removal).

Coracoclavicular Fixation. Is the more popular procedure and is accomplished more commonly by the insertion of a screw from the distal clavicle into the base of the coracoid process. It can also be done using a cerclage technique with wire, synthetic tape, or autogenous tendon or fascia wrapped around the clavicle and beneath the coracoid process. The

Table 9–4. Types, Pathoanatomy, and Presentation of Acromioclavicular Injuries

Type	Pathoanatomy	Presentation	Treatment
Type I	Sprain of acromioclavicular (AC) ligament AC joint intact	Tenderness to palpation at AC joint; no deformity Mild pain with shoulder range of motion (ROM)	Ice; protect until painless, full ROM (usually around 2 weeks) Surgery: Not indicated Prognosis: Excellent
Type II	AC ligaments torn AC joint subluxated and widened slightly; may have *slight* vertical separation Coracoclavicular (CC) ligaments sprained	Moderate to severe pain at AC joint to palpation and with shoulder ROM Outer end of clavicle may be slightly superior to acromion	Can splint but good results with "skillful neglect": sling 10–14 days or until comfortable, then rehabilitation Avoid heavy lifting or contact sports for 8–12 weeks Surgery: not indicated acutely Prognosis: good—some long–term problems
Type III	AC joint dislocated Clavicle relatively displaced upward CC ligaments torn CC interspace *25%–100% > normal shoulder* Deltoid and trapezius muscles torn and detached from distal end of clavicle	Arm adducted against body and supported to relieve pain in AC joint Shoulder complex is depressed Distal clavicle may tent the skin superiorly Pain with ROM, especially abduction	Early surgical repair dependent on level of activity Indicated in patients with (1) extreme prominence of distal clavicle, (2) who do heavy work, or (3) frequent or prolonged overhead work Otherwise "skillful neglect" Procedure: AC repairs vs. CC repairs Prognosis: depends on activity level
Type IV	Type III plus clavicle anatomically displaced posteriorly into or through the trapezius muscle	Like type III but examination of seated patient from above shows that the clavicle is inclined posteriorly compared with the uninjured shoulder	If distal clavicle can be manipulated out of the trapezius muscle it may be treated closed followed by figure-of-eight bandage. Otherwise, surgical reduction and repair is necessary

Table 9–4. Types, Pathoanatomy, and Presentation of
Acromioclavicular Injuries (*Continued*)

Type	Pathoanatomy	Presentation	Treatment
			Procedure: open reduction/internal fixation (ORIF) if seen early Prognosis: poor if left displaced
Type V	Type III plus gross disparity between clavicle and scapula CC interspace between *100%–300% > normal shoulder* Deltoid and trapezius detached from the distal half of clavicle	Like an exaggerated type III: the distal end of the clavicle appears to be grossly superiorly displaced towards the base of the neck More pain than Type III, especially over distal half of clavicle due to muscle and soft tissue disruption	Surgical repair (ORIF) Prognosis: poor if not treated
Type VI	AC joint dislocated and clavicle displaced inferior to the acromion or coracoid process CC interspace is reversed in subcoracoid type or decreased in subacromial type	Superior aspect of the shoulder is flattened Acromion is prominent and there is a step-down to the superior surface of the coracoid on palpation Swelling from associated injuries may mask contours	Open reduction and internal fixation Prognosis: must be reduced

goal is to restore anatomic relationships to allow the ligaments to heal, or to overcorrect and fuse the clavicle to the coracoid.

Indications. If the distal acromion is very prominent, the patient is a heavy laborer, if occupation demands repeated use of the arm with the shoulder abducted or flexed to 90 degrees, if the clavicle is unreducible, closed, or if rupture of the coracoclavicular ligament is associated with a distal clavicle fracture.

Contraindications. If none of above conditions are met, the patient will probably do worse with surgery, even if anatomic reduction is achieved. Surgery may be deferred on noncompliant patients because failure of fixation devices is possible if activity is not controlled and rehabilitation protocols are not followed postoperatively.

TECHNIQUE OF SURGICAL ASSISTING

Familiarity with the use of fixation screws is important. Exposure, gentle traction to avoid injury to the subclavicular vessels and nerves, and assisting with fixation are primary roles of the PA.

PEDIATRIC CONSIDERATIONS

Distal clavicle fractures in children and adolescents under age 15 years are actually fractures through the physis and, therefore, are pseudodislocations rather than a true acromioclavicular separation. All heal without functional sequelae but, for severe displacement, surgical reduction with internal fixation is indicated for cosmetic reasons. Fixation may be removed in 4 to 6 weeks and rehabilitation started.

OBSTETRICAL CONSIDERATIONS

Consult obstetrics and anesthesia if surgery is necessary. Use caution in performing x-rays and prescribing analgesics.

PEARLS FOR THE PA

Request radiographs of the acromioclavicular joint rather than the shoulder. The acromioclavicular joint requires one third to one half the x-ray penetration required for the glenohumeral joint, so films using the shoulder technique will be overpenetrated (dark) and small fractures may be overlooked.

Sprains: Ankle
Richard E. Donnelly, PA-C, BS, BS

DEFINITION

A complete or partial disruption of ligamentous structures around or about the ankle joint. This includes medial and lateral aspects of the ankle, as well as interosseous connections between the tibia and fibula. Ankle sprains are usually categorized as minor ligamentous injuries (grade I), incomplete ligamentous tears (grade II), complete disruption of the ligaments and high ankle sprain disruption of the interosseous ligament (grade III).

HISTORY

Symptoms. Patients with an ankle sprain describe a popping or tearing sensation in the ankle. Occasionally, there is an audible noise. Frequently, they remember only pain and loss of support. Pain and swelling occur immediately following the injury. Depending on the severity, typically those patients with grade II or grade III injuries have difficulty weight bearing or walking on the injured ankle, although this is not always the case.

General. The injuries occur during running, while cutting, or landing from a jump (usually from landing on another athlete's foot). Patients who can remember describe an inversion, plantar flexion, or internal rotation mechanism. The mechanism of injury must be ascertained (e.g., inversion or eversion), as well as the type of activity engaged in at time of injury.

Age. Ankle sprains may occur in all ages, but occur most often in the second to fourth decades of life in active individuals.

Onset. Sudden inversion or eversion of the ankle while engaged in some type of running or jumping activity.

Duration. Six to eight weeks if treated adequately.

Aggravating Factors. Continued activity on the injured extremity or return to activity before healing is complete.

Alleviating Factors. Nonweight bearing, elevation, ice, and compression of injured ankle.

Associated Factors. High ankle injuries or syndesmotic injuries must be ruled out on all ankle sprains. The syndesmosis is the ligamentous complex between the tibia and fibula that stabilizes the ankle and maintains the integrity of the mortise. If injured, widening of the mortise occurs, and instability of this complex ensues. Pain that continues beyond the expected 6 to 8 weeks of healing time or extends into the anterodistal leg between the tibia and fibula should cause suspicion of a high ankle sprain.

PHYSICAL EXAMINATION

General. The patient may appear in relatively acute distress, guarding the involved ankle. Neurovascular status must be evaluated distal to the injury.

Orthopedic. Ecchymosis and swelling are likely to be present at the time of initial examination and may be found distal to the area of injury. Palpation over the injured ligament elicits point tenderness, with generalized low-grade tenderness in the surrounding area. The majority of time the ankle is limited in dorsiflexion, plantar flexion, and inversion/eversion. An anterior drawer sign usually is positive with complete ruptures, grades II and III. Meticulous examination with fingertip palpation of all structures potentially involved in an ankle sprain often leads the examiner to the correct clinical diagnosis. With thorough examination, one may find involvement of the peroneal or posterior tibial tendons. Avulsion or hairline fractures of the fibula, tibia, calcaneus, fifth metatarsal, cuboid, or talus and subtle neurologic injuries can also be detected. With medial ankle sprains, the examiner must exclude syndesmotic injury, lateral ligamentous injury, and high fibular fractures or proximal tibiofibular joint injury. Patients with syndesmotic injuries have well-localized anterolateral ankle pain located over the anterior syndesmosis of the ankle and are more precisely localized than in cases of severe lateral ankle sprains.

PATHOPHYSIOLOGY

The lateral ligamentous complex of the ankle consists of three ligaments: the anterior talofibular, the calcaneofibular, and the posterior talofibular. The medial ligamentous complex consists of the medial collateral ligaments, a strong fan-shaped or deltoid-shaped ligament complex that provides stability to the medial talocrural joint. The stability of the ankle is tied together by the interosseous ligament between the tibia and fibula, known as the syndesmotic complex. The most common ligament disruption involves the anterior talofibular ligament. Most are midsubstance tears, but avulsion of the talus and fibula can occur. The second most common injury is a combination rupture of the anterior talofibular and calcaneofibular ligaments. The medial ankle complex and syndesmotic complex are the least common ligamentous injuries.

DIAGNOSTIC STUDIES

Laboratory
CBC, Full Chemistry Profile, PT, PTT. As routine preoperative screen.

Radiology
Ankle X-rays. Three views are preferred: AP, lateral, and mortise. Stress views show integrity of the ligament structures and of ankle mortise.
MRI. To confirm an acute deltoid ligament tear.

Other
Arthrography. To confirm an acute deltoid ligament tear.

DIFFERENTIAL DIAGNOSIS

Traumatic
Ankle Fractures. Seen on ankle x-ray.
Tendon Ruptures. Such as the posterior tibial and peroneal tendons. Differentiated on physical examination.

Infectious
Infection of the Joint. Must be ruled out when swelling of the ankle is present with or without pain and with no history of specific trauma.

Metabolic

Gout and Pseudogout.   Periodic, acute attacks of joint swelling and pain without history of a specific injury. Elevated serum uric acid levels with gout.

Neoplastic.   Not applicable.

Vascular

Deep Vein Thrombosis.   Regardless of the severity of injury, prolonged swelling must be investigated with vascular studies, especially if it occurs above the ankle.

Congenital.   Not applicable.

Acquired.   Not applicable.

TREATMENT

Medical.   Nonoperative treatment is the mainstay for the vast majority of ankle sprains. This initially consists of rest, ice, compression, and elevation (RICE). Traditionally, grade I and II injuries get excellent results with this form of treatment. Conservative treatment is also indicated for most cases of grade III ankle sprains, which may require cast immobilization for a 3- to 6-week period in addition to RICE. Mobilization is begun, usually when pain and swelling have improved. An elastic brace, lace-up brace, plastic stirrup brace, or taping is used for protection during this period. During this time, the patient is allowed to bear weight as tolerated, based on swelling and discomfort. Crutches and assisting aids are discontinued as soon as the patient can tolerate their absence. The next phase involves physical therapy with range-of-motion exercises, peroneal strengthening, and Achilles tendon strengthening. Once pain and swelling allow, proprioceptive training with wobble board, tilt board, or mini-trampoline is instituted. Ankle protection is required for approximately 3 to 4 weeks longer for unstable injuries.

Treatment of deltoid ligament injuries depends on the associated injuries. If the fibula is fractured and reduced and is stable or the syndesmosis is reduced and stabilized, there is no need to repair the deltoid. Casting these injuries for 8 to 10 weeks typically results in sufficient healing of the deltoid. The previously mentioned mobilization phases can be instituted. Treatment of acute stable syndesmosis injuries must be taken care of quickly, while arranging studies for proper diagnosis. This includes the RICE formula, then casting for 8 to 10 weeks.

Surgical.   If frank diastasis with or without fracture is evident, the patient is taken to the operating room as soon as the soft-tissue swelling allows for open reduction and internal fixation, if necessary.

Indications.   Acute repair in athletes is recommended if there is a history of mementary talocrural dislocation with complete ligamentous disruption, the presence of a clinical anterior drawer sign, a stress inversion test with 10 degrees or more of tilt on the affected side, or clinical or presence of an osteochondral fracture. Widening of the mortise is also indication for repair.

Contraindications. Inadequate trial of conservative therapy.

TECHNIQUE OF SURGICAL ASSISTING

Exposure, traction during repair, immobilization, and postoperative follow up are primary roles of the PA.

PEDIATRIC CONSIDERATIONS

Always rule out growth plate injuries by using comparison x-rays. Treatment is the same as in adults.

OBSTETRICAL CONSIDERATIONS

No surgical treatment during pregnancy. Use caution in performing x-rays and prescribing analgesics.

PEARLS FOR THE PA

Ankle sprains are the most common injury in sports.

Rest, ice, compression, and elevation (RICE) is the mainstay of treatment.

Rule out associated fracture (e.g., fibula).

Sprains: Biceps Tendon Ruptures
John W. Bullock, PA-C, BA, BS

DEFINITION

Disruption of either the proximal (long head) or distal (at the bicipital tuberosity of the radius) tendinous attachments of the biceps.

HISTORY

Symptoms. For proximal tears of the long head, the patient feels something snap in the shoulder. When the arm is observed, an unfamiliar lump is seen that soon becomes ecchymotic from subcutaneous bleeding. For distal ruptures, the patient may have acute pain in the antecubital fossa associated with ecchymosis and swelling, along with moderate weakness of elbow flexion and more marked weakness of supination.

General. 97% of biceps tendon ruptures are proximal (at the shoulder) and 3% are distal.

Age. Proximal (long head): middle aged (35 years) and older. Distal: young adult to active middle aged. Males more affected than females.

Onset. Proximal: usually involves minimal trauma. Sudden "pop" in shoulder. Distal: sudden, during force overload with elbow in mid flexion.

Duration. Proximal: most improved by 2 to 3 weeks; strength returns in 8 to 12 weeks. Distal: see surgical repair below.

Intensity. Variable.

Aggravating Factors. History of prior symptoms, steroid injections.

Alleviating Factors. Time.

Associated Factors. Rotator cuff tears. Proximal: associated with subacromial impingement and is often attritional.

PHYSICAL EXAMINATION

General. The patient may present in acute pain with guarding of the elbow.

Orthopedic. In proximal (long head) tears, as the muscle belly contracts unopposed, it forms a firm ball of muscle in the lower part of the upper arm (the "Popeye sign").

PATHOPHYSIOLOGY

Proximal. Can be the end result of chronic biceps tendinitis (which is often secondary to impingement).

Distal. Sudden overload with forearm supinated and elbow in partial flexion.

DIAGNOSTIC STUDIES

Laboratory

CBC, Full Chemistry Profile, PT, PTT. As routine preoperative screen.

Radiology

MRI. Can demonstrate the ruptured tendon (however, the diagnosis of both proximal and distal injuries is primarily made clinically).

DIFFERENTIAL DIAGNOSIS

The sudden onset, history, and characteristic appearance are diagnostic.

TREATMENT

Medical. Generally, long head of the biceps tendon ruptures need no intervention apart from reassurance and explanation. The short head of the biceps hypertrophies to compensate. Function and movement of the shoulder is minimally affected.

Surgical. Distal ruptures require surgical repair to reattach the tendon to the radial tuberosity. This is most often done using a two-incision (Boyd-Anderson) technique. Postoperatively, the elbow is immobilized in flexion and supination for 6 to 8 weeks.

Indications. Distal tendon rupture.

Contraindications. None unique to this condition.

TECHNIQUE OF SURGICAL ASSISTING

The PA assists with the reanastomosis of the tendon to the radial tuberosity and with immobilization and follow-up postoperatively.

PEDIATRIC CONSIDERATIONS

Not applicable.

OBSTETRICAL CONSIDERATIONS

Distal ruptures require repair. Consult obstetrics and anesthesia. Use caution in performing x-rays and prescribing analgesics.

PEARLS FOR THE PA

When a patient presents with a long head of the biceps tendon rupture, the issue of least concern is elbow weakness.

Most proximal biceps ruptures are associated with shoulder pathology and, if suspicious, additional tests should be made to assess the adequacy and integrity of the rotator cuff.

A high percentage of patients who present with a spontaneous rupture of the long head of the biceps tendon have an associated rotator cuff tear.

Sprains: Digits

Richard E. Donnelly, PA-C, BS, BS

DEFINITION

Soft-tissue injuries of digits can involve jammed fingers, sprains, ligament tears, dislocations, subluxations, and avulsion fractures. The injuries may be subtle and unrecognized by the practitioner.

HISTORY

Symptoms. Pain, swelling, and deformity.

General. Injuries to the digits of the hand are caused by a blow to the end of the finger by upward, twisting, or side-to-side force. This usually occurs when the patient is engaged in some sport activity, with a higher incidence with sports that use some type of ball. Avulsions may occur with heavy lifting or when the patient forcibly grasps an object (e.g., the shirt of a fellow football player). Crush injuries may result in lacerations of tendons that cause progressive deformities. With job-related injuries, a careful history as to place, time, and how the injury occurred is important. Document the dominant hand and any pre-existing limitations or abnormalities of the hands. Note a history of systemic diseases (e.g., rheumatoid arthritis) or medication use (e.g., prednisone).

Age. Any, but occurs more often in the teens to mid to late thirties. More frequent in males than females.

Onset. Sudden onset with initiation of injury.

Duration. The injury may take 1 to 6 weeks or longer to heal with proper treatment.

Intensity. Depends on injury.

Aggravating Factors. Continued activity, improper treatment, prone to reinjury.

Alleviating Factors. Reduction of dislocation and immobilization.

Associated Factors. Rheumatoid arthritis and other connective tissue diseases.

PHYSICAL EXAMINATION

General. Neurovascular status must always be assessed by capillary refill, pallor, cyanosis, and sensory/motor testing of the digit.

Orthopedic. Finger sprains and dislocations can be deceptive, with a number of hidden injuries being possible. These injuries include tendon avulsions, mallet finger, boutonniere deformity, flexor profundus avulsions, or phalangeal fractures. Systematically evaluate the finger, regardless of how unimpressive the sprain or dislocation initially appears. Palpate all areas for tenderness, determine active and passive range of motion, and perform stress testing to evaluate for instability or loss of tendon function. It may be necessary to perform an accurate ligament examination under digital block. The joint should be stressed passively in all planes and then allowed to be moved by the patient to determine active stability. Sometimes the ligamentous injury is so severe that the joint subluxates or dislocates during active motion under digital block. If the joint is dislocated, check for lateral stability after reduction. ROM of the proximal interphalangeal (PIP) and distal interphalangeal (DIP) joints should be tested. The DIP is tested by immobilizing the proximal and middle phalanges to test the extensor and flexor digitorum longus. In open fractures, soft-tissue damage is an index to the likelihood of infection or other complications.

PATHOPHYSIOLOGY

The pathophysiology of soft-tissue injuries of the finger is no different than any other ligament, tendon, or soft-tissue injury of other joints. All involve some degree of tearing of soft tissue, if not complete tearing. These injuries are more intricate due to the fine dexterity needed in these special appendages to carry out daily activities.

DIAGNOSTIC STUDIES

Laboratory
CBC, Full Chemistry Profile, PT, PTT. As routine preoperative screen.
Rheumatoid Factor. As indicated to evaluate for rheumatoid arthritis.
Radiology
Plain X-rays. AP, lateral, and oblique views are minimum to evaluate for fracture. If reduction is done, a postreduction series is necessary to make sure no avulsion fractures were created with reduction and that the reduction was successful. A piece of bone lodged at one of the pulleys of the tendon in the finger or in the palm may be seen in flexor tendon avulsions.

DIFFERENTIAL DIAGNOSIS

Traumatic
Avulsion and Compression. Can be easily missed.
Infectious
Joint Infections. May occur with blunt trauma. Bites from human teeth can be very serious. Erythema and discharge may be seen; elevated WBC.
Metabolic
Rheumatoid Arthritis. Positive rheumatoid factor.
Neoplastic
Tumor. Resulting in a pathologic fracture; seen on radiographic studies.

Vascular. Not applicable.
Congenital. Not applicable.
Acquired. Not applicable.

TREATMENT

Medical. Proper care of fractures depends on identifying the type and extent of fracture injury. Generally, fractures of the hand and finger should not be kept in an extreme position for longer than 10 days. Certain unstable finger, most metacarpal, and phalangeal fractures may be adequately controlled in the functional position. Most hand fractures should not be immobilized for over 3 weeks, and early ROM helps prevent disabling stiffness.

Mallet Finger. Prompt recognition of the extensor tendon avulsion allows closed treatment with a dorsal splint, used for 5 or 6 weeks.

Boutonniere Deformity. If there is doubt about the integrity of the tendon, the joint should be immobilized in an extension cast for 3 to 6 weeks, which ensures healing and prevents flexion contracture of the joint. This treatment can be applied 6 to 12 weeks after initial injury.

Distal Interphalangeal Joint Dislocation. Splint for 2 to 3 weeks. Early ROM for mobilization.

Proximal Interphalangeal Joint Dislocation. Reduced by gentle traction in the direction of the deformity under digital block. Apply a small amount of cotton between the adjacent finger and the injured finger and buddy tape them together and apply a dorsal splint to immobilize and prevent hyperextension while allowing active flexion of the finger. The splint can be discontinued after 1 to 2 weeks and the patient can continue protected full flexion of the finger, which is still taped.

Metacarpophalangeal (MCP) Joint Dislocation. May be difficult to reduce in a closed manner. MCP joint dislocation of the thumb can be reduced in a closed manner by pushing the proximal phalanx distally until it can be flexed forward easily over the metacarpal head. Closed reduction by pulling should not be attempted on the fingers, because this only tightens the structures on each side of the metacarpal head. Closed reduction of the MCP joint can be attempted by gentle pressure on the proximal end of the proximal phalanx and opposing pressure on the metacarpal head under local block.

Fracture of the Proximal Phalanx. Fractures of the proximal phalanx are usually volar angulated, owing to the intrinsic tendinous pull across the fracture and are often stable in full flexion of the MCP joint.

Spiral Fractures of the Proximal Phalanx. These often have a rotary component, so that the finger rotates under or on top of an adjacent finger during flexion. Check for rotation when reduced and in flexion to make sure the reduction remains stable. The PIP, DIP, and nail bed should all line up with adjacent fingers.

Surgical. Deformities associated with fractures that cannot be reduced anatomically require open reduction and internal fixation.

Flexor Tendon Avulsions. Prompt repair of the avulsed tendon restores normal grip to the injured finger. Successful repair can be accomplished up to about 3 weeks after the injury. Delayed recognition may leave the patient with some degree of permanent functional impairment.

Boutonniere Deformity. If an avulsion fracture is present, refer the patient for operative repair.

Avulsion Fractures. Avulsion fractures often appear innocent, and only x-ray stress views of the joint demonstrate instability. Often, these fractures, along with condylar fractures of the finger, require open reduction and internal fixation.

Indications. Fractures that involve growth centers or joints surfaces, fractures that are open (through the skin), markedly displaced, badly comminuted, segmental, or unstable (those that will not stay reduced). Most require care by an orthopedic or hand surgeon.

Contraindications. Inability to tolerate anesthesia.

TECHNIQUE OF SURGICAL ASSISTING

Exposure and gentle retraction in repairing tendons and ligaments are important roles of the PA. A knowledge of surgical anatomy is imperative when assisting with these procedures.

PEDIATRIC CONSIDERATIONS

Obtain consultation with a hand surgeon if there is any suspicion of underlying injury.

OBSTETRICAL CONSIDERATIONS

No surgical treatment during pregnancy. Use caution in performing x-rays and prescribing analgesics.

PEARLS FOR THE PA

Always assess neurovascular status.

Tendon avulsions, mallet finger, boutonniere deformity, flexor profundus avulsions, or phalangeal fractures all may occur with digit trauma. A high index of suspicion needs to be maintained.

Sprains: Epicondylitis of the Elbow

Carrie Gunn-Edel, PA-C

DEFINITION

Epicondylitis (also known as "tennis elbow") is divided into two types.

Lateral Epicondylitis. Inflammation or small tears of fibers that attach the extensor carpi radialis brevis muscle to the lateral humeral epicondyle.

Medial Epicondylitis. Inflammation of the fibers that attach the flexor carpi radialis and less frequently flexor digitorum superficialis to the medial humeral epicondyle.

HISTORY

Symptoms. Patients complain of pain over the lateral epicondyle and extensor muscle mass when lifting objects with the palm down, when playing racket sports, or with throwing and wringing motions.

General. Tennis elbow occurs 7 to 10 times more often on the lateral than on the medial side. Typically, patients are active recreational sports enthusiasts who play at least three or four times per week. Symptoms usually appear after a fairly vigorous activity sequence.

Age. Commonly seen in patients aged 30 to 50 years, but may occur at any age. Most common in third to fifth decades, with a range of 12 to 80 years and an equal male to female ratio.

Onset. Commonly occurs after repetitive use of wrist and arm or lifting with the palm side of the hand facing down. Most commonly symptoms have a gradual, insidious onset. Acute onset may be associated with a direct blow to one of the epicondylar areas or a sudden extreme effort or activity.

Duration. May be chronic if not treated. Resolved 90% to 95% of the time with medical management.

Intensity. Mild to moderate pain. Occasional intense pain with point tenderness or range of motion.

Aggravating Factors. Motion, overuse of arm, lifting or grasping items.

Alleviating Factors. Rest, anti-inflammatories, forearm band.

Associated Factors. Athletics, repetitive work.

PHYSICAL EXAMINATION

General. The patient is usually in no distress.

Orthopedic. Tenderness to palpation over the involved humeral epicondyle and radiocapitellar ligament, aggravated by wrist extension if lateral and by wrist flexion if medial side is injured. Occasionally, both are painful. Grip strength is decreased as a result of pain on attempts to stabilize the wrist in extension. Straightening fingers may elicit pain, as may pronating and supinating the forearm. In severe cases any elbow movement can be uncomfortable.

PATHOPHYSIOLOGY

The lesion in tennis elbow is due to a tear in the common extensor or flexor origin at or near the respective epicondyle. The normal tendon fibers are disrupted by a characteristic invasion of fibroblasts and vascular granulation-like tissue of angiofibroblastic hyperplasia. The tendon appears hypercellular, degenerative, and microfragmented. These tears occur in degenerated tendon fibers and are produced by mechanical overload in sports or at work. Tears range from microscopic to gross rupture or avulsion.

DIAGNOSTIC STUDIES

Laboratory
CBC, Full Chemistry Profile, PT, PTT.   As routine preoperative screen.
Radiology
Elbow X-ray.   PA, lateral, oblique views may demonstrate lateral exostosis, bone chips, or calcific deposits over the lateral epicondyle.

DIFFERENTIAL DIAGNOSIS

Traumatic
Synovitis.   Differentiated by history and physical examination.
Fractures of the Distal Humerus.   Differentiated by x-ray.
Loose Bodies in Elbow Joint.   Differentiated by history and physical examination.
Ulnar Nerve Neurapraxia.   Is commonly associated with tennis elbow and is manifest by numbness in the distribution of the ulnar nerve.
Infectious.   Not applicable.
Metabolic
Rheumatoid Arthritis.   Positive rheumatoid factor.
Osteoarthritis.   Differentiated by history, physical examination, and x-ray.
Neoplastic.   Not applicable.
Vascular.   Not applicable.

Congenital

Malformed Elbow Joint. Differentiated by history, physical examination, and x-ray.

Acquired

Radial or Cubital Tunnel Syndrome. May have symptoms of numbness and weakness. May cause symptoms similar to lateral epicondylitis.

TREATMENT

Medical. Initial treatment consists of rest, ice, and NSAIDs, followed by an exercise program to strengthen the forearm and hand muscles. Forearm support band, and heat and ultrasound treatments may also be beneficial.

In more severe cases, up to three local injections of cortisone and lidocaine may be given. Forearm splint with the wrist in slight extension and supination may be used in recalcitrant cases. Changing to "palm up" lifting and analyzing sport technique and form are necessary to prevent relapse. Wrist curls to strengthen forearm extensors and proper stretching exercises are indicated after initial recovery is well under way.

Surgical. Surgery is indicated in the few cases that do not respond to conservative therapy. There are four types of operations.

1. The treatment of choice is repair of the extensor and flexor origin after excision of torn tendon, granulation tissue, and part of the epicondyle.
2. Relieve tension on common extensor and flexor origin by fasciotomy or by direct release by dissection of the origin from the respective epicondyle or by lengthening the extensor carpi radialis brevis tendon distally (only 50% of cases relieved of pain).
3. Attention toward the radial nerve. Denervate the outside of the elbow by severing sensory fibers or decompressing the posterior interosseous nerve.
4. Intra-articular procedure with partial or complete division of the orbicular ligament, reshaping the radial head (or synovectomy), occasionally used in combination with fasciotomy or release of the extensor origin. Usually not warranted, because the lesion is extra-articular.

Indications. Surgery is necessary 5% to 10% of the time when medical management is not effective.

Contraindications. Inadequate trial of medical management (must take patient's lifestyle into consideration when deciding time frame). Minimum of 6 weeks and three attempted cortisone injections.

TECHNIQUE OF SURGICAL ASSISTING

Providing appropriate exposure.

PEDIATRIC CONSIDERATIONS

Not common in children.

OBSTETRICAL CONSIDERATIONS

No surgical treatment during pregnancy. Use caution in performing x-rays and prescribing analgesics.

PEARLS FOR THE PA

The pain of tennis elbow is experienced when the patient lifts objects with the palm down.

Symptoms are due to a tear of the common extensor or flexor tendon.

Treatment of choice is conservative.

Sprains: Frozen Shoulder
John W. Bullock, PA-C, BA, BS

DEFINITION

Restriction of active and passive range of shoulder motion in all planes due to contracture and loss of compliance of the glenohumeral joint capsule. The specific cause is unknown. (Note: the common term "adhesive capsulitis" is a misnomer because arthroscopic examination of patients with primary frozen shoulder shows an absence of any intra-articular adhesions.)

HISTORY

Symptoms. Nonspecific, aching discomfort around the shoulder. Typically, pain is referred to the area of the deltoid insertion and is worse at the limits of motion. Increasing shoulder discomfort is associated with a slowly progressive shoulder stiffness.

The views expressed in this material are those of the author and do not reflect the official policy or position of the United States Government, the Department of Defense, or the Department of the Air Force.

General. The initial severe pain decreases as the disease passes through three phases until functional motion returns. The freezing (acute) phase lasts 3 to 9 months, a frozen phase (interim) lasts 4 to 12 months, and the thawing (resolution) phase lasts 12 to 42 months.

Age. Usually between 40 and 70 years of age. Uncommon under 40. More common in females.

Onset. Insidious.

Duration. Usually a self-limiting condition that resolves in 12 to 24 months. However, symptoms can last as little as a few weeks or as long as 42 months.

Intensity. Varies according to the phase of the disease. Freezing phase: severe pain at rest and any attempted motion. Frozen phase: pain gives way to increasing stiffness. Thawing phase: pain resolves as mobility increases.

Aggravating Factors. Vigorous attempts at restoring ROM early in the disease. Prolonged immobilization.

Alleviating Factors. Pain tends to be inversely proportional to the amount of flexibility. After the acute phase, gentle ROM exercises and stretching help.

Associated Factors. Predisposing factors include age, immobility, insulin-dependent diabetes mellitus, middle age, cervical disc disease, hyperthyroidism, cardiothoracic surgery, intrathoracic disorders (such as tuberculosis or Pancoast tumor), intracranial pathology, personality disorder, severe emotional stress, or depression. However, a direct causal relationship has not been established.

PHYSICAL EXAMINATION

General. The patient may present with an obvious limitation of movement of the affected shoulder.

Orthopedic. Look for loss of passive glenohumeral motion on the affected side. External rotation is usually lost first, followed soon after by forward flexion, abduction, and internal rotation. There is a solid endpoint to motion, which is painful as the limits of motion are reached. The key to the diagnosis is this asymmetric limitation to passive motion, which is painful.

Functional loss of motion is more important than absolute numbers, so compare the affected shoulder to the unaffected side. The shoulder ROM as recommended by the American Society of Shoulder and Elbow Surgeons should include measurement of:

- Active and passive forward elevation (flexion). Measure angle between arm and thorax.
- Passive external rotation, arm by side, elbow 90 degrees. Measure angle between forearm and sagittal plane.
- Active internal rotation, arm behind back, tip of thumb to highest spinous process. Note level reached.
- Active abduction (lateral). Measure angle between arm and trunk.
- Independent glenohumeral motion.

PATHOPHYSIOLOGY

Idiopathic frozen shoulder is a primary inflammatory condition that involves the capsule and synovium. Although arthroscopy shows an absence of intra-articular adhesions, it often shows a vascular reaction around the biceps long head tendon as it opens into the subscapularis bursa. Intra-articular glenohumeral synovitis with capsular contracture has been described. Surgical exposure in several recalcitrant cases also showed significant contracture of the coracohumeral ligament and rotator interval. The specific cause is unknown.

DIAGNOSTIC STUDIES

Laboratory
CBC, Full Chemistry Profile, PT, PTT. As routine preoperative screen. Used only to evaluate for predisposing conditions.
Radiology
Shoulder X-ray. AP and lateral radiographs taken in the plane of the scapula plus a supraspinatus outlet view to evaluate acromial pathology are the minimum necessary. These generally are consistently normal except for mild osteopenia in long-standing cases.
Arthrogram. Of the affected shoulder shows restricted capacity for contrast, a small subscapular recess, and obliteration of the inferior hanging axillary fold.
Cervical Spine X-ray. If indicated by history and physical examination. Look for spondylosis.

DIFFERENTIAL DIAGNOSIS

Traumatic
Fractures. Of the glenoid or proximal humerus are visualized on x-ray.
Posterior Dislocation. Suspected on physical examination and visualized on x-ray.
Rotator Cuff Injury. Positive drop arm test (see topic rotator cuff).
Tendinitis. Often secondary to impingement. May have a positive Yergason's maneuver (elbow flexed and externally rotated causes pain if the bicep tendon is involved).
Bursitis. Of the subacromial region can cause pain and reduced active movement of the shoulder.
Infectious
Septic Joint. Should be considered if the pain is severe and there are signs of acute inflammation, swelling, and erythema.
Metabolic
Metabolic Bone Disease. Associated with bone pain, proximal muscle weakness, and secondary symptoms of hypercalcemia.
Polymyalgia Rheumatica. Systemic condition that is manifested by stiffness in the proximal limb muscles.

Fibromyalgia. Chronic, systemic process that involves multiple sites (nonarticular); may cause stiffness.

Shoulder Arthritis. Degenerative changes seen on x-ray.

Neoplastic

Tumors. Affecting the cervical spine, shoulder, or intrathoracic contents may cause shoulder pain and stiffness. Radiographic studies identify the lesion.

Vascular

Avascular Necrosis. Most often associated with changes on x-ray. Comparison x-ray views are often helpful.

Thoracic Outlet Syndrome. Entrapment of the brachial plexus and vascular structures (see topic thoracic outlet).

Congenital. Not applicable.

Acquired

Postoperative Stiffness. History of surgery.

Other

Cervical Radiculopathy. Due to spondylosis or herniated disc; may cause shoulder area pain. Usually has associated numbness, weakness, and reflex change in a dermatomal distribution (see topic cervical and lumbar intervertebral disc disease).

Reflex Sympathetic Dystrophy. Is manifest by swelling, pain, color changes, and temperature fluctuation of the skin.

TREATMENT

It is thought that all patients will get better if left alone, but the amount of residual stiffness, disability, and pain is variable, and many patients are not willing to wait the months or years to see whether their syndrome will resolve.

Medical. Therapy is based on the stage of the disease. There is a wide variation of management and treatment continues to be a matter of debate, but the following common approach has been shown to be safe and effective.

Freezing Phase. During this phase, the shoulder generally responds poorly to many of the usual forms of treatment, including manipulations, injections, anti-inflammatory medication, heat, rest, ultrasound, acupuncture, and vigorous physical therapy. Patients tend to become emotionally depressed because they are told they "aren't working hard enough" to keep their shoulder from freezing further. Partially because of the inexorable progress of the disease and, possibly, because of increased inflammation caused by vigorous attempts at movement, the harder the patients work, the stiffer they get.

The treatment in this phase is reassurance that the patient will get better and support with pain control (medication, sling, consider a TENS unit) as well as a sedative at night, if necessary, to ensure adequate rest. Encourage the patient to use the arm as normally as possible within his or her comfort level. Pendulum-type exercises should be done for 1 to 2 minutes every 1 to 2 hours while the patient is awake. If the patient awakens at night with pain, pendulum exercises done for 1 to 2 minutes can supplement or even supplant analgesics for night pain.

Frozen Phase. Encourage the patient to use the arm within the limit of range of comfort. The patient should be seen regularly (aproximately once a month) for monitoring. Gentle home therapy is encouraged. Stretching, concentrating on passive forward elevation and external rotation, is started.

Thawing Phase. Motion of the shoulder gradually returns and patients are quite optimistic during this phase. Regular pendulum exercises, frequent stretching, and frequent ROM exercises (again, dictated by comfort) are started. The patient is encouraged to stretch in whatever direction seems stiff. Forceful exercise is to be avoided. Formal physical therapy can be very helpful in educating the patient and correcting abnormal shoulder girdle mechanics (the patient has been substituting scapulothoracic motion for glenohumeral motion for months now and must "re-educate" the shoulder). As motion increases (around 150 degrees of forward elevation, 45 degrees of external rotation, and internal rotation to the 12th vertebra), stretching in abduction may start.

In general, the less aggressive the physical therapy and the more naturally the patient uses the arm within the range of comfort, the shorter the period of pain and limited motion.

Surgical

Hydraulic Distention (Brisement). May be performed in conjunction with an arthrogram of the shoulder and consists of introducing progressively larger increments of fluid (normal saline or contrast) mixed with lidocaine in an attempt to disrupt the capsular contracture. The distention is continued until free extravasation occurs, noted by a sudden drop in resistance to further injection. ROM exercises are started while the anesthetic is still active.

Arthroscopic Débridement. The specific role of arthroscopy in frozen shoulder has not been established. Some of the benefit may be a brisement effect.

Manipulation Under General Anesthesia. May be indicated in patients who have persistent pain and have failed to regain greater than 90 degrees of active/passive range of motion or 0 degrees of external rotation after prolonged (3 to 6 months) physical therapy. Manipulation works by tearing the inferior capsule and is best done in the late frozen phase. The affected shoulder is stabilized by placing one hand over the deltoid and acromion while the manipulation is performed with the other hand, which grasps the patient's arm just distal to the axilla while the patient's forearm rests on the manipulator's forearm. The hand must hold the arm proximally to minimize the risk of humerus fracture. External rotation is addressed initially, followed by abduction, forward flexion, adduction, and internal rotation. Intra-articular steroids are usually instilled, along with a local anesthetic; physiotherapy starts the same day as manipulation.

Open Release. Rarely indicated and is associated with a high degree of residual stiffness. May be used when there is a high risk of fracture of the humerus (severe osteopenia on radiographs), concomitant dislocation or fracture, or failure of simple manipulation.

Indications.   Initial conservative management is ideal but if no progress is being made, pain is persistent, and functional motion is not returning despite a well-supervised physiotherapy program, then a more aggressive approach is indicated.

Contraindications.   Insulin-dependent diabetics have a lower success rate with manipulation, a relative contraindication.

TECHNIQUE OF SURGICAL ASSISTING

Assistant is not necessary.

PEDIATRIC CONSIDERATIONS

Not a disease of children.

OBSTETRICAL COMPLICATIONS

No surgical treatment during pregnancy. Use caution in performing x-rays and prescribing analgesics.

PEARLS FOR THE PA

If the patient does not improve, order a true axillary view of the shoulder to rule out unreduced posterior shoulder dislocation.

The length of the period of immobility is a significant factor in the development of frozen shoulder.

Early, gentle mobilization must be encouraged.

Ultimately, although there may be objective residual loss of motion, there is rarely any subjective functional impairment.

Sprains: Knee
Kent W. Wallace, PA-C, ARNP

DEFINITION

Injuries to the four primary stabilizing ligaments of the knee, the anterior cruciate ligament (ACL), posterior cruciate ligament (PCL), lateral collateral ligament (LCL), and the medial collateral ligament (MCL).

HISTORY

Symptoms. Symptoms occur with different levels of activity in all the ligamentous injuries around the knee. An audible pop at the time of injury is characteristic of an ACL tear. The mechanism of injury for ACL tears is usually one of deceleration with flexion and rotation. Hyperextension of the knee and hyperflexion with a violent contraction of the quadriceps mechanism has also been shown to be sufficient to tear the ACL. The most common complaints following ACL injuries are pain and giving way. Pain is usually related to activity, but may occur with acute injury. Giving way is described as the knee either buckling or feeling as if it would not hold the patient's weight and is as common as pain. Swelling is the next most common complaint, and is generally mild and occurs with activity.

The most common reported mechanism for injury in isolated PCL is the classic dashboard injury. The knee is in a flexed position, approximately 90 degrees, and a posterior force is applied to the proximal tibia as the knee strikes the dashboard. This can also happen in other types of deceleration injuries.

MCL injuries usually result from some type of valgus force, such as a clipping injury, whereas LCL injuries are most commonly caused from a varus type of force.

General. The most frequent injury of the knee after meniscal injury is ligamentous injuries. They vary from minor to severe, and can be an inconvenience or moderately disabling. The mechanisms of injury with its associated sounds and symptoms are extremely valuable in assessing and obtaining an accurate history.

Age. Teens to adults; adolescent injuries are uncommon.

Onset. Usually acute, resulting from some type of varus, valgus, rotational, or hyperextension injury.

Intensity. Complete disruption of the ACL or PCL usually has minimal pain. Pain is usually from joint effusion. MCL and LCL are initially moderately painful.

Aggravating Factors. Twisting or cutting maneuvers and abrupt deceleration. Also prolonged descent (e.g., stairs, hills) is very aggravating.

Alleviating Factors. Modify activity level to avoid the above modalities is helpful. Prophylactic functional bracing may be helpful as well.

Associated Factors. Multiple ligamentous injuries, meniscal pathology, and osteochondral injury.

PHYSICAL EXAMINATION

General. Inspect for visual signs such as joint effusion, abrasions, old scars, or bruising. The state of the skin may give information about the direction, force, and mechanism of the present injury or past history.

Orthopedic. Inspect the shape of the joint, upper and lower limb, in regard to the general alignment as well as atrophy or swelling (localized or diffuse).

As a baseline, examine the uninjured knee first. The palpatory examination of the knee involves a subtle gradient of applied force. Palpate anatomical structures, noting pain, effusion, induration, gaps in the underlying soft tissue, and stability of structures. This must be done with the patient's full knowledge and co-operation. Once palpation is complete, have the patient actively move the well knee first through a full range of motion, then have the patient move the injured extremity within the bounds of comfort, noting any limitations, pops, clicks, or instability. Stability is best evaluated with flexion and extension of the knee.

Collateral ligaments are best examined at hyperextension, neutral, and 30 degrees of flexion. If the knee is stable in hyperextension, the medial and lateral capsuloligamentous structures and the PCL are intact. Laxity in hyperextension to varus or valgus forces are signs that may indicate disruption of major ligamentous structures. In hyperextension, if the knee joint is lax to valgus force, the medial capsuloligamentous structures and the PCL may be interrupted. If the knee is lax to varus force, the arcuate complex and PCL may be disrupted. Varus and valgus stress applied in hyperextension, zero degrees, and 30 degrees of flexion best determine medial and lateral capsular injuries. The patellae should be examined for excursion; the patient will indicate by apprehension if tenderness, pain, or instability exist.

Adjunct tests include the Lachman and pivot shift. The Lachman test is specific, reliable, and minimally painful to the patient. With the knee flexed at 30 degrees and the patient relaxed, the lower leg is drawn forward on the upper leg by firmly stabilizing the femur with one hand and drawing the tibia forward with the other hand. Increased anterior excursion with this test is pathognomonic of a torn ACL. The end point should be graded or described as mild (1+), moderate (2+), or severe (3+ [described as 1 + Lachman]). The pivot shift test is performed with the knee in full extension. The tibia is internally rotated with one hand grasping the foot. The other hand applies a mild valgus stress at the level of the knee joint. Then, with flexion of the knee to approximately 20 to 30 degrees, and firmly maintaining the valgus stress, a pathologic slip should be felt. This reproduces the dysfunction that the patient recognizes if he or she has a pivot shift. The pivot shift also should be graded as described above (e.g., 1 + pivot shift).

PATHOPHYSIOLOGY

This would best be described as the end result of pathomechanics plus the amount of force applied to cause injury to the knee ligaments. Flexion, extension, and rotational forces place the knee under extreme conditions; as such, the stress applied with sports or high-impact accidents puts the knee at risk. Forces that go beyond the tensile strength of the tendons that hold the knee together cause the knee to give way. With increased laxity, degenerative changes usually occur because of the ligamentous insufficiency.

DIAGNOSTIC STUDIES

Laboratory
CBC, Chemistry Profile, PT, PTT. For preoperative evaluation.
Radiology
Knee X-rays. An AP, lateral, patellar-trochlear (skyline, merchant, and others), and notch views make up a complete series. Radiographs are mostly used to exclude fractures that involve the femoral condyle and tibial plateau regions, as well as to exclude tibial eminence avulsion fractures.
Other
MRI. Ligamentous tears can be evaluated in a noninvasive fashion.

DIFFERENTIAL DIAGNOSIS

Traumatic
Fractures, Patellar Dislocations, Meniscal Injuries. Differentiated on physical examination and radiographic studies.
Infectious. Not applicable.
Metabolic. Not applicable.
Neoplastic. Not applicable.
Vascular
Osteochondritis Dissecans. Avascular necrosis of the femoral condyle. Comparison x-rays should be obtained.
Congenital. Not applicable.
Acquired. Not applicable.

TREATMENT

Medical. Conservative treatment includes immobilization, functional bracing, and aggressive rehabilitation of the quadriceps and hamstrings.
Surgical. Primary repair of torn ligament, with secondary ligamentous reconstruction as indicated. The procedure can be open or performed through an arthroscopic approach.
Indications. Functional instability from either ACL or PCL injury, triad injuries (ACL, MCL, medial meniscus tear), grade II to grade III MCL tear, instability with LCL injury; patient with chronic ACL disruption who has been functioning satisfactorily develops symptoms after sustaining a nonrepairable meniscal tear.
Contraindications. Open growth plates, age, underlying medical conditions.

TECHNIQUE OF SURGICAL ASSISTING

Familiarization with the surgical procedure is essential. Competency in preparation of grafts for ligamentous reconstructions.

PEDIATRIC CONSIDERATIONS

Due to skeletal maturity, injuries in children and adolescents are uncommon. Injuries tend to begin in the teens.

OBSTETRICAL CONSIDERATIONS

No surgical treatment during pregnancy. Use caution in performing x-rays and prescribing analgesics.

PEARLS FOR THE PA

Examine the uninjured knee initially to obtain a baseline.

ACL: Deceleration, with flexion and rotation or hyperextension/ hyperflexion.

PCL: Classic dashboard injury (deceleration).

MCL: Valgus force.

LCL: Varus force.

Sprains: Patellofemoral Disorders
Kent W. Wallace, PA-C, ARNP

DEFINITION

Conditions involving the extensor mechanism of the patellofemoral pathomechanics that are usually associated with pain of varying intensity and may become debilitating at times, associated with signs and symptoms of patellar laxity. Terms such as patellofemoral syndrome, chondromalacia (softening and deterioration of the articulating surface of the patellae), subluxation, and malalignment are all used to describe some type of pain without details of their genesis.

HISTORY

Symptoms.   Patients usually have symptoms of anterior or retropatellar knee pain, associated with cracking, buckling, locking, and catching. Symptoms of quadriceps weakness are often noted and patients may demonstrate signs of patella instability.

General. Patellofemoral articulation and biomechanics are among the most complex and poorly understood in the musculoskeletal system. Even the classification of patellofemoral disorders is confusing. A basic understanding of the surface anatomy and pathophysiology of the underlying problem are extremely helpful.

Causes of patellofemoral pain can be divided into three categories:

Local: Acute trauma, repetitive trauma/overuse syndrome, posttraumatic sequelae, patellofemoral dysplasia, osteochondritis dissecans, and synovial plica.

Distant: Increased Q angle, gynecoid pelvis, femoral anteversion, genu valgum, genu varum, genu recurvatum, tibia vara, external tibial torsion, and pronated forefoot.

Systemic: Congential hyperlaxity and obesity.

Age. Patellofemoral problems are more common in adolescent females, but may be seen in all age groups. Chondromalacia patellae is found in all age groups, especially adults.

Onset. Acute onset (usually less than a month in duration) of anterior knee pain is generally associated with traumatic events such as patella contusions, dislocation, subluxation, or osteochondral fractures. Insidious onset (slow to start and ongoing) is generally seen with inflammatory disorders such as patella tendinitis, inflammation of the synovial plica, or other synovial impingement phenomena. Chondromalacia patellae frequently has a very insidious onset.

Duration. Once symptoms occur, it may take 4 to 6 weeks for the patient to become pain free. Sometimes it may take several months for symptoms to diminish completely. Both the duration and the intensity can be highly variable.

Intensity. Initially, the symptoms may cause little functional impairment, but as symptoms and pain increase, the condition becomes more debilitating.

Aggravating Factors. Stair climbing, running, descent (e.g., stairs, hills), prolonged sitting, and bicycling.

Alleviating Factors. Decreasing the aggravating factors, rest, weight loss, McConnell taping.

Associated Factors. Ligamentous laxity, patella alta, patella baja, obesity, occupation, femoral anteversion, and external tibial torsion. More frequently, problems are seen in the weekend athlete.

PHYSICAL EXAMINATION

General. For the physical examination to be properly performed, the patient should be wearing shorts throughout the examination so that the involved and contralateral limb can be fully inspected. Examination takes place in the standing, sitting, supine, and prone positions and begins with observation of the standing patient. Observe for any effusion of the knee joint, wasting of the quadriceps, atrophy of the vastus medialis obliquus (VMO), and anatomical differences of the patellae.

Orthopedic. Document the overall alignment of the leg standing, sitting, and supine, measuring varus, valgus, and Q angle (the angle between the line of application of the quadriceps force and the direction of the patellar tendon, normally 20 degrees or less) of the leg. Evaluating abnormalities such as femoral anteversion and tibial torsion are important as well. The thigh circumference should be measured (7 inches above the lateral joint line). The examiner should attempt to push the patellae both medially and laterally to assess stability compared with the opposite side. The patient may contract the quadriceps with fear that the patellae will dislocate (positive patellar apprehension test). Observation of the patella tracking and glide should be noted as the knee flexes and extends. Palpate for crepitus over the anterior patella and note any mechanical tracking abnormalities. Palpate the medial and lateral retinacular tissue, inferior pole of the patellae, and medial and lateral synovial plicas for pain or discomfort. Perform the downward compression test, looking for pain. The passive glide test is done with the knee flexed at 30 degrees and the quadriceps relaxed as the patella is pushed medially and laterally to evaluate tracking. Medial deviation of one quadrant or less is consistent with contracted lateral retinaculum. Lateral deviation of greater that two quadrants is consistent with a laxity or ruptured medial retinaculum.

PATHOPHYSIOLOGY

Usually the pathomechanics precedes the pathophysiology of the patellofemoral disease. This may be trauma to the patellae, patellofemoral tracking problems, quadriceps atrophy, or increased Q angle. All may lead to the pathophysiological changes such as cellular degeneration, fissuring and cracking of the articulating cartilage, and possibly subsequent degenerative changes.

DIAGNOSTIC STUDIES

Laboratory
CBC, ESR, Rheumatoid Profile. May be helpful when inflammatory arthropathies are suspected.
Radiology
Knee X-rays. AP, lateral, and merchant views are essential for evaluation. Tunnel view to rule out loose bodies is helpful.
Bone Scan, CT and MRI Scan. Are generally reserved for unusual disorders or other occult disease processes.

DIFFERENTIAL DIAGNOSIS

Traumatic
Patella Fracture. Seen on x-ray.
Osteochondral Injury. Seen on x-ray.

Infectious

Joint Infection.   Should be considered if the pain is severe and there are signs of acute inflammation, swelling, and erythema.

Metabolic

Rheumatoid Arthritis.   Positive rheumatoid factor.

Osteoarthritis.   Systemic and degenerative joint condition. Joint degeneration seen on x-ray.

Neoplastic

First-degree Osteosarcoma.   In adolescence may present as chondromalacia patellae.

Vascular.   Not applicable.

Congenital

Absence of (or Shallow) Patellofemoral Groove, Hypoplastic Patellae, Congenital Hyperlaxity.   Seen on physical examination and/or radiographic studies.

Acquired.   Not applicable.

TREATMENT

Medical.   NSAIDs, physical therapy, home exercise program, bracing, orthotics, lifestyle modification, stretching of the quadriceps, iliotibial band, and hamstrings are all forms of conservative therapy that should be considered before surgical intervention is entertained. A minimum of at least 4 to 8 weeks of conservative treatment should be attempted.

Surgical.   Proximal or distal patella realignment, lateral retinacular release, diagnostic and operative arthroscopy, and possible patellectomy. Less common are ORIF for patella fractures and tendon repair/reconstruction for primary tendon ruptures.

Indications.   Patella instability or malalignment, patellofemoral pain syndrome and/or chondromalacia of the patellae, osteoarthritis or rheumatoid arthritis, as well as failed conservative therapy.

Contraindications.   Active reflex sympathetic dystrophy, underlying medical conditions.

TECHNIQUE OF SURGICAL ASSISTING

Be familiar with the clinical presentation of the problem. Intraoperative traction, exposure, and assistance with alignment are primary responsibilities of the PA.

PEDIATRIC CONSIDERATIONS

Open growth plates, Osgood-Schlatter disease, external tibial torsion, femoral anteversion, patella alta, and Siding-Larsen-Johansson disease are conditions encountered in the pediatric population. Referral to a pediatric specialist in orthopedics is recommended.

OBSTETRICAL CONSIDERATIONS

No surgical treatment during pregnancy. Use caution in performing x-rays and prescribing analgesics.

PEARLS FOR THE PA

Patellofemoral problems are more common in adolescent females.

Always compare examination findings with the uninvolved knee.

Patellar disorders are due to trauma, patellofemoral tracking problems, quadriceps atrophy, or increased Q angle.

Sprains: Rotator Cuff Tears
John W. Bullock, PA-C, BA, BS

DEFINITION

Disruption of any or all of the musculotendinous complex that makes up the rotator cuff of the shoulder (subscapularis, supraspinatus, infraspinatus, and teres minor muscles).

HISTORY

Symptoms. Patients typically present with impingement symptoms (see topic shoulder impingement syndrome) with accompanying weakness. With smaller tears this may only be noticeable with prolonged use of the arm above shoulder level, but with a large tear the patient may not be able to raise the arm at all. Pain may be worse at night and may awaken the patient from sleep.

General. Tears of the rotator cuff are the most common cause of shoulder pain in patients older than 40 years.

Age. Usually over 30 years old, but typical patient is over 40 years old. Equally involves males and females, dominant and nondominant shoulders.

Onset. May be insidious or sudden; 50% have no history of trauma. In the younger patient, full-thickness tears may present with a history of sudden, unexpected loading of the arm followed by shoulder weakness (this presentation is less typical in older patients, because the older the patient, the more likely the cause is attritional rather than acute trauma).

Duration. Varies: The patient may have several years of chronic tendinitis symptoms or can have onset associated with overuse or a specific event.

Intensity. Varies from completely asymptomatic to incapacitating.

Aggravating Factors. Working or holding arms above shoulder level.

Alleviating Factors. Early in the course, holding the arm adducted helps.

Associated Factors. Narrowing of the supraspinatus outlet due to acromioclavicular or subacromial osteophytes or anatomical variants.

PHYSICAL EXAMINATION

General. The patient may be asymptomatic or present in acute distress.

Orthopedic. Pain from subacromial impingement may cause muscle inhibition that mimics the weakness of a cuff tear; a test to distinguish the two is essential. The impingement injection test consists of an injection of 10 ml of 1% lidocaine into the subacromial space. If the pain disappears with the space anesthetized, it is diagnostic of subacromial impingement. If, however, weakness (especially external rotation of the shoulder with the arm adducted) remains, it is suspicious for a full-thickness rotator cuff tear. It is also useful in conjunction with the drop arm test, in which the patient holds his or her arms abducted and internally rotated while trying to resist the examiner's downward force on the arm. The test is positive if the arm suddenly drops due to weakness in abduction.

Atrophy in the infraspinatus and supraspinatus fossae can be seen when viewing the patient from behind. There is also often a discrepancy between active and passive motion. The best clinical sign of a full-thickness tear of the rotator cuff is weakness of external rotation. With the arm at the side and the elbow flexed 90 degrees, the patient is asked to resist internal rotation by the examiner. With full-thickness tears there is often a giving way by the patient, and even in partial tears there is weakness on the affected side. The examiner may be able to feel subacromial crepitants or a palpable defect in the rotator cuff. With large tears, the patient may not be able to initiate flexion or abduction of the arm. The deltoid muscle, acting unopposed because the rotator cuff is no longer able to effectively stabilize the humeral head against the glenoid, causes the shoulder to shrug as abduction or forward elevation is attempted. This is a classic finding with large tears that probably will not be present with smaller tears.

PATHOPHYSIOLOGY

There is increasing evidence that the primary set up for cuff tears is aging, which makes the cuff susceptible to attrition and degeneration and less resistant to sudden loads. It has been demonstrated that the presence of rotator cuff defects both in cadavers and in autopsy specimens from patients with no history of shoulder symptoms was age related and that no rotator cuff defects were detected before the fifth decade of life. After that, the incidence of tears "to some degree" was 33% in the fifth decade, 20% in the sixth decade, 100% in the seventh decade, and 99% in the eighth and ninth decades. With increasing age and disuse, less force is required to tear the cuff (Fig. 9–1).

DIAGNOSTIC STUDIES

Laboratory
CBC, Full Chemistry Profile, PT, PTT.   As routine preoperative screening.

Radiology
Standard Views (AP Views of the Shoulder with the Arm in Internal and External Rotation).   Plain radiographs can only give indirect evidence of the presence of rotator cuff disease. In younger patients, bony avulsion of the tuberosity may be seen; in all patients, one should look at the adequacy of the supraspinatus outlet.

On standard views, cuff arthropathy is demonstrated as marked cephalad migration of the humeral head with an acromiohumeral interval of less than 7 mm, humeral head osteopenia and possible collapse, cyst formation, sclerosis of the underside of the acromion, and/or degenerative glenohumeral arthritis.

Special Views (30-Degree AP Caudad Tilt View, Supraspinatus Outlet View).   Are ordered in addition to the standard views to evaluate proliferative changes of the acromion and acromioclavicular joint that cause narrowing and impingement at the supraspinatus outlet.

Arthrogram.   Reveals full-thickness tears as contrast leaks from the joint into the subacromial or subdeltoid areas. Very accurate in demonstrating the presence or absence of a full-thickness tear of the rotator cuff in patients who have not had previous surgery. Disadvantages are that the procedure is invasive, pain may last 1 to 2 days, and inability to demonstrate partial thickness tears other than at articular surface.

MRI Arthrograms.   Fat-suppressed, T1-weighted images have achieved a sensitivity and specificity of up to 100% in detecting full-thickness and partial-thickness tears. Especially useful in evaluating patients who have undergone previous rotator cuff surgery.

Ultrasonography.   Can reveal the thickness of various components of the cuff and the extent of cuff defects. More operator-dependent than MRI.

A Note on Special Imaging Studies.   Imaging studies beyond plain films are not necessary or cost effective unless they will change the treatment of

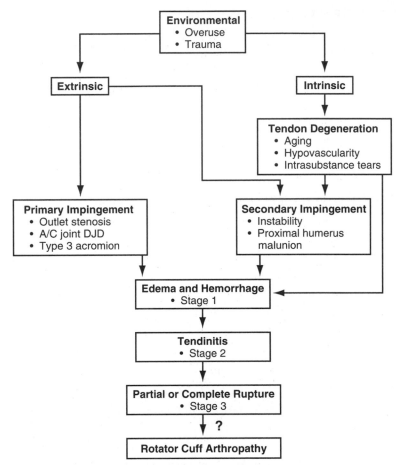

Figure 9–1. Flowchart showing etiology of rotator cuff disease. (From Frymoyer JW, ed: Orthopaedic Knowledge Update 4. Chicago: American Academy of Orthopaedic Surgeons, 1993, p. 304.)

the patient. For example, patients younger than 40 years of age without a major injury are unlikely to have significant cuff defects. Conversely, older patients with weak external rotation whose plain films show the humeral head in contact with the acromion need nothing else to establish the diagnosis. Cuff imaging is primarily needed only for those situations where the results would change the management of the patient (e.g., 47-year-old patient with weakness of flexion and external rotation after a major fall on the outstretched arm).

DIFFERENTIAL DIAGNOSIS

Traumatic
Posttraumatic Glenohumeral Arthritis, Acromioclavicular Arthritis. Differentiated on physical examination and radiographic studies.
Infectious
Joint Infection. Should be considered if the pain is severe and there are signs of acute inflammation, swelling, and erythema.
Metabolic
Gout, Pseudogout. Periodic, acute attacks of joint swelling and pain without history of a specific injury. Elevated serum uric acid levels with gout.
Psoriatic Arthritis. More commonly seen with pustular or erythrodermic psoriasis. Associated with skin lesions. Arthritis may involve the hands, feet, sacroiliac, hip, or cervical spine.
Rheumatoid Arthritis. Positive rheumatoid factor.
Neoplastic
Bone Tumors. Presence of bony destruction or lesion on MRI or plain film evaluation.
Vascular. Not applicable.
Congenital. Not applicable.
Acquired
Cervical Radiculopathy. Presence of motor, sensory, and reflex change in a dermatomal distribution.
Acute Calcific Tendinitis. Most commonly involves the supraspinatous tendon; seen on radiographs.

TREATMENT

Medical. The vast majority of patients with partial rotator cuff tears can be managed successfully without surgery. Most symptomatic, complete rotator cuff tears are chronic or are an acute extension of a pre-existing tear in a degenerative tendon. Despite long-standing symptoms, approximately 50% of these patients can be successfully managed nonoperatively (depending on the patient's age, activity level, and expectations).

Therapy should address the natural decrease of pain with time and the rehabilitation of the remaining rotator cuff muscles, the three portions of the deltoid muscle, and the scapular stabilizers (the trapezius and serratus anterior muscles). It should emphasize stretching in internal rotation, cross-body adduction, and elevation. After a comfortable, normal ROM is re-established, gentle progressive strengthening of the cuff muscles is started. Activity modification is important, avoiding repeated motions in which the humerus makes a greater than 10-degree angle above the scapular spine. Exercises should not be painful or exacerbate symptoms.

Physiotherapy modalities (e.g., ultrasound) can augment the total rehabilitation program. Such modalities work by creating increased tissue temperature, thereby causing hyperemia, which has the potential to increase healing in small tears. Variations include phonophoresis, which uses ultrasound to deliver topical medications to deeper tissues. Iontophoresis is like phonophoresis except that it uses electrical rather than ultrasonic energy. Corticosteroid injections have widespread use but there is no significant benefit over physiotherapy, nonsteroidal anti-inflammatory medications, or acupuncture. The adverse effects of corticosteroids on local tissues, including tendons, delays healing and decreases the quality of the rotator cuff tendon. Therefore, if local corticosteroids are used, they must be used judiciously (no more than three injections at least 6-week intervals), especially in acute cases in which partially torn fibers may be healing.

NSAIDs may be of benefit in attritional tears that involve chronic inflammation. Their analgesic effect is helpful.

Surgical. The goal of surgery is to relieve pain and, if possible, improve the strength and muscular balance of the shoulder. A good quality cuff needs to be present for best results. The best candidates are those patients with a traumatic tear in which a physiologically sound cuff has been torn acutely by a substantial injury. In contrast, the older patient with a large, attritional tear of long standing has little to work with. Repairing the tear does not restore the quality of the tendon tissue and a retear is likely in the face of sudden or large loads. The patient must be educated and have realistic expectations before surgery and be prepared for a lengthy recovery period.

Technique. Specific procedures vary. Each cuff tear is approached as unique, based on configuration, location, and quality and quantity of tissue. Therefore, the following description is a generalization.

For a cuff tear, usually an anterosuperior approach is used. An inferior or anterior acromioplasty is usually included in the procedure because decompression to allow clearance for the rotator cuff to pass within the subacromial space is an important component of rotator cuff surgery. Decompression and débridement, as well as certain repairs, can be done arthroscopically.

The actual cuff repair follows several principles. The overlying bursa and degenerative distal tendon stump are excised. The greater tuberosity of the humerus is trimmed, as are the frayed, fragmented tendon edges. The tissue is evaluated for quality and quantity and, if possible, mobilized and reattached to a bony trough made near the greater tuberosity. In larger tears, subscapularis transposition, biceps utilization, and infraspinatus transposition or advancement may be necessary.

In massive tears, repair may be impossible. If significant cuff tear arthropathy (e.g., glenohumeral degeneration) is present, a hemiarthroplasty may be necessary. If the cuff can be repaired, thereby giving added stability, a total shoulder arthroplasty is preferred.

Indications. For extremely active patients, the diagnosis of an acute cuff tear should lead to early surgical repair. Less active patients are treated conservatively for at least 3 months, with surgery if there is no improvement. For inactive or physiologically old patients, surgical treatment should be undertaken only to relieve pain.

Contraindications. Stiff shoulder, noncompliant patient.

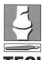

TECHNIQUE OF SURGICAL ASSISTING

Exposure, traction, and assisting with reattachment are primary intraoperative roles of the PA. Coordinating physiotherapy and following the patient's progress during conservative therapy are nonoperative responsibilities.

PEDIATRIC CONSIDERATIONS

Full-thickness tears are rare in children and uncommon in people younger than 40 years of age because the young, healthy cuff is highly resistant to disruption or degeneration. More likely is an avulsion of the bone from the greater tuberosity.

OBSTETRICAL CONSIDERATIONS

No surgical treatment during pregnancy. Use caution in performing x-rays and prescribing analgesics.

PEARLS FOR THE PA

Suspect rotator cuff tear in a first-time anterior shoulder dislocation in a patient older than 40 years.

The more experienced surgeon places more emphasis on conservative management.

A rupture of the long head of the biceps tendon may also be present with a full-thickness rotator cuff tear.

Over half of the patients with a rotator cuff tear on one side also have one on the other.

Sprains: Tibialis Posterior
Richard E. Donnelly, PA-C, BS, BS

DEFINITION

The tibialis posterior tendon functions as a powerful invertor of the foot and supports the longitudinal arch. Loss of this support causes a painful planovalgus foot deformity (flat foot), evidenced by progressive hindfoot valgus, loss of the longitudinal arch, and abduction of the forefoot. In time, degenerative hindfoot changes and lateral impingement develop. A spectrum of disease exists involving the tibialis posterior tendon.

HISTORY

Symptoms

Stage I.   Pain symptoms are mild to moderate, poorly localized, involve the medial hindfoot, and deformity has not occurred. The patient may have aching along the medial aspect of the hindfoot exacerbated by physical activity. Usually, the patient has reduced his or her activities.

Stage II.   Evolution occurs over several months; the symptoms progressively increase to the point that pain may be present during and after cessation of weight bearing. The location of pain has not changed, and mild deformity may be noticed by the patient.

Stage III.   Progression occurs over a few years; the location of pain has changed to the lateral ankle as well as the medial ankle, localizing more in the sinus tarsi region and often resulting in significant disability for the patient. Progressive loss of function ensues with progressive, unilateral acquired flatfoot deformity that becomes fixed.

General.   Can be seen with traumatic ankle injury in the physically active individual. It is, however, a diagnosis that is often missed. Prior acute trauma of a substantial degree usually cannot be recalled by the patient. Instead, there is a progressive, unilateral loss of the longitudinal arch, with subsequent heel valgus and forefoot abduction.

Age.   Any age, but is seen almost exclusively in adults, usually occurring in those over the age of 40 years; women more often than men.

Onset.   The onset has been insidious without an inciting episode being related.

Duration.   May occur over a few months to several years, progressively getting worse in pes planus, hindfoot valgus, and forefoot pronation deformity.

Intensity.   Usually mild pain and discomfort in stage I; progressively gets worse with time as the deformity progresses to where, in the later part of stage III, the pain shifts to the ankle as the deformity becomes fixed.

Aggravating Factors.   Obesity may be an aggravating factor but has not been proven. Increased activity and allowing the condition to go untreated in the earlier stages.

Alleviating Factors.   Early conservative treatment in stage I with good arch supports and ankle compression brace. Early tendon débridement and synovectomy in stage I if conservative treatment fails.

Associated Factors.   Obesity may contribute to the progression of the disease; higher incidence in rheumatoid patients.

PHYSICAL EXAMINATION

General.   Patients with stage I disease may be in no acute distress. Those with stage II and III may exhibit guarding of the involved foot.

Orthopedic. The point of maximal tenderness corresponds to the area of pathology and is usually where the tendon passes around the tip of the medial malleolus to the insertion on the navicular. Swelling is best appreciated by viewing the hindfoot from a posterior vantage point while the patient is standing, paying specific attention to the inferior medial malleolus area of the affected foot and comparing it with the unaffected foot. Swelling is present even in the mildest of cases. Alignment of the hindfoot/forefoot is normal in stage I because the tendon is of normal length.

Testing for strength of the tibialis posterior tendon is done with the single heel rise test with the patient facing away from the examiner. The patient is asked to rise up on the ball of the affected foot while holding the other foot off the ground. The patient may use a door or a wall for balance. A positive heel rise test is the inability to go up on the forefoot or raise the heel off the ground. In stage I, the heel rise test is normal. In stage II, the tendon may be disrupted and secondary changes are developing. Swelling and tenderness have also progressed and are more pronounced. The single heel rise test becomes abnormal because the tendon has been elongated and weakened. With elongation of the tibialis posterior tendon, the initial heel inversion is weak and the patient either rises up incompletely without locking the heel or does not go up on the ball of the foot at all. The absence of the initial heel inversion is important in making the diagnosis of a stage II tendon elongation. Another helpful diagnostic sign is that of too many toes. When viewing the hindfoot from the posterior aspect, more toes are seen lateral to the ankle than are seen on the opposite normal foot. As the heel goes into more resting eversion or valgus, and the forefoot goes into abduction, more toes are seen laterally on the affected foot. The number of extra toes seen is a recordable measurement of the degree of deformity. In stage III, the tendon is elongated or ruptured, the hindfoot is moderately or severely deformed, and physical findings are most significant. Pressing on the sinus tarsi reproduces the pain symptoms, as does forcefully pressing the foot into the deformed position. Hindfoot valgus and forefoot abduction will be moderate to severe. The single heel rise shows absence of locking of the hindfoot and complete inability to rise up on the ball of the foot. The too many toes sign will be more apparent, and the patient is usually aware that the foot has become quite flat.

PATHOPHYSIOLOGY

The tibialis posterior muscle forms part of the deep posterior compartment of the calf. Arising from the interosseous membrane and adjacent posterior surfaces of the tibia and fibula, the large muscle units of the tibialis posterior converge onto its tendon in the distal third of the leg. The tendon has a very short excursion, and the muscle is quite powerful. This muscle-tendon unit is the main dynamic stabilizer of the hindfoot against valgus (eversion) deformity and is considered the principal invertor of the foot. It contributes to the elevation of the longitudinal arch by insertions into the inferior aspect of the navicular bone, the medial and intermediate cuneiform bones, and the bases of the second, third, and fourth metatarsal bases.

Disorders are manifest by inflammation about the tendon or longitudinal split tears within the tendon substance. The tendon may be mildly enlarged, with a bulbous configuration with fluid around the tendon sheath and peritendinitis present. A relatively mild elongation of the tendon decreases its function significantly. Elongation of the tendon leads to lateral rotation of the calcaneus, cuboid, navicular, and distal part of the foot. This results in abduction of the forefoot and valgus angulation of the calcaneus. The talus becomes plantar flexed without support of the sustentaculum tali, and occasionally the deltoid ligament becomes stretched. Adhesions form around the tendon in its sheath and the tendon undergoes a change to firmness in its consistency.

In stage III, the bony projection at the anterior margin of the posterior facet of the talus impinges on the superior aspect of the calcaneus in the sinus tarsi region. The talus becomes plantar flexed without support of the sustentaculum tali, and occasionally the deltoid ligament becomes stretched. Insufficiency is associated with peritalar subluxation/dislocation with lateral impingement of the calcaneus upon the fibula.

DIAGNOSTIC STUDIES

Laboratory
CBC, Full Chemistry Profile, PT, PTT. As routine preoperative screening.

Radiologic
Foot and Ankle X-rays. A minimum of three views is required. Usually, in stage I the x-rays are normal, with no loss of the longitudinal arch. In stage II, mild changes are noted, and in stage III, these changes have progressed with moderate loss of the longitudinal arch. Usually joint narrowing of the subtalar joint is present with osteophyte formation. In the sinus tarsi region, on the calcaneus, a white sclerotic region appears (white sign), which also indicates degenerative changes and impingement.

Technetium-99 Bone Scan. Shows, on the delayed views at this stage, uptake of the isotope at the site of the sinus tarsi region.

MRI. Shows fluid around the tendon in all stages; in stages II and III longitudinal tears may be seen in the tendon as it turns under the medial malleolus and extends distally.

DIFFERENTIAL DIAGNOSIS

Traumatic
Tendon/Ligamentous Injury. Differentiated by physical examination.

Infectious. Infection with any type of swelling, pain, and inflammation must be ruled out.

Metabolic. Always keep rheumatological disease in mind.

Neoplastic
Tumors. Physical examination can rule out tumor. Tumors are very rare in this area.
Vascular. Not applicable.
Congenital
Pes Planus Deformity. Seventeen percent of the population is born with this asymptomatic condition.
Acquired
Reflex Sympathetic Dystrophy. Is manifest by swelling, pain, color changes, and temperature fluctuation of the skin.

TREATMENT

Medical. Treatment for stage I tibialis posterior tendon difficulties should initially be nonoperative. An NSAID-type agent should be used for several weeks. A simple orthosis in the shoe, an elastic ankle brace, or avoiding aggravating footwear may be helpful. Decreasing or ceasing of sports or recreational activities that exacerbate the pain is recommended. Injected steroids should be avoided due to the risk of tendon weakness and subsequent rupture. Stage II may be treated similarly or with a more extensive shoe insert such as a UCBL orthosis.

Surgery
Stage I. Surgical treatment would be appropriate after continued inflammation after 3 months of conservative treatment. Intervention during stage I is successful in stopping the inflammation and tendon degeneration that would otherwise proceed to stage II. Surgical treatment involves opening the tendon sheath from the musculotendinous junction to its insertion. This release is followed by a synovectomy and débridement of the flaps of tendon, if present. Any longitudinal split tears can be sutured with a burying-of-the-knot technique. The roof of the tendon sheath is removed particularly distal to the medial malleolus so that it will not reconstitute itself.

Stage II. Surgical treatment of stage II with elongated tendon and mildly deformed hindfoot has been the substitution transfer of adjacent tendons. The most common transfer is that of the flexor digitorum longus to substitute the tibialis posterior tendon. Patients do not always get relief of the deformity, but usually get relief of pain symptoms.

Stage III. When the amount of deformity that exists in stage III is present, surgical intervention is indicated. Tendon transfers in the presence of this amount of deformity have not been effective. The most reliable procedures have been realignment of the hindfoot, followed by an arthrodesis procedure. Arthrodesis is an effective procedure because it does correct the static hindfoot deformity to some degree and provides predictable pain relief. Hindfoot motions in the subtalar joint are then absent and the ability to adapt to uneven surfaces is lost.

Indications. Surgical treatment of stage I is undertaken if conservative measures are not successful. In stage II, surgery is indicated if deformity is progressing or if symptoms interfere with normal activity. Stage III surgery is indicated to correct the deformity.

Contraindications. Relative in the older or less active population. Inability to undergo anesthesia.

TECHNIQUE OF SURGICAL ASSISTING

The PA assists with opening the tendon sheath, synovectomy, and débridement. Traction is maintained on tears and reanastomoses during suturing.

PEDIATRIC CONSIDERATIONS

Because this is a degenerative disease, it is rare in children and adolescents.

OBSTETRICAL CONSIDERATIONS

No surgical treatment during pregnancy. Use caution in performing x-rays and prescribing analgesics.

PEARLS FOR THE PA

The tibialis posterior tendon is a powerful invertor of the foot and loss of support leads to flat feet.

Hindfoot valgus and forefoot abduction deformities may occur with long-standing disease.

Injected steroids should be avoided due to the risk of tendon weakness and subsequent rupture.

Sprains: Wrist
Carrie Gunn-Edel, PA-C

DEFINITION

Trauma that causes complete or partially torn ligaments in the wrist joint.

HISTORY

Symptoms. Characterized by pain, edema, disability, and often ecchymosis, depending on the degree of injury to ligaments.

General. Occurs following a traumatic extension or flexion event of the wrist. Determine mechanism of injury and forces affecting the upper extremity at the time of acute event. Most patients are involved in an activity such as skate boarding, inline skating, basketball, volleyball, or other sports that require the use of the hands.

Age. Occurs in all ages, but more often in the second through fourth decades.

Onset. Immediately following trauma.

Duration. The majority of the time is acute, but chronic sprains may occur with overload or overuse. Ligamentous injuries may require 6 to 9 months to heal with conservative treatment.

Intensity. Moderate to severe pain immediately after traumatic event. Mild to moderate pain postinjury while wrist is at rest and immobilized.

Aggravating Factors. Motion of wrist against resistance or with the wrist in a dependent position.

Alleviating Factors. Immobilization, elevation, analgesics.

Associated Factors. Athletics.

PHYSICAL EXAMINATION

General. Inspect for areas of erythema or warmth that suggest an infectious process. Anhidrosis is indicative of neurologic injury. Evaluation for neurologic and vascular insufficiency is crucial.

Orthopedic. Observe and compare the wrists for swelling, ecchymosis, or gross deformity. Determine the functional status of the hand by asking the patient to perform simple maneuvers. Palpate the bones of the wrist, distal radius and ulna, hand, and digits for tenderness, deformity, or subluxation to rule out associated injury. Palpate all tendons and soft tissue for tenderness. Perform this examination with the patient's hand medially and laterally rotated, with the fist clenched and extended, and with the fingers independently flexed. Employ active resistance in all directions to elicit tenderness that may localize specific tendon or bone involvement.

PATHOPHYSIOLOGY

The wrist is comprised of a multiplicity of bones, tendons, and ligaments that allow the patient to perform the intricate functions of the hand. It is an active, mobile structure and is relatively unprotected from injury. Trauma can cause disruption of the ligaments about the wrist and sometimes cause avulsion of the ligament, demonstrated as an avulsion fracture. Tendons may stretch or tear with sufficient flexion, extension, or rotation. The small bones of the wrist (navicular, lunate, triquetrium, pisiform, trapezium, trapezoid, capitate, and hamate) may fracture with sufficient force.

DIAGNOSTIC STUDIES

Laboratory
CBC, Full Chemistry Profile, PT, PTT. As routine preoperative screening.
Radiology
Wrist X-ray (AP/Lateral/Oblique). Repeat in 10 to 14 days. Specialized x-rays with varied views when indicated (e.g., lateral flexion/extension views, radial/ulnar deviation views, clenched fist views, carpal tunnel views).
Wrist Arthrogram, Trispiral Tomogram, CT Scan, MRI. Are performed as indicated for continued symptoms.
Other
Three-phase Bone Scan. 72 hours after injury confirms a suspected fracture.

DIFFERENTIAL DIAGNOSIS

Traumatic
Carpal Instability. Instability of the wrist noted on physical examination.
Fracture. Seen on x-ray.
Infectious. Not applicable.
Metabolic
Gout, Pseudogout. Periodic, acute attacks of joint swelling and pain without history of a specific injury. Elevated serum uric acid levels with gout.
Neoplastic
Pathologic Fractures. Fracture and lesion seen on x-ray.
Vascular. Not applicable.
Congenital. Not applicable.
Acquired
Ganglion. Developed following traumatic event; palpable.
Carpal Tunnel Syndrome. Associated with numbness, weakness, and pain in the distribution of the median nerve (see topic carpal tunnel syndrome).

TREATMENT

Medical. For acute sprains, rest, immobilization, elevation, and ice pack for the first 24 to 48 hours. For chronic sprains, the patient is instructed to soak the wrist briefly in warm water each day while doing gentle ROM exercises. Referral to a hand therapist may be required for ultrasound, passive/active ROM exercises, edema control, and intermittent splinting. Occasionally, the use of short-acting steroid injection into the injured ligament is used.

Surgical. Generally none. Wrist arthroscopy is performed if extensive ligament injuries occur that cause instability of the wrist. Surgery is the most efficient way to evaluate the triangular fibrocartilage complex (TFCC).

Indications. When diagnostic tests are unable to show incomplete ligamentous injuries or full- or partial thickness cartilaginous defects and osteochondral fractures.

Contraindications. When diagnostic tests are negative for extensive ligament injuries and stability is maintained.

TECHNIQUE OF SURGICAL ASSISTING

Surgery is generally not required for wrist sprain. If extensive injuries are present, arthroscopy is the treatment of choice. Arthrotomy is not recommended. Primary wound healing must be complete before rehabilitation can begin.

PEDIATRIC CONSIDERATIONS

Always rule out growth plate injuries by using comparison x-rays. Treatment is the same as in adults.

OBSTETRICAL CONSIDERATIONS

No surgical treatment during pregnancy. Use caution in performing x-rays and prescribing analgesics.

PEARLS FOR THE PA

Ligamentous injuries of the wrist may require 6 to 9 months to heal with conservative treatment.

Referral to a hand specialist is recommended for specialized therapy or if associated injury or loss of function exists.

Further Reading

Adams JC: Outline of Fractures, ed 7. New York, Churchill Livingstone, 1978.

Jackson DW, et al: The Anterior Cruciate Ligament: Current and Future Concepts. New York, Raven Press, 1993.

Beaty JH: Fractures of the head and neck of the femur in children: A current concepts review. J Bone Joint Surg [Am] 76:283–294, 1994.

Browner B: Skeletal Trauma, Fractures, Dislocations, Ligament Injuries. Philadelphia, W.B. Saunders, 1992.

Canale ST: Fractures of the hip in children and adolescents. Orthop Clin North Am 21:341–352, 1990.

Chapman MW: Operative Orthopaedics. Philadelphia: J.B. Lippincott, 1993.

Crenshaw AH (ed): Campbell's Operative Orthopaedics, ed 8. Philadelphia, Mosby Year Book, 1992.

Dee R: Principles of Orthopaedic Practice. New York, McGraw-Hill, 1989.

Donnelly RE, Saltzman CL, Kile TA, Johnson KA: Modified chevron osteotomy for hallux valgus. Foot Ankle Int 15:642–645, 1994.

Esses SI: Textbook of Spinal Disorders. Philadelphia, J.B. Lippincott, 1995.

Feagin JA, et al: The Cruciate Ligament. New York, Churchill Livingstone, 1988.

Frandsen PA, Andersen E, Madsen F, et al: Garden's classification of femoral neck fractures: An assessment of inter-observer variation. J Bone Joint Surg [Br] 70:588–590, 1988.

Frymoyer JW (ed): Orthopaedic Knowledge Update 4. Chicago, American Academy of Orthopaedic Surgeons, 1993, pp 304–312.

Gould JS: The Foot Book. Baltimore, Williams & Wilkins, 1988.

Green DP: Operative Hand Surgery, vol. 3, ed 3. New York, Churchill Livingstone, 1993.

Henry JH: Patellofemoral problems. Clin Sports Med 2:1989.

Hurst JW: Medicine of the Practicing Physician, ed 3. Butterworth-Heinemann, 1992.

Iannotti JP (ed): Rotator Cuff Disorders: Evaluation and Treatment. Park Ridge, IL, American Academy of Orthopaedic Surgeons, 1991.

Johnson KA: Surgery of the Foot and Ankle. New York, Raven Press, 1989.

Johnston O: Further studies of the inheritance of hand and foot anomalies. Clin Orthop 8:146–160, 1956.

Jupiter JB (ed): Flynn's Hand Surgery, ed 4. Baltimore, Williams & Wilkins, 1991.

Labus JB (ed): The Physician Assistant Medical Handbook. Philadelphia, W.B. Saunders, 1995.

Mann RA, Coughlin MJ: Surgery of the Foot and Ankle. St Louis, Mosby, 1993.

Marcus RE, Goodfellow DB, Psister ME: Tendon rupture in sports injuries. Orthopedics, 18:715–721, 1995.

Matsen FA, et al: Practical Evaluation and Management of the Shoulder. Philadelphia, W.B. Saunders, 1994.

Miller MD: Review of Sports Medicine and Arthroscopy. Philadelphia, W.B. Saunders, 1995.

Netter F (ed): Musculoskeletal System, Part III—Trauma, Evaluation, and Management. CIBA Collection of Medical Illustration, Vol. 8. W. Caldwell, NJ, Cisa-Geigy, 1993.

Nuber G, Bowen M: Acromioclavicular joint injuries and distal clavicle fractures. J Am Acad Orthop Surg 5:11–18, 1997.

Rakel RE: Textbook of Family Practice. Philadelphia, W.B. Saunders, 1995.

Richards R: Acromioclavicular Joint Injuries. Instructional Course Lectures, vol. 42. Chicago, American Academy of Orthopaedic Surgeons, 1993.

Roberts C, Rosenblum S, Uhl R, Fetto J: Surgical treatment of Achilles tendon rupture. Orthop Rev 18:513–516, 1989.

Rockwood CA, Green DP, Bucholz RW, Heckman JD: Fractures in Adults, ed 4. Philadelphia, Lippincott-Raven, 1996.

Rockwood CA, Wilkins KE: Fractures in Children. Philadelphia, J.B. Lippincott, 1991.

Rothman RH, Simeone FA, et al: The Spine, ed 3. Philadelphia, W.B. Saunders, 1992.

Rowe CR (ed): The Shoulder. New York, Churchill Livingstone, 1988, pp 155–163.

Schwartz GR: Principles and Practice of Emergency Medicine. Malvern, PA, Lea & Febiger, 1992.

Scuderi GR et al: The Patellae. New York, Springer-Verlag, 1995.

Turner JA, Ersek M, Herron L, et al.: Surgery for lumbar spinal stenosis: Attempted meta-analysis of the literature. Spine 17:1–8, 1992.

Weinstein SL, Buckwalter JA: Turek's Orthopaedics: Principles and Their Application. Philadelphia, J.B. Lippincott, 1994.

United States Department of Commerce—Geographic Area Series: Economic and Statistical Administration, Bureau of Census. U.S. Government Printing Office, Washington, D.C., November 1994, page 11.

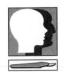

Chapter **10**

Plastic and Reconstructive Surgery

Blepharoplasty

Major William A. Mosier, PA-C, EdD, USAF

DEFINITION

Reconstruction, restoration, or cosmetic surgery of the eyelids.

TECHNIQUE

The technique of blepharoplasty involves a combination of skin removal and fat excision. The most important factors to consider are degree of brow ptosis, excess upper (or lower) lid skin, orbital fat in the upper lid, palpebral fat of the lower lid, degree of actinic dermatitis, and possible the dislocation of lacrimal gland.

Preoperative Assessment and Ophthalmologic Examination. A medical history must be taken to assess for indications of eye disease, pre-existing eyelid abnormalities, previous eye surgery, or systemic conditions that can contribute to eyelid abnormalities (e.g., diabetes mellitus, hypertension, and thyroid disease). An ophthalmic examination is absolutely necessary to rule out any ocular pathology prior to performing surgery.

Preoperative Surgery Preparation. Meticulous care must be taken to avoid getting prep solution in the eyes due to the possibility of corneal damage. Saline solution must be readily available to irrigate the eyes. Ophthalmic ointment applied prior to the preparation can be protective.

Cornea Protection. Protection of the cornea from desiccation, irritation, and trauma is an essential responsibility of the surgical team. It is imperative to administer saline drops in the conjunctival sac periodically during the procedure. The use of a plastic contact protective shell should be used to prevent desiccation and injury to the cornea. Instruments should never be passed over the eyes. Gauze and cotton should not touch the cornea. At the termination of the surgery, saline solution should be used to irrigate the conjunctival sacs to wash out any foreign body particles. When applying dressing, ensure that the eyelids are closed to protect the cornea.

Anesthesia. Local anesthesia is usually used. Topical anesthetic drops are often used to diminish corneal reflexes. Nerve block to the eyelids is also useful. Avoid deep injection of anesthetic, which can rupture small blood vessels and cause a retrobulbar hematoma.

Incisions. Incisions for lower eyelid blepharoplasty may be transconjunctival if no skin excision is needed. Incisions may also be subciliary, immediately below the lower eyelid lashes. Incision for upper eyelid blepharoplasty is usually performed in the supratarsal skin fold.

Procedure. Both upper eyelids are revised first. A modest elliptical excision of any excess skin is usually sufficient. The skin excision above the brow should be wider at the lateral two thirds than at the medial one third. Also of importance is the placement of the suture line for the standard upper eyelid incision. The lowermost line of the ellipse should lie within 7 mm above the ciliary margin. This allows the final scar to fall within the supratarsal folds. Because the final suture line tends to displace upward, it should be placed at a level lower than its intended destination. Removal of the medial fat pockets should be accomplished through a stab wound in the orbital septum. Suturing is with a subcuticular suture of nylon that can remain in place for up to 5 days.

Correcting the lower eyelid is the most difficult part of blepharoplasty, and operating technique varies widely. Complete hemostasis using fine, needle-tipped forceps and cautery must be maintained throughout the procedure to prevent a hematoma.

In the patient with only moderate protrusion of periorbital fat and minimal skin excess, an incision 3 mm below the ciliary margin is usually carried through the skin and orbicularis muscle, creating a skin–muscle flap. The orbital septum can then be incised and excess fat removed from the appropriate compartments. The amount of fat removed is determined by the degree of fat protrusion observed when pressure is gently applied to the globe.

In a patient with excessive fat protrusion and moderate amounts of excess skin, the fat is removed first. The excess fat is removed either through an incision, splitting the orbicularis muscle, or by making multiple stab wounds through the muscle and orbital septum. The majority of excess fat is found in the medial fat compartment. It should be cautioned that fat removal from the lateral pocket must always be conservative to prevent postoperative contour depression.

An accurate determination of the amount of skin to be excised is imperative in order to avoid a marked contracture and eversion of the eyelids (ectropion) caused by excessive resection. When suturing, avoid undue tension on the skin flap because vertical or horizontal foreshortening of the lower eyelid margin can result in buckling of the tarsus with either ectropion or excessive tearing (epiphora). The entire skin flap must be approximated, with exactness, to the contours of the wound bed. Then interrupted, fine silk sutures should be used to stitch the wound edges.

Postoperative Care. Bandaging the eyes after the procedure is usually not necessary. If bandages are not used, it is important to make sure that the cornea is covered and that the eyes remain well lubricated with an ophthalmic ointment until the anesthesia has worn off. If bandages are used, it is important to ensure that the eyelids are in their proper position under the dressing. The dressing should be removed on the second postoperative day. Ice compresses should be applied, starting on day two and

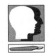

continuing for an additional two days. Most interrupted sutures are removed on the fourth postoperative day. Sutures left longer can result in the formation of epithelial tunnels. Sterile strips of adhesive tape can be placed across tension lines of the incision to ensure wound agglutination.

The patient should avoid strenuous activity and prolonged reading or watching television for at least 1 week postoperatively. The patient should be instructed to use liquid tears when the eyes feel dry or scratchy. The patient should also be informed that a sensitivity to light and bruising usually resolve.

INDICATIONS

Indications for blepharoplasty can be put into two categories: cosmetic enhancement and reconstructive surgery due to congenital deformities, trauma, or tumors.

CONTRAINDICATIONS

The only real contraindications for blepharoplasty would be a preexisting condition that would put the patient's vision at risk if the procedure were performed, or the inability to undergo anesthesia.

COMPLICATIONS

The overall complication rate is low. However, excessive fat excision results in a sunken look around the eyes. Excessive lower lid skin excision can result in an ectropion in patients with inadequate lower lid tone. The inability to completely close the eyes (lagophthalmos) can be caused by excision of too much skin from the upper eyelids. Inclusion cyst formation, often caused by employing through-and-through skin sutures, can be markedly reduced by using subcuticular sutures in the upper eyelids. This does not apply to the lateral margins.

Complications that are annoying to the patient, and are rather common, include blurred vision, ecchymosis of the eyelids, epiphora, hematomas, numbness, and eyelash alopecia. They all usually resolve without treatment.

ROLE OF THE PA

Having oxygen available and maintaining a clear airway is absolutely essential. Preoperative assessment, patient education, and postoperative care are always important responsibilities for the competent surgical PA.

Breast Reconstruction

Patricia Podres, PA-C, and
Angela Ballard, PA-C, BS

DEFINITION

It is a devastating event when a woman is informed she has breast cancer. Treatment for breast cancer is either lumpectomy and radiation or mastectomy with possible subsequent adjuvant chemotherapy. The fear of mastectomy is lessened for a woman when she is informed of the many reconstructive possibilities available. Once the patient and general surgeon decide on a mastectomy as their choice of treatment, the patient is then referred to a plastic surgeon to discuss the reconstructive possibilities.

TECHNIQUE

The timing of reconstruction is very important. The factors influencing whether the reconstruction is done immediately following a mastectomy or in a delayed manner are the judgment of the surgeon, the stage of the disease, and the patient's desires. In cases when chemotherapy is required, an immediate reconstruction does not delay healing nor postpone the initiation of chemotherapy.

There are basically two types of breast reconstruction. One type involves the use of the patient's own tissue (autogenous) from various sites on the body; the other involves the use of an implant device with or without a tissue expander. An implant is rarely used alone without a tissue expander in delayed reconstruction. In an immediate setting, there are situations when an implant can simply be placed subpectorally and complete a reconstruction. In the delayed setting and some immediate settings due to insufficient tissue, an expander is placed subpectorally with the intention of placing a series of saline injections to inflate the expander over an extended period of time (usually 4 to 6 weeks) during office visits. Once the expansion process is complete, the physician may choose to leave the expander in place to serve as the breast mound or, as in most cases, the patient is returned to the operating room, where the expander is removed and a permanent implant is placed. The final stage of breast reconstruction is the nipple/areola reconstruction, followed by tattooing.

There are multiple donor sites for autogenous tissue breast reconstruction with each providing its own amount of fat and skin tissue. These sites include the abdomen, buttock, lateral thigh, back, and hip. Each has its own indications as well as advantages and disadvantages.

The most common type of reconstruction is the transverse rectus abdominis myocutaneous (TRAM) flap. This procedure involves harvesting an island of skin and fat of the abdomen, along with a segment of the rectus muscle, which serves as its blood supply. This tissue is either tunneled up under the upper abdominal skin and brought out onto the chest still attached to the rectus muscle, or it is completely detached, incorporating its own blood supply from the rectus muscle; these arteries and veins are reanastomosed to blood vessels in the axilla or on the chest wall.

The use of buttock tissue, known as gluteal reconstruction, is an option that involves harvesting skin and fat from the buttocks based on the inferior or superior gluteal muscle and its blood supply and transferring this tissue to the chest wall defect, where it is reanastomosed microscopically to the axillary or chest vessels.

The use of lateral thigh tissue for breast reconstruction, known as the lateral transverse thigh flap (LTTF), involves transferring excess skin and fat from the "saddlebag" area of the thigh, with its blood supply, based on the lateral circumflex system to the chest and reattaching it microscopically to the vessels of the axilla or chest wall.

The use of the latissimus muscle from the back was used primarily before the introduction of the TRAM flap, but required use of an implant as well. Now, however, with the appropriate patient, skin, fat, and muscle can be harvested and tunneled through the axilla onto the chest wall. There is a resulting scar on the back following this procedure. However, even more recently, this procedure can be performed endoscopically, thus drastically reducing the size of the scar.

The hip flap, known as Ruben's flap, allows use of the tissue in the "love handle" region. This involves using fat and skin of the hip based on the deep circumflex iliac system and transferring this tissue onto the chest wall, where it is reanastomosed to the vessels in the axilla or on the chest.

In all of the above procedures, once the tissue is placed on the chest wall, shaping plays a vital role in the reconstruction. It can be a very time-consuming effort to achieve symmetry with the opposite breast or even to simulate bilateral breasts. In some cases, if the vasculature of the flap is vigorous and the shape is impeccable, nipple/areola reconstruction can be performed immediately. However, in most cases the nipple reconstruction is usually performed secondarily as an outpatient procedure, with a tattooing procedure following approximately 2 months after the nipple reconstruction.

Postoperative Care.   Recovery for breast reconstruction usually entails a 2- to 5-day hospital stay with ambulation beginning on the first day following the procedure. All procedures involve the use of drains in the operative sites that stay in place in the patient for up to 2 weeks. Total rehabilitation time is approximately 6 weeks. At that time, most patients can resume normal activity.

Implant/expander patients should be informed to avoid direct blows to the tissue expander, keep the incision line clean and dressed, apply antibiotic ointment as ordered, and not use a heating pad over the expander. The patient should also be aware that it is normal for the tissue to be slightly swollen and bruised. Suture removal should be scheduled.

INDICATIONS

The indications for all types of reconstruction, in addition to following mastectomy, include correction of chest wall defects, congenital defects, and trauma.

TRAM. This is the flap of choice for most patients, provided the patient has not had an abdominoplasty and has an adequate volume of abdominal tissue.

Gluteal Reconstruction. This procedure is used only when there is a lack of tissue in other sites.

LTTF. Patients with previous abdominoplasty or TRAM, minimal abdominal tissue, generous "saddlebag" deformity, and preference of patient.

Latissimus Muscle. Previous TRAM or abdominal surgery, high-risk patients (e.g., morbid obesity, diabetes), decreased complexity of surgery, minimal surgery time, hardiness of the flap, and patient choice.

Ruben's Flap. Include previous TRAM or abdominal surgery, generous available tissue, inadequate tissue in other areas, and aversion to implants.

CONTRAINDICATIONS

TRAM. Inadequate amount of tissue and disruption of blood supply from previous abdominal surgery.

Gluteal Reconstruction. Inadequate tissue volume, flap complexity due to inexperience of the surgeon, unacceptable donor defect to a specific patient and surgeon, and possible need for a balancing procedure on the opposite buttock.

LTTF. Inadequate thigh tissue, complexity of the surgery based on limited surgeon experience, unacceptable donor defect and scar, and the need for balancing procedure on the opposite thigh.

Latissimus Muscle. Include possible undesirable scar, inadequate flap volume, and possible need for an implant.

Ruben's Flap. Include insufficient tissue, previous liposuction, increased technical complexity, surgeon's lack of experience with this technique, need for revision of donor site with secondary procedure, and the need for a balancing procedure on the opposite hip.

COMPLICATIONS

Risks include hematoma, unequal breast size (which is normal even in nonoperated breasts), tissue slough, vascular occlusion resulting in loss of the flap, fat necrosis resulting in lumping or draining, scars that widen or change, numbness or pain, fluid collection, and the possible need for blood transfusion.

ROLE OF THE PA

The physician assistant's role in breast reconstruction begins with the initial interview with the patient, at which time the appropriate flap decision is made in conjunction with the surgeon and patient. The PA will prep, drape, prepare the appropriate donor site and, depending on experience and under the supervision of the surgeon, may begin harvesting the flap while the surgeon begins preparation of the breast site and vessels. The PA assists with the microscopic portion of the procedure and with closing. The PA may then apply dressings, write the postoperative orders and operative note, and usually accompanies the patient to the recovery room. The flap is monitored postoperatively in the inpatient and outpatient setting, and in the case in which tissue expanders are used, the PA or physician is responsible for the task of expansion.

Face Lift

Major William A. Mosier, PA-C, EdD, USAF

DEFINITION

Reconstructive surgery on the face for elevating sagging tissues and eliminating wrinkles and other signs of aging.

TECHNIQUE

Preoperative Instructions to Patients. The patient should be instructed to wash hair, face, and neck with a disinfectant solution the night prior to the surgical procedure.

Premedication. The preoperative combination of a tranquilizer, a hypnotic, and a narcotic are useful to assist the patient in becoming and remaining calm for the duration of the procedure.

Anesthesia. Local anesthesia is adequate in conservative procedures, although general anesthesia is an option (90% of patients undergo the procedure under local anesthetic).

Positioning the Patient for the Procedure. The patient should be positioned on the operating table with head and shoulders elevated from the table. This allows access to the area around the ears and nape of the neck. The hair is combed back and upward and parted to accommodate the incisions.

Sterilization. The skin of the area to undergo the procedure must be washed with a disinfectant solution and then draped with sterile towels and sheets.

Incisions. Cuts are to be curved and angular. The intent of this is to eliminate wrinkles without conspicuous scarring. Incisions should be concealed in the hairline and in the folds of the ear. Incisions made in the temporal region should be within the hairline and should be angled from anterior to the superior part of the ear up into the scalp. Care must be taken to avoid the superficial temporal artery and vein.

Preauricular incisions should be made immediately anterior to the tragus. It is essential in this area to enact closure without tension on the tissue.

Lobule incisions should be made in the lobular fold that is created by the attachment of the lobule to the cheek. In the patient without lobules separate from the cheek, it is best to create lobules by stitching the medial cut edges of the lobule together. Then the facial flap should be fixed superiorly and medially under the reconstructed lobule.

The postauricular incision should be positioned no more than 4 mm lateral to the postauricular sulcus, directly on the posterior surface of the auricle.

The incision at the nape of the neck should be immediately inside the margin of the hair, starting at the mid portion of the mastoid bone, moving down to the nape region.

Undermining.   Undermining, mostly performed in the subdermal fatty layer, is the most important component of the face lift technique. Undermining in the temporal region is usually carried out with an incision at the margin of the hairline on the temporal fascia at a plane deeper than the rest of the face and neck. Beginning dissection, anterior to the ear, the platysma muscle is observed. The level of dissection should be lateral to the platysma due to its support of cranial nerve VII (facial nerve). Proceeding anteriorly into the cheek, the branches of the facial nerve become progressively more superficial.

Undermining should not be carried to the commissure, the nasolabial line, nor the mentum due to increased risk of hematoma and injury to facial nerve branches. Deep penetration at this incision site may cause damage to the upper branches of the facial nerve. This incision may also cause a loss of hair follicles and interfere with blood supply to the follicles.

Undermining the forehead region is easier, but is only modestly effective at eliminating furrows and wrinkles.

The orbital region is usually not undermined because the pull subsequent to undermining the temporal region often accomplishes adequate tightening of the skin around the orbits. When this is not adequate, wrinkles are best resolved by implementing a separate technique confined to the eyelids.

The skin of the neck should be undermined at the plane external to the platysma muscle. The skin should be raised postauricular down into the nape of the neck and forward along the lateral neck submandibularly.

Postoperative Care.   Diet should be restricted to liquid consumption for at least 3 days to minimize movement of the new tissue bed. The patient may be discharged by the third postoperative day and should be taught exercises to relax the facial muscles. Rehabilitation should include cautioning the patient against excessive and exaggerated use of the mimetic muscles to avoid reproducing wrinkles.

INDICATIONS

Face lifting is a corrective procedure for correcting deformities of the face and neck. Example applications are for correcting bags, bulges, skin folds, heavy lines, sags, and chin or throat wattles.

CONTRAINDICATIONS

Historically, surgeons were discouraged from correcting physiognomic irregularities of the face, regardless of severity because cosmetic surgery was considered frivolous and immoral. However, since the early part of the twentieth century, cosmetic surgery has become more acceptable as a treatment of choice for its psychological value in terms of self-esteem and self-image. The only contraindication would be related to the physical condition of the patient, such as immune compromise or medical conditions that would prohibit the use of anesthesia.

COMPLICATIONS

Complications of face lift occur in direct proportion to the aggressiveness of undermining and the ability to control bleeding. Hematoma is the most frequently occurring complication. Bleeding can be controlled by using epinephrine during local anesthetic injection, controlling hypertension, and elevation of the head and neck. Although large hematomas need to be evacuated, small hematomas spontaneously absorb. Skin necrosis is caused by excessive undermining that interferes with blood supply. Loss of hair may result from using a hairline incision in the temporal region. Hair loss may also result from excessive tension on the temple flap and by undermining that interferes with the blood supply to the hair follicles. Infection and facial nerve paralysis are also potential complications.

ROLE OF THE PA

The PA may serve as a first assistant in face lift procedures. It is important for the PA to assist in tightening and fixing of the areas being undermined by stretching the skin and using the fingertips in a centripetal fashion. When the PA is responsible for adjusting tension, it is important to be aware of the delicacy of the tissue being pulled against.

Facial Lacerations

J. Jeffrey Heinrich, PA-C, EdD, and
Bruce Fichandler, PA

DEFINITION

A minor laceration is defined as a wound that is without complicating circumstances (e.g., associated deep structure injury). A facial laceration is a traumatic wound that disrupts the normal anatomical features of this important aesthetic unit.

TECHNIQUE

It is important to have a good understanding of the historical and physical characteristics associated with any laceration. One should establish the mechanism of injury and the time that has elapsed since injury. Physical assessment should include location, size, depth, extent of debris, and the amount of soft-tissue damage. Injury to vital facial structures should be carefully evaluated and properly documented.

Closure is the goal in the management of any wound in order to minimize deformity and to prevent infection. Wound closure may be obtained in one of three ways:

1. First intention (primary) closure, using edge to edge approximation, a skin graft, or flap
2. Secondary intention (spontaneous healing), which allows the wound to contract or re-epithelialize by itself
3. Third intention (delayed) closure, using edge-to-edge approximation, a skin graft, or a flap after it is established that the wound is no longer contaminated.

In the vast majority of cases, facial lacerations are closed primarily. There are two basic exceptions to primary closure: significant contamination or extensive deep structure injury.

Management of the clean wound starts with local anesthesia to ensure patient comfort. This is followed by cleansing, débriding, hemostasis, and atraumatic closure. In an attempt to minimize scarring, intradermal sutures should be used. This is followed by placement of skin sutures, which assist in the meticulous approximation of the wound edges, leading to the best possible result. Interrupted sutures are recommended for the intradermal closure and a continuous suture is recommended for the skin closure.

Wound healing begins immediately following closure of the facial laceration. The first phase of healing is the inflammatory stage, and this continues for approximately 24 to 48 hours following wound closure. This phase represents the common findings of redness, swelling, and pain.

The second phase is the collagen phase, which lasts 42 to 60 days following the wound closure. Collagen synthesis and increased tensile strength of the scar are the hallmarks of this phase.

The third phase is scar maturation. This phase represents the remodeling of the collagen fibers and is clinically thought to last 9 to 15 months.

INDICATIONS

The obvious indication for repairing a facial laceration is to restore the aesthetic unit to mirror its original appearance as closely as possible. Nevertheless, patients should be advised that scarring is inevitable with any facial laceration. The best results are uniformly achieved by immediate repair and meticulous approximation of the wound edges. One must carefully assess for deep structure injury, such as injuries to the facial nerve, parotid duct, and so on. Of particular note is the need to pay attention to the anatomical landmarks, such as the vermilion border, the eyebrow, and the eyelid. Failure to repair these areas correctly may leave the patient with a very significant deformity. Unless the PA is familiar with how to repair lacerations in these areas, it is best to consult a specialist.

CONTRAINDICATIONS

Facial lacerations are of secondary concern when the patient has airway problems, significant bleeding, or an intracranial injury. Only when deep structure injuries are demonstrated to be nonexistent or are corrected should facial lacerations be surgically closed. When there are deep structure injuries, facial lacerations should be managed by a specialist and not by the primary care PA. The same is true if the lacerations is greater than 8 hours old because significant levels of bacteria may be present. If aggressive débridement is necessary, consultation may be appropriate. It is not uncommon to consult a plastic surgeon for wound closure to give the patient the best possible result.

COMPLICATIONS

Although scarring is inevitable, it is the most common complication with a facial laceration. Scar revision is possible following a reasonable amount of time for scar maturation. The most common early complication following wound closure is infection. The rich blood supply of the face makes this anatomical region more forgiving; therefore, the infection rate is low. Hematoma, excessive soft-tissue trauma, and a compromised vascular supply can all contribute to poor wound healing and the dreaded complication of soft-tissue loss secondary to necrosis. Proper technique minimizes this complication. Inadequate nutrition, the use of steroids, and chronic illnesses such as diabetes mellitus represent some of the systemic elements that may negatively impact wound healing.

ROLE OF THE PA

A minor laceration is commonly cared for by a PA in the office or emergency department. A PA, however, should not primarily close a facial laceration greater than 8 hours old due to the risk of infection. The PA caring for a patient with a facial laceration should carefully evaluate the whole patient and establish the proper treatment plan.

Free Flap
Patricia Podres, PA-C, and
Angela Ballard, PA-C, BS

DEFINITION

A free flap is the transfer of muscle, skin, fat, or fascia (with its own blood supply) to a distant site on the body. The procedure is performed in order to cover the defect of either an open or closed wound with exposed bone, tendon, or unstable scar.

Microsurgery is required to anastomose the artery and veins of the flap to the artery and veins at the site of the wound.

TECHNIQUE

Initiation of the surgery involves débridement and exploration of the wound site with dissection of an adequate uninjured recipient artery and vein. The next step of the surgical process involves the proper choice of flap to close the defect: myocutaneous (e.g., free rectus), fasciocutaneous (e.g., temporalis), osteomyocutaneous (e.g., scapular, fibular), or muscle (rectus, gracilis, latissimus). In addition, the size and thickness of the flap needed must be taken into consideration in order to decide from which site on the body the flap is to be harvested. The flap must be dissected carefully with its supporting vasculature. Example: Latissimus dorsi along with the thoracodorsal artery and vein.

After the flap is harvested and transferred to the defect, a vascular supply must be re-established. At this point, the artery and vein must be anastomosed to the vessels in the defect using microvascular technique under microscopic magnification. The suture used in this anastomosis is usually a 9-0 or 10-0 Prolene or nylon. Following adequate perfusion of the flap, the microscope is removed from the field, and the flap is inset into the defect and sutured in place carefully in order not to obstruct the blood flow. At this time, if a muscle flap has been used, as opposed to a cutaneous flap, a skin graft must be harvested from the buttocks or thighs to provide skin coverage. The graft is meshed and placed on top of the flap and secured with sutures or staples.

Postoperative Monitoring. The first 24 hours are usually the most critical in ensuring flap viability. Monitoring of the flap is carried out by several different methods. The amount and color of the drainage of the flap is closely watched. The color and temperature of the flap itself and any swelling is closely followed. Doppler of the vessels ensures the competency of the new anastomoses. Finally, bleeding from the flap with a needle stick helps determine the health of the flap by the quickness of the return and the color of the blood.

INDICATIONS

The procedure is performed in order to cover the defect of either an open or closed wound with exposed bone, tendon, or unstable scar.

CONTRAINDICATIONS

Contraindications to free flap include inadequate vasculature at the wound site, generally poor patient vascular status (due to peripheral vascular disease, diabetes mellitus, etc.), radiation injury to the involved area that destroys both tissue and vasculature, unstable complications of diabetes mellitus, and inexperience in microvascular surgery.

COMPLICATIONS

Risks include hematoma, tissue slough, vascular occlusion resulting in loss of the flap, fat necrosis resulting in lumping or draining, scars that widen or change, numbness or pain, fluid collection, and the possible need for blood transfusion.

ROLE OF THE PA

The role of the PA begins in the preoperative phase with the history and physical examination, as well as screening of the patients. Detailed explanation of the procedure, expected outcomes, possible complications, and postoperative course requirements are also the PA's responsibility to the patient.

In the operative suite, in addition to all prepping and draping, the PA's role includes proper positioning of the patient for adequate access to the wound and the proposed flap site. During the surgery, the PA allows a two-team approach with the PA and surgeon working together to begin the flap harvest, débride the wound, and dissect adequate recipient vessels. In tandem, the surgeon and the PA work under the microscope, preparing the vessels and anastomosing them. After the anastomosis is complete, the PA and the surgeon close the donor defect and inset the flap. Upon closing the donor site and placing the appropriate type and number of drains, the proper size and thickness of skin graft (if needed) is harvested, placed on the wound, and secured. Together, the sterile dressings are applied and the patient is taken to the recovery room. The PA is responsible for the postoperative notes and orders.

Postoperatively, the approximate hospital stay is 5 to 7 days, during which the PA follows the patient and flap daily, assesses flap viability, monitors drain output, alters medications, and changes dressings as needed.

Rhinoplasty

Major William A. Mosier, PA-C, EdD, USAF

DEFINITION

Reconstructive, restorative, or cosmetic surgery of the nose.

TECHNIQUE

Nasal plastic surgery is the most technically challenging of all procedures in plastic surgery. Correcting each nose with the same technique (cookbook approach) is not possible. There are at least four basic surgical approaches that should be understood if one is to be able to adequately treat any one individual nose with rhinoplasty. This is due to the wide variation in size, shape, direction of alar cartilage, subcutaneous tissue, and overlying skin on the tip structure of patients.

Aesthetic rhinoplasty is most commonly performed using local anesthesia on an outpatient basis. Patient dissatisfaction is more frequent with nasal surgery than with any other cosmetic procedure. This is mostly due to the extended healing process.

There are two basic approaches to rhinoplasty: open structure rhinoplasty and closed structure rhinoplasty. The closed technique does not allow nasal structure changes to be made under direct visualization. This is why many surgeons prefer the open structure approach, especially for the complicated problems of the nasal tip. In open structure rhinoplasty, more emphasis is placed on reshaping the nasal contour than on reducing it. The open approach permits precise tissue debulking on the undersurface of the nasal skin, thus allowing better draping of the skin–soft-tissue envelope (S–STE) over the lower third of the nose.

Preoperative Assessment. Preoperative assessment should include evaluation for the following: adenoid hypertrophy, allergic rhinitis, cold symptoms, deviated septum, foreign body, fractures, polyps, tumors, and turbinate hypertrophy.

Patient Education. Patients should be informed that nasal packing may require mouth breathing for up to 3 days postoperatively. Depending on edema resolution and gradual tissue softening, satisfactory results may take up to 1 year. For this reason, preoperative patient education about realistic expectations and timeliness for final results is important.

Anesthesia.   Careful titration of anesthetic agents and close monitoring of vital signs is imperative with open structure rhinoplasty because the procedure may take 2 hours or more to complete. Rhinoplasty is usually done under local anesthesia, although general anesthesia may be used in special cases where the patient is extremely apprehensive. Local anesthetic injections of 1:1 mixture of 2% lidocaine HCl with 1:1000 epinephrine in combination with nasal packs of a 10% cocaine solution combined with 1:1000 epinephrine reduce bleeding and shrink tissue to facilitate good visualization of nasal structures (epinephrine overdose can result in headache, hypertension, nervousness, palpitations, respiratory distress, restlessness, or tachycardia; close cardiac monitoring is essential). It is key to remember to keep the total dosage as low as possible. Excellent infiltration can be achieved with no more than 10 mL of anesthesia using a 27-gauge needle.

The first area to infiltrate is the dorsum of the nose. Next, field blocks immediately lateral to the pyriform aperture are performed. Intraforaminal blocks are useful and the base of the nose is infiltrated last, near the nasal spine, with no more than 2 mL of solution. It is most appropriate to wait 5 minutes for the anesthesia to take effect before commencing with the surgery. During the waiting period, the nose can be packed with 1-inch gauze soaked in saline to prevent blood and debris from draining into the posterior pharynx during the procedure.

Positioning the Patient.   The operating table should be elevated so that the patient's head is above the heart. This diminishes bleeding during the operation. A foot plate is also useful to prevent the patient from sliding down the table.

Preoperative Preparation.   Nasal vestibule hair should be trimmed and the external nares cleaned with a sterilizing solution. Draping must be done in a manner that does not obscure the forehead and chin so that the facial contours, in relation to the nose, can be appreciated during the procedure.

Incisions.   When using the open approach, a number 15 scalpel blade can be used to make an incision through the subcutaneous tissue to the level of the medial crura. The midcolumellar incision should then be connected, inside the nose, to bilateral columellar marginal incisions that begin at the inferior aspect of the medial crura. Care must be taken not to cut the underlying cartilage.

Undermining.   Through the incision, the skin overlying the columella and nasal tip is dissected away from the alar cartilage bilaterally. This allows for modification of the alar and nose tip cartilage under direct visualization. The extent of undermining depends on the redraping required and the exposure needed to perform the surgery.

Resectioning.   Revisions in the bony pyramid of the nose are performed by using an osteotome to rasp the dorsum of the nose to reduce a nasal hump. It can also be applied to the infrastructure of the nasal bones arising from the maxilla for narrowing the nose.

Typical Surgical Steps. Typical surgical steps include septum revision, sculpturing of lateral cartilage, nasal tip revision, nasal length shortening, lowering of the nasal bridge, nasal bone fracturing (if indicated), and upper lateral cartilage refinement.

Closure and Suturing. Suturing varies, depending on the revisions performed. Often, a 4-0 chromic catgut suture, with the knot tied inside the nose, incorporating muscle and alar base, is used to relieve tension from the skin sutures. However, marginal incisions are often closed with 6-0 chromic catgut. To reduce suture scars, sutures can be removed by the fourth postoperative day. When the skin sutures are removed, the wound is then best supported with Steri-Strips for 1 week.

Dressing, Packing, and Splinting. Tight, intranasal packing is *not* necessary except in the rare cases where a wide, submucous resection that requires bilateral elevation of mucoperichondrial flaps is performed. If packing is used, it should be removed by the second postoperative day, except when extensive septal reconstruction has been performed. In that case, packing should be removed by the fourth postoperative day. Sterile paper tape is applied when indicated. A malleable splint can be placed over the taping or directly on the skin to approximate skin flaps to bone. A splint can also help prevent hematoma formation under skin flaps. A nasal splint should usually be left in place for 10 days. Premature removal of a splint can elevate skin flaps, and thus prolong healing. Unless contraindicated, antibiotics are routinely used.

Postoperative Care. Due to the drying of mucous membranes, the inside of the nose may undergo a crusting that can be very uncomfortable for the patient. This usually begins once the packing is removed and can continue for 3 weeks. Moistened cotton swabs may be used to soften and loosen the crust. The patient should be encouraged to use a humidifier at night until the crusting has resolved. The patient is instructed *not* to blow the nose until the second postoperative week.

The patient should also be alerted to the possibility that, as blood clots dissolve (around the fifth postoperative day), bleeding may occur. In this case, the patient should be instructed to sit upright, very gently pinch the lower third of the nose, apply an ice pack if needed, and call the surgeon if the bleeding does not stop within a few minutes.

The patient should avoid strenuous physical activities for at least 3 weeks postoperatively. The patient should be further informed that ecchymosis may take as long as 4 weeks to subside and that residual edema may persist for up to 2 years.

INDICATIONS

Typical reasons for requesting rhinoplasty are for reducing overall nose size, reshaping the tip, and removing a hump. Breathing difficulty, requiring nasal-septal reconstruction (septorhinoplasty), may accompany these complaints. In that case, a simple operation may be used to correct the combination of problems.

CONTRAINDICATIONS

The main contraindications are pre-existing conditions that would put the patient at risk during the surgical procedure, such as the inability to undergo anesthesia.

COMPLICATIONS

The most common complications of rhinoplasty are hemorrhage or epistaxis. However, they are not serious complications and usually resolve without any problem. The most serious frequent complication is an uneven thickening of the nose tip and dorsum, caused by thickening scar tissue.

ROLE OF THE PA

Facilitating good exposure at the operating site, achieving hemostasis efficiently, and handling tissue appropriately are the hallmarks of a competent surgical PA. Additional, procedurally specific duties include making sure that the airway is clear and that oxygen is available. Preoperative assessment, patient education, and postoperative care are important components of the surgical PA's responsibilities.

Skin Grafting

Bruce Fichandler, PA, and
J. Jeffrey Heinrich, PA-C, EdD

DEFINITION

A skin graft is a section of skin harvested from one location on the body (donor site) and transplanted to another location on the body (recipient site). There are three types of skin grafts: autograft (same patient), allograft (same species), and xenograft (different species).

Skin grafts may also be defined by thickness. A split-thickness skin graft includes the epidermis and a portion of the dermis. This category may be further subclassified as a thin or a thick split-thickness skin graft based on how far into the dermis one harvests. In contrast, a full-thickness skin graft includes the epidermis and all of the dermis.

TECHNIQUE

Skin grafts are taken by using either a free-hand knife (e.g., Watson) or a dermatome machine. A free-hand knife is used most commonly for harvesting either small amounts of skin or skin from irregular surfaces. Similar to a straight razor, but with a guard to control the depth, a free-hand knife is moved in a back-and-forth slicing motion to obtain the skin graft.

Dermatome machines include the manually operated Padgett drum dermatome, as well as a variety of gas- or electric-driven devices. They are useful for taking larger amounts of skin, as well as for obtaining a more uniform depth than the free-hand method.

Prior to obtaining the skin graft, the area may be prepared with a lubricant such as saline or mineral oil to facilitate the movement of the dermatome over the surface. One should avoid harvesting over joint surfaces, the dorsum of the hand, the face, and areas of known thin skin such as the medial thighs.

The grafts may be sutured and then treated in either an open or closed dressing technique. Those favoring the open technique use the opportunity to provide constant attention to the graft site, watching for the development of any seromas or hematomas. These must be incised or drained in order to put the skin back in contact with the wound. A compressive dressing is used to help hold the graft against its recipient site in an attempt to prevent the collection of a seroma or hematoma. Such a dressing should either be changed within the first 24 to 48 hours, when care can be given to any development of a seroma or hematoma, or not until 7 to 10 days, by which time the graft would have taken. Great care must be taken in any dressing change so as not to lift up the graft with the removal of the dressing and disrupt the tenuous attachment of the graft to the underlying bed.

The donor site is treated by covering the area with either a medicated or a biologic dressing. The donor site heals by re-epithelialization in 10 to 14 days, depending on the depth taken. The site may be used again, bearing in mind that dermis does not regrow and the site may be used only a finite amount of times depending on the amount of dermis removed each time.

INDICATIONS

A skin graft is indicated in those instances in which the skin deficit, either traumatically or surgically created, is deemed to be too large for spontaneous wound closure. This would include those wounds in which the time for closure would be generally more than 2 to 3 weeks or in which spontaneous closure would likely result in greater cosmetic distortions or functional deficits (e.g., across joint surfaces).

Split-thickness skin grafts are by far the most frequently used type of skin graft. They are used for coverage of large areas of body surface involvement, generally take better than a full-thickness skin graft, and allow for repeated harvesting of the donor site if additional skin is necessary. Because there is no transfer of hair follicles in the skin graft, the patient does not get growth of hair at the recipient site.

A full-thickness skin graft has the advantages of less contraction than a split-thickness graft, and generally a better color match. In addition, because it is thicker, it can provide more padding, which is useful in an area such as the finger tip. A full-thickness skin graft is a hair-bearing transfer and can be used to reconstruct areas such as the eyebrow. Furthermore, a full-thickness graft is usually of such a size that the donor site can be closed primarily, with less likelihood for scarring than a split-thickness donor site. Postoperative management of the donor site is generally easier and may be treated like any other surgical incision site.

Size is the major limiting factor for selecting a full-thickness skin graft in order for the donor site to be closed primarily. Occasionally, a full-thickness skin graft will be taken to cover a wound, and a split-thickness skin graft is used to cover the donor site of the full-thickness graft.

CONTRAINDICATIONS

Full-thickness skin losses of less than 2 cm^2 generally close in sufficient time such that skin grafting is not required. Other contraindications include a recipient site that is poorly vascularized, a recipient site with a high level of bacteria, when there is exposed tendon without paratendon coverage, or if there is a bone exposed without periosteum. In addition, those wounds that are heavily irradiated frequently result in failure of the skin graft and other means of coverage may need to be considered.

COMPLICATIONS

Failure of the skin graft to take in the recipient site is the major complication. This can occur as a result of any one or a combination of the following factors:

1. Shear forces between the recipient bed and the graft
2. Hematoma or seroma between the graft and the recipient site
3. Infection

Regrafting of some or all of the wound is occasionally required.

ROLE OF THE PA

The PA assists with both the harvesting and application of the skin graft.

Further Reading

Cohen KI, Diegelmann RF, Lindblad WJ (eds): Wound Healing: Biochemical and Clinical Aspects. Philadelphia, W.B. Saunders, 1992.
Elliott LF (ed): Autogenous tissue breast reconstruction. Clin Plast Surg 21:2, 1994.
Hartrampf CR Jr, Michelow BJ (eds): Hartrampf's Breast Reconstruction with Living Tissue. New York, Raven Press, 1991.
Smith JW, Aston SJ (eds): Grabb and Smith's Plastic Surgery. Boston, Little, Brown, 1991.

Chapter 11

Thoracic Surgery
Bronchial Obstruction
Lyle W. Larson, PA-C, MS

DEFINITION
Bronchial obstruction is a clinical finding that encompasses a wide variety of causes. Obstruction (or threatened obstruction) may be viewed as occurring from one of two causes: extrinsic or intrinsic. The location of the obstruction is just as important as the cause.

HISTORY
Symptoms. Dependent upon the source of obstruction, may include fever, exertional dyspnea, croup, malaise, weight loss, cyanosis, or hemoptysis. Dysphagia or hematemesis may also be presenting complaints.

General. Extrinsic causes include mediastinal tumor (e.g., thymoma), intrathoracic goiter, aortic aneurysm, foreign body aspiration, and esophageal cancer.

Intrinsic causes include epiglottitis, croup, tracheal tumors, tracheal stenosis, vocal cord paralysis, asthma (reactive airway disease), endobronchial granuloma, bronchiectasis, tuberculosis, bronchial stenosis, chronic occlusive pulmonary disease (COPD), and emphysema.

Age. Variable from infancy to late adulthood, depending on cause.

Onset. Sudden onset to insidious, depending on cause.

Duration. Intermittent to continuous, depending on cause.

Intensity. Asymptomatic to life-threatening, depending on cause and the location of the obstruction.

Aggravating Factors. Underlying pulmonary disease (e.g., fibrosis) and cardiac disease (e.g., ischemia, valvular heart disease, or arrhythmia).

Alleviating Factors. Bronchial relaxation; removal of offending source of obstruction.

Associated Factors. Reactive airway disease.

PHYSICAL EXAMINATION
General. Dependent upon the source of the obstruction, the patient may appear acutely ill (e.g., with sepsis), cachectic, lethargic, tachypneic, or present with acute respiratory distress.

Pulmonary. The hallmark of bronchial obstruction includes wheezing, consolidation of lung distal to the obstruction, cough, shortness of breath, exertional dyspnea, and stridor if obstruction is high. Auscultation should be performed over the upper airway and lungs to evaluate for wheezing or reduced or absent breath sounds. Percussion should also be performed to evaluate for consolidation. Croup may be evident. Rapid, shallow respi-

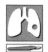

rations, bronchial or bronchovesicular sounds, bronchophony, egophony, and/or whispered pectoriloquy are often present; tactile fremitus may be increased.

Cardiac. Auscultation of the heart and palpation of pulses may reveal an arrhythmia, which may signify atrial fibrillation. A complete examination should be performed to evaluate congestive heart failure (CHF) as a source for the respiratory symptoms. Physical signs of CHF include peripheral edema, resting tachycardia, displaced point of maximal intensity, diminished S1, presence of S3 (if not in atrial fibrillation), murmur of mitral regurgitation, orthopnea, and wheezing (cardiac asthma).

Gastrointestinal. An abdominal examination should be performed to evaluate any symptoms of dysphagia or hematemesis. Cough associated with swallowing is an ominous physical finding. Any change in esophageal motility may lead to an aspiration pneumonitis in the unobstructed lung.

Head, Eyes, Ears, Nose, and Throat (HEENT). The throat should be observed for epiglottitis (see Pediatric Considerations), which constitutes a pulmonary emergency. If an extrinsic cause is suspected, neck examination should be performed with attention to lymph nodes, placement of the trachea (deviation), thyroid, or any palpable masses.

PATHOPHYSIOLOGY

Extrinsic (external) causes of bronchial obstruction may occlude the bronchus by compression (mass effect) or by direct obstruction (e.g., foreign body aspiration). The location of the obstruction may suggest a cause.

Intrinsic (internal) causes of bronchial obstruction may be multifocal. The most common forms of obstruction include asthma (reactive airway disease) and COPD, including emphysema. Their mechanisms differ, because asthma has an intermittent and reversible course, whereas COPD and emphysema do not. Other forms of airway obstruction include invasive masses, infectious processes, and iatrogenic causes (e.g., tracheal stenosis from prolonged or difficult intubation).

DIAGNOSTIC STUDIES

Laboratory

Arterial Blood Gases. Are performed to assess the degree of pulmonary compromise. The patient may be hypoxic or found to be retaining CO_2. Metabolic compensation may provide a clue to the duration of the obstruction.

Chemistry Panel. Used to rule out metabolic disturbances that may contribute to the obstruction. A low albumin level or the presence of hyponatremia may point to volume overload, whereas elevated blood urea nitrogen (BUN) and creatinine levels may indicate renal insufficiency.

Complete Blood Count. If the WBC is elevated with a left shift, cultures should be performed to identify the causative source.

Skin Test for Tuberculosis. Should be routinely performed, especially in the high-risk (e.g., immunocompromised) patient.

Skin Tests for Mycotic Infections. May be considered to evaluate for conditions such as coccidiomycosis or blastomycosis.

Blood Cultures. If sepsis is suspected.

Radiology

Chest X-ray. Is used to evaluate the entire bronchial tree as well as lung parenchyma; also to rule out foreign body or mediastinal mass.

CT of the Chest. Can provide a more definitive look at the bronchial tree and can quantitate the degree of obstruction.

Other

Tomograms of the Neck. Can identify and quantitate tracheal stenosis.

Pulmonary Function Studies. To further assess the degree of pulmonary compromise and differentiate between pure obstructive versus mixed obstructive/restrictive components.

Ventilation/Perfusion (V-Q) Scan. Performed to rule out pulmonary embolus (as indicated).

Electrocardiogram (ECG). Is done if there is observed or suspected arrhythmia, chest pain, infarct hypertrophy, or cardiomegaly.

DIFFERENTIAL DIAGNOSIS

Traumatic

Pulmonary Contusion. Associated with localized tenderness; varying degrees of consolidated in anatomically unrelated lobes.

Infectious

Empyema. The patient has fever, malaise, loculated fluid on CT of the chest; air-fluid levels on chest x-ray.

Pneumonia. Differentiated on chest x-ray with the classic appearance of pneumonia.

Viral Pleurisy. Diffuse rub present on examination without specific findings on chest x-ray.

Metabolic

Anaphylaxis. Associated with symptoms of urticaria or shock.

Atelectasis. Classic appearance on chest x-ray. Rales or rhonchi heard on auscultation.

Neoplastic

Metastatic Disease. Chest x-ray/CT of the chest shows lesion(s) and possibly adenopathy.

Vascular

Pulmonary Embolus. Hemoptysis, chest pain, anxiety, sense of impending doom. May have evidence of a deep vein thrombosis (e.g., calf swelling, positive Homan's sign).

Aortic Aneurysm. Of the thoracic region may show a widened mediastinum on chest x-ray; may be hyper- or hypotensive.

Acute Myocardial Infarction. Chest pain with or without radiation; ECG changes consistent with ischemia or infarct; complete heart block.

Cardiac Tamponade. "Water bottle" heart on chest x-ray; jugular venous distention; narrow pulse pressure; pulsus paradoxus.

Congenital. Not applicable.

Acquired. Not applicable.

TREATMENT

Medical. Treatment for intrinsic obstruction, as a result of narrowing of large and small airways due to spasm of smooth muscle, edema, or inflammation of the bronchial mucosa, is directed toward the cause. Agents that may be used include:

- Beta agonists (albuterol, 2 to 4 mg tid to qid; metaproterenol, 20 mg tid to qid)
- Anticholinergics (racemic epinephrine nebulizer PRN; ipratropium, 2 puffs qid)
- Methylxanthines (theophylline, 100 to 300 mg tid or qid; aminophylline, 200 mg tid or qid)
- Steroids (beclomethasone, 2 puffs tid or qid; triamcinolone, 2 puffs tid or qid)
- Cromolyn sodium (200 mg PO qid or 20 mg inhaled qid)

Inhaled beta agonists are used for acute exacerbations such as those seen with asthma. Infectious processes such as tuberculosis require more directed therapy, with or without surgical intervention. Intrinsic diseases caused by tumor invasion or obstruction require therapy directed toward the specific cause. Supportive therapy with oxygen is often necessary.

Management of extrinsic disease is directed at the correct diagnosis and management of the offending cause.

Surgical. Bronchoscopy, whether flexible or rigid, is the procedure of choice in making a diagnosis and relieving obstruction when an intrinsic mass or foreign body is suspected. Flexible bronchoscopy offers advantages of visualizing the distal bronchial tree, whereas rigid bronchoscopy is better suited for removing foreign objects and dilatation of stenotic areas. Either method permits biopsy and excision of a suspicious lesion. Thoracotomy may be required in certain instances to relieve the obstruction.

Indications. To provide definitive diagnosis of the cause of the compression and relieve the compression through therapeutic intervention.

Contraindications. The inability to protect the airway through intubation or tracheostomy if complications occur.

TECHNIQUE OF SURGICAL ASSISTING

The PA assists with opening and closure of the chest cavity. Airway patency (which may require a double-lumen tube) must be assured throughout the procedure. Depending on the cause, the PA provides suctioning to keep the field and airway clear of any obstruction. Chest tube thoracostomy is often required, because the lung is frequently deflated for the procedure. Postoperative care of the chest tube and its eventual removal are primary responsibilities of the PA.

PEDIATRIC CONSIDERATIONS

Epiglottitis should be managed only by those experienced with advanced airway management, with emergency airway capabilities readily available.

OBSTETRICAL CONSIDERATIONS

If a bronchial obstruction is present in the pregnant patient, close monitoring of the patient's oxygen level is crucial to avoid critical hypoxia, which may threaten both the mother and fetus.

PEARLS FOR THE PA

Understanding of medications, including inhalers, and their use is paramount in managing this disorder.

A prearranged back-up plan must be available for exacerbations and complications.

Annual influenza immunizations are recommended.

Greater morbidity occurs with repeated hospitalization, nocturnal exacerbations, mechanical ventilation, and steroid dependence.

The more proximal the cause, the sooner treatment should be implemented.

Chest Wall Tumors
Lyle W. Larson, PA-C, MS

DEFINITION

Chest wall tumors encompass a broad range of both primary and metastatic neoplasms of the soft tissues and thoracic skeleton, as well as primary neoplasms invading the thorax from lung, pleura, mediastinum, and breast.

HISTORY

Symptoms. Patients are initially asymptomatic; however, chest wall pain inevitably occurs with continued growth. With involvement of bone,

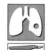

periosteum, or pleura, pain may be continuous. Less common symptoms include weight loss, fever, adenopathy, brachial plexus neuropathy, and symptoms from the source of invading neoplasm (e.g., pulmonary symptoms from lung, and pulmonary or cardiovascular symptoms from mediastinal involvement).

General. History should be obtained as to prior trauma to the area, previous radiation therapy, or neoplasm elsewhere, because these conditions may present with similar symptoms to chest wall tumors.

Age. The median age for benign tumors is 26 years and the median age for malignant tumors is 40 years. Male:female ratio is 2:1, except for desmoid tumor, which is 1:2.

Onset. Generally present as slow-growing masses.

Duration. Progressive unless treated.

Intensity. Initially asymptomatic. Pain is more common in malignant tumors, but cannot be used for differential diagnosis.

Aggravating Factors. Deep breaths rarely increase symptoms, except with advanced disease.

Alleviating Factors. Not applicable.

Associated Factors. Not applicable.

PHYSICAL EXAMINATION

General. Palpation reveals a firm mass, usually fixed to the chest wall, with or without fixation to skin or subcutaneous tissue.

By the time the patient with a chest wall tumor presents to the surgeon, many have had radiation therapy and may present with a postradiation necrotic ulceration.

Musculoskeletal. Localized musculoskeletal pain may be present with involvement of surrounding structures. With rib tumors, a mass may not be present on examination but appears on chest x-ray.

PATHOPHYSIOLOGY

There are a large number of tumors that may affect the chest wall. The most frequently encountered benign tumors are listed in Table 11–1 and the malignant tumors are listed in Table 11–2.

DIAGNOSTIC STUDIES

Laboratory

Electrolytes. Performed as part of the baseline evaluation in anticipation of a metastatic work-up.

CBC with Differential. Elevated WBC may be present with infectious causes such as empyema necessitatis or secondary infection (e.g., area of radiation necrosis).

Text continued on p. 466

Table 11-1. Benign Tumors

Tumor	Occurrence	Chest X-ray	Histology	Treatment
Chondroma	Most common benign tumor of chest wall Usually arises in ribs near costochondral junction May grow to enormous size Often painful	Lobulated density which displaces but does not replace bony cortex	Mature hyaline cartilage with areas of calcification and myxoid degeneration	Local, wide excision
Fibrous dysplasia	Associated with trauma Occurs most commonly over posterior rib, but can arise anywhere	Central fusiform mass with thin cortex and no calcification	Trabeculae with "fishhook" appearance; no transition from coarse fibers to lamellar bone	Local, wide excision
Osteochondroma	Rare; occurs early in 1st–2nd decade of life Solitary lesion that rarely progresses to malignancy Multiple lesions have a higher frequency of progression to malignancy	Focally radiolucent area surrounded by osteosclerotic tissue	Cartilaginous cap covering mature bone	Local, wide excision

Eosinophilic granuloma	Peak incidence, 5–15 years A disease of the lymphoreticular system Solitary or multifocal Occurs at metaphysis or diaphysis of bone	Osteolytic lesions	Eosinophils, neutrophils, giant cells, Langerhans cells	Resection or radiotherapy
Desmoid	3rd to 4th decade of life Reported to grow after trauma Growth associated with estrogen Often dull aching Mass fixed to underlying tissue but not skin	No radiographic findings	Sheets of fibroblasts with abundant, well differentiated collagen and without encapsulation May spread along fascial planes	Wide, local excision (wider than other lesions given ability to spread along fascial planes) Tamoxifen reported to decrease size and symptoms (related to sensitivity to estrogen)

Table 11–2. Malignant Tumors

Tumor	Occurrence	Radiology	Histology	Treatment
Chondrosarcoma	Most common malignant primary chest wall tumor 50% of all malignant neoplasms 25% of all primary chest wall tumors 80% arise in ribs, 20% in sternum Frequent local recurrence with late metastasis Most are solitary lesions Often present for 12–18 months prior to presentation	Lobulated mass arises in medullary bone with cortical destruction Stippled calcification pattern common	Varies from poorly differentiated to well differentiated lesion indistinguishable from benign chondroma	Wide local excision with margins of at least 4 cm Chest wall reconstruction often required Extremely resistant to radio- and chemotherapy
Ewing sarcoma	Most patients 5–30 years of age Most common chest wall malignancy in children 8%–22% of chest wall malignancies in adults Patients may present with progressive chest wall pain with or without a chest wall mass	Characteristic "onion peel" produced by new layers of periosteal bone formation Bony destruction Wide cortex and medullary bone also common	Neuroectodermal tumor with a neurohistogenesis	Resection of entire rib with partial or complete resection of adjacent ribs Chest wall reconstruction often necessary Postoperative external beam irradiation chemotherapy (doxorubicin, dactinomycin, cyclophosphamide, vincristine) to control distant disease

	Clinical features	Radiographic findings	Histology	Treatment
Osteosarcoma	Usually confined to one rib, but may include others Occurs at 10–15 years, again after age 40 Presents as painful mass Accounts for small number of rib-based tumors Association with prior irradiation after 10-year latency	Classic "sunburst" pattern of new periosteal bone formation Periosteal elevation (Codman's triangle sign)	Eosinophilic staining with glassy appearance	Preoperative chemotherapy with doxorubicin, high-dose methotrexate, cisplatin Wide, local excision Chest wall reconstruction may be needed
Plasmacytoma	Mean age of occurrence 60 years Ribs > clavicles > sternum Often with soft-tissue invasion	Osteolytic changes with pericostal opacities	Sheets of plasma cells Hypervascular Amyloid present in 25% of cases	High-dose irradiation (5,000–6,000 cGy) Wide, local excision Chemotherapy only if progressive
Soft-tissue sarcomas	Primary soft-tissue sarcomas uncommon Includes fibro-, lipo-, rhabdomyo-, dermato-, and angiosarcomas	Usually nonspecific; however, sarcomas tend to metastasize to lungs	Varies with origin of tumor	Wide, local excision Possible chest wall reconstruction Radiotherapy and chemotherapy have no prognostic value for high-grade sarcomas

Liver Function Tests, Alkaline Phosphase. To rule out primary hepatic tumor or metastasis.

Radiology

Chest X-ray. Findings vary (see Table 11–2).

CT of the Chest. To differentiate tissue planes, document extension of tumor, and identify metastasis.

MRI of the Chest. Further refinement of CT findings, but the role as a primary imaging technique is controversial.

Bone Scan. To rule out metastasis.

Other

Incisional Biopsy. To make diagnosis; however, not recommended for all chest wall tumors.

Excisional Biopsy. Often needed to make diagnosis.

Needle Biopsy. Used in rare instances.

DIFFERENTIAL DIAGNOSIS

Traumatic

Chest Wall Trauma. May be associated with the formation of fibrous dysplasia and desmoid tumors.

Rib Fracture. Usually a history of trauma or hard coughing. Chest x-ray reveals the fracture. Old, healed fractures may be associated with irregular borders. Bone scan may be required to differentiate from neoplasm.

Infectious

Pneumonia. Causing chest wall symptoms. Chest x-ray positive for infiltrate.

Metabolic. Not applicable.

Neoplastic

Metastasis. Differentiated by biopsy.

Vascular. Not applicable.

Congenital. Not applicable.

Acquired

Localized Pleurisy. Causing chest wall symptoms. Chest x-ray negative for lesion.

Neuritis. May present with chest wall tenderness. Negative chest x-ray differentiates.

TREATMENT

Medical. Radiation therapy (see Tables 11–1 and 11–2) and chemotherapy (see Tables 11–1 and 11–2).

Surgical

Excisional Biopsy. Is used to determine the diagnosis and serves a threefold purpose: to remove the mass, provide adequate tissue for an accurate diagnosis, and allow earlier institution of adjuvant therapy (if indicated). If the resulting lesion is benign, often no further intervention is necessary. If the lesion proves malignant, the patient should undergo further resection.

Chest Wall Resection.   Is essential to the successful management of malignant chest wall tumors, and the extent of the dissection should be wide. High-grade malignancy involving bone should have the entire bone and any involved structures (lung, pericardium, thymus, muscle) removed. If the sternum or manubrium are involved, the corresponding bilateral costal arches should be removed as well.

Chest Wall Reconstruction.   Is often necessary following chest wall resection. Considerations for reconstruction are centered around the ability of the thorax to continue to support respiration and protect the underlying organs. Other considerations include the location, size, and depth of the defect, condition of local and surrounding tissue, and the general condition of the patient. Skeletal defects are corrected with or without methyl methacrylate–impregnated Prolene, Gore-Tex, or Marlex mesh. Soft-tissue defects are closed using muscle flaps (latissimus dorsi, pectoralis major, rectus abdominis) or omentum.

Indications.   For definitive diagnosis and removal of tumor.

Contraindications.   None.

TECHNIQUE OF SURGICAL ASSISTING

Chest wall resection requires meticulous technique to prevent tumor extension, and full-thickness excisions with wide margins are necessary. The assistant must be proficient with techniques of bone resection, muscle mobilization, and assistance with resection of underlying structures (e.g., lung, pleura, and thymus). Reconstruction often requires a high degree of creativity, and often a multidisciplinary surgical team is necessary.

PEDIATRIC CONSIDERATIONS

Because many of the tumors occur in childhood, always consider chest wall tumors in the differential diagnosis in a child with chest wall pain. Avoid radiation to the thyroid in young patients.

OBSTETRICAL CONSIDERATIONS

Special considerations may be necessary when treating the desmoid tumor with tamoxifen. As always, the risk versus benefit of any treatment, to the mother *and* fetus, should be weighed and treatment plans made accordingly.

PEARLS FOR THE PA

The keys to success in the treatment of chest wall tumors include early diagnosis as well as aggressive surgical resection.

Lung Cancer
Lyle W. Larson, PA-C, MS

DEFINITION

Lung cancers are primary neoplasms of lung parenchyma and are generally divided into two broad categories: small cell carcinoma and nonsmall cell carcinoma (including squamous cell, adenocarcinoma, and large cell carcinoma). Other less common neoplasms involving lung parenchyma include lymphoma, sarcoma, and blastoma. Classification is important, because the therapeutic approach to each category differs. Ninety to ninety-five percent of all lung tumors are malignant.

HISTORY

Symptoms. Chest pain, shoulder or arm pain, superior vena cava syndrome (e.g., tearing in the eyes, swelling of the eyelids, face, neck, arms, upper chest, proptosis, Horner's syndrome, red, edematous face), productive or nonproductive cough, hemoptysis, hoarseness, wheezing, dyspnea, voice change, dysphagia, back pain, exercise limitation, malaise, weight loss, anorexia, fatigue.

General. Presentation is varied and unpredictable. Exposure to asbestos, smoking, industrial hazards (mining, volatile chemicals), tuberculosis, and radon may be implicated. Previous history of breast carcinoma or lymphoma should be elicited. Approximately 25% of symptoms are directly related to the tumor itself, 30% of presenting symptoms are related to metastasis, and 30% present with systemic symptoms of malaise, weight loss (>5% body weight), and anorexia.

Age. Any age, but greatest occurrence between 50 and 70 years. Males more often than females.

Onset. Variable.

Duration. Continuous and progressive unless treated.

Intensity. Variable; however, progressive disease may result in chronic, relentless pain, particularly with metastasis.

Aggravating Factors. Underlying disease such as pneumonia, atelectasis, or consolidation.

Alleviating Factors. None.

Associated Factors. Exposure to asbestos, smoking, industrial hazards (mining, volatile chemicals), tuberculosis.

PHYSICAL EXAMINATION

General. The patient may appear malnourished, have a wasting appearance. Evaluate supraclavicular nodes for enlargement.

Pulmonary. The patient may have no specific objective findings or may have an examination consistent with lung consolidation. Auscultation may reveal bronchial breath sounds with late inspiratory crackles. Percussion is dull over an airless area. Increased tactile fremitus and transmitted voice sounds help to differentiate from atelectasis, effusion, or hemothorax.

PATHOPHYSIOLOGY

Squamous Cell Carcinoma. Arises from hyperplastic, metaplastic bronchial basal cells, typically located in major bronchi (lobar or first segmental bronchus of upper lobes). It exfoliates easily and is expectorated in sputum. The tumor tends to obstruct the bronchus as it grows into and through the bronchial wall. Symptoms generally occur with segmental collapse. The tumor tends to remain localized, is highly amenable to resection.

Adenocarcinoma. Arises from peripheral bronchioles and begins as a solitary nodule. The tumor does not exfoliate into the bronchus, so sputum is not helpful. Peripheral location helps with detection and accessibility with percutaneous biopsy. The bronchiolar variant is unique because the tumor grows along the alveolar septum; is often multifocal with lymph node metastasis common.

Large Cell Carcinoma. Undifferentiated with no consensus on histogenesis; clinically aggressive.

Small Cell Carcinoma. Related to smoking and arises from hyperplastic bronchial basal cells in major lobar or segmental bronchi. Has a 25% presence in the peripheral lung and often presents with metastasis. Focal areas of squamous or glandular differentiation are common. Tumor is sensitive to a combination of chemotherapy and radiation therapy.

DIAGNOSTIC STUDIES

Laboratory

Full Chemistry Profile. Including alkaline phosphatase, liver function studies, calcium, phosphate, magnesium. Used for metastatic screening and to establish a baseline prior to treatment.

Complete Blood Count. To evaluate for anemia.

Radiology

Chest X-ray. Used for identification and localization of tumor and to evaluate for the presence of pleural effusions, atelectasis, and consolidation.

CT Scan of the Chest. To provide information about the tumor, including single or multiple lesions, size, structure, relationship to surrounding structures, lung parenchyma, pleura, and presence or absence of adenopathy.

MRI of the Chest. Provides no distinct advantage over CT, but may help differentiate neurogenic invasion.

Other

Pulmonary Function Studies. To evaluate the degree of pulmonary compromise and assist with decision making regarding the extent of pulmonary resection.

Bronchoscopy. To assist with diagnosis of bronchial invasion and to perform biopsies.

Mediastinoscopy. Is used to sample mediastinal lymph nodes.

Bone Scan, CT Scan of Head and Abdomen. Performed as metastatic screening studies.

DIFFERENTIAL DIAGNOSIS

Traumatic. Not applicable.

Infectious

Granuloma. May present as a single lesion. Comparison with prior x-rays is indicated when possible.

Fungal. Infections such as coccidiomycoses, histiomycoses may present as pulmonary lesions. Differentiated by a history of exposure or travel to an endemic area or positive skin test. Immunosuppressed patients are at higher risk; chest x-ray is worse than symptoms suggest.

Tuberculosis. May present with pulmonary lesions. TB test is positive; patient responds to treatment with antituberculosis drugs.

Pneumonia. May present with consolidation. Follow-up chest x-ray is necessary in high-risk individuals to rule out underlying lesion. CT of the chest is performed as indicated to rule out a lesion.

Metabolic. Not applicable.

Neoplastic

Metastatic Disease. From a distant source may localize in the lung and diagnosis may be made on biopsy. Full metastatic screening is mandatory.

Vascular. Not applicable.

Congenital. Not applicable.

Acquired. Not applicable.

TREATMENT

Medical

Chemotherapy. Either as a single agent, or in combination for susceptible lesions.

Radiation Therapy.   Performed after histologic confirmation for susceptible lesions.

Supportive Care.   Including pain control for unresectable lesions or in those with metastasis.

Small Cell Lung Cancer.   Is usually disseminated and requires systemic therapy. Tends to be highly responsive to chemotherapy; however, relapse rate is high.

Nonsmall Cell Lung Cancer.   Responds poorly to chemotherapy and surgical resection is preferred. Postoperative radiation therapy is helpful.

Surgical.   Principles of surgical intervention include the complete removal of the tumor and associated lymph nodes, avoidance of tumor spillage (spread), and confirmation of clear margins whenever possible.

The surgical approach is usually by way of a posterolateral thoracotomy, with entry into the pleural space achieved through the fifth intercostal space, with or without rib resection. The location of the lesion(s) dictates the choice of procedure. Procedures include:

Wedge resection: Removal of wedge of lung

Segmental resection: Resection of segment of specific lobe of lung

Lobectomy: Removal of specific lobe of lung

Pneumonectomy: Removal of entire lung

Care must be taken to avoid damage to other structures in the chest (e.g., vagus, phrenic, and recurrent laryngeal nerves, thoracic duct, and heart and great vessels).

Staging is performed using tissue obtained through biopsy or open thoracostomy using the Tumor, Node, Metastasis Staging System (TNM) listed in Tables 11–3 and 11–4.

Indications.   Surgery is used for both diagnostic and therapeutic management.

Contraindications.   Metastatic disease, because not all lesions will be able to be resected.

TECHNIQUE OF SURGICAL ASSISTING

Standard technique for surgical assisting centers around a clear understanding of the anatomy of the chest wall and intrathoracic contents, as well as the various specialty instruments (staplers, etc.) used in lung resection.

PEDIATRIC CONSIDERATIONS

Not applicable.

OBSTETRICAL CONSIDERATIONS

Not applicable.

Table 11–3. TNM Staging System

Tumor (T)

TX	Occult disease, malignant cells present without identifiable tumor
T1	Tumor less than or equal to 3 cm in diameter, surrounded by lung or visceral pleura, but not proximal to a lobar bronchus
T2	Tumor greater than 3 cm, or with involvement of main bronchus at least 2 cm distal to carina, visceral pleural invasion, or associated atelectasis or obstructive pneumonitis extending to the hilar region but not involving the entire lung
T3	Tumor invading chest wall, diaphragm, mediastinal pleura, or parietal pericardium; or tumor in main bronchus within 2 cm but not invading the carina, or atelectasis or obstructive pneumonitis of entire lung
T4	Tumor invading mediastinum, heart, great vessels, trachea, esophagus, vertebral body, or carina; or ipsilateral malignant pleural effusion

Nodes (N)

N0	No regional lymph node metastasis
N1	Metastases to ipsilateral peribronchial or hilar nodes
N2	Metastases to ipsilateral mediastinal or subcarinal nodes
N3	Metastases to contralateral mediastinal or hilar nodes, or to any scalene or supraclavicular nodes

Distant metastasis (M)

M0	No distant metastasis
M1	Distant metastasis present

Table 11–4. Stages

Occult	TX N0 M0
Stage I	T1–2 N0 M0
Stage II	T1–2 N1 M0
Stage IIIa	T3 N0–1 M0
	T1–2 N2 M0
Stage IIIb	T4 N0–2 M0
	T1–4 N3 M0
Stage IV	TX–4 N0–3 M1

PEARLS FOR THE PA

It is the practitioner's responsibility to prove that any solitary pulmonary nodule is not malignant.

Presentation is varied and unpredictable.

Environmental exposures such as asbestos, smoking, industrial hazards (mining, volatile chemicals), tuberculosis, and radon may be implicated in the development of lung cancer.

Pneumothorax
Lyle W. Larson, PA-C, MS

DEFINITION

A pneumothorax is an accumulation of air between the surfaces of the visceral and parietal pleura with secondary lung collapse. There are three basic types of pneumothorax: spontaneous (occurring without obvious cause), traumatic, and tension (intrathoracic air volume sufficient to cause hemodynamic compromise).

HISTORY

Symptoms.   Dyspnea to severe respiratory distress. Chest pain may be present. Symptoms may be similar to myocardial infarction, pulmonary embolism, pleurisy, rib fracture(s), hepatitis, cholecystitis, esophagitis, or aortic dissection and must be ruled out.

General.   Spontaneous pneumothorax may occur following sudden changes in intrathoracic pressure (playing musical instrument, vigorous exercise, stretching, diving, flying) sufficient to rupture a known or unknown superficial lung bulla.

Traumatic pneumothorax occurs following penetrating trauma to the thorax, rib fracture, or perforation of the diaphragm, lung, trachea, bronchus, or esophagus.

A tension pneumothorax occurs when the source of air leak is under greater pressure than the lung and mediastinal structures, allowing for complete collapse of the affected lung and movement of mediastinal contents toward the contralateral side.

Age.   Variable, depending on cause. Spontaneous pneumothorax is most common in males 20 to 40 years of age.

Onset. Sudden.
Duration. Continuous.
Intensity. Asymptomatic to cardiovascular collapse.
Aggravating Factors. Symptoms aggravated with movement, respirations, and cough, persistent air leak greater than 48 hours, pneumomediastinum, or hemothorax.
Alleviating Factors. Reabsorption of air, administration of O_2.
Associated Factors. More frequent in young, tall, thin males.

PHYSICAL EXAMINATION

General. Patients may be observed experiencing dyspnea or tachypnea or may be in acute respiratory distress. Vital signs may reveal a tachycardia. Tension pneumothorax may present with a weak, rapid pulse, neck vein distention, or tracheal deviation.
Pulmonary. Percussion is hyperresonant or tympanic over the affected area, breath sounds are decreased or absent, and there is no transmission of tactile fremitus or transmitted voice.
Cardiovascular. Findings include tachycardia, displaced point of maximal intensity, jugular venous distention.

PATHOPHYSIOLOGY

Perforation of the visceral pleura allows air from the lung to enter the potential pleural space, which is normally less than atmospheric pressure. This may occur from trauma or spontaneous rupture from an emphysematous bullae. Penetration of the chest wall, diaphragm, mediastinum, trachea, bronchus, or esophagus may also allow the influx of air into the pleural space.

As the apex of the lung is displaced by intrapleural air, lung compliance decreases, with subsequent decreases in the functional residual capacity, ventilatory capacity, and oxygenation.

DIAGNOSTIC STUDIES

Laboratory
Arterial Blood Gases. To evaluate the presence and extent of pulmonary compromise.
Radiology
Chest X-ray. Shows an absence of lung markings in the affected area. These usually occur in the apex, but may also be present laterally and inferiorly along the diaphragm. A mediastinal shift to the contralateral side is seen in tension pneumothorax. Bullae may also be present.

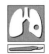

CT Scan of the Chest.   Is usually unnecessary to make a diagnosis of pneumothorax, but may help to identify multiple, small bullae.

DIFFERENTIAL DIAGNOSIS

Traumatic
Pulmonary Contusion.   No evidence of pneumothorax on chest x-ray.
Infectious.   Not applicable.
Metabolic
Pleurisy.   No evidence of pneumothorax on chest x-ray.
Neoplastic.   Not applicable.
Vascular
Aortic Dissection.   Differentiated on chest CT scan or aortogram.
Congenital.   Not applicable.
Acquired.   Not applicable.

TREATMENT

Medical.   Observation may be all that is necessary if the patient is asymptomatic, has normal arterial blood gasses, and the pneumothorax occupies less than 20% of the affected side. Supplemental oxygen and bedrest may hasten the reabsorption of air.

Surgical.   A tube thoracostomy is performed to remove air from the pleural space, allowing the affected lung to re-expand. The patient is placed in the supine position, and the chest wall is prepped and draped. The preferred site of chest tube placement is through the fourth or fifth intercostal space in the midaxillary line; however, the anterior axillary line is acceptable. The site of incision and proposed tube tract are infiltrated with 1% lidocaine to include the periosteum and pleura. A 2-cm incision is made over the inferior border of the rib over which the tube will course and is carried down to the superficial fascia. A subcutaneous tunnel is then formed with blunt dissection using a Kelly or Vanderbilt clamp and the pleural space is entered over the superior margin of the rib above the incision site. Once the pleura is entered (a gush of air is often heard on relief of a tension pneumothorax), it is spread open for approximately 1 cm. A finger is then inserted into the pleural cavity to confirm entry and break any adhesions present. The tube is then inserted superiorly, using a clamp to direct its course superiorly and posteriorly along the chest wall. The tube is then attached to an appropriate waterseal apparatus with suction, and the tube is secured in place with suture and dressed with an air-occlusive dressing.

For recurrent pneumothoraces, pleurodesis may be performed. Intrapleural administration of doxycycline or bleomycin via a chest tube may stimulate pleural adhesions, allowing the lung to adhere to the chest wall and obliterate any potential space. Alternatively, talc may be used; however, this requires general sedation and thoracoscopy to effectively coat the pleura.

Blebs and bullae are resected either by thoracoscopy or thoracotomy. Either approach must allow the surgeon to visualize the bleb or bulla, which is then resected following stapling of adjacent healthy lung parenchyma. Chest tubes are mandatory afterward, because air leaks across the staple line are common.

Indications.   Symptomatic pneumothorax with respiratory or cardiovascular compromise.

Contraindications.   None; however, anticoagulated patients may pose an increased risk for hemothorax.

TECHNIQUE OF SURGICAL ASSISTING

A surgical assistant not usually required for tube thoracostomy; however, an assistant is necessary for thoracoscopic surgery or thoracotomy. Postoperative follow-up of the chest tube is essential to confirm that the lung has re-expanded.

With thoracoscopic techniques, the assistant must be capable of manipulating thoracoscopic instruments including the camera, electrocautery, suction, stapler, and instruments for visualization and retraction.

PEDIATRIC CONSIDERATIONS

Not applicable.

OBSTETRICAL CONSIDERATIONS

Not applicable.

PEARLS FOR THE PA

Re-expansion pulmonary edema may occur following re-expansion of large pneumothoraces.

For recurrent pneumothorax, rule out bronchopleural fistula.

Surgery is usually indicated following two episodes of spontaneous pneumothorax on the ipsilateral side.

Think pneumothorax in any young, tall, thin male with acute shortness of breath.

Pulmonary Contusion
Lyle W. Larson, PA-C, MS

DEFINITION

Blunt trauma to the thorax and lung parenchyma that does not alter alveolar architecture.

HISTORY

Symptoms. Shortness of breath, productive cough, wheezing, tachypnea, or respiratory distress.

General. History of blunt trauma or nonpenetrating missile injury. Contusion may not be seen on initial chest x-ray; as such, it may be missed with initial evaluation.

Age. Variable.

Onset. Immediate, with symptoms of shortness of breath or hypoxia occurring within minutes to hours.

Duration. Variable, depending on extent of injury.

Intensity. Minor discomfort to life-threatening hypoxia, depending on degree and severity of the blunt trauma.

Aggravating Factors. Hypoxia may be severe enough to require intubation and mechanical ventilation.

Alleviating Factors. Not applicable.

Associated Factors. Pulmonary contusion is a major risk factor for adult respiratory distress syndrome (ARDS).

PHYSICAL EXAMINATION

General. Chest wall discomfort is usually present on palpation. Evaluate for multi-trauma.

Pulmonary. Consolidation may be present with decreased breath sounds on auscultation, dullness to percussion, and positive bronchophony, egophony, or whispered pectoriloquy. Cough may be observed to be nonproductive or may produce blood-tinged sputum.

PATHOPHYSIOLOGY

Pulmonary contusion consists of a diffuse infiltration of blood and proteinaceous fluid within intact alveoli. Can cause significant shunting (blood passing through pulmonary capillaries is not exposed to ventilated alveoli, and as such, is not oxygenated) and resultant hypoxia.

DIAGNOSTIC STUDIES

Laboratory
Arterial Blood Gases.   To evaluate the presence or extent of pulmonary compromise.
Radiology
Chest X-ray.   Reveals diffuse density in lung parenchyma, but may not be seen for 24 to 48 hours following initial traumatic event; also used to rule out fractures of the bony thorax.
Other
Pulmonary Function Tests.   Are usually not indicated, but may be helpful if symptoms persist or if there is underlying COPD.

DIFFERENTIAL

Traumatic.   Not applicable.
Infectious
Occult Pneumonia.   Associated with fever, elevated WBC, and pulmonary infiltrate on chest x-ray.
Metabolic.   Not applicable.
Neoplastic.   Not applicable.
Vascular.   Not applicable.
Congenital.   Not applicable.
Acquired.   Not applicable.

TREATMENT

Medical.   Consists of supportive measures, including oxygen and bedrest. Intubation and mechanical ventilation are used if hypoxia is severe, but should not be performed prophylactically.
Surgical.   If contusion is seen at the time of thoracotomy for other reasons, the surgeon should resist the temptation to excise the contused portion, because function inevitably returns.
Indications.   None.
Contraindications.   Not applicable.

TECHNIQUE OF SURGICAL ASSISTING

Not applicable.

PEDIATRIC CONSIDERATIONS

Not applicable.

OBSTETRICAL CONSIDERATIONS

Not applicable.

PEARLS FOR THE PA

Pulmonary contusions occur as a later finding following trauma to the chest.

Consider a repeat chest x-ray in 24 to 48 hours if respiratory compromise following trauma does not improve or worsens.

Further Reading

Fraser RG, Pare JAP: Diagnosis of Diseases of the Chest, ed 3. Philadelphia, W.B. Saunders, 1989.

Gibbon JH, Sabiston DC, Spencer FC: Surgery of the Chest, ed 5. Philadelphia, W.B. Saunders, 1990.

Griffith F, Pearson MD: Thoracic Surgery. New York, Churchill-Livingstone, 1995.

Shields TW: General Thoracic Surgery, ed 3. Philadelphia, Lea & Febiger, 1989.

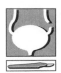

Chapter 12

Urologic Surgery
Benign Prostatic Hypertrophy
Rita Altman, PA-C, BA, BS

DEFINITION

Hyperplasia of prostate tissue that is benign. May result in urethral obstruction, thereby causing blockage of urination and sometimes complete urinary retention. Severe cases eventually may result in hydronephrosis or upper urinary tract dysfunction.

HISTORY

Symptoms.   Obstructive symptoms: urinary frequency, nocturia, decreased stream, hesitancy, post-void dribble, incomplete emptying, or hematuria.

General.   Obtain a history of prior or recurrent urinary tract infections (UTIs).

Age.   Men older than age 45 years. Fifty-one percent incidence in men 60 to 69 years old.

Onset.   Gradual enlargement of the prostate over several years; only in men with testes.

Duration.   Microscopic benign prostatic hypertrophy (BPH) increases with age in all male populations, suggesting that all men will develop symptomatic BPH if they live long enough.

Intensity.   Ranges from mild to severe.

Aggravating Factors.   Obstructive symptoms, urinary retention, recurrent UTIs.

Alleviating Factors.   Catheter placement for retention, medical treatment, surgical treatment.

Associated Factors.   May be associated with recurrent UTI, prostatism and, in severe cases, renal failure.

PHYSICAL EXAMINATION

General.   Hypertension, tachycardia, tachypnea may be early signs that the patient has severe obstruction or renal failure.

Gastrointestinal.   Palpate the kidney for tenderness and the bladder for distention.

Genitourinary.   Rectal examination may reveal a large, smooth surface with definable right and left lobes of the prostate; consistency can be soft or firm depending on whether there are glandular or fibromuscular contents.

PATHOPHYSIOLOGY

Changes of BPH occur in the periurethral glands around the verumontanum, possibly due to an abnormal accumulation of dihydrotestosterone.

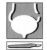

After initial hypertrophy, other changes may occur, such as resistance of the prostatic urethra, decompensation of the detrusor muscle, or degeneration of nerve cells. No BPH exists in men castrated prior to puberty. No relation to cancer has been established. Not genetically or environmentally influenced.

DIAGNOSTIC STUDIES

Laboratory
Urinalysis.   With or without culture; to rule out infection, stones, upper/lower tract pathology.
Prostate-Specific Antigen (PSA).   Screen for malignancy, provide baseline (normal, 0 to 4 ng/mL).
CBC with Differential.   Rule out infection.
Creatinine, BUN.   Provide baseline, check renal function.
Radiology
Ultrasound.   Measure bladder and prostate volumes; check for residual urine.
Other
Simple Uroflow.   Volume urinated is more than 125 mL; normal flow greater than 20 mL/s; mild obstruction, 11 to 15 mL/s; moderate to severe obstruction, less than 11 mL/s.
Pressure/Flow Studies.   Conducted with a catheter in the bladder and rectum; reveals high pressures (more than 60 cm H_2O with low flows less than 11 mL/s).
Residual Urine.   Via catheter or ultrasound; should be less than 100 mL.
Cystoscopy.   To rule out other causes of obstruction and to evaluate anatomy and urethral length. May show trabeculations (markings in the bladder that indicate long-term increased pressure).
AUA Symptom Score.   One of the most valuable tools in assessing patients' symptoms. Scores: 0 to 7, mild (watchful waiting); 8 to 20, moderate (medical and/or surgical intervention); greater than 20, severe (should seek treatment before totally obstructed).

DIFFERENTIAL DIAGNOSIS

Traumatic.   Not applicable.
Infectious
Prostatitis.   Prostate may be tender; WBC or RBC may be found on urinalysis; may have associated fever or elevated serum WBC.
Metabolic
Neuropathic Bladders.   History of conditions such as diabetes or alcoholism.

Neoplastic
Prostate Cancer. Asymmetric prostate, significantly elevated PSA. Ultrasound, biopsy, or both used to differentiate.
Bladder Cancer, Renal Tumor. Prostate may feel normal, RBC in urine, PSA normal; additional diagnostic studies differentiate.
Vascular. Not applicable.
Congenital: Not applicable.
Acquired
Medications. Causing retention or urinary symptoms of frequency, urgency (e.g., anticholinergics, antihistamines, allergy pills).
Other
Urethral Stricture, Defects of Bladder Neck (Anatomical and Functional). No BPH identified on physical examination; diagnostic studies differentiate.

TREATMENT

Medical. Alpha$_1$ blockers, 5-alpha reductase inhibitors, luteinizing hormone-releasing hormone (LH-RH) agonists may be used to reduce prostate size. Close follow-up and monitoring of renal function is essential in order to prevent complications of increased prostate size.

Surgical
Transurethral Resection of Prostate (TURP). Removes the obstructing, adenomatous portion of the prostate via the urethra using a resectoscope and electrocautery. This is performed by resecting the bladder neck fibers between 5 and 7 o'clock and resection of the hyperplastic gland in quadrants.

Complications include TUR syndrome, which occurs due to the high degree of irrigation fluid under pressure, thereby causing absorption of fluid via the venous sinuses. If resection is prolonged, it may lead to increased fluid absorption, resulting in hypervolemia and hyponatremia that causes cerebral edema and seizures. Incidence of TUR syndrome is 2%. Using continuous flow resectoscopes and diuretics (mannitol and furosemide [Lasix]) reduces this risk. Other complications include retrograde ejaculation (100%), failure to void (6.5%), hemorrhage (4%), clot retention (3%), and UTIs (2%). Late complications include bladder neck contractures (up to 25%), impotence (30%), and incontinence (<10%).

Transurethral Incision of the Prostate (TUIP). Similar to TURP; two deep incisions are made at 5 and 7 o'clock, extending from ureteric orifices to the sides of the verumontanum. TUIP has fewer complications of retrograde ejaculation, bladder neck contracture, and saves operative time and postoperative recovery time.

Hyperthermia (Laser, Microwave, High-Frequency Radio Waves). Includes laser prostatectomy, microwave hyperthermia, and transurethral needle ablation.

Laser Prostatectomy. An outpatient procedure used for glands smaller than 60 g (varying kinds of laser, some FDA approved, many being investigated). Advantages include technical simplicity and decreased complications of intraoperative fluid absorption, bleeding, retrograde ejaculation, impotence, and incontinence. The main disadvantage is that the catheter is left in longer than with a TURP.

Microwave Hyperthermia. Heat-induced tissue damage used in area of transition zone to a temperature of 42 to 45°C. Experimental in the United States.

Transurethral Needle Ablation (TUNA). Under trial. High-frequency radio waves are used to cause thermal injury to prostate.

Transurethral Balloon Dilatation (TUBD). Noncompliant balloons are used to dilate prostate under pressure.

Open Prostatectomy. Ten percent (BPH) have supra- or retropubic approach; indication is a prostate gland larger than 60 g. Also popular if the abdomen requires exploration for other reasons.

Indications. Moderate to severe obstruction.

Contraindications. Consider open prostatectomy if prostate size is larger than 60 g. Evaluate cardiac condition prior to surgery. Patients older than 80 years are at greatest risk of morbidity/mortality.

TECHNIQUE OF
SURGICAL ASSISTING

An assistant is not ordinarily utilized.

PEDIATRIC CONSIDERATIONS

Not applicable.

OBSTETRICAL CONSIDERATIONS

Not applicable.

PEARLS FOR THE PA

If left untreated, BPH may lead to blockage of urination and possible hydronephrosis of upper urinary tract dysfunction.

Prostate examination reveals large, smooth surface with definable right and left lobes and a soft or firm consistency.

Bladder Carcinoma
Gerard J. Marciano, RPA-C

DEFINITION

Malignant neoplasm of the urinary bladder, usually epithelial in origin.

HISTORY

Symptoms.   Painless, gross hematuria; flank pain if hydronephrosis is present.

General.   Male-to-female ratio, 2:1. Environmental and occupational history needs to be obtained for to ascertain exposure to potential carcinogens.

Age.   Average age of onset is 65 years.

Onset.   Insidious or acute.

Duration.   Indefinite, pending treatment.

Intensity.   Progressive.

Aggravating Factors.   Progression to hydronephrosis with associated flank pain.

Alleviating Factors.   Appropriate treatment.

Associated Factors.   Carcinogens may include rubber, dyes, paint, aluminum, gas, leather; associated occupations include kitchen workers and clerical workers.

PHYSICAL EXAMINATION

General.   Initially unremarkable; later, if disease becomes extensive, there may be signs associated with metastases.

Urologic.   Initially unremarkable; later, thickening, mass, or both may be found on rectal or vaginal examination. Percuss costovertebral angle for tenderness, which may suggest upper urinary tract pathology.

PATHOPHYSIOLOGY

Ninety-eight percent of tumors are epithelial in origin; 80% are papillary lesions. Spread occurs by local extension via lymphatic and hematogenous routes. Distant metastases (in order of decreasing frequency) are to pelvic nodes, lungs, bones, and liver.

DIAGNOSTIC STUDIES

Laboratory

Urinalysis.   Hematuria and pyuria are usually present.

CBC.   Anemia of chronic disease may be noted.

Chemistry Profile. May show azotemia secondary to impairment of renal function due to obstruction.

Radiology
IVP or Retrograde Cystourethrogram. Early finding is that of a filling defect in the bladder. Late findings include hydronephrosis.

Other
Cystoscopy. Used for direct visualization and biopsy.

DIFFERENTIAL DIAGNOSIS

Traumatic
Renal Injury. May cause hematuria, but it is usually associated with pain.

Infectious
Pyelonephritis and Cystitis. May cause hematuria, but it is usually associated with pain.

Metabolic
Urolithiasis. Associated with pain.

Neoplastic
Renal or Ureteral Tumor. May cause painless hematuria.

Vascular. Not applicable.

Congenital. Not applicable.

Acquired
Foreign Bodies. Noted on imaging studies or physical examination.

TREATMENT

Medical. Intravesical chemotherapy, usually following transurethral resection of bladder tumor (TURBT).

Surgical
TURBT. Procedure in which the tumor is resected and fulgurated via cystoscopy.

Cystectomy. In the presence of more extensive disease, via suprapubic incision, the bladder is isolated and excised, the local area including lymphatics is explored, and a suprapubic cystostomy or ileal conduit is brought externally to provide drainage of the urinary tract.

Indications. Painless hematuria is always an indication for diagnostic/therapeutic cystoscopy.

Contraindications. Marked systemic disease states.

TECHNIQUE OF SURGICAL ASSISTING

In cystoscopy and TURBT, the PA frequently remains outside the sterile field, except for sterile gloves, and assists with instrumentation. For an open procedure, the PA may provide first or second assistance with hemostasis, retraction, opening, and closing.

PEDIATRIC CONSIDERATIONS

Rarely seen.

OBSTETRICAL CONSIDERATIONS

Evaluation of risk versus benefit of diagnostic studies and subsequent therapy must be made for both maternal and fetal well being.

PEARLS FOR THE PA

In the presence of gross hematuria ALWAYS irrigate the bladder until it is clear of clots, because the mere presence of blood in the bladder may cause further bleeding.

Cardinal symptom is painless, gross hematuria.

Hydrocele (Newborn and Adult)
Rita Altman, PA-C, BA, BS

DEFINITION

Collection of fluid surrounding the testis and possibly along the spermatic cord.

HISTORY

Symptoms.   Scrotal mass, usually nonpainful, soft or tense; fluid is clear or yellow.

General.   Congenital hydroceles are diagnosed at birth. Adult hydroceles may develop rapidly secondary to local injury, or as a slow-growing mass as fluid collects around the testis.

Age.   Communicating hydrocele is seen in infants and young boys; chronic hydrocele is seen in men older than 40 years.

Onset.   Present at birth or, in adults, acute with trauma or progressive with increased fluid accumulation.

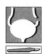

Duration.   Ninety percent of congenital hydroceles spontaneously resolve by 1 year of age. Adult hydrocele is ongoing until repaired.

Intensity.   Usually painless; the heavy bulkiness can be uncomfortable.

Aggravating Factors.   If accompanied by acute epididymal infection, it can become painful.

Alleviating Factors.   None, except definitive surgery in adults.

Associated Factors.   Local injury, radiation, acute nonspecific epididymitis, or orchitis; it may also accompany neoplasm. Sometimes associated with an indirect inguinal hernia.

PHYSICAL EXAMINATION

General.   Patients may have fever if concurrently infected.

Genitourinary.   Testicular examination reveals a scrotal mass, nontender to palpation, with positive transillumination. In young boys, the cystic mass may be small and soft in the morning, but by nighttime it becomes large and tense.

PATHOPHYSIOLOGY

Hydrocele results from a collection of fluid within the tunica/processus vaginalis. The communicating hydrocele (infants and young boys) is caused by a patent processus vaginalis that is continuous with the peritoneal cavity.

DIAGNOSTIC STUDIES

Laboratory

Urinalysis and/or Culture.   Usually negative, unless accompanied by infection.

White Blood Count.   Usually negative, unless accompanied by infection.

Radiology

Sonography.   Is used if the diagnosis is questionable.

Other

Transillumination.   Of scrotal fluid is the definitive diagnostic tool.

DIFFERENTIAL DIAGNOSIS

Traumatic

Hematocele, Other Traumatic Injury.   Does not transilluminate.

Infectious

Epididymitis.   Usually painful; may have hydrocele present.

Orchitis.   Painful; fever.

Metabolic.   Not applicable.

Neoplastic
Testicular Tumor. Firm, noncystic.
Vascular
Varicocele. Does not transilluminate.
Congenital. Not applicable.
Acquired
Inguinal Hernia. May accompany a communicating hydrocele. Evidence of abdominal contents in scrotum during Valsalva or crying.
Spermatocele. Freely movable cystic mass that lies above the testicle.

TREATMENT

Medical. None.
Surgical. Through an inguinal incision, high ligation of the patent processus vaginalis is made at the internal inguinal ring. Loupes are helpful, and a bloodless field is necessary. After opening hydrocele sac, the fluid is drained. Perform a subcuticular closure with absorbable suture to avoid staple removal in pediatric patients.
Indications. Tense or large, bulky hydrocele (uncomfortable or embarrassing to the patient) or bowel in the sac. In pediatrics, surgery is performed if the hydrocele does not spontaneously close before age 1 year.
Contraindications. Surgery is contraindicated if none of the indications are present.

TECHNIQUE OF SURGICAL ASSISTING

An assistant may not be necessary when performing an adult hydrocelectomy, but one is usually utilized on a pediatric case. In bilateral cases (e.g., communicating hydrocele with bilateral inguinal hernias), the PA works in tandem with the surgeon (opening or closing) to expedite the smoothness and efficiency of the case.

PEDIATRIC CONSIDERATIONS

Communicating hydrocele is continuous with the peritoneal cavity as noted earlier. If it is large, bowel may be found in the contents. Most close spontaneously before 1 year of age. If bowel is suspected in the sac, surgical correction is indicated.

OBSTETRICAL CONSIDERATIONS

Not applicable.

PEARLS FOR THE PA

Transillumination is the definitive diagnostic tool for hydrocele.

In pediatric patients, most communicating hydroceles close spontaneously before 1 year of age.

In young boys, the mass may be reduced in the morning and increase in size during the day.

Hypospadias
Rita Altman, PA-C, BA, BS

DEFINITION

Occurs when the urethral meatus opens on the ventral side of the penis, proximal to the tip of the glans penis.

HISTORY

Symptoms. Most newborns or young boys are asymptomatic; older males may have difficulty in directing urinary stream; stream "spraying."

General. May have difficulty having intercourse if chordee (curvature of the penis) is present; infertility may result. Congenital deformity that occurs in 1 of every 300 male births.

Age. Congenital. Urethral development begins at approximately 8 weeks *in utero* and is completed at 15 weeks *in utero*.

Onset. At birth; diagnosed at delivery.

Duration. Indefinite unless repaired.

Intensity. Ranging from no symptoms to moderate symptoms, depending on the type and severity of hypospadias.

Aggravating Factors. None.

Alleviating Factors. None.

Associated Factors. Estrogens and progestins given during pregnancy are known to increase the incidence; possible familial pattern; severe hypospadias is associated with bilateral cryptorchidism, which may represent problems of intersex.

PHYSICAL EXAMINATION

Genitourinary. Examination of the penis reveals meatus opening on the ventral side of penis, and/or undescended testes, bifid scrotum, or ambiguous genitalia/feminization. Epispadias (urethra displaced dorsally) is more rare and involves both males and females.

PATHOPHYSIOLOGY

Hypospadias results from incomplete fusion of the urethral folds *in utero*. There are several types of hypospadias, depending on location, and ranging from mild (glandular opening) to severe (perineal opening). Seventy percent are distal penile or coronal.

DIAGNOSTIC STUDIES

Laboratory
Buccal Smear and Karyotyping.   Should be performed in severe cases (penoscrotal or perineal) to rule out intersex.
Radiology
Renal Ultrasound and Intravenous Pyelogram.   Not generally necessary unless there is an indication of other congenital deformities of the upper tracts.
Other
Urethroscopy and Cystoscopy.   Rarely indicated.

DIFFERENTIAL DIAGNOSIS

Traumatic.   Not applicable.
Infectious.   Not applicable.
Metabolic.   Not applicable.
Neoplastic.   Not applicable.
Vascular.   Not applicable.
Congenital
Intersex Problems.   Must be considered.
Acquired.   Not applicable.

TREATMENT

Medical.   None.
Surgical.   Vascular flaps, occasional free skin grafts, and the foreskin are used to form the neourethra from the proximal opening to the glans penis. An artificial erection is produced by injecting saline to check for chordee (ventral bending and bowing of the penile shaft) before the surgical repair of the hypospadias; and chordee is repaired if necessary. An urethral catheter (8 Fr) is inserted and sutured to the glans and kept in place for 1 week. A double diaper is used, with the catheter placed between the diaper layers in order to keep the draining urine away from the wound.

A small Tegaderm dressing is wrapped around the penis and kept on for 1 day. There are more than 150 methods of corrective surgery for hypospadias that have been described in the literature. Complications include infection, loss of skin flap, damage to urethra, urethral stricture, fistulas, diverticulum.

Indications. Repair hypospadias at approximately 8 to 12 months of age.

Contraindications. None.

TECHNIQUE OF SURGICAL ASSISTING

The assistant usually wears loupes to keep the field of vision in synchrony with that of the surgeon. A bloodless field is crucial, with use of Weck sponges (not suction) and delicate instruments (Bishop-Harmon forceps) to provide countertraction. Simultaneous closing of flaps is carried out by the surgeon and assistant.

PEDIATRIC CONSIDERATIONS

This is a congenital condition.

OBSTETRICAL CONSIDERATIONS

Amniocentesis should be performed as indicated to evaluate for genetic abnormalities.

PEARLS FOR THE PA

Early diagnosis of hypospadias leads to normal growth and development of babies treated surgically.

Avoid immediate circumcision of newborns with hypospadias because the skin may be useful for future reconstruction.

Prostate Cancer
Rita Altman, PA-C, BA, BS, and
Robert McNellis, PA-C, MPH

DEFINITION

A generally slow-growing malignant neoplasm of the acinar cells of the prostate gland that can lead to urinary obstruction or metastases. Most common cancer in American men (32%); second most common cause of cancer deaths (38,000/yr); 200,000 new cases are diagnosed in the United States each year.

HISTORY

Symptoms. Usually asymptomatic, but may cause urinary obstructive symptoms. In more advanced (metastatic) disease, bone pain and weight loss may exist.

General. Often an incidental finding during rectal examination or transurethral resection of the prostate. Commonly has already spread beyond the prostate locally or distantly. Many are diagnosed by routine prostate-specific antigen (PSA) blood tests.

Age. Males older than 40 years of age; mean age 60 to 70 years.

Onset. Slow-growing and insidious in most cases; sometimes aggressive and rapidly progressive.

Duration. Early treatment may eliminate obstructive symptoms, but if there is more extensive disease (e.g., metastatic: bone metastasis), then the symptoms may remain indefinitely. May have clinically inapparent foci of carcinoma for 50 years.

Intensity. Depends on severity of disease; severe obstructive symptoms may result in painful urinary retention. Once metastasized is very progressive.

Aggravating Factors. Exogenous testosterone, high-fat diet, infectious agents (bacterial and viral), medications (anticholinergics, which can increase retention).

Alleviating Factors. Castration (medical or surgical).

Associated Factors. Genetic predisposition, hormonal influence, dietary factors, environmental factors, and infectious agents. African Americans have a 50% greater incidence than caucasian Americans.

PHYSICAL EXAMINATION

General. Shortness of breath, anemia, lymphadenopathy, and weight loss suggest metastatic disease.

Genitourinary. A digital rectal examination and palpation of the prostate must be performed; note any irregularity, asymmetry, enlargement, or hard, palpable nodules. Suspicious lesions should be biopsied.

Lymphatic. Palpate any enlarged nodes.

Musculoskeletal. Pathologic fractures may suggest metastases.

Neurologic. Complete assessment is indicated to rule out any changes that could be secondary to metastatic disease.

PATHOPHYSIOLOGY

Prostate cancers are adenocarcinomas of acinar cells. The prostate gland normally atrophies between the fifth and seventh decade. Premalignant changes often occur in the active glands rather than in atrophic tissue. There may be an association of carcinoma and androgenic stimulation. Seventy percent of prostate cancers arise in the peripheral zone of the prostate; 15% to 20% in the central zone; 10% to 15% in the transitional zone. Generally, the disease progresses at a very slow rate within the prostate, and then extends beyond the prostate by local, lymphatic, and hematogenous spread (Table 12–1).

DIAGNOSTIC STUDIES

Laboratory
Urinalysis.   Check for hematuria, rule out infection.

Prostate-Specific Antigen (PSA).   Normal, 0 to 4 ng/mL. Age corrected PSA rises 0.04 ng/mL per year in normal individuals without cancer and 0.02 ng/mL in men with BPH, such that a man 70 to 79 years old with a PSA of 6.5 ng/mL can be normal. PSA blood test is performed as a baseline, as well as post-prostatectomy to detect recurrent disease.

CBC and Chemistry Profile.   To evaluate for any abnormal white/red cell count, renal or liver function abnormality.

Prostatic Acid Phosphatase.   Less reliable indicator of carcinoma in the prostate, but elevation may indicate metastatic spread.

Radiology
Transrectal Ultrasound.   Carcinoma appears as hypoechoic lesions in prostate.

Bladder Ultrasound.   Performed if obstructive symptoms are present; check for residual.

Abdominal/Pelvic CT/MRI.   Used in clinical staging when the PSA is over 10 ng/mL and the Gleason sum score is greater than 7. May reveal enlarged lymph nodes indicative of metastasis.

Bone Scan: May indicate metastatic lesions in bone.

Other
Prostate Biopsy.   Pathologic confirmation of disease; allows for grading (often on a Gleason scale from 2 to 10, lower score is well differentiated, higher score is poorly differentiated).

Pelvic Lymphadenectomy.   Is performed for staging purposes for a Gleason sum score greater than 7 or PSA over 10 ng/mL. Pelvic lymphadenectomy can be performed laparoscopically or during open radical retropubic prostatectomy.

Cystoscopy.   Is usually performed to assess damage to the bladder, residual urine, bladder stones and tumor, and for determination of prostate size, location, and urethral integrity.

Table 12–1. A Comparison of Two Staging Systems for Prostate Cancer

TNM Staging System		AUA (Modified Jewett Staging System)
T_x	Primary tumor cannot be assessed	
T_0	No evidence of primary tumor	
T_{1a}	Tumor incidental histologic finding in ≤5% of tissue resected	Stage A_1 — Focal
T_{1b}	Tumor incidental histologic finding in >5% of tissue resected	Stage A_1 — Diffuse
T_{1c}	Nonpalpable tumor identified by needle biopsy (e.g., because of elevated PSA)	Stage B_0
T_{2a}	Palpable, half a lobe or less	Stage B_1 — Palpable, less than one lobe and <1.5 cm in size
T_{2b}	Palpable, less than half of one lobe but not both lobes	
T_{2c}	Palpable, involves both lobes	Stage B_2 — Palpable, involving both lobes and >1.5 cm in size
T_{3a}	Unilateral, extracapsular extension	Stage C_1 — No involvement of seminal vesicles
T_{3b}	Bilateral, extracapsular extension	
T_{3c}	Tumor invades seminal vesicles	Stage C_2 — Tumor invades one or both seminal vesicles
T_{4a}	Tumor invades bladder neck, external sphincter, or rectum	
T_{4b}	Tumor invades levator muscles, or is fixed to the pelvic sidewall	
N_x	Regional lymph nodes cannot be assessed	
N_0	No regional lymph node metastases	
N_1	Metastases in a single lymph node ≤2 cm in greatest dimension	Stage D_1 — Regional metastases to pelvic lymph nodes or ureteral obstruction causing hydronephrosis
N_2	Metastases in a single lymph node >2 cm but ≤5 cm in greatest dimension or multiple nodes, none >5 cm in greatest dimension	
N_3	Metastases in a lymph node >5 cm in greatest dimension	
M_x	Presence of distant metastases cannot be assessed	
M_0	No distant metastases	
M_{1a}	Nonregional lymph nodes	Stage D_2 — Metastases to distant nodes, bones, lungs, and other soft tissues
M_{1b}	Bone	
M_{1c}	Other sites	

From Tanagho EA, McAninch JW (eds): Smith's General Urology, ed 14. Norwalk, CT, Appleton and Lange, 1995, p. 409.

DIFFERENTIAL DIAGNOSIS

Traumatic.   Not applicable.
Infectious
Prostatitis.   Will have tender, indurated prostate.
Prostatic Tuberculosis.   Positive TB test, biopsy to rule out prostate cancer.
Metabolic
Calculi, Renal Failure.   May cause or result from urinary obstruction. Prostate examination normal.
Paget's Disease, Bladder Disease.   Biopsy to rule out prostate cancer.
Neoplastic
Benign Prostatic Hyperplasia.   Elevated PSA and enlarged gland but generally smooth and symmetric. Best differentiated by pathology.
Prostatic Cysts.   Biopsy to rule out prostate cancer.
Vascular.   Not applicable.
Congenital.   Not applicable.
Acquired
Fibrosis Secondary to Previous Biopsies.   Biopsy to rule out prostate cancer.

TREATMENT

Medical.   Treatment depends on the stage of the disease. Disease that is confined to the prostate (stage A or B) is most commonly treated with radical prostatectomy or radiation therapy along with neoadjuvant drug therapy. Disease with local invasion (stage C) is treated similarly, with significantly reduced effectiveness. Disease with distant metastasis (stage D) is treated with hormonal manipulation using orchiectomy, antiandrogens, LH-RH agonists, or estrogens. Cytotoxic chemotherapy is of little help. Palliative measures are given in advanced disease.

Surgical.   There are three types of radical prostatectomies: retropubic, suprapubic (rarely used), and perineal. With the retropubic approach, a lymphadenectomy can be performed via the same incision; otherwise it can be done laparoscopically. There tends to be more blood loss with this approach and transfusion may be necessary. Using the perineal approach, it is important to accurately position the patient into an exaggerated lithotomy position.

Radical prostatectomy is curative for carcinoma restricted to the prostatic capsule. Accurate clinical staging by pelvic lymph node dissection is important. Dissection may be done through low abdominal incision or laparoscopically. The nodes may be examined by frozen section to detect metastases. If several nodes are positive, the patient is unlikely to benefit from prostatectomy; if nodes are negative, the urologist may proceed with the prostatectomy. The Walsh technique has been successful in maintaining potency. The prostate is resected retrograde beginning at the urethra, working back to the bladder neck. Dissection is carried out close to the prostatic capsule to preserve the neurovascular bundle. The vesicourethral anastomosis is completed.

Complications include blood loss; infection; injury to nerves, ureter, or rectum; deep vein thrombosis; pulmonary embolism; and urinary retention. Long-term complications include bladder neck contracture, incontinence, and impotence. Side effects of orchiectomy include transient hot flashes and psychological trauma.

Indications. Stage A2, B, sometimes stage C. Locally confined prostate cancer can be effectively treated by radical prostatectomy with a long-term survival of 80% to 90%. Metastatic cancer is better treated by total androgen ablation (either by radical orchiectomy or injections of LH-RH agonists).

Contraindications. High-risk surgical patient (e.g., severe cardiac impairment) and those with metastatic disease.

TECHNIQUE OF SURGICAL ASSISTING

The keys to assisting in a radical prostatectomy are suction (due to the sometimes excessive blood loss), exposure, and retraction. As in all surgeries, make use of both hands to enhance the flow of the surgery. If the patient is obese, visualization may be challenging when identifying anatomical structures (e.g., neurovascular bundle, seminal vesicles, and vas deferens).

PEDIATRIC CONSIDERATIONS

Not applicable.

OBSTETRICAL CONSIDERATIONS

Not applicable.

PEARLS FOR THE PA

It is beneficial to do rectal examinations on all men over the age of 40 or 50 years.

Well-differentiated cancers do well, poorly differentiated do poorly.

Rule out other causes of obstructive symptoms or urinary retention, but if there is a high PSA and/or positive physical findings, think cancer and do a biopsy.

Natural history of disease is not well understood.

Stress Urinary Incontinence
Robert McNellis, PA-C, MPH

DEFINITION

Involuntary loss of urine caused by failure of the bladder to store, failure of the sphincter to function, or a combination of both.

HISTORY

Symptoms. Leakage of urine during stress (sneezing, coughing, or straining).

General. A full medical, surgical, and review of systems history should be obtained; note medications taken, prior trauma, pelvic or urinary tract surgery, number of vaginal deliveries, medical conditions (e.g., neuromuscular disorders or diabetes mellitus), prior UTIs, and abnormal bowel habits. In males, obtain a sexual history of erectile or ejaculatory dysfunction. A voiding or incontinence diary that records frequency, timing, and episodes is helpful.

Age. Typically, multiparous females aged 45 to 70 years.

Onset. Postmenopausal.

Duration. Episodic.

Intensity. May remain mild or may have increasing frequency and volume over years.

Aggravating Factors. Full bladder; certain medications may affect bladder function.

Alleviating Factors. Frequent urination.

Associated Factors. Medications (anticholinergics, psychotropics, antihistamines, or adrenergics), prior trauma, pelvic or urinary tract surgery, difficult or uncontrolled vaginal deliveries, neuromuscular disorders, diabetes mellitus, recurrent UTIs. In males, erectile or ejaculatory dysfunction.

PHYSICAL EXAMINATION

General. When the bladder is full, the patient should be asked to cough while in both supine and upright positions, to evaluate for incontinence. Digital pressure applied to the paraurethral tissues in an anterior direction through the vagina re-establishes the urethrovesical angle and prevents stress incontinence.

Gastrointestinal. Examine kidneys for enlargement, bladder for distention, flanks for costovertebral angle tenderness. Rectal examination is performed and anal sphincter tone and perianal sensation documented.

Genitourinary. Pelvic examination is performed to evaluate for cystocele or urethrocele.

Neurologic. Lower extremity motor and sensory function and reflexes should be evaluated. A complete neurologic examination should be performed to search for other manifestations of neurogenic dysfunction (e.g., multiple sclerosis or diabetic neuropathy).

PATHOPHYSIOLOGY

Stress incontinence is caused by the descent of the bladder neck and internal sphincter from their normal intra-abdominal position. This causes obliteration of the normal urethrovesical angle, which normally provides resistance at the bladder outlet. Intra-abdominal pressure exerts force on only the bladder, no longer the sphincter, allowing intraluminal bladder pressure to overcome sphincter resistance and thereby causing leakage.

DIAGNOSTIC STUDIES

Laboratory
Urinalysis and Urine Culture. To rule out UTI.
Urodynamic Studies. Cystometrogram records voiding and filling pressures in the bladder and can differentiate between stress incontinence and detrusor instability.
Sphincter Electromyography. Provides evidence of sphincter dysfunction.
Radiology
Voiding Cystourethrogram. Evaluates bladder neck and urethra, reveals descent of stress incontinence or detects sphincter incompetence.
Other
Cystoscopy. In selected patients to evaluate intravesical pathology. Upper tract evaluation not routine part of incontinence work-up.

DIFFERENTIAL DIAGNOSIS

Traumatic
Spinal Cord Trauma or Transection. History of trauma and evidence of paralysis with involuntary bladder contractions.
Infectious
Poliomyelitis. History of disease with overflow incontinence.
Metabolic
Diabetes Mellitus or Tabes Dorsalis. Loss of bladder sensation and decreased bladder contractility.
Neoplastic
Brain Tumors. Detrusor hyperreflexia with incontinence.
Vascular. Not applicable.

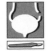

Congenital

Ectopic Urethral Orifice.   Incontinence in spite of normal voiding.

Acquired

Neurogenic Bladder.   History neurologic disorder (e.g., multiple sclerosis).

TREATMENT

Medical.   Mild cases may be treated with pelvic floor exercises (Kegel exercises) to strengthen the pelvic musculature. Oxybutynin chloride or ephedrine may help by causing detrusor relaxation. A new approach uses the injection of Teflon paste into the periurethral tissues.

Surgical.   Restoration of the bladder neck and urethra to the proper anatomical position may be achieved by several different procedures.

Marshall-Marchetti-Kranz Procedure.   Uses an anterior abdominal approach. The bladder and urethra are dissected off the posterior aspect of the symphysis pubis. Sutures are placed into the vaginal fascia on either side of the bladder neck and the urethra. These sutures are then placed in the posterior aspect of the symphysis to reposition and anchor the bladder superiorly and anteriorly.

Stamey, Raz, and Other Procedures.   These procedures use a combined vaginal and suprapubic approach to suspension. Sutures are placed through a vaginal incision into tissue on each side of the bladder neck. The bladder neck is supported by a Dacron graft (Stamey) or blunt dissection with suture reinforcement (Raz). The bladder neck sutures are passed into a suprapubic incision. Suspension sutures are then tied over the anterior rectus fascia. A cystoscope is used to confirm proper suture placement and check for bladder penetration.

Indications.   Moderate to severe urinary stress incontinence.

Contraindications.   None.

TECHNIQUE OF SURGICAL ASSISTING

Maintain a clear surgical field, keep suture material organized, and assist with suspension.

PEDIATRIC CONSIDERATIONS

Stress incontinence is generally not a disorder of childhood. Enuresis in children may indicate a psychiatric disorder, developmental delay, or regression. The family history may be positive for similar problems. Support, counseling, and avoidance of punishment for the behavior may be of benefit. If enuresis continues, psychiatric referral may be required.

OBSTETRICAL CONSIDERATIONS

Deliveries should be controlled and defects immediately repaired when possible to lessen the incidence of significant pelvic organ trauma.

PEARLS FOR THE PA

Always perform a full evaluation to rule out other causes of incontinence (e.g., neurologic disorder, pelvic organ anomalies, medical conditions, medications, etc.).

Surgery is successful in 80% of cases.

Testicular Torsion
Rita Altman, PA-C, BA, BS

DEFINITION

Twisting of the spermatic cord, causing strangulation of the blood supply to the testis. It is a true surgical emergency and, if not corrected immediately, will cause damage to the testis within 3 to 4 hours.

HISTORY

Symptoms
Neonates. Asymptomatic.
Infants. Present with scrotal a mass caused by swelling and inflammation of the scrotum.
Older Males. Severe pain in one testicle, followed by swelling and inflammation of the scrotum. Pain often radiates into the abdomen with associated nausea and vomiting.
General. On occasions, the patient may have moderate scrotal swelling and little or no pain. Due to the severity of this condition, it is imperative to rule out torsion. Fifty percent of testicular torsions occur during sleep.
Age. Infants to adolescent males.
Onset. Sudden.
Duration. Until medical treatment is sought and cord is detorsed.
Intensity. Severe in most cases.
Aggravating Factors. Elevation of the scrotum.
Alleviating Factors. None until detorsion.

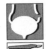

Associated Factors. Trauma; congenital abnormality of the tunica vaginalis or spermatic cord.

PHYSICAL EXAMINATION

General. The patient may be in significant distress.

Genitalia. Swollen, tender testicle retracted upward and may lie horizontal when patient stands. Very difficult to examine the patient due to pain. Test Prehn's sign by gently lifting the scrotum above the symphysis pubis. With torsion, this test is positive because the pain is greatly increased.

Abdominal. May have some lower abdominal tenderness on palpation.

PATHOPHYSIOLOGY

Testicular torsion is due to anomalous development of the tunica vaginalis. The testis rotates within the tunica. Spasm of the cremaster muscle causes the patient's left testis to rotate counterclockwise and the right testis to rotate clockwise (from the viewpoint of the foot of the bed). With vascular occlusion there can be ischemic death of the testis and epididymis.

DIAGNOSTIC STUDIES

Laboratory

Urinalysis. Screen for leukocytes, hematuria, bacteriuria to rule out other causes of testicular pain.

CBC. Leukocytosis may develop rapidly.

Radiology

Doppler. Absence of arterial flow signifies torsion unless proven otherwise. Hypervascularity may represent an inflammatory lesion.

Scintillation Scan. Accurate in 90% to 100% of cases. Twisted testis or avascular trauma cause decreased vascularity, whereas a tumor causes increased vascularity.

DIFFERENTIAL DIAGNOSIS

Traumatic

Direct Trauma to Testicle. Differentiated by scintillation scan.

Infectious

Acute Epididymitis. Rare before puberty; fever, pain relieved with elevation of scrotum.

Metabolic. Not applicable.

Neoplastic

Testicular Tumor. Usually painless.

Vascular. Not applicable.

Congenital. Not applicable.

Acquired
Inguinal Hernia. Usually painless, may be felt on inguinal examination.

TREATMENT

Medical. If patient is seen a few hours after onset, attempts can be made for manual detorsion under local anesthetic, but immediate surgical exploration and detorsion is essential.

Surgical. Bilateral surgical fixation should be considered in all cases in order to prevent subsequent torsion. If the torsion persists for more than 24 hours, preservation is doubtful. If it persists more than 48 hours, orchiectomy is advised.

Complications include wound infection, nerve damage, torsion of contralateral side (if not repaired concurrently).

Indications. Emergency detorsion within 12 hours of onset yields good results.

Contraindications. None.

TECHNIQUE OF SURGICAL ASSISTING

The assistant provides delicate countertraction and holds the testicle after detorsion while suture fixation is being conducted. Bilateral fixation is highly recommended due to contralateral abnormal attachments.

PEDIATRIC CONSIDERATIONS

This condition usually occurs in young boys.

OBSTETRICAL CONSIDERATIONS

Not applicable.

PEARLS FOR THE PA

Although torsion is uncommon, always consider it in the differential diagnosis for testicular pain in a young man.

Positive Prehn's sign (lifting the scrotum above the symphysis pubis) greatly increases the pain.

Testicular Tumor

Rita Altman, PA-C, BA, BS

DEFINITION

Malignant neoplasm of the testes, of which 90% to 95% are germ cell tumors.

HISTORY

Symptoms. Painless enlargement of the testicle, slightly more common on the right side.

General. Malignant tumors are rare (0.2% for caucasian males in the United States).

Age. 20- to 40-year-old men have the highest incidence. Also noted in infancy (0 to 10 years), and late adulthood (60 years of age and older).

Onset. Gradual sensation of heaviness in the testicle; 10% asymptomatic.

Duration. Continues until treatment is sought.

Intensity. Ranges from mild to severe. Ten percent of patients have acute testicular pain that may be associated with hemorrhage or infarction, and 10% present with metastatic symptoms (back pain, dyspnea, anorexia, nausea and vomiting, bone pain, lower extremity swelling).

Aggravating Factors. Prolonged sitting, biking, and exercise can intensify the testicular pain if tumor is present.

Alleviating Factors. Definitive treatment.

Associated Factors. Cryptorchid testis; exogenous estrogen to the pregnant mother. Scandinavian men have a much higher incidence and Japanese men have a much lower incidence than American men. In the United States, caucasian men have 75% higher incidence than African-American men.

PHYSICAL EXAMINATION

Chest/Pulmonary. Gynecomastia is present with some types of testicular tumors; also, hemoptysis may be present in metastatic disease of the lungs.

Gastrointestinal. Palpate for any retroperitoneal masses that indicate advanced disease.

Genitalia. Firm, nontender testicular mass or diffuse enlargement of the testicle. A hydrocele may also be present. Transilluminate the testes to fully evaluate.

Lymphatic. Assess involvement, especially supraclavicular, scalene, and inguinal nodes.

PATHOPHYSIOLOGY

Germ cell tumors comprise approximately 95% of all testicular tumors. It is thought that the congenital factor of undescended testes as well as acquired factors play a major role in the development of tumor. During embryonal development, the germ cells normally differentiate into spermatocytes. Sometimes they can take an abnormal pathway, resulting in seminomas, which are embryonal carcinomas. These can further differentiate into teratomas and even further into choriocarcinomas or yolk sac tumors (the most common in infants and children). Most of the tumor types spread via lymph nodes, except choriocarcinoma, which spreads hematogenously to the lung. Otherwise, the retroperitoneum is the most common metastatic site, followed by lung, liver, brain, bone, kidney, adrenal, gastrointestinal tract, and spleen (Table 12–2).

DIAGNOSTIC STUDIES

Laboratory

Urinalysis. Screen for leukocytes, hematuria, bacteriuria to rule out infection, stones, etc.

Serum Biomarkers. Human chorionic gonadotropin (βhCG), alpha-

Table 12–2. Clinical Staging of Testicular Tumors

T—Primary Tumor	
TX	Cannot be assessed.
T0	No evidence of primary tumor.
Tis	Intratubular cancer (CIS).
T1	Limited to testis.
T2	Invades beyond tunica albuginea or into epididymis.
T3	Invades spermatic cord.
T4	Invades scrotum.
N—Regional Lymph Nodes	
NX	Cannot be assessed.
N0	No regional lymph node metastasis.
N1	Microscopic lymph node metastasis.
N2a	Metastasis in <5 nodes, or any node >2 cm.
N2b	Metastasis in >5 nodes, or any node >2 cm.
N3	Extranodal invasion.
N4	Unresectable retroperitoneal metastasis.
M—Distant Metastasis	
MX	Cannot be assessed.
M0	No distant metastasis.
M1	Distant metastasis present.

From Tanagho EA, McAninch JW (eds): Smith's General Urology, ed 14. Norwalk, CT, Appleton and Lange, 1995, pp. 436–437.

fetoprotein (AFP), lactate dehydrogenase (LDH) may suggest the presence of tumor.

CBC.   To evaluate for infection or anemia.

Chemistry Profile.   In advanced disease to evaluate for abnormal liver function tests or renal failure.

Radiology

Scrotal Ultrasound.   To identify the presence of the tumor.

Chest Film; CT Scan of Abdomen and Pelvis.   Used to assess the two most common sites of metastasis, lung and retroperitoneum.

DIFFERENTIAL DIAGNOSIS

Traumatic

Hydrocele.   May accompany a tumor. Ultrasound is indicated to evaluate for tumor.

Hematocele.   Differentiated by ultrasound.

Infectious

Epididymitis.   Enlarged, tender epididymis that is separate from the testis. Positive history of acute onset of fever, urethral discharge, and dysuria.

Epididymo-orchitis, Granulomatous Orchitis.   Differentiated by ultrasound.

Metabolic.   Not applicable.

Neoplastic

Benign Epidermoid Cyst.   Testicle is not usually enlarged; cysts are small and well defined.

Vascular

Hematocele, Varicocele.   Differentiated by scrotal ultrasound.

Congenital.   Not applicable.

Acquired

Spermatocele, Testicular Torsion.   Usually painful, whereas tumor usually is painless.

TREATMENT

Medical.   Combined treatment with radiation, chemotherapy, and surgery, depending on the type and staging of the tumor.

Surgical.   An inguinal approach is mandatory so that the scrotal lymphatics are not disturbed. An inguinal incision is used, cutting down to the external ring and exposing the spermatic cord, to help mobilize the cord and keep it retracted. Blunt dissection is used to mobilize the testis from the scrotum. The cord is ligated inside the internal inguinal ring with a large, permanent suture. Secure sutures are required because the most serious complication arises from cord stump bleeding. The vas deferens is ligated separately. A testicular prosthesis may be used for cosmetic reasons and sutured in place. Usually done as an outpatient procedure.

Complications include bleeding and wound infection (rare). For lymphadenectomy, there can be significant morbidity, especially in regard to fertility.

Indications. Almost all testicular tumors require radical orchiectomy, and some require retroperitoneal lymph node dissection (if they have spread) for surgical staging and potential cure.

Contraindications. None.

TECHNIQUE OF SURGICAL ASSISTING

The assistant uses countertraction for exposure and helps identify and protect the ilioinguinal nerve. Be sure to use a noncrushing clamp on the spermatic cord to avoid potential tumor spread via veins or lymphatics. The PA assists with closure of the incision (with dissolvable sutures) after copious irrigation.

PEDIATRIC CONSIDERATIONS

Peak age is 2 years. The pediatric population represents 2% of all testicular tumors, with a greater incidence of benign tumors. Observe for virilization signs. Yolk sac is the most common pediatric tumor (47%), followed by Leydig cell (18%), teratoma (14%), and Sertoli cell (10%).

OBSTETRICAL CONSIDERATIONS

Exogenous estrogen taken by the pregnant woman may lead to the development of testicular neoplasms.

PEARLS FOR THE PA

Twenty-five percent of tumors are misdiagnosed as epididymitis.

Always consider cancer in the differential diagnosis of an enlarged testicle.

Urolithiasis
Gerard J. Marciano, PA-C

DEFINITION

Aggregation of crystalloid material (kidney stone) within the urinary tract, frequently leading to obstructive uropathy.

HISTORY

Symptoms.   Sudden onset of flank, low back, or abdominal pain, relieved by movement, that radiates to the scrotum or labia.

General.   Obtain a history of prior kidney stones, full past medical history, and review of systems for conditions and medications that may predispose to stone formation.

Age.   Variable.

Onset.   Acute.

Duration.   Variable/intermittent.

Intensity.   Severe; comparable to childbirth.

Aggravating Factors.   Prior history of stone formation, irritable bowel syndrome, gout, familial renal disease, certain medications (e.g., diuretics), sedentary lifestyle.

Alleviating Factors.   Analgesia, stone passage, or treatment.

PHYSICAL EXAMINATION

General.   Patients may present with marked pain and distress (a writhing patient), with diaphoresis, tachypnea, tachycardia, and fever in the presence of obstruction or infection.

Urological.   Decreased bowel sounds, palpable kidney in the presence of severe hydronephrosis; palpable bladder with bladder neck obstruction, or costovertebral angle tenderness.

PATHOPHYSIOLOGY

Urinary tract pain is secondary to obstruction and the distention that develops proximal to the obstruction. Table 12–3 lists types of kidney stones.

DIAGNOSTIC STUDIES

Laboratory

Urinalysis.   Macroscopic or microscopic hematuria, bacteriuria, pyuria, or crystals.

Table 12–3. Types of Kidney Stones

Type of Stone	Age/Gender/Cause
Calcium phosphate	30–50 years of age/males
Calcium oxalate	30–50 years of age/males
Magnesium ammonium phosphate (struvite/Staghorn calculus)	Associated with infection
Cystine	Rare/genetic
Uric acid	
Xanthine	

Radiology
IVP. Delay or nonvisualization acutely; hydronephrosis (late).
Tomogram. Extravasation of dye secondary to a tear due to increased pressure.
Ultrasound. Used in patients who are allergic to the contrast agent, pregnant, or have a history of chronic renal failure; may show obstruction or hydronephrosis.
Retrograde Cystourethrogram and CT Scan. Rarely used.

DIFFERENTIAL DIAGNOSIS

Traumatic
Abdominal, Back, Perineal Injury. May cause pain and hematuria.
Infectious
Pyelonephritis. Fever, painful costrovertebral angle tenderness, positive urine culture, proteinuria and hematuria, or elevated BUN/creatinine may be present.
Metabolic
Cholelithiasis. May have elevated liver enzymes and a tender right upper quadrant on examination.
Neoplastic
Calcified Tumor or Lymph Nodes. Seen on IVP and found on physical examination, respectively.
Vascular. Not applicable.
Congenital. Not applicable.
Acquired. Not applicable.

TREATMENT

Medical. Calcium phosphate stones are treated by decreasing calcium in diet, directly and indirectly, by restricting calcium, sodium, fat, and refined carbohydrates. The patient is adequately hydrated orally or intravenously. Teas and juices are avoided and all urine is strained to detect the passage of the stone.

Patients with cystine, uric acid, or xanthine stones are given a low purine diet, the urine is alkalinized, and allopurinol given as indicated.

Surgical. The types of surgery are determined by the location of the stone. Magnesium ammonium phosphate (struvite) stones require excision of the Staghorn calculus.

Kidney. Nephrectomy, open lithectomy, or extracorporeal shock wave lithotripsy (ESWL) is used for stones occurring in the kidney. ESWL is ultrasonic fragmentation of a large stone in the urinary tract under fluoroscopic guidance, followed by irrigation to remove the particulate remnants of the stone.

Ureter. If the stone is localized to the ureter, a small basket or balloon

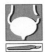

may be inserted via cystoscopy and the stone removed. ESWL also may be used. Stent placement may be required as indicated to relieve hydronephrosis.

Bladder.   Transurethral irrigation can be employed to remove small stones, or, by using cystoscopy and fluoroscopic guidance, the stone can be fragmented by electrohydraulic lithotripsy and irrigated from the bladder. Open, suprapubic surgical excision is sometimes required.

Urethra.   Stones in the urethra may be irrigated or removed by cystoscopic guidance if small, but usually require open, surgical removal.

Indications.   Intractable UTI, progressive renal disease, urinary obstruction, persistent pain.

Contraindications.   To ESWL include infections and pacemakers; contraindications for other surgeries are the same as with any surgical procedure (e.g., patient unable to tolerate anesthesia).

TECHNIQUE OF SURGICAL ASSISTING

For cystoscopic procedures, assisting is frequently limited to maintaining sterility in the passage of instrumentation. For an open surgical procedure, assistance is required for hemostasis, retraction, opening and closing.

PEDIATRIC CONSIDERATIONS

Rule out congenital anomalies.

OBSTETRICAL CONSIDERATIONS

Consider the diagnosis of urolithiasis with severe, recurrent pyelonephritis or UTI. Diagnosis is made by ultrasound. Treat with appropriate, nonteratogenic analgesics and fluids.

PEARLS FOR THE PA

A writhing patient in pain has a kidney stone until proven otherwise.

Urinary tract pain is secondary to obstruction and the distention that develops proximal to the obstruction.

Intravenous pyelogram (IVP) is the diagnostic study of choice.

Varicocele
Rita Altman, PA-C, BA, BS

DEFINITION

Dilated, tortuous testicular veins within the spermatic cord.

HISTORY

Symptoms. A boggy feeling in scrotum; may be asymptomatic.
General. Usually found in men who seek medical attention because they have difficulty conceiving; left side is more common.
Age. Most common in adolescent boys and young men.
Onset. Gradual onset.
Duration. Lasts until treatment.
Intensity. May be painful in sexually active men.
Aggravating Factors. Valsalva maneuver increases the dilatation of vessels; exercise without scrotal support.
Alleviating Factors. Lying down, wearing scrotal support apparel (e.g., jock strap); definitive treatment.
Associated Factors. Low sperm count; infertility; renal tumor (older men).

PHYSICAL EXAMINATION

Genitalia. Examine the patient in a warm environment using Valsalva's maneuver with the patient supine as well as standing. Palpate the spermatic cord. If there is an increased thickness of the cord, discrete pulse during Valsalva, or a smaller left testis with a boggy feeling in scrotum (bag of worms), then it is highly indicative of varicocele. The veins above and posterior to the testis may look like a mass when the patient stands, but this disappears in the supine position. Varicocele does not transilluminate.

PATHOPHYSIOLOGY

Varicocele is found in 10% of young men. It is the most common diagnosis made in an infertile man due to decreased concentration and motility of the sperm. The pampiniform plexus above the testis becomes involved due to incompetent or absent valves, which are more common in the left internal spermatic vein. Over time, it becomes difficult for the veins of the plexus to drain, causing dilatation.

DIAGNOSTIC STUDIES

Laboratory
Semen Analysis.   To evaluate for low count and motility.
Hormone Levels.   Gonadotropin and testosterone levels are usually normal. Follicle-stimulating hormone (FSH) may be elevated.
Radiology
Scrotal Ultrasound.   Useful in documenting size of varicosities; may demonstrate reflux.
Other
Venography.   Most specific method of identifying varicoceles, but invasive, higher risk, and expensive.

DIFFERENTIAL DIAGNOSIS

Traumatic
Scrotal Injury.   History of trauma; associated with pain.
Infectious
Epididymitis.   Usually painful; may have hydrocele present.
Metabolic.   Not applicable.
Neoplastic
Testicular Tumor.   Firm, noncystic; "bag of worms" not palpated.
Epididymal Cysts.   Differentiated on ultrasound; "bag of worms" not palpated.
Vascular.   Not applicable.
Congenital.   Not applicable.
Acquired
Hydrocele.   Scrotal mass, nontender to palpation, positive transillumination.
Spermatocele.   Freely movable cystic mass that lies above the testicle.

TREATMENT

Medical.   Trial of scrotal support is used in patients with chronic pain. Percutaneous therapy using a balloon catheter or sclerosing agents may be used to occlude the veins.
Surgical.   Ligation of internal spermatic veins at or above the internal ring. The procedure can be done by laparoscopy or via an inguinal open approach or a scrotal approach. The latter is the least popular approach due to the numerous veins and the risk of arterial injury. The procedure is done as an outpatient procedure and has minimal risk.
Indications.   Infertility (usually greatly improves semen quality and increases the chance of conception).
Contraindications.   None.

TECHNIQUE OF SURGICAL ASSISTING

An assistant is used, especially during a laparoscopic approach. The assistant aids in controlling the camera as well as using the laparoscopic instruments. As always, the concepts of countertraction and suction apply. Doing a laparoscopic procedure is very similar to a virtual reality game. Always watch the screen and not your hands. After the vessels are located, tied-off, and cut, look for bleeding and coagulate.

PEDIATRIC CONSIDERATIONS

May be clinically evident at puberty. The only recommended treatment is for severe varicoceles with loss of testicular volume. Not all patients become infertile, so only those at high risk for testicular dysfunction should be treated.

OBSTETRICAL CONSIDERATIONS

Not applicable.

PEARLS FOR THE PA

Varicocele feels like a bag of worms.

If sudden onset in an older man, it may be a late sign of a renal tumor.

Further Reading

Hardy J (ed): Hardy's Textbook of Surgery, ed 2. Philadelphia, J.B. Lippincott, 1988.
Tanagho EA, McAninch JW (eds): Smith's General Urology, ed 14. Norwalk, CT, Appleton and Lange, 1995.
Walsh PC, Retik AB, Stamey TA, Vaughan ED (eds): Campbell's Urology, ed 6. Philadelphia, W.B. Saunders, 1992.

Chapter **13**
Vascular Surgery
Diseases of the Aorta
Deborah A. Opacic, PA-C, MMS

DEFINITION

Diseases of the aorta may be classified as aneurysmal or dissecting. They are classified as fusiform where the aneurysm encompasses the entire circumference of the aorta and assumes a spindle shape. Saccular aneurysms involve only a portion of the circumference, in which there is a neck and an asymmetric outpouching of the aorta. Dissecting aneurysms occur with a tear in the intima of the vessel, which permits a column of blood to dissect along the media of the vessel. Aortic dissection is most frequently seen in the ascending aorta, but may be seen at the aortic arch, isthmus, descending, and abdominal aorta.

HISTORY

Symptoms. The patient can present with chest or severe back pain. Depending on the area of dissection, it can compromise blood flow to a specific organ, causing hemiplegia, transient blindness, or aortic regurgitation. Other presentations include epigastric pain, bronchial obstruction, vomiting, hematemesis, or melena (if there is involvement of the mesenteric arteries). If the renal arteries are involved, oliguria or hematuria may be present. Hoarseness can occur with stretching of the recurrent laryngeal nerve. Involvement of the stellate ganglion can cause Horner's syndrome.

General. A history of hypertension; syndromes such as Marfan's, Ehlers-Danlos, or Turner's; bicuspid aortic valve; coarctation of the aorta; giant cell arteritis; atherosclerosis; syphilis; cystic medial necrosis; collagen vascular disease; or trauma to the chest wall should be obtained.

Age. Usually seen in the fifth to seventh decades.

Onset. Progressive symptoms or acute with rupture.

Duration. Enlargement with eventual rupture possible.

Intensity. May be asymptomatic or life-threatening with rupture or vascular compromise.

Aggravating Factors. Smoking; deficiency of collagen or elastin in the arterial wall.

Alleviating Factors. Blood pressure control.

Associated Factors. Aortic dissection occurs in those individuals who are predisposed to degeneration of the elastic and smooth muscle components of the aortic media with factors such as age, hypertension, pregnancy, Marfan's syndrome, Ehlers-Danlos syndrome, bicuspid aortic valve, coarctation of the aorta, Turner's syndrome, giant cell arteritis, or blunt chest trauma. Other causes include atherosclerosis, syphilis, and cystic medial necrosis.

513

PHYSICAL EXAMINATION

General. The patient may appear normal or present with life-threatening hemorrhagic shock.

Cardiovascular. Including systemic hypertension, 20% of the patients that present with systemic hypotension have a proximal dissection. Thirty percent to forty percent of patients have a unilateral reduction in the arterial pressure and pulse in an extremity. If the dissection ruptures into the pericardium, there can be jugular venous distention or pulsus paradoxus, along with muffled heart sounds and a pericardial friction rub. Auscultation can reveal aortic regurgitation. Dullness to percussion of the left chest is noted if there is a hemothorax.

Auscultation should be performed of the carotid, abdominal aorta, and femoral arteries to evaluate for a bruit. Palpation of the abdominal aorta may reveal lateral pulsations, which are indicative of an aneurysm. Measurements should be taken during the examination to ascertain the approximate size of the aneurysm.

Neurologic. A full neurologic examination is indicated if the cerebral vessels appear to be involved or if there is involvement of the spinal cord. Focal abnormalities may be identified.

PATHOPHYSIOLOGY

Aortic dissection occurs in those individuals who are predisposed to degeneration of the elastic and smooth muscle components of the aortic media by factors such as advanced age, hypertension, pregnancy, Marfan's syndrome, Ehlers-Danlos syndrome, bicuspid aortic valve, coarctation of the aorta, Turner's syndrome, giant cell arteritis, and blunt chest trauma. The most frequent causes of aneurysm formation include atherosclerosis, aortic dissection, and collagen vascular disease.

There are three types of aortic dissection.

Stanford type A (Debakey type I & II) begins at the ascending aorta and extends to the aortic arch; causes include syphilis, and cystic medial necrosis

Stanford type A (Debakey type I & II) begins at the ascending aorta and ends before the innominate artery; causes include congenital, Marfan's syndrome, and syphilis

Stanford type B begins distal to the left subclavian artery and involves only the descending aorta; causes include syphilis, atherosclerosis, dissection, or trauma

The infrarenal abdominal aorta is the most common site of abdominal aneurysms. The most common cause is atherosclerosis. The risk of aneurysmal rupture approaches 80% once the dilatation reaches 6 cm. With an elevated blood pressure (diastolic) of greater than 100 mm Hg, the risk of rupture is compounded. Surgical repair at this point can prolong patient survival.

DIAGNOSTIC STUDIES

Laboratory
Electrolytes. May show abnormal blood urea nitrogen (BUN) and creatinine levels if renal artery stenosis is present.

Cardiac Isoenzymes. Used to rule out myocardial infarction.

Arterial Blood Gases. Are performed to evaluate for acidosis in patients with renal compromise.

CBC. Used to evaluate the presence or extent of anemia. Anemia may be profound in those in whom the aneurysm has ruptured.

Radiology
Chest X-ray. May reveal a widened mediastinum, deviated trachea, or pleural effusion.

CT of the Chest or Abdomen. Performed with contrast to determine the presence and extent of aneurysmal dilatation. Adequate hydration must be ensured prior to giving contrast in order to avoid worsening or potentiation of renal insufficiency.

MRI of the Chest or Abdomen. Superior to CT in determining the presence and extent of aneurysmal dilatation.

Aortogram. The definitive diagnostic test to determine the presence and size of the aneurysm.

Other
Electrocardiogram (ECG). Can reveal left ventricular hypertrophy or low voltage suggestive of pericardial effusion.

Transesophageal Echocardiogram. Can be an extremely useful diagnostic tool; may reveal a pericardial effusion, aortic insufficiency, as well as identify aneurysmal dilatation or dissection.

DIFFERENTIAL DIAGNOSIS

Traumatic
Traumatic Aneurysm. Most originate distal to the left subclavian artery.

Infectious
Syphilitic or Mycotic Aneurysms. Least likely to originate in the ascending aorta. Historical information and serology may reveal the origin.

Metabolic. Not applicable.

Neoplastic
Neoplasm. No bruit heard on auscultation. Widened mediastinum on chest x-ray suggests mediastinal adenopathy. CT/MRI identifies lymphadenopathy or tumor.

Vascular
Takayasu Arteritis. Presents with systemic findings. Patients may complain of jaw pain or syncope. Most frequent aneurysms are in the descending thoracic aorta.

Congenital
Marfan's Syndrome. Aneurysms typically involve the ascending aorta. Additional physical findings such as acromegaly may be evident.

Acquired. Not applicable.

TREATMENT

Medical. First and foremost is to control systolic blood pressure and to maintain the lowest pressure that will perfuse end organs adequately (mean arterial pressure, 80 to 90 mm Hg). Beta blockers are the drug of choice both to reduce the force of myocardial contraction and to decrease the heart rate. Additional agents include alpha methyldopa, reserpine, nitroprusside, or trimethaphan. The patient should be monitored for any advancement of the aneurysm by performing a detailed neurologic examination, assessing for renal dysfunction, bowel ischemia, pain, or acidosis. If the dissection only involves the distal aorta, the patient can be treated medically with beta blockade. The patient should be followed with a contrast CT or ultrasound every 6 months. Prophylactic beta-blocker therapy should be considered in patients with connective tissue disease abnormalities such as Marfan's or Ehlers-Danlos syndrome to minimize the risk of dissection.

Surgical. A left posterolateral thoracotomy or laparotomy is performed. Bypass is implemented to protect blood supply to the spinal cord and kidneys. The aorta is appropriately occluded proximal and distal to the aneurysm or dissection. The aneurysm is widely opened and the anterior wall is excised, followed by removal of the inner lining of the aneurysm. There is usually no need to remove the entire abnormal segment. A Dacron prosthesis is used for reconstruction with a continuous suture for the anastomosis. The sac remaining from the aneurysm can then be used to surround the graft.

Complications of this procedure can include hemorrhage, paradoxical hypertension, paraplegia, thrombosis, distal embolization, renal, mesenteric ischemia, infection, chylothorax, or recurrent nerve paralysis.

Indications. Aortic insufficiency (acute or severe), tamponade, leakage of the aneurysm, occlusion of a major systemic artery, severe pain, uncontrollable hypertension, progressive enlargement of the aneurysm, or if a pulsatile mass greater than 6 cm is noted on abdominal examination. Without surgical intervention, these patients can die within 48 hours. If there is a proximal dissection, the mortality rate of those treated medically is 65% to 80%. If the patient is operated on immediately, the mortality rate can be reduced to 10% to 30%.

Contraindications. Critical coronary artery disease, severe pulmonary or renal insufficiency, or any major complication of dissection.

TECHNIQUE OF SURGICAL ASSISTING

The PA acts as the first or second assistant, and assists with the incision, tissue retraction, ensuring adequate hemostasis, preparing arterial grafts (as indicated), and wound closure. Pre- and postoperative care are significant responsibilities of the surgical PA.

PEDIATRIC CONSIDERATIONS

Not applicable.

OBSTETRICAL CONSIDERATIONS

See Pathophysiology.

PEARLS FOR THE PA

Adequate blood pressure control is imperative.

Frequent physical evaluation is essential with dissecting aortic aneurysms in order to note any advancement.

Carotid Atherosclerotic Disease
Deborah A. Opacic, PA-C, MMS

DEFINITION

Stenotic, occlusive diseases of the aortic arch, carotid, or vertebral arteries.

HISTORY

Symptoms. Depending on the area of the occlusion, the patient may present with monocular vision loss (amaurosis fugax), motor deficits involving the functional loss of one or more of the extremities, sensory loss (including paresthesias), speech or language difficulties, unsteadiness, vertigo, sudden loss of the motor function of the lower extremities not associated with loss of consciousness, confusion, memory disturbance, headache, diplopia, dysarthria, dysphasia, or bowel or bladder incontinence. Patients can also present with asymptomatic bruits.

General. Twenty percent of the patients with bruits on examination progress to a stroke. Transient ischemic attacks (TIAs) are the leading predictors of stroke occurrence.

Age. Incidence increases with advancing age.

Onset. Slow and progressive, stepwise (e.g., with repeated TIAs), or acute with stroke.

Duration. Progressive.

Intensity. Patients may be asymptomatic, present with transient symptoms, or have significant or life-threatening disabilities with a stroke.

Aggravating Factors.   Failure to seek treatment or recognize symptoms such as systemic hypertension, TIAs.

Alleviating Factors.   Anticoagulation, antiplatelet therapy, blood pressure control.

Associated Factors.   Hypertension, peripheral vascular disease in other vessels, smoking, family history, hyperlipidemia, diabetes mellitus, and age greater than 70 years.

PHYSICAL EXAMINATION

General.   The patient may appear normal or have overt neurologic deficits if he or she is experiencing a TIA or has had a completed stroke.

Cardiovascular.   All of the pulses must be evaluated for evidence of flow reduction and bruits. Reduction of the right subclavian and common carotid pulsation may indicate disease involving the innominate artery. If the carotid pulsation is diminished, disease involving the common carotid is suspected. Diminished pulsation of the temporal artery may be an indication of external carotid obstruction. Auscultatory evidence of bruits at the lower neck level signify disease that may involve the common carotid. If heard at the supraclavicular fossa, consider subclavian disease. A bruit at the angle of the mandible may signify obstruction at the carotid bifurcation. The blood pressure must be checked in both arms to rule out subclavian arterial obstruction. A complete cardiac examination should be performed to rule out any coexisting pathology.

Neurologic.   A complete and thorough neurologic examination should be performed to evaluate for any current or residual focal deficits.

Ophthalmologic.   A detailed examination of the eyes is performed with attention to the fundi to evaluate for any evidence of emboli or thrombosis. Unilateral arcus senilis may be present, which can be an indicator of carotid disease involving the opposite side. Xanthelasma *of the eyelid* is associated with hypercholesterolemia.

PATHOPHYSIOLOGY

The majority of these lesions are attributable to atherosclerosis, with the greatest percentage occurring at the carotid bifurcation. The second highest pathological entity is that of fibromuscular dysplasia. Reduced cerebral blood flow is due to the stenosis or secondary to an embolus or thrombus. Any condition that increases blood turbulence (e.g., cardiac murmur, vessel ulceration, uneven plaque) can lead to thrombus formation.

DIAGNOSTIC STUDIES

Laboratory
Chemistry Profile.   Used as a baseline prior to surgery. BUN and creatinine levels may be elevated in patients with concurrent renal artery stenosis.

CBC.   To evaluate for elevated hemoglobin and hematocrit, which may contribute to the formation of thromboemboli.

Platelets.   Elevation, which may contribute to the formation of thromboemboli.

Prothrombin Time.   Used as a baseline prior to the institution of anticoagulation, and monitored for patients on warfarin (Coumadin).

Partial Thromboplastin Time.   Used as a baseline prior to the institution of anticoagulation, and monitored for patients on heparin.

Radiology

Angiography.   The definitive test for arterial stenosis. Should include the aortic arch, carotids, and vertebral arteries. Angiography is performed if the noninvasive tests suggest hemodynamically significant stenosis or if surgery is contemplated.

CT/MRI of the Brain.   Performed if there has been a neurologic event or physical finding. CT/MRI is used to evaluate for the presence or extent of a new stroke. Old, unrecognized strokes can also be seen. In the acute setting, an infarct may not be recognized; repeat imaging studies should be performed after several days. Hemorrhages or neoplasms may be identified as a source of the patient's symptoms.

Xenon Cerebral Blood Flow Studies.   Can also determine reserve flow in areas of question.

Other

Carotid Duplex Ultrasound.   Should be performed if a bruit is heard or if the patient has experienced neurologic symptoms. Used as a noninvasive screening test for stenosis.

Transcranial Doppler.   Used to evaluate cerebral blood flow. Can be useful for posterior circulation (vertebral) evaluation.

Oculoplethysmography (OPG).   Is a good indicator of hemodynamically significant internal carotid stenosis.

DIFFERENTIAL DIAGNOSIS

Traumatic

Head Injury.   History of injury. Area of trauma can be identified through CT/MRI.

Infectious

Cerebral Abscess.   The patient may be septic, have an elevated WBC, fever. Appearance on CT/MRI is that of a well-defined lesion with ring enhancement.

Metabolic

Hyponatremia, Hypercalcemia, Hypoxia.   May cause neurologic symptoms with or without carotid artery lesions present. Identified on serum chemistry analysis, ABG, or pulse oximetry.

Neoplastic

Intracerebral Neoplasms.   May present with symptoms of stroke/TIA. CT/MRI likely shows the lesion.

Vascular
Intracerebral Hemorrhage. May present with symptoms of stroke/TIA. CT/MRI can identify the bleed.
Subarachnoid Hemorrhage. Due to any cause (aneurysm, arteriovenous malformation) may present with symptoms of stroke/TIA. After the hemorrhage has occurred, the patient may suffer vasospasm, which can cause transient neurologic symptoms. Atherosclerotic disease may give rise to intracerebral aneurysm formation.
Congenital
Aneurysmal Dilatation. Can result in intracerebral hemorrhage.
Acquired
Illicit Drug Use. May cause transient neurologic symptoms such as lethargy. Drugs that increase blood pressure or vasospasm may lead to stroke. Drug screen positive.
Other
Seizure. May present with transient, unexplained neurologic symptoms. Electroencephalogram (EEG) is frequently positive, CT/MRI usually negative, and the patient responds to anticonvulsant therapy.

TREATMENT

Medical. In patients with minimal stenosis (<30% reduction in vessel diameter), treatment is begun with anticoagulants (warfarin, heparin) or antiplatelet regimens (aspirin, ticlopidine [Ticlid]). Thrombolysis can be considered in those patients with unstable neurologic symptoms in whom there is a risk of recurrent embolization. Agents that are used include streptokinase and tissue plasminogen factor.

Surgical. The most common site of stenosis is the internal carotid at the origin. A longitudinal arteriotomy is made above and below the plaque at the level of the bifurcation. The plaque is then dissected out and the vessel is then flushed with heparin and saline. Primary closure of the vessel is performed.

Low-dose aspirin or anticoagulation may be given postoperatively with thromboembolectomy.

Indications. The patient who has experienced TIAs with no permanent neurological defects, a long life expectancy, nonclassic symptoms (e.g., syncope, dizziness) along with a high-grade (>80%) stenosis, or a hemodynamically significant carotid lesion or ulceration. Prophylactic carotid endarterectomy has been shown to benefit those individuals with multiple areas of unilateral internal carotid artery stenosis, along with the complete occlusion of the internal carotid artery on the contralateral side.

Contraindications. Less than 4 weeks following a stroke due to the risk of causing hemorrhage into newly injured brain tissue.

TECHNIQUE OF SURGICAL ASSISTING

The PA acts as the first or second assistant, and assists with the incision, tissue retraction, ensuring adequate hemostasis, preparing arterial grafts (as indicated), and wound closure. Pre- and postoperative care are significant responsibilities of the surgical PA.

PEDIATRIC CONSIDERATIONS

Not applicable.

OBSTETRICAL CONSIDERATIONS

Not applicable.

PEARLS FOR THE PA

Twenty percent of the patients with bruits on examination progress to a stroke.

TIAs are the leading predictors of stroke occurrence.

Renal Atherosclerotic Disease
Deborah A. Opacic, PA-C, MMS

DEFINITION

Stenotic, occlusive diseases of the renal arteries.

HISTORY

Symptoms.   Patients may present with hypertension, symptoms related to peripheral vascular disease, or symptoms of renal insufficiency such as malaise, volume overload, dyspnea, orthopnea, and reduced urinary output.

General.   The patient may have been diagnosed with a recent rise in blood pressure.

Age.   Associated with atherosclerosis in males greater than age 50 years; in females, it is most often associated with fibrous dysplasia.

Onset.   Recent acceleration in blood pressure.

Duration.   Continued rise in blood pressure.

Intensity.   The hypertension may be severe and resistant to medical therapy.

Aggravating Factors.   Smoking, oral contraceptives, ethanol.

Alleviating Factors. Dietary restriction of fats and sodium to lower serum lipid levels and intravascular volume.

Associated Factors. Smoking, hypercholesterolemia, and fibrous dysplasia have been identified in patients with renal stenosis. Abdominal aortic or peripheral vascular disease.

PHYSICAL EXAMINATION

General. Vital signs may reveal a markedly elevated systemic blood pressure.

Cardiopulmonary. Findings consistent with fluid overload such as rales, jugular venous distention, and peripheral edema may be present if the renal compromise is significant enough to cause a reduction in the glomerular filtration rate.

Vascular. Abdominal or flank bruits may be heard on physical examination. Diminished peripheral pulses suggest diffuse vascular disease.

PATHOPHYSIOLOGY

The most common cause of renal vascular disease is atherosclerosis, typically occurring at the ostia, with involvement of the left renal artery affected most often. There is a high association of renal artery stenosis found in patients with documented peripheral vascular disease and diseases of the abdominal aorta. In young, hypertensive individuals, the leading cause is fibromuscular dysplasia.

DIAGNOSTIC STUDIES

Laboratory

Serum Electrolytes. Hypokalemia may be present with hyperaldosteronism.

Catecholamine/17 Hydroxyketosteroid. Elevated in Cushing's disease and with pheochromocytoma.

Renin/Angiotensin. May be elevated in renovascular disease.

Urine Electrolytes. Identify renal parenchymal disease or an excess in potassium secretion in hyperaldosteronism.

Radiology

Rapid-sequence Excretory Urography. Reveals a small kidney with delayed excretion of contrast material on the affected side.

Isotope Renography. I^{131} and Tc^{99} (DTPA) are used to indirectly measure renal plasma flow and glomerular filtration rate.

Split Renal Function Studies. Performed to identify which kidney is affected.

Captopril Renal Scanning. Used to detect elevated plasma renin levels following administration.

Digital Subtraction Angiography. Used in the evaluation of peripheral vascular disease by including an aortic flush to evaluate the renal arteries.

Renal Duplex Sonography. Noninvasive study used to detect the presence or degree of renal artery stenosis.

DIFFERENTIAL DIAGNOSIS

Traumatic
Renal Contusion. Can be associated with gross hematuria, flank pain, and tenderness.

Infectious
Pyelonephritis. Associated with flank and bladder tenderness, fever, dehydration, pyuria, WBC casts and bacteria in the urine.

Metabolic
Hyperaldosteronism. Associated with hypertension, hypokalemia, metabolic alkalosis, muscle weakness, and cramping.

Cushing's Disease. Associated with hypertension, truncal obesity, moon facies, virilism in females, muscle wasting, and weakness observed in the presence of increased steroids.

Pheochromocytoma. Associated with hypertension, palpitations, diaphoresis, elevated catecholamines, and an abnormal mass on imaging studies.

Parenchymal Renal Disease. Associated with hypertension, abnormal urinary sediment, anemia, and symptoms of renal failure previously identified.

Neoplastic
Renal Tumors. A flank mass may be able to be palpated, there may be associated fever as well as bone pain as a manifestation of metastatic disease. CT/MRI identifies the mass.

Vascular
Essential Hypertension. Renal studies normal.

Congenital
Coarctation of the Aorta. Associated with hypertension, inconsistent blood pressure readings between the upper and lower extremities. A soft bruit may be noted to be the loudest in the back; femoral pulses may be delayed.

Acquired
Volume Dependent Hypertension. Hypertension subsides with diuresis.

TREATMENT

Medical. Pharmacologic treatment is contraindicated unless the patient is critically ill or when surgery is contraindicated. Thrombolytic therapy for renal artery stenosis remains experimental.

Surgical. High-grade stenosis or occlusion from atherosclerosis is treated by bypass grafting or endarterectomy. Fibromuscular stenosis or the renal artery can be amenable to balloon angioplasty.

Prior to the actual operative procedure, any antihypertensive medication must be reviewed with caution in that associated perioperative vasomotor collapse can be associated with the general anesthesia. In the case of the severely hypertensive patient, concomitant treatment must be monitored extremely closely along with notifying the anesthesiologist of the need of antihypertensive treatment. Alpha methyldopa often has been used in such a scenario.

The two most common procedures encountered are the thromboendarterectomy, with a patch graft to minimize the amount of narrowing at the suture line, or bypass grafting from the aorta to the renal artery distal to the stenosis. Additional procedures include a splenorenal anastomosis, implantation of the renal artery directly into the aorta, and resection of the stenotic area with end-to-end reanastomosis or with a graft interposition. With the bypass procedure and prior to clamping, the patient is given 50 mg of heparin. Mannitol may be given during the procedure to stimulate osmotic diuresis.

Postoperative complications may include excessive diuresis as well as systemic hypertension. Close monitoring of the patient's volume status and myocardial function is warranted.

Indications. Patients with documented renovascular hypertension or renal insufficiency secondary to renal artery lesions.

Contraindications. Those patients in whom anesthesia cannot be safely performed.

TECHNIQUE OF SURGICAL ASSISTING

The PA acts as the first or second assistant, and assists with the incision, tissue retraction, ensuring adequate hemostasis, preparing arterial grafts (as indicated), and wound closure. Pre- and postoperative care are significant responsibilities of the surgical PA.

PEDIATRIC CONSIDERATIONS

Not applicable.

OBSTETRICAL CONSIDERATIONS

Not applicable.

PEARLS FOR THE PA

Include renal artery stenosis in the differential diagnosis in a patient with hypertension.

Frequently associated with fibrous dysplasia in females.

There is a high association of renal artery stenosis with peripheral vascular disease and diseases of the abdominal aorta.

Arteriosclerosis Obliterans
Deborah A. Opacic, PA-C, MMS

DEFINITION

Arteriosclerosis obliterans is a disease process that consists of the narrowing of large and medium-sized vessels in a segmental pattern with "skip areas." It is identified most commonly in the lower extremities; however, the cranial vessels can also be involved. Involvement of the upper extremities is uncommon; an example is the subclavian steal syndrome.

HISTORY

Symptoms.   Patients with peripheral arterial disease can present with any number of symptoms, ranging from end-organ disease (e.g., stroke) if the stenosis is significant enough or, as in the case of aneurysmal dilatation, completely asymptomatic. With arteriosclerosis, the individual can complain of calf pain or cramping induced by exercise (claudication), rest pain, atrophic changes in the limb, coldness of the limb, paresthesias, or even tissue necrosis manifesting as ulceration or gangrene. If the area of involvement is comprised of the inflow tract, the patient may complain of claudication in the buttocks or of impotence. Outflow involvement may manifest as thigh pain. Calf pain may result from involvement of any branch of the arterial system. Foot pain can result from the smaller vessels such as the tibial or peroneal vessels.

General.   Most patients with peripheral occlusive disease have associated diffuse atherosclerosis, elevated systemic blood pressure, along with signs or symptoms of heart disease. Family history of vascular disease may be present.

Age.   More common in the older male.

Onset.   Progressive as stenosis becomes worse over time, or acute with arterial occlusion.

Duration. Progressive.

Intensity. Symptoms may resolve with rest. Increased activity may cause significant occlusion.

Aggravating Factors. Symptoms increase with walking or exercise.

Alleviating Factors. Antiplatelet therapy, smoking cessation.

Associated Factors. Smoking, hyperlipidemia, diabetes mellitus.

PHYSICAL EXAMINATION

General. Decreased hair growth, pallor, and atrophy of the involved extremity may be present. Complete cardiac and neurologic examinations are performed to identify coexisting disease.

Vascular. Must include a thorough inspection, palpation of the peripheral pulses, and auscultation for bruits. Dependent rubor along with visible ulceration is consistent with advanced disease. Absent pulses signify obstruction occurring proximal to the pulse. A palpable thrill signifies severe stenosis. With Leriche syndrome, a form of isolated aortoiliac disease, one can present with claudication of the lower back, buttocks, or thigh or impotence.

PATHOPHYSIOLOGY

Arterial disease of the lower extremity, depending on the vessel involved, can be divided into inflow, outflow, runoff, and small vessel disease. The larger vessels, such as the aortic, iliac, and common femoral arteries, are classified as inflow disease. Diseases of the femoral and popliteal systems comprise the outflow tract. The smaller vessels, such as the tibial and peroneal, comprise the runoff vessels. The small vessel diseases are made up of the arterioles and others not previously mentioned.

Extracranial involvement usually includes the carotid and vertebrobasilar systems. The most common sites are the superficial femoral and the distal aorta at its bifurcation. The majority of the vascular diseases are acquired through atherosclerosis and are considered to be chronic. Diabetes mellitus is known to potentiate the development of the disease. The atheromatous plaques develop in the vessel intima and are associated with thrombosis. These lesions are segmental and can be multiple. The degree of stenosis identified as causing impedance to flow with exercise has been found to be 60%.

The majority of arterial disorders are due to an obstruction of blood flow due to either thrombus, embolus, or atherosclerosis. Aneurysmal dilatation can remain silent until a thrombus or rupture occurs. Trauma with resultant arterial disruption can lead to hemorrhage or acute arterial occlusion.

DIAGNOSTIC STUDIES

Laboratory
Chemistry Profile.   BUN and creatinine levels are elevated with renal disease. Elevated serum glucose suggests the presence of diabetes mellitus.
CBC.   Identifies polycythemia vera or coexisting infection.
Lipid Profile.   Evaluated as a risk factor for atherosclerotic disease.
Platelets.   To rule out a coagulopathy or hypercoagulable state.

Radiology
Arteriography.   Remains the gold standard but should not be used in the routine evaluation of vascular disease. This should be reserved for those patients in whom surgery is contemplated. Indications for cerebrovascular arteriography as well as surgery are those individuals who have suffered TIAs or a stroke and have significant recovery of function. Risks with invasive arteriograms include thrombosis, embolus, arteriovenous fistula, hemorrhage, stroke, and allergy to contrast media.

Other
Doppler Ultrasound (along with measurement of distal limb pressure).   Is one of the least invasive and can be used for routine evaluation and for screening.

ABI (Ankle, Brachial Index).   Is obtained by dividing the ankle systolic pressure by the arm systolic pressure. Those individuals with claudication most often fall between an ABI of 0.5 to 1.0. Those patients with rest pain have been found to fall below 0.5. Pressure readings of less than 30 mm Hg signify significant disease.

$TCPO_2$.   Can be used in determining the oxygenation of peripheral tissues.

Plethysmography.   Is most commonly used in evaluating the digits.

OPG.   Cerebrovascular diseases can be identified.

DIFFERENTIAL DIAGNOSIS

Traumatic
Limb Injury.   Patient has a history of trauma.
Infectious.   Not applicable.

Metabolic
Diabetes Mellitus.   Elevated serum glucose; patient may have a known history of diabetes.

Raynaud's Phenomenon.   Symptoms secondary to a mixed connective tissue disease.

Neoplastic
Erythromelalgia.   Manifested by a burning pain in the hands or feet. Erythema is usually triggered by elevated temperatures.

Myeloproliferative Disease.   Can be ruled out by the CBC identifying erythrocytosis, thrombocytosis, or leukocytosis.

Vascular
Acrocyanosis.   Is most common in females, not associated with pain; peripheral pulses full.
Congenital.   Not applicable.
Acquired
Buerger's Disease.   Occurs in the younger male with a significant smoking history. Arteriogram reveals distal segmental occlusions.
Other
Spinal Stenosis.   Claudication of the cauda equina relates to nerve root compression, due to spinal stenosis, which is worsened by increased activity. Pulses are strong and easily detectable.
Acrocyanosis.   Pulses are strong and easily detectable.

TREATMENT

Medical.   The level of intensity or the degree of functional impairment is usually what dictates the level of diagnostic evaluation as well as the aggressiveness of treatment. The intensity can be subdivided into several distinct categories: life-threatening, limb- or organ-threatening, functional disability, and asymptomatic.

Medical management is reserved for those patients who are asymptomatic or minimally functionally impaired or who are not good surgical candidates, such as those with comorbid conditions of coronary disease, chronic obstructive pulmonary disease, or renal insufficiency. Individuals who present with recent onset of symptoms would also be candidates for medical therapy. Referral of candidates with even moderate claudication should be considered for catheter-based intervention. Dietary management is encouraged to control cholesterol and glucose levels, in addition to lipid lowering and hypoglycemic agents. Patients must also be counseled on the benefits of exercise on improving blood flow as well as encouraged to stop smoking. Meticulous skin care and hygiene is also an important component of patient education.

There are a number of alternative treatments short of surgical intervention. Catheter-based devices such as balloon angioplasty and laser-assisted angioplasty are available. There is, however, an associated 35% failure rate with these procedures, necessitating a second procedure within a year. Rotational atherectomy, stent placement, thrombolysis, as well as proximal and distal reconstruction are also options. There may be a reduction of proximal vessel surgeries because the lesions that are located in the iliac vessels are amenable to these techniques. This has been accompanied by an increase in peripheral reconstructive surgeries.

Surgical.   Antimicrobial prophylaxis should include drugs that cover *Staphylococcus aureus, S. epidermidis,* and *Escherichia coli.* Frequently given antibiotics include methicillin, cefazolin, and cefuroxime.

If the disease is extensive enough, the bypass can consist of a prosthetic material such as in aortoiliac disease. Autogenous saphenous vein grafting can be done if the femoral, popliteal, or tibial vessels are involved. Localized disease of the superficial femoral artery can be managed with an endarterectomy; however, if the disease is more significant and involves a greater area, then a saphenous vein graft is appropriate. The diameter of the graft should be at least 4 mm to be considered acceptable. Complications of this procedure are related to the coexisting atherosclerotic diseases that involve the coronary vessels and the extracranial vessels, resulting in myocardial infarction or stroke. Perioperative risk of an myocardial infarction is at 3% to 55%. Limb loss during the immediate perioperative period is 5%, which can extend to 10% during the late postoperative period. Patency in 5 years for aortofemoral grafts can be 90%; femoral-popliteal, 60% to 75%; and femoral-tibial grafts, 50%. Prosthetic grafts have a patency rate of less than 50% to the knee in 5 years.

Complications may include the compartment syndrome with the femoral-popliteal bypass. If the pressure in the compartment exceeds much more than 30 mm Hg, it may compromise perfusion to the local nerves and muscle, requiring a fasciotomy. Ileus is a common postoperative complication with abdominal procedures (abdominal aortic, iliac) that can be reduced with the placement of a nasogastric tube and suction until there is return of peristalsis.

Indications. Rest pain is indicative of severe vascular compromise and an indication for surgery. Surgical intervention is saved for those individuals who are either life threatened, limb threatened, or have a markedly limited functional capacity. Surgery can also be considered prophylactically in those patients who have an aneurysmal dilatation to prevent a rupture or thrombosis. Patients with a critical carotid stenosis may also warrant the procedure to minimize their risk of a devastating stroke. Patients with occlusive disease may require reconstructive surgery and may undergo endarterectomy if the vessel is accessible.

Contraindications. Comorbid conditions such as critical coronary artery disease, cerebrovascular disease, renal insufficiency, or pulmonary insufficiency. In the case of a femoral-popliteal bypass, contraindications would include extensive aneurysmal disease of the aorta.

TECHNIQUE OF SURGICAL ASSISTING

The PA acts as the first or second assistant, and assists with the incision, tissue retraction, ensuring adequate hemostasis, preparing arterial grafts (as indicated), and wound closure. Pre- and postoperative care are significant responsibilities of the surgical PA.

PEDIATRIC CONSIDERATIONS

Not applicable.

OBSTETRICAL CONSIDERATIONS

Not applicable.

PEARLS FOR THE PA

Rest pain signifies significant stenosis, warranting surgical intervention.

Associated cardiovascular disease must be ruled out.

Acute Arterial Occlusion: Embolism, Thrombosis
Deborah A. Opacic, PA-C, MMS

DEFINITION

Acute occlusion of the arterial supply to an organ or extremity by an emboli, thrombus, or trauma.

HISTORY

Symptoms. Sudden onset of pain, paresthesias, weakness, or paralysis. If the embolus is at the aortic bifurcation, the patient can present with shock, abdominal pain, nausea, and vomiting.
General. Associated with the six Ps: pain, pallor, paresthesias, paralysis, pulselessness, polar.
Age. Variable, depending on the cause.
Onset. Sudden.
Duration. Progression may lead to gangrene or necrosis if not recognized and treated.
Intensity. Severe, and in the case of the abdominal aorta, catastrophic.
Aggravating Factors. Inaccurate diagnosis.
Alleviating Factors. Early diagnosis and treatment.
Associated Factors. Hypercoagulable states.

PHYSICAL EXAMINATION

General. If acute, the patient is in significant distress and exhibits hypertension and tachycardia.
Cardiac. If the embolus is of a cardiac source, the patient may have a detectable murmur or irregular heart rate.
Vascular. The patient has a cool extremity with cyanosis and pulselessness. The muscles are soft shortly after the occlusion, followed by edema

and necrosis. The presence of stiff muscles indicates that tissue necrosis has occurred. The carotid, femoral, and aorta should be auscultated for bruits.

PATHOPHYSIOLOGY

Arterial emboli tend to lodge at the arterial bifurcation. The clots can be caused by plaques in the aorta and cholesterol emboli. Thrombus can be associated with platelet or fibrin debris, cholesterol from atheromatous plaques, aneurysm, trauma, or iatrogenic from arterial lines or repeated arterial blood sticks. The origin of emboli is most often the left side of the heart. Atrial fibrillation, mural thrombi that are associated with a myocardial infarction (MI) or ventricular aneurysm have also been identified as causative agents. Arterial diseases may manifest by plaques or ulcerations. Venous disease may be associated with a paradoxical embolus through an atrial-septal defect or patent foramen ovale, as well as foreign bodies such as catheters. The abdominal aorta can occlude at any one of its branches; splanchnic artery occlusion causing intestinal ischemia, celiac occlusion presenting with mesenteric occlusion, renal artery occlusion leading to renal failure, and occlusion at the aortic bifurcation.

DIAGNOSTIC STUDIES

Laboratory
Full Chemistry Profile. BUN and creatinine elevation may signify renal insufficiency.
CBC/Platelets. To rule out polycythemia vera.
Protein C&S, Antithrombin III, PT/PTT, Lupus Anticoagulant, Anticardiolipin, Fibrinogen. To rule out hypercoagulable states.
Radiology
Arteriogram. The arteriogram can delineate the area of occlusion as well as possible access for thrombolytic therapy. The golden period for thrombolysis is considered to be 4 to 6 hours. If needed, intraoperative angiography can be performed.
Other
Doppler. To identify the degree of obstruction and to evaluate a venous or arterial cause.
TCPO$_2$. To identify the degree of tissue hypoxia or reduction in blood flow.
Echocardiogram. Performed if there is a suspicion of a cardiac source.

DIFFERENTIAL DIAGNOSIS

Traumatic
Knee Injuries. Injuries to the popliteal artery may be present.
Infectious
Sepsis. Presents most often with systemic effects as opposed to an isolated area. Positive blood culture; fever.

Endocarditis. May present with multiple septic embolic sites. Positive blood culture; fever.
Metabolic
Systemic Lupus. Associated with hypercoagulable states.
Neoplastic
Adenocarcinoma. Associated with hypercoagulable states.
Vascular
Deep Venous Thrombosis. Arteriogram or Doppler differentiates arterial from the venous cause.
Congenital
Deficiency of Antithrombin III/Protein C&S/Fibrinogen. Serologic evaluation of these compounds reveals the deficiency.
Acquired. Not applicable.
Other
Sur Contra. Hemodynamic instability; critical coronary artery disease. Limb may be deemed nonviable.

TREATMENT

Medical. Pharmacological treatment consists of streptokinase or urokinase IV or intra-arterial 250,000 IU bolus, followed by 100,000 IU for 72 hours (IV). Do not elevate the extremity, because this may reduce perfusion. Thrombolysis is most effective if utilized before 72 hours. Percutaneous transluminal angioplasty can also be considered.

Surgical. Embolectomy may be performed using a Fogarty balloon catheter that is introduced via a femoral cutdown. The catheters are placed both proximal and distal to the level of occlusion. The balloon is then inflated and the catheter is withdrawn to retrieve the embolic debris. This is done with extreme caution so as not to cause further intimal disruption, dissection, perforation, or the development of an arterial venous fistula. The incision is made directly over the uppermost level of the occlusion. The vessel is isolated and 5000 units of heparin is administered IV. A longitudinal arteriotomy is made and the clot or embolus is removed. An intraoperative angiogram may be considered to ensure patency and complete removal of the occlusion. The heparin should be continued for 6 hours and then warfarin (Coumadin) initiated.

Indications. Anesthesia or paralysis.

Contraindications. Inability to tolerate anesthesia; coagulopathy.

TECHNIQUE OF SURGICAL ASSISTING

The PA acts as the first or second assistant, and assists with the incision, tissue retraction, ensuring adequate hemostasis, preparing arterial grafts (as indicated), and wound closure. Pre- and postoperative care are significant responsibilities of the surgical PA.

PEDIATRIC CONSIDERATIONS

Not applicable.

OBSTETRICAL CONSIDERATIONS

Not applicable.

PEARLS FOR THE PA

Most arterial emboli originate from a cardiac source.

Muscle necrosis and clot propagation are minimized if embolectomy is performed within 6 hours of the onset of ischemia.

Thoracic Outlet Syndrome
Deborah A. Opacic, PA-C, MMS

DEFINITION

Hand, arm, shoulder, or neck pain or paresthesias occurring secondarily to the compression of the neurovascular structures at the thoracic outlet by bony structures. The symptoms are caused by compression of the subclavian artery, vein, or the brachial plexus due to a congenital or acquired structural process of the bones and muscles of the chest in the area of the thoracic outlet. The signs and symptoms are the result of varying degrees of compression of the brachial plexus, subclavian artery, or vein.

HISTORY

Symptoms.   The patient may present with muscle weakness and paresthesias involving the affected extremity. Occasional pallor can occur with certain movements if the arterial supply is compromised. There may also be edema if there is significant vascular congestion or compression.

General.   Inquire as to the history of any previous neck or chest trauma. Determine if there are any specific movements of the extremity or neck that may precipitate the pain or numbness.

Age.   Most common in females aged 35 to 50 years.

Onset.   May be insidious; exacerbated with movement.

Duration.   Variable if position dependent.

Intensity.   Mild to moderate pain and paresthesias with movement.

Aggravating Factors. Abduction of the affected extremity.
Alleviating Factors. Avoidance of aggravating movements.
Associated Factors. Presence of a cervical rib.

PHYSICAL EXAMINATION

General. Appearance of the patient is unremarkable.
Vascular. The Adson maneuver is performed by asking the patient to take a deep breath while extending the neck and rotating the head toward the affected side. A positive response is noted when the radial pulse is obliterated. The hyperabduction (Allen) test can also be performed by having the patient hyperabduct the arm to 180 degrees, which will in turn reproduce the symptoms as well as obliterate the radial pulse. Inspect the hand for evidence of atrophy (thenar and hypothenar areas). Motor, sensory, and deep tendon reflex testing is performed and compared between the extremities to rule out radiculopathy or neuropathy as a cause of the symptoms.

PATHOPHYSIOLOGY

Symptoms are caused by compression of the subclavian artery as it crosses over the first rib by a cervical rib, fibrous bands, or prominent scalenus muscle. The lower roots of the brachial plexus may also be compressed. Neurovascular compression can occur adjacent to the clavicle or over the first rib by overexaggerating posterior extension of the shoulder. The neurovascular bundle at the area of the scapula can be compressed through hyperabduction of the arm.

DIAGNOSTIC STUDIES

Laboratory
Chemistry Profile, CBC, PT/PTT. Performed as part of the routine preoperative screen.
Radiology
Chest X-ray. May reveal an extra or cervical rib.
Cervical Spine Films. Performed to help rule out cervical stenosis or arthritis.
MRI of the Cervical Spine. Performed to rule out other pathologies such as herniated cervical disc, spinal stenosis, or spinal cord tumor.
Angiogram. May be required to identify compression of the subclavian artery or significant intravascular disease.
Other
EMG/NCV. Performed as indicated to rule out neural compression syndromes, neuropathy, or radiculopathy.

DIFFERENTIAL DIAGNOSIS

Traumatic

Tendinitis/Bursitis. Distinguishable by pain extending over the humerus, bicipital groove; x-rays may reveal calcification of the bursa/tendons.

Infectious. Not applicable.

Metabolic

Multiple Sclerosis (MS). Waxing and waning neurologic symptoms. Positive MRI of the brain or cerebrospinal fluid studies for MS.

Neoplastic

Spinal Cord Tumor. Positive long tract signs (e.g., Babinski), painless weakness of the lower extremities; MRI positive for lesion.

Tumors Involving the Brachial Plexus. May be seen on chest x-ray; CT/MRI may be required. EMG/NCV may be helpful in determining the cause of the compression.

Vascular

Acute Emboli or Thrombosis. Identified through Doppler imaging, venogram, or arteriogram.

Congenital

Developmental Anomalies. Such as an abnormal first thoracic rib or abnormal insertion or position of the scalene muscle may give rise to thoracic outlet symptoms.

Acquired

Carpal Tunnel Syndrome. Differentiated on electromyography and nerve conduction (EMG/NCV) studies.

Ulnar Nerve Compression. Differentiated on electromyography and nerve conduction studies.

Cervical Nerve Root Compression. Positive radicular signs of numbness, weakness or reflex change in a dermatomal distribution. Positive MRI for herniated cervical disc or EMG/NCV evidence of denervation.

TREATMENT

Medical. Nonsteroidal anti-inflammatory drugs (NSAIDs) may be given to help reduce the symptoms. Physical therapy may be helpful to enhance range of motion and develop strategies that help the patient to avoid aggravating positions.

Surgical. The procedure usually includes surgical removal of the first rib and any fibrous bands through a transaxillary approach between the pectoralis major and the latissimus dorsi. The first rib is identified through blunt dissection while protecting the T1 nerve root. Arterial disease may require an endarterectomy.

Complications of the procedure may include pneumothorax, hematoma, transient injury to the brachial plexus or the long thoracic nerve, axillary or subclavian vessels.

Indications. Surgery is indicated if there is a failure of conservative therapy, intractable pain, neurologic deficits, or loss of function.

Contraindications. Inadequate trial of conservative therapy, inability of the patient to undergo anesthesia or coagulopathy. This procedure is reserved most often in those patients with a cervical rib or obvious subclavian artery obstruction.

TECHNIQUE OF SURGICAL ASSISTING

The PA acts as the first or second assistant, and assists with the incision, tissue retraction, ensuring adequate hemostasis, preparing arterial grafts (as indicated), and wound closure. Pre- and postoperative care are significant responsibilities of the surgical PA.

PEDIATRIC CONSIDERATIONS

Not applicable.

OBSTETRICAL CONSIDERATIONS

Not applicable.

PEARLS FOR THE PA

Symptoms of upper extremity or neck pain and paresthesias occur secondarily to the compression of the neurovascular structures at the thoracic outlet by bony structures.

Surgery is performed for thoracic outlet syndrome only when absolutely necessary.

Varicosities
Deborah A. Opacic, PA-C, MMS

DEFINITION

Dilated, enlarged, or tortuous superficial veins.

HISTORY

Symptoms. Aching, heaviness, swelling, and increased warmth of the limbs.

General. Depending on the organ system involved, the patient may present with cardiac, renal, or hepatic failure.

Age. Increases with advancing age; females more affected than males.

Onset. Gradually increased appearance of vessels or symptoms.

Duration. Progressive.

Intensity. Variable, depending on the degree of vascular dilatation, swelling, and the level of the patient's immobility.

Aggravating Factors. Age and local vascular damage. May worsen with menses; extended periods of standing or sitting, stasis, trauma, low cardiac output, or hypercoagulability.

Alleviating Factors. Leg elevation, stocking support.

Associated Factors. Congenital weakness of the vessels, absence of the valve leaflets, hypervolemic states, hormonal changes with pregnancy, ascites, or occupations that are associated with prolonged periods of standing or sitting.

PHYSICAL EXAMINATION

General. Inspection identifies any visible patterns of varicosities.

Vascular. A positive Homan's sign is suggestive of thrombophlebitis. Palpate for superficial veins or tender cords. Visible edema or skin color changes are consistent with venous stasis. The Trendelenburg test is done to evaluate the presence of superficial or deep vein involvement. This is performed by elevating the affected limb to evacuate the veins of blood. Pressure is then placed by hand or tourniquet to the saphenofemoral junction. With the patient standing, varicosities are observed for filling. If the perforating vessels are incompetent, there is rapid filling. The pressure is then released and rapid filling of the saphenous vein is observed if the saphenofemoral valve is incompetent.

Cardiac. Full evaluation is essential to rule out a cardiac source as a cause for lower extremity edema.

PATHOPHYSIOLOGY

The lower extremities are prone to a variety of disorders because of the gravitational condition of being upright as well as the increases of hydrostatic pressure. Varicosities are the distended, tortuous, superficial vessels that have incompetent valves. Nearly 20% of the population is affected. There are two divisions when considering venous diseases, primary or secondary. Primary causes refer to a disorder of the superficial veins of the lower extremities, thought to be due to primary valvular weakness or weakness of the vessel wall. A positive family history is common. Secondary varicosities are related to deep venous insufficiency associated with edema, skin discoloration or ulceration, and a loss of valvular competence.

DIAGNOSTIC STUDIES

Laboratory
Chemistry Profile.   Performed to evaluate renal function, electrolytes, and albumin or to rule out systemic pathology.
CBC.   To identify infection for hyperviscosity.
Platelets.   To evaluate for hyperviscosity or coagulopathy.
Radiology
Contrast Venography.   The standard imaging technique for evaluation of the venous system. Descending venography is utilized in localizing incompetent valves of the iliofemoral system.
Other
Doppler Ultrasound.   To locate any areas of obstruction or thrombosis.
Impedance Plethysmography.   To isolate valvular incompetence or obstruction.

DIFFERENTIAL DIAGNOSIS

Traumatic.   Not applicable.
Infectious
Cellulitis.   Is usually identified by additional signs of inflammation such as increased erythema and warmth.
Metabolic
Renal Insufficiency.   Appropriate historical information along with evaluation of urinary sediment and electrolytes may isolate the pathology.
Neoplastic
Lymphadenopathy.   Lymphatic obstruction may be demonstrated through physical examination or by the diagnosis of coexisting, primary malignancy.
Vascular
Cardiac Failure.   May cause lower extremity edema. Evaluation for congestive heart failure or other cardiac sources is essential.
Congenital.   Not applicable.
Acquired.   Not applicable.

TREATMENT

Medical.   Instruct the patient to avoid long periods of sitting or standing, knee-high stockings, and to wear support hose when exercising or walking. In severe cases excision or sclerotherapy (for isolated large veins) may be indicated for vessels that are symptomatic or for recurrent ulceration.
Surgical.   With the aid of a vein stripper, the vessel is removed distal to proximal.
Complications can include hematoma, hypesthesia (manifested as patchy numbness), infection, or early recurrence.

Indications. Cosmetic reasons, if the patient is increasingly symptomatic, anatomic progression, prophylactic treatment, and finally stasis ulceration.

Contraindications. Hemodynamic instability, presence of disorders that prolong or prohibit adequate healing (e.g., severe peripheral vascular disease, diabetes mellitus, long-term steroid use).

TECHNIQUE OF SURGICAL ASSISTING

The PA acts as the first or second assistant, and assists with the incision, tissue retraction, ensuring adequate hemostasis, preparing arterial grafts (as indicated), and wound closure. Pre- and postoperative care are significant responsibilities of the surgical PA.

PEDIATRIC CONSIDERATIONS

Not applicable.

OBSTETRICAL CONSIDERATIONS

Transient varicosities may be associated with pregnancy. No therapy is usually necessary, although the patient may be instructed to use support hose or limit long periods of sitting or standing.

PEARLS FOR THE PA

Do not assume that the cause of peripheral edema is uniquely dependent or a manifestation of peripheral vascular disease.

Systemic illness such as renal, cardiac, neoplastic, or nutritional conditions may be the source.

Further Reading

Moore WS (ed): Vascular Surgery: A Comprehensive Review, ed 4. Philadelphia, W.B. Saunders, 1993.

Sabiston DC, H Kim Lyerly (eds): Sabiston's Essentials of Surgery, ed 2. Philadelphia, W.B. Saunders, 1994.

Schwartz SI (ed): Principles of Surgery, ed 6. New York, McGraw-Hill, 1994.

Chapter **14**
Procedures
Casting Techniques
Nancy Anderson, PA-C

DEFINITION

Immobilization of a body part due to fracture or subluxation to allow realignment and healing.

TECHNIQUE

Casting. Is primarily performed by Orthopedics and is not usually done in the acute situation due to potential complications of edema. Support may be added to an existing, worn, or broken cast in the emergency room. Cast material is rolled over the existing cast for reinforcement. Casts that are too tight may be split to allow for edema. A cast is "bivalved" by cutting through the cast, padding the opposing sides, and rewrapping with an Ace bandage.

Splinting. General instructions: Pad the limb well with cast padding for comfort, apply the splint material, cover the splint with an Ace bandage (allows for expansion due to edema), and mold into desired position.

Common Splints

Leg. Jones long-leg splint. Is used for knee immobilization. Splints are applied medial and lateral from the groin to just proximal to the malleoli. The line is usually extended for weightbearing or flexed up to 45 degrees for non-weightbearing.

Sugar tong/stirrup splint: Is a continuous U-shaped splint used to prevent inversion/eversion of the foot. This splint runs medial and lateral from the level of the tibial tubercle and is continued across the plantar hindfoot.

Posterior splint: Runs from the toes on the plantar foot surface, up the posterior lower leg, to the knee. Keep the foot 90 degrees to the lower extremity (neutral). Used for foot or ankle injuries.

Arm. The position of function has the wrist dorsiflexed to 35 degrees with the fingers flexed (as if holding a glass).

Posterior splint (elbow): Apply the splints on the dorsal forearm extending posteriorly on the upper arm and flex the elbow to 90 degrees. Extend the plaster to support the wrist.

Posterior splint (wrist): Apply the splints from the metacarpophalangeal (MCP) joints to just below the elbow. Allow the fingers and MCP joints to be free.

Volar splint: Apply from the palmar crease to below the elbow. Keep the MCP joints free.

Sugar tong: Runs from the palmar crease proximally on the volar surface, around the flexed elbow, and back on the dorsal forearm to just below the MCP joints. Used to decrease pronation and supination.

Gutter splints: These run from the palmar crease to just below the elbow on either the radial or ulnar aspect of the forearm. Used for radial or ulnar injuries.

Thumb spica: Circumferentially splint the thumb in full extension on the end of a radial gutter splint. Used for navicular injuries.

INDICATIONS

Necessity of immobilization due to fracture, dislocation, or significant soft tissue injury.

CONTRAINDICATIONS

Significant laceration necessitating frequent inspection, compartment syndrome.

COMPLICATIONS

If the cast or splint is applied too tightly, or if edema develops subsequent to the application of the cast or splint, the distal vascular supply may be interrupted, causing cyanosis, peripheral nerve injury, or loss of the affected area. Infection may occur within the casted or splinted area if an abrasion or laceration is unrecognized. Pressure sores may result if incorrectly applied.

Chest Tube Thoracostomy
Jack Pike, PA-C, BS

DEFINITION

Insertion of a tube into the pleural space for decompression.

TECHNIQUE

Materials: Thoracostomy tray, assorted chest tubes (usually #24, 28, 32), Pleurovac, povidone-iodine solution, gown, gloves.

Position the Patient: For anterior tube placement, the patient is supine with the head of the bed elevated 30 to 45 degrees. For lateral tube placement, the patient is placed into the lateral decubitus position with the involved side up.

Determine the placement of the tube; prep and drape.

Plan the incision to be one interspace below the rib where the tube will actually be placed.

Infiltrate the skin along a line parallel to the rib. Using a long needle, extend the lidocaine superiorly in the direction that the tube will be tracked. The final area to be anesthetized will be the pleura where the tube will be placed. In anesthetizing and placing the tube, avoid the intercostal neurovascular bundle that lies on the inferior aspect of each rib (Fig. 14–1).

Incise the skin over the anesthetized wheal and then create a tunnel superiorly toward the intercostal space using a Kelly clamp.

Enter the pleural space, with the Kelly clamp over the superior aspect of the rib. Spread the clamp to create an opening where the tube will be placed.

Place a finger into the pleural space to confirm that the chest has been entered and to check for adhesions (Fig. 14–2). The chest tube is placed by either grasping the tip of the tube with the Kelly clamp and inserting it into the pleural space (Fig. 14–3), withdrawing the clamp and directing the tube further into the pleural space, or leaving the trocar in the chest tube, placing the tube in the same way as above, removing the trocar after entering the pleural space. The clinician placing the tube must take care to have control of the trocar as it enters the pleural space in order to avoid iatrogenic trauma.

After placing the tube, ensuring that all of the holes in the tube are within the pleural space, secure it to the chest wall with heavy suture material.

Cover with a sterile dressing of petroleum gauze and sponges.

Obtain a chest x-ray to ensure tube position and evacuation of air and/or fluid.

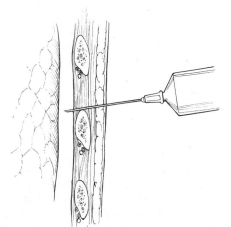

Figure 14–1. Insert the needle over the superior aspect of the rib to avoid the neurovascular bundle that lies on the inferior aspect of the rib. (From Rakel RE: Saunders Manual of Medical Practice. Philadelphia, WB Saunders, 1996.)

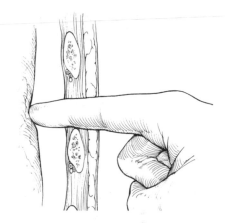

Figure 14–2. Place a finger into the pleural space to confirm that the chest has been entered and to check for adhesions. (From Rakel RE: Saunders Manual of Medical Practice. Philadelphia, WB Saunders, 1996.)

INDICATIONS

Pneumothorax, hemothorax, hydrothorax, or chylothorax, severe chest trauma patients with instability and unknown injuries, instillation of chemotherapy agent after effusion removal.

CONTRAINDICATIONS

Essentially none, but small pneumothoraces may spontaneously resolve without chest tube insertion; patients with bleeding dyscrasias need to be managed cautiously due to the possibility of hemorrhage.

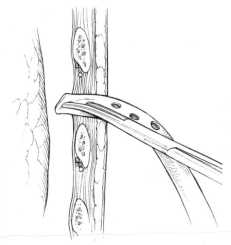

Figure 14–3. Grasp the chest tube with a Kelly clamp and insert the tube into the pleural space. (From Rakel RE: Saunders Manual of Medical Practice. Philadelphia, WB Saunders, 1996.)

COMPLICATIONS

Hemorrhage, laceration of the lung, infection, cardiac injury, subcutaneous placement, re-expansion pulmonary edema.

Emergency Cricothyrotomy
Jack Pike, PA-C, BS

DEFINITION

Urgent access to the airway through the cricothyroid cartilage due to acute respiratory compromise.

TECHNIQUE

Materials: Knife blade and handle, tracheostomy tube (or pediatric endotracheal tube or large gauge angiocatheter), bag-valve ventilation unit, and oxygen.

Anesthesia is not required as, by definition, a patient requiring emergency cricothyrotomy does not need local anesthesia.

The patient is positioned supine with head extended. Palpate the cricothyroid membrane between the thyroid and cricoid cartilages (Fig. 14–4). Make a vertical incision in the midline over the cricothyroid membrane and incise the membrane horizontally. Place the blunt end of the knife handle, or an instrument such as a Delaborde dilator, through the cricothyrotomy and enlarge the opening. Place the tracheostomy tube or endotracheal tube through the opening, inflate the cuff, and ventilate. Secure the tracheostomy tube to the skin with suture and/or umbilical tapes.

INDICATIONS

Emergency tracheotomy is indicated when respiratory obstruction is too severe to allow time for an orderly tracheotomy, when an endotracheal tube and equipment are unavailable, or when risk of brain damage is increased by waiting even a few minutes.

CONTRAINDICATIONS

None.

COMPLICATIONS

Hemorrhage, esophageal perforation, failure to achieve tracheostomy.

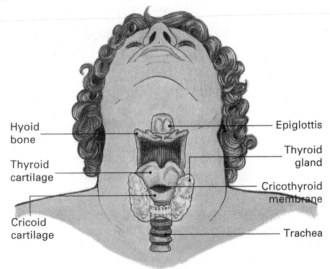

Hyoid bone

Thyroid cartilage

Cricoid cartilage

Epiglottis

Thyroid gland

Cricothyroid membrane

Trachea

Figure 14–4. Anatomic landmarks used when palpating for the cricothyroid membrane. (From Bledsoe BE, Porter RS, Shade BR: Brady Paramedic Emergency Care, 3rd ed. Upper Saddle River, NJ, Prentice-Hall, 1996, p. 270.)

Endotracheal Intubation

Jack Pike, PA-C, BS

DEFINITION

The method of obtaining an airway by using a tube placed in the trachea.

TECHNIQUE

Materials: Assortment of endotracheal (ET) tubes, 10-ml syringe, laryngoscope with straight or curved blades, malleable stylet, bag-valve-mask unit with oxygen source, suction capability.

Hyperventilate the patient, if possible, using the bag-valve-mask and 100% oxygen.

Suction the oropharynx, remove dentures, and other possible obstructions.

Standing at the patient's head, hold the laryngoscope with the left hand and open the mouth with the right. Advance the laryngoscope into the right side of the mouth while moving the patient's tongue to the left, aiming for the base of the tongue in the midline (Fig. 14–5). If using a straight blade, the tip is placed into the vallecula, looking for the glottic opening. If using a curved blade, the tip is placed under the epiglottis. With the vocal cords visualized, place the ET tube, under direct vision, through the cords, advancing the cuff approximately 2 cm past the cords into the trachea (Fig. 14–6).

If using a stylet, remove it, inflate the cuff, and ventilate the patient.

Assess for presence of bilateral breath sounds. If clear, then secure the tube to the patient with tape.

It is not uncommon for the tube to be inserted too far, usually into the right main-stem bronchus. If breath sounds are unequal, pull the tube out 1 cm and listen again.

If gurgling sounds are heard, the tube may be in the esophagus, and should be removed so that the patient can be hand-ventilated before a second attempt is made to intubate.

Chest x-ray should be performed to evaluate the position of the ET tube.

INDICATIONS

Cardiopulmonary arrest, respiratory insufficiency, unresponsive patient with compromised airway, severe head and neck trauma, burns, or to hyperventilate a patient with elevated intracranial pressure.

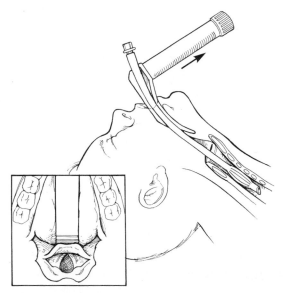

Figure 14–5. View during placement of laryngoscope (curved blade). (From Rakel RE: Saunders Manual of Medical Practice. Philadelphia, WB Saunders, 1996.)

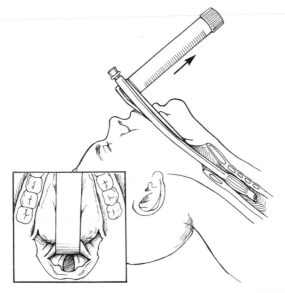

Figure 14–6. View during placement of laryngoscope (straight blade). (From Rakel RE: Saunders Manual of Medical Practice. Philadelphia, WB Saunders, 1996.)

CONTRAINDICATIONS

Essentially none, as the urgency of obtaining an airway supersedes other considerations. A tracheostomy may be elected if the patient's upper airway is obstructed (e.g., from a foreign body, mass lesion, or trauma) or if long-term intubation is required.

COMPLICATIONS

Unilateral (usually right main-stem bronchus) intubation, esophageal intubation, tracheal trauma, hemorrhage, erosion of the trachea (long term).

Internal Jugular Cannulation
Jack Pike, PA-C, BS

DEFINITION

Cannulization of the internal jugular (IJ) vein. The IJ vein arises from the base of the skull posterior to the internal carotid artery (ICA) and lateral to the common carotid. It lies medial to the sternocleidomastoid (SCM) muscle superiorly, crossing deep to the muscle, and emerges at the triangle between the two heads of the SCM.

TECHNIQUE

Patient Position. Supine, 10 to 20 degrees Trendelenburg, head turned to opposite side, roll between scapulae (Fig. 14–7). There are three approaches to the IJ: central, anterior, and posterior.

Central Approach. After prepping and draping, locate the triangle formed by the two heads of the SCM (if possible, have patient lift his or her head to locate the triangle).

Insert a #22-gauge finder needle with syringe at the apex of triangle formed by the two heads.

Aim the needle parallel to the clavicular head, toward the ipsilateral nipple at a 45-degree angle until the vein is entered. If inserted more than 3 cm with no blood return, withdraw the needle and try a new angle. Be careful proceeding medially, because the carotid artery can be punctured.

When the IJ is located, use the 18 gauge needle with syringe to puncture the vein.

Remove the syringe and, using Seldinger technique, pass the guidewire. It should advance easily. If resistance is encountered, DO NOT force it. Try again.

Withdraw the needle, leaving the guidewire. Nick the skin with a #11 blade, slide a dilator over the wire to enlarge the tract, and remove the dilator.

Advance the catheter over the wire and into position; remove wire, flush and cap all ports, and suture catheter to skin. Place sterile dressing.

Obtain chest x-ray.

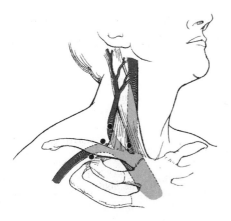

Figure 14–7. Correct patient positioning for internal jugular cannulation. (From Rakel RE: Saunders Manual of Medical Practice. Philadelphia, WB Saunders, 1996.)

Anterior Approach. Retract the carotid artery medially from anterior border of the SCM.

Introduce the needle at the midpoint of the anterior border of the SCM at the point halfway between mandible and clavicle.

Aim the needle 30 to 45 degrees toward the ipsilateral nipple.

Use Seldinger technique (as described above) for the remainder of venous access.

Posterior Approach. Insert the needle under the SCM at the junction of the middle and lower thirds of the posterior border, aiming anteriorly to the suprasternal notch at a 45-degree angle to sagittal and horizontal planes. The vein should be entered within 5 cm.

If venous blood is encountered, follow Seldinger technique (as described above) for remainder of venous access technique.

INDICATIONS

Vasopressor administration, central venous pressure (CVP) monitoring, emergency IV route, hyperalimentation.

CONTRAINDICATIONS

Thrombosis of veins, coagulopathy.

COMPLICATIONS

Arterial puncture, hemorrhage, pneumothorax, air embolus, thoracic duct injury (left-side approach), neural injury (brachial plexus), infection, thrombosis.

Norplant: Insertion and Removal
Paul Taylor, PA-C, BS

DEFINITION

Norplant (a progestin-only birth control device) insertion is a minor surgical procedure, performed under local anesthesia. Using a trocar, implants are placed under the skin on the inside of a woman's upper arm in a fan-shaped pattern. Norplant acts by inhibiting ovulation, thickening and decreasing the amount of cervical mucus, and by creating a thin, atrophic endometrium.

TECHNIQUE

Insertion

Obtain informed operative consent.

Using the width of four to five fingers, measure up from the inside elbow crease. The fan pattern of implants will be on the medial aspect of arm.

Use the provided template to mark the pattern—the better the insertion, the easier the removal.

Position the patient on her back with her preferred arm at a right angle on the table.

Using sterile technique, clean and drape the field desired with Betadine or Hibiclens.

Inject the local anesthetic slowly: lidocaine and sodium bicarbonate mixed 10 to 1 (injection at base of fan and along insertion sites).

Using blade provided in Norplant kit, make a 2- to 3-mm incision at the fan base.

Special care should be given to subdermal insertion, as opposed to intradermal or into deeper tissue. With the plunger firmly placed in the trocar, insert subdermally underneath the first line in the fan, pull upward (tenting the skin), while advancing the trocar to the black line.

The trocar should remain in the incision (under the skin) between insertion of each implant. This allows for insertions in the same plane.

Once the trocar is positioned (advanced to the black line), remove the plunger without moving the trocar. Place an implant in the barrel and replace the plunger without applying pressure to the implant. With slight pressure on the implant, using the plunger, the tip can be felt at the end of the trocar. Slowly withdrawing the trocar, not moving the plunger, the implant will be placed. Be careful not to push on the plunger while removing the trocar. The Norplant inserts are flexible and will bow at the time of insertion.

Repeat this process underneath each line in the pattern. Attempt to place each Norplant insert in the same plane, depth, and distance from the incision. Remember, proper placement is key to each removal.

After all six implants are placed, manipulation is possible to move an unsatisfactorily placed insert.

Clean and dry the incision site. Steri-Strips are necessary to approximate the edges of the skin. Cover with a 4 × 4 gauze and wrap arm. Tell the patient the warning signs of infection and to return to clinic as needed.

Removal

Obtain informed consent.

Palpate inserts and mark the incision site. It is best if the incision is made at the base of the fan just over the proximal end of the implants; implants may also be marked for reference during removal.

Using sterile technique, clean and drape the desired field.

Use a generous amount of local anesthesia (e.g., lidocaine and sodium bicarbonate).

An incision of 8 mm to 1 cm should provide adequate exposure. Dissect to the level of the implants and use forceps to release adhesions.

With the finger, apply pressure to the distal end of the implant and push toward the incision. If unsuccessful, a small curved hemostat may help to trap and grasp the insert.

Do not pull hard with the hemostat, because inserts will break.

With a blade or gauze, remove the scar tissue covering the end of the Norplant.

All inserts may not be removed using this techique. Ultrasound and fluoroscopy have proven to be effective in the location and removal of difficult implants.

Approximate the edges of the skin with Steri-Strips, wrap, and gauze.

Nonsteroidal anti-inflammatory drugs (NSAIDs) may be necessary for pain control.

Contraceptive effects wear off quickly after removal, with a median time to conception of 1 month.

INDICATIONS

Patients in whom Norplant may be preferred include those who are breast-feeding (as Norplant is a progestin-only device, it may be used in these women), older women (low failure rates), young women (low failure rates, reversibility), women who cannot take estrogen (e.g., history of breast cancer), history of deep vein thrombosis, and compliance problems with birth control pills or barrier methods.

A single act leads to long-term use (5 years), with high levels of effectiveness (year 1, 99.1%; year 2, 99.5%; year 3, 98.8%; year 4, 98.4%; year 5, 99.6%).

Reduces the risk of ectopic pregnancy (1.3 per 1,000).

Higher continuation rate compared to other hormonal contraceptives.

Noncontraceptive benefits include decreased menses or no menses, decreased anemia, reduced menstrual cramps and pain, less pain associated with ovulation (Mittelschmerz), and decreased risk of endometrial cancer, ovarian cancer, and pelvic inflammatory disease.

CONTRAINDICATIONS

Known or suspected pregnancy, unexplained or abnormal uterine bleeding, anticonvulsant use, active thrombophlebitis, suspected breast cancer.

COMPLICATIONS

Weight gain, as progestin-only methods increase appetite.

Menstrual cycle disturbance is the most frequent reason for discontinuation.

Potential for pain and anxiety at time of insertion and removal; scar on inner upper arm.

Anticonvulsants make Norplant failure rates rise to unacceptable levels (except valproic acid).

Local inflammation or infection at site of implants.

Increased frequency of ovarian cysts, because Norplant suppresses the hypothalamic pituitary axis, particularly follicle-stimulating hormone (FSH).

Other complications include headaches (16% to 18%), breast tenderness (6% to 7%), nausea (5% to 8%), and dermatitis (4% to 8%).

Cost at insertion ranges from $500 to $700; removal takes more time and the charge is usually greater. However, implants may be paid for by Medicaid, by the Norplant Foundation, or by the patient's health insurance. Most major HMOs in the United States have decided to pay for all or part of the cost.

Intrauterine Devices (IUDs): Insertion and Removal
Paul Taylor, PA-C, BS

DEFINITION

Device inserted into the uterus for the purpose of birth control. The mechanism of action is not completely understood, but is thought to immobilize sperm (interferes with migration of sperm from vagina to the fallopian tube) and speed transport of the ovum through the fallopian tube. Local affects on the endometrium are not well understood.

TECHNIQUE

It is initially determined that the patient is:
- six weeks postpartum and breast-feeding
- six weeks postpartum, no menses, not breast-feeding, negative pregnancy test
- status post first trimester abortion (immediately to within 3 weeks)
- without a contraindication and has a negative pregnancy test
- within 6 days of unprotected intercourse, if the woman desires a postcoital contraceptive device

Insertion. These instructions generally apply to all IUDs, but specifically to the Copper T38OA.

The easiest time of insertion is during menses, but may be inserted anytime during the cycle.

Explain the procedure to the patient, answer questions, obtain an informed consent.

Perform a bimanual examination to determine the position of the uterus (increased risk of uterine perforation if in the retroflexed position).

Insert speculum and view cervix. Use an antiseptic solution to thoroughly clean the cervix (e.g., Betadine or Hibiclens) using Q-tip swabs.

Using a tenaculum, grasp the anterior lip of the cervix 1.5 to 2.0 cm from the os.

Using the tenaculum for gentle retraction, sound the uterus. A depth of 5 cm or greater is necessary for proper insertion. An endometrial biopsy curette is the most user-friendly; centimeters are well marked.

Load the IUD into the inserter barrel under sterile conditions. Do not bend the arms of the T earlier than 5 minutes prior to insertion.

Introduce the push rod from the opposite end of the insertion tube, being careful not to dislodge the IUD. Adjust the movable flange on the tube so that it matches the sounded depth of the uterus. This is best done by holding the endometrial biopsy curette parallel (without touching) to the insertion tube.

Introduce the insertion tube through the cervical canal into the uterine fundus. Again, gentle traction on the tenaculum aids in straightening the cervical canal. Insert the tube to the flange.

DO NOT FORCE THE INSERTION OR TOUCH VAGINAL SIDE WALLS.

Insert/eject the IUD by holding the push rod in place and sliding the insertion tube away from the IUD. This releases the arms of the T.

Slowly withdraw the insertion tube and push the rod from the cervix and vagina.

Cut the IUD strings long so that they are inside the vagina but easily felt by the patient.

Follow-up visit 1 week following the next menses to check IUD position and make sure strings are in place. Expulsion rate is higher with first menses postinsertion.

Removal.   Removing at the time of menses or at midcycle may be easiest.

Using forceps, always apply gentle, steady traction and remove slowly while grasping the string.

If necessary, a tenaculum may be used to steady the cervix or straighten the cervical canal. For difficult removals, use laminaria or cervical dilators.

If no strings are visible, probe the cervical canal with narrow forceps. If the strings are absent or entirely within the uterine canal, an ultrasound or x-ray may confirm the location.

If the IUD is in the uterine cavity, alligator forceps, a hook, uterine packing forceps, or a Novak curette may be used to grasp the strings or the IUD itself.

INDICATIONS

Patients best suited for IUD placement are parous women in a monogamous relationship with no history of sexual transmitted diseases (STD). IUDs have a high level of effectiveness (98.5% to 99.2%), lack of associated systemic metabolic side effects, a single act leads to long-term use (10 years), are less expensive than other methods per year, and may be placed "the morning after" to prevent pregnancy.

CONTRAINDICATIONS

Acute pelvic inflammatory disease (PID) or history of PID, uterine abnormalities, postpartum endometritis, untreated cervicitis or vaginitis, history of ectopic pregnancy, multiple sexual partners, and those who are immunocompromised.

COMPLICATIONS

Increased risk of PID, higher risk of human immunodeficiency virus (HIV) (users vs. non-users), dysmenorrhea (10% to 15%), expulsion between 2% and 10% during the first year, may be painful to place.

Uterine perforation (1 in 1000) occurs at the time of insertion or late due to erosion. Erosion usually occurs at one of three sites: uterine fundus, body of the uterus, or cervical wall. A simple perforation may only require standard removal of IUD and antibiotic coverage. Complicated perforations involving the bowel may require abdominal surgery.

Early IUD warning signs include late menses, abnormal spotting, abdominal pain, infection, vaginal discharge, malaise (fever, chills, nausea), or a missing string.

Lumbar Puncture
James B. Labus, PA-C

DEFINITION

Technique of accessing the subarachnoid space or obtaining cerebrospinal fluid (CSF) in the lumbar region.

TECHNIQUE

The patient is placed in the lateral decubitus position, usually with the legs drawn up to the chest.

The procedure can also be performed in the sitting position, because this distends the lumbar subarachnoid space and increases the success of obtaining CSF on the first needle pass.

The entire lumbar area is exposed to identify landmarks and to note any scoliosis.

The patient should be positioned so that the spine is as close to 90 degrees as possible.

The proposed puncture site is localized, commonly at the L4–L5 interspace, which is usually at the level of the iliac crest.

The area is prepped and draped in a sterile fashion.

Local anesthetic is injected by creating a skin wheal, continuing the injection between the spinous processes.

The tray is prepared (connecting the manometer, arranging tubes, preparing the spinal needle) while the anesthetic is working.

The spinal needle is advanced (bevel up) after rechecking landmarks, patient position, and the site of the anesthetic injection.

The spinal needle (with the stylet in place) is advanced in the midline, between the spinous processes, in a slightly cephalad direction.

Loss of resistance may be felt when the needle encounters the epidural space. At this point the stylet may be removed to check for CSF flow. If none is obtained, the stylet is replaced and the spinal needle advanced further.

A second loss of resistance will be felt when the dura is punctured. Again the stylet is removed to check for CSF flow.

If no CSF flow is obtained, the needle is withdrawn to the skin and another attempt is made. If additional attempts are unsuccessful, the patient may be placed in a sitting position or another interspace attempted. Do not move the spinal needle back and forth while deep, because this can cause laceration of epidural veins or dura.

Once CSF has been obtained, check the opening pressure with the manometer (the sitting patient will have to lie down while needle position is guarded for adequate pressure measurements) and record. Do not aspirate CSF.

Four tubes of CSF are obtained for study. Tube 1 is for Gram stain, cell count, culture and sensitivity; tube 2 for glucose and protein; tube 3 for special studies; and tube 4 for cell count or special studies.

After the CSF has been collected, the closing pressure is measured with the manometer and recorded. The stylet is replaced and the spinal needle withdrawn.

The patient is instructed to lie flat for approximately 1 hour and remain sedentary for the remainder of the day to prevent spinal headache.

A small dressing is applied to the puncture site.

INDICATIONS

To obtain spinal fluid to test for infections (meningitis), subarachnoid hemorrhage, demyelinating disease (e.g., multiple sclerosis), cytology for tumor spread, or to reduce CSF pressure. This approach is also used to inject myelographic dye or medications (antibiotics or chemotherapeutic agents), perform anesthetic procedures (epidural or spinal), or to insert catheters for spinal fluid drainage.

CONTRAINDICATIONS

Infection at the proposed puncture site, sepsis, epidural abscess (may convert to meningitis), tethered cord, or bleeding dyscrasia. If there is any indication of a cerebral mass lesion (e.g., papilledema) or spinal cord mass lesion, CT/MRI scan of the brain or cord should be performed prior to performing the procedure.

COMPLICATIONS

Meningitis, epidural hematoma, epidural abscess, spinal headache, pain at the puncture site, spinal cord injury (if tethered or if puncture is performed too high), or inability to obtain CSF.

Percutaneous Muscle Biopsy
Roderick S. Hooker, PA

DEFINITION

Obtaining a sample of striated muscle for the purpose of pathologic examination.

TECHNIQUE

Obtaining an adequate amount of muscle for the pathologist is a relatively simple procedure and does not require an open biopsy approach. The procedure is more yielding than the historically used Bergstrom needle, and is as adequate as an open muscle biopsy, but with considerably less morbidity. The procedure described is for the vastus lateralis (lateral quadriceps but is applicable to the deltoid, biceps, pectoral, or rectus femoris.

With the patient supine, the site of penetration is the belly of the muscle, half way between the trochanteric prominence and the knee.

A mark is made on the skin with the end of a swab, then cleansed and prepped in the usual manner. The area is infiltrated with 20 mL of bupivacaine 0.5%. Initially a wheal is made in the skin with 5 mL of bupivacaine. Then the anesthetic is injected into the muscle down to the periosteum and fanning out in a cone-shaped distribution so the site is well infused.

A 1-cm stab wound is made through the skin, nicking the fascia lata. In a heavy set or muscular patient, the scalpel may have to penetrate 4 cm.

An intervertebral rongeur (cutting, no teeth) is inserted, with the mouth of the rongeur closed, well into the wound and advanced in a rotating fashion until well into the muscle. The rongeur is then opened and closed tightly. This should obtain 4 mm of tissue.

Although one pass is usually adequate, two or three passes produces ample tissue for almost any study. Closure is performed with Steri-Strips and a small dressing. Codeine or hydrocodone helps with postprocedural analgesia.

INDICATIONS

The main criterion for muscle biopsy is an inflammatory or neuromuscular disease (e.g., muscle weakness) where a direct histopathologic diagnosis will be more helpful than indirect tests such as clinical examination or electromyographic studies.

CONTRAINDICATIONS

Essentially none, although patients with bleeding dyscrasias should be corrected before any invasive procedure is performed.

COMPLICATIONS

Infection, inability to diagnose the condition with the tissue provided, vascular or nerve injury.

Subclavian Line Insertion
Deborah A. Opacic, PA-C, MMS

DEFINITION

Insertion of a catheter into the subclavian vein for central venous access.

TECHNIQUE

Place the patient in the Trendelenburg supine position.
   Place a towel between the patient's shoulders.
   Turn the patient's head away from the procedure.

Identify the following landmarks:
- Just lateral to the midclavicular line at the junction of the medial third of the clavicle
- Lateral to the insertion of the clavicular head of the sternocleido-mastoid

Apply a local anesthetic (e.g., 1% lidocaine) from the skin to the clavicle.

Insert the central line needle (bevel up) to within 5 cm by walking under the clavicle and aiming toward the midpoint, staying closely to the undersurface of the clavicle, parallel to the floor. This is done while gently aspirating on a syringe to confirm venous return.

Remove the syringe with a hemostat (so the needle does not torque) and have the patient perform the Valsalva maneuver while covering the hub (to prevent influx of air) and introduce the J wire with the tip toward the heart, maintaining the needle in the same position. There should be minimal resistance with the advancement.

Remove the needle and enlarge the site with a scalpel.

Introduce the dilator over the wire from 3 to 4 cm while controlling the wire.

Remove the dilator and introduce the catheter over the wire to 15 cm on the right and 18 cm on the left.

Remove the wire and check for blood return through all ports, then flush with sterile saline.

Suture and dress.

Obtain a chest x-ray to rule out a pneumothorax and to ensure accurate positioning in the superior vena cava.

INDICATIONS

Emergency intravenous (IV) route, hyperalimentation, vasopressor administration, central venous pressure measurement, rapid volume resuscitation, transvenous pacemaker, Swan-Ganz catheter placement, IV access if unable to obtain a peripheral route, infusion of hypertonic or irritable solutions, or hemodialysis.

CONTRAINDICATIONS

Vein thrombosis, coagulopathy, or untreated sepsis.

COMPLICATIONS

Arterial puncture, pneumothorax, air embolus, malpositioning dysrhythmias, and with a posterior IJ approach—Horner's syndrome.

Management of Nosebleeds

Carroll F. Poppen, PA-C

DEFINITION

The treatment and management of acute epistaxis varies with the site and severity of the bleeding. Often, pressure over the nose by pinching is enough to curtail anterior septal oozing. Approximately 90% of all nosebleeds may occur from the anterior nasal septum (Little's area or Kiesselbach's plexus). Have the patient sit upright and lean forward slightly while applying gentle pressure over the nasal ala for approximately 10 minutes. If this bleeding continues, the application of a vasoconstrictor such as 1% Neo-Synephrine and a topical anesthetic (4% topical lidocaine) will slow or stop the hemorrhage.

TECHNIQUE

Cauterization.   When the bleeding site can be seen, the vessel should be cauterized. Topical application of silver nitrate can be very successful in sealing the vessel. If available, electrocautery by a hyfrecator or suction cautery unit can seal vessels that are not amenable to topical silver nitrate application. Care should be taken not to cauterize both sides of the nasal septum at the same level, for this may cause a septal perforation to occur.

Hemostatic Agents.   A number of agents are commercially available (e.g., Oxycel, Surgicel) for application directly over the bleeding site. These agents dissolve in the nose and do not require removal. Often, a thin layer of this material over the cautery site can add extra security for prevention of another bleed or be placed over the cautery site prior to packing the nose.

Packing.   Adequate lighting and suction are a must. Before the nose is packed, the mucus membranes must be adequately decongested and anesthetized. This can be accomplished with 1% Neo-Synephrine and 4% topical lidocaine pledgets. Begin by preparing the packing material, which is usually 72 inches long and 1/2-inch wide, by applying an antibiotic ointment such as Cortisporin, Polysporin, or Bacitracin through the gauze. Use a bayonet forceps for layering the gauze strips, first beginning at the floor of the nose and layering another strip on top of the previously inserted gauze until the entire nasal cavity is filled. Apply several strips of tape to cover the nostril and use a folded gauze pad as a "drip pad" to collect minor secretions. Consider removing the pack in 5 to 7 days and cover the patient with an appropriate antibiotic that will protect him or her from a staphylococcal infection.

Persistent oozing may require a compression dressing for control. This can usually be achieved by packing the anterior nasal cavity with petrolatum-impregnated gauze or insertion of a commercially available cellulose pack. Allow the pack to remain for 3 to 5 days. If an infection is a concern, institute appropriate antibiotic coverage.

Posterior Pack. This requires the use of an assistant and often a phenol palatine block for patient comfort.

After adequate anesthesia, begin by passing a catheter through the affected nostril and out the mouth. Tie the free ends of a previously fabricated adenoid tampon, and pull the catheter back out of the nose.

By applying tension to the silk sutures and guiding with the finger, secure the tampon into the nasopharynx and choana.

While the assistant provides traction, pack the nasal chamber with Vaseline-impregnated gauze (as previously described) and finish by tying the silk sutures from the nasal pharyngeal pack around a dental roll.

Complete the procedure by applying a drip pad and cover the patient with an appropriate antistaphylococcal antibiotic.

Hospitalization for comfort and observation is required.

Consider removing the packing in 5 to 7 days.

Balloon Pack. Several types of balloon packs are commercially available and come with insertion instructions. Another alternative is to use a Foley catheter.

Insert the catheter through the affected nostril until its presence can be seen in the posterior oropharynx. Inflate with 10 to 15 mL of water, then apply traction, causing the balloon to fit securely over the nasal choana.

While an assistant snugly holds the catheter in place, pack the nose with a Vaseline-impregnated gauze (as previously described).

Apply liberal packing around the ala and secure the folded catheter with an umbilical clamp.

INDICATIONS

Continued bleeding despite treatment with pressure, vasoconstrictors, or topical anesthetics.

CONTRAINDICATIONS

Basilar skull, significant facial, sinus, or nasal fractures. Otorhinolaryngology, neurosurgery, or craniofacial surgery consultation is indicated in these cases.

COMPLICATIONS

Cauterizing both sides of the nasal septum at the same level may cause septal perforation. Patient sensitivity or allergy to antibiotics or the topical agents applied.

Consider referral to an otorhinolaryngologist if the bleeding continues after appropriate packing and bedrest have been tried.

Thoracentesis

Jack Pike, PA-C, BS

DEFINITION

Puncture or intubation (chest tube) of the pleural space for the purpose of decompressing the lung by removing fluid or for diagnostic purposes.

TECHNIQUE

Materials: Usually done with sterile, disposable thoracentesis tray, gloves, Betadine solution. Review current chest x-ray for location of fluid.

Position: Sitting up with arms supported on a bedside table or tray and pillow (Fig. 14–8).

Locate fluid level by percussion and egophony. Thoracentesis will be performed about one to two interspaces below the determined fluid level but should not go lower than eighth intercostal space.

Anesthetize the skin using a 25-gauge needle and then insert needle perpendicularly into the deeper tissues to the rib.

Upon finding the rib, walk the needle over the top of the rib and penetrate the pleura keeping negative pressure with the syringe (Fig. 14–9).

On penetration of the pleura and subsequent return of pleural fluid, inject anesthesia through the pleura and as the needle is being withdrawn.

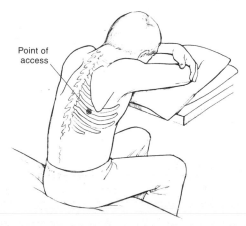

Point of access

Figure 14–8. Correct patient positioning for thoracentesis. (From Rakel RE: Saunders Manual of Medical Practice. Philadelphia, WB Saunders, 1996.)

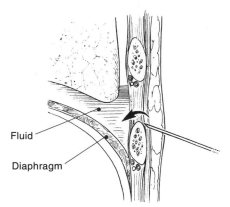

Figure 14–9. The needle is advanced over the superior aspect of the rib into the pleural space while applying negative pressure to the syringe. (From Rakel RE: Saunders Manual of Medical Practice. Philadelphia, WB Saunders, 1996.)

Fluid

Diaphragm

Using the combination of a catheter-over-needle mounted on a syringe, re-enter the pleura, again keeping negative pressure. The needle is then removed and the catheter is advanced into the chest cavity and hooked up to a stopcock to allow for removal of the fluid into a container while preventing air from entering (Fig. 14–10).

After completion, place a small dressing and lay the patient down. Order a follow-up chest x-ray to assess for pneumothorax.

INDICATIONS

Drainage of pleural fluid that compromises respiratory or cardiovascular function; to obtain pleural fluid for diagnostic purposes (e.g., empyema, chylothorax).

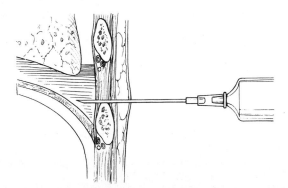

Figure 14–10. Pleural fluid is aspirated using a needle or catheter. (From Rakel RE: Saunders Manual of Medical Practice. Philadelphia, WB Saunders, 1996.)

CONTRAINDICATIONS

Pleural scarring, previous pleural ablation, bleeding dyscrasia.

COMPLICATIONS

Pneumothorax, hemothorax, lacerations/punctures of spleen and liver.

Saphenous Vein Harvesting
Jack Pike, PA-C, BS

DEFINITION

Removal of the greater saphenous vein from the leg for use as a bypass graft (usually coronary artery).

TECHNIQUE

Having made the decision to harvest the greater saphenous vein (Fig. 14–11) and after prepping and draping, the leg is abducted anterolaterally with the knee flexed about 45 degrees.

If the ankle is chosen as a starting point, then an incision is made over the posterior edge of the distal tibia and carried down to the deep saphenous vein. (The author prefers to avoid carrying the incision down over the medial malleolus, because this is painful for the patient postoperatively).

After isolating the vein, the incision is carried cephalad using a knife or scissors. Staying above the vein and keeping the scissors tips up, the tissue planes are divided in a vertical fashion to avoid creating flaps.

Superficial veins will need to be ligated or clipped as the incisions are lengthened.

There are several ways to approach incisions in the leg: to create one long incision or to make several linear incisions over the vein, leaving skin bridges of various sizes. Although the author does not believe that leaving skin bridges in the lower leg or thigh provides any advantage in the healing process, assuming no skin flaps are present, it is thought that leaving a skin bridge over the medial knee area significantly reduces patient discomfort in the postoperative period.

As the vein is exposed and dissected out in the lower leg, care should be taken to avoid the saphenous nerve.

The vein may divide just below the knee into two similarly sized branches that come together above the knee. It is usually better to pursue the anterior branch, unless the posterior branch is significantly larger.

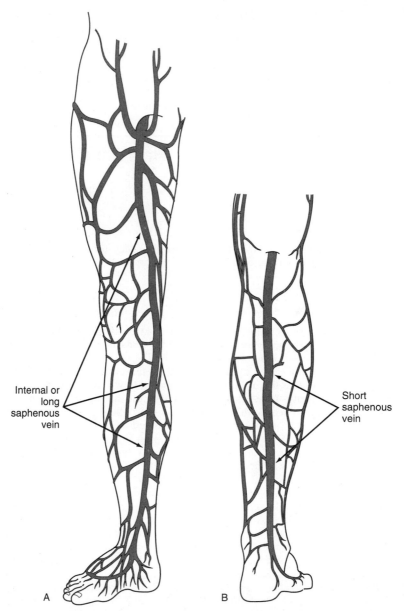

Internal or
long
saphenous
vein

Short
saphenous
vein

A   B

Figure 14–11. Anatomic location of the (A) long (internal)
and (B) short saphenous veins.

In the thigh, be observant to pursue the deeper branch of the saphenous vein while avoiding the superficial branch, which may not be suitable in size. If the entire vein is needed, lengthen the incision to a level just distal to the penetration of the fascia lata and termination in the femoral vein.

After exposing the length of vein needed, begin isolating the vein from its bed and side branches. The author prefers to use either an umbilical or vascular tape to retract the vein anteriorly during dissection.

Venous branches are usually hemoclipped distally and either tied proximally at the time of dissection or later, during vein preparation.

After completing isolating the vein from its bed, leaving both ends still attached, the vein is removed, taking care to identify which is the distal end.

A "Christmas tree" type or another similar connector is inserted into the distal end and secured with a ligature.

The proximal end is removed after clamping and tying the remaining vein stump and the vein is removed to an area for completion of preparation.

Finally, if the incision is to start in the groin, knowing the landmarks and making incisions carefully can prevent large flaps of skin which could cause significant morbidity in the healing process. Two methods can be used. One is to locate the femoral artery and make the incision medial to the artery over the femoral vein. This incision should really be a curvilinear or oblique incision in order to follow the saphenous vein in its pathway distally. Another method is to locate the symphysis pubis, measure two fingerbreadths over from the lateral edge of the pubis, then two fingerbreadths down and make the same type of incision at that location.

All leg incisions are closed with absorbable synthetic suture; skin incisions can be stapled. If there are flaps, caution should be taken in placing deep sutures that can diminish vascularity to the flaps. A better approach would be to place Jackson-Pratt drains or a Hemovac and just close a superficial layer and skin or just skin.

It cannot be stressed enough that the integrity of the vein is a cardinal goal during removal and preparation because one of the foundations of successful grafting is good vein quality. The manner in which the operator handles the vein during removal, preparation, and storage prior to use can minimize damage such as intimal disruption, contraction damage to smooth muscle, and disruption of extracellular matrix. Although there may be some disagreement as to what particular methods are harmful, most agree that overdistention of the vein and venous spasm during preparation are not positive steps.

Prior to surgery, the surgeon should stand the patient and examine the legs to determine which side might have the better vein for harvesting. Superficial varicosities do not necessarily portend poor saphenous vein quality but may adversely influence wound healing, and choosing a leg without varicosities would be best. If both legs seem good, then it is up to the surgeon to decide. Some believe that using the patient's nondominant side is better for postoperative ambulation because many people tend to use their dominant leg first in climbing stairs, so that not having a tender, healing wound, especially at the knee, would be less burdensome.

Very often, what makes the decision is what side of the patient that the scrub nurse stands during surgery so as to make it easy for everyone to do their job.

INDICATIONS

Removal of the saphenous vein is a very common procedure used for coronary artery bypass surgery. It also is harvested for peripheral revascularization procedures and stripped for severe varicosities.

CONTRAINDICATIONS

Although the greater saphenous vein is the preferred conduit for most revascularization procedures, occasionally other veins must be used if the greater saphenous has already been harvested or stripped, or if severe varicosities exist. The next preferable conduit would be the lesser saphenous vein, which is located on the posterior aspect of the lower leg. Following that, removal of the cephalic vein from the arm would be carried out. If the saphenous vein is unsuitable for use, the internal mammary artery may be chosen for coronary bypass procedures. Infection of the leg may prohibit the vein from being harvested.

COMPLICATIONS

Damage of the vein during harvesting, pain at the harvest site, infection, peripheral nerve or arterial injury.

Wound Care
Jack Pike, PA-C, BS

DEFINITION

Wounds of the body are a situation that all PAs encounter. Obtaining a working knowledge of the principles of wound healing can improve treatment results, help the patient and family understand what to expect, and allow for a deeper appreciation and interpretation of the pathophysiology of other diseases.

NORMAL WOUND HEALING

Wound healing is a complex process by which virtually all wounds heal in the same sequence; often with varying time frames, but always in the order that nature demands. As the clinician utilizes proper and timely treatment techniques, the process is facilitated to allow satisfactory outcomes. Wound healing is divided into three phases: substrate (or inflammatory), proliferative, and maturation.

Inflammatory Phase.   Lasts up to 4 days. Immediately following injury, there is a short period of vasoconstriction followed by vasodilation that floods the wound with leukocytes, erythrocytes, and platelets. The leukocytes, mainly polymorphonucleocytes (PMN) and mononuclear cells, clean up the debris of dead cells and other foreign material to prepare the wound for fibroblast infiltration during the next phase. Additionally, a fibrin clot is formed as an initial barrier and to render a small amount of strength to the wound.

Proliferative Phase.   Lasts 3 days to 3 weeks. The second phase of wound healing involves the continuing migration of epithelial cells into the wound to form a barrier that prevents further bacterial invasion into the wound. Fibroblasts, arising from the adventitia of the local capillaries and blood vessels in the area, invade the wound using the fibrin clot as a temporary buttress upon which to build. Fibrinolysis is initiated to dissolve the fibrin clot as fibroblasts synthesize collagen. Collagen is a large protein that is initially laid down in a random pattern in which the wound strength begins to increase.

Maturation Phase.   Duration of 2 weeks to 18 months. The final phase, which is often disconcerting to uninformed patients, is the period of time in which there are pronounced changes in the bulk, form, color, and strength of the scar. Patients must understand that scar revision should not be carried out, or decided upon, until the maturation process is complete.

FACTORS IN WOUND HEALING

Local Factors

Foreign Material.   Proper débridement is necessary.

Infection.   Prolongs the inflammatory phase.

Ischemia.   Oxygen needed for collagen synthesis and other cellular functions.

Temperature.   Warm environments favor healing.

Systemic Factors

Diabetes Mellitus.   Hyperglycemia inhibits PMN phagocytosis and decreases collagen accumulation. Diabetics often have sensory deprivation that leads to pressure sores from being unable to sense pressure changes and ischemic pain.

Anemia.   Decreases oxygen supply to wound.

Nutrition.   Protein deficiency retards vascularization and healing, but not unless proteins are significantly low.

Vitamin Deficiency: Vitamin C is necessary in the formation of the collagen molecule; vitamin A enhances immunity and collagen production; vitamin E enhances absorption of vitamin A and improves PMN function; zinc deficiency impairs nucleic acid synthesis among other wound healing factors.

TECHNIQUE

WOUND EVALUATION

It is imperative to take an adequate history from the patient (e.g., when the injury occurred, how it happened, where the injury took place). These questions help determine the course of action to be taken at that time, as well as appropriate diagnostic studies needed.

The location of the injury on the body helps the clinician do the appropriate system examination as well as decide if consultants are needed. Neurovascular and motor function are imperatives in the evaluation, especially in the facial area and hands.

Wound Class

Clean. Typically elective surgical cases, not in the mouth, gut, genitourinary (GU) or respiratory system.

Clean Contaminated. As above, but includes mouth, gut, GU, respiratory system.

Contaminated. Lacerations, open fractures, elective cases with spillage from above systems.

Dirty or Infected. Perforated viscus, abscess, grossly contaminated wounds.

Local Anesthesia

Local anesthesia is essential for proper débridement and exploration of the wound, but should not be used before sensory evaluation is performed.

Types of Anesthesia

- Lidocaine without epinephrine, which has rapid onset and low toxicity with normal use amounts (maximum dose is 4.5 mg/kg)
- Lidocaine with epinephrine (a vasoconstrictor) prolongs anesthesia time; never to be used on digits or penis (maximum dose is 7 mg/kg)
- Marcaine, an alternative anesthetic, has a slower onset of action but lasts up to 10 hours

Anesthetic Techniques

Local. When the anesthetic is injected directly into the area where the procedure or repair will occur.

Field Block. Anesthetic is injected around the area to be worked on.

Digital Block. Used to numb an entire finger or toe.

Regional Block. Used to anesthetize a larger area, such as an arm or below the waist, than an epidural block would achieve.

Sutures

- Absorbable sutures are usually used for layers beneath the skin or mucosal surfaces.
- Chromic or plain suture absorbs quickly (7 to 10 days); tensile strength gone quickly.
- Synthetic sutures cause less inflammatory response; tensile strength lasts longer.
- Nonabsorbable sutures are usually for skin and subcutaneous pull-out sutures.

- Silk is inexpensive but very tissue reactive; holds knots well.
- Monofilaments (nylon, propylene, steel wire) have prolonged tensile strength and low tissue reaction, but require more "throws" to secure knot.

Needles
- Taper-cut needle has a round body with a sharp point; used on easily penetrated tissue.
- Cutting needle has a beveled needle with sharp cutting edges (can be forward or reverse cutting) used on more dense tissue (e.g., skin, fascia).

PRINCIPLES OF WOUND CLOSURE

In order to achieve the best possible result for the patient, the wound is to be closed in layers, ensuring that each layer (e.g., peritoneum, fascia, fat, dermis, and epidermis) is matched to itself. Except for the scalp, hand, and feet, there exists little excuse for one-layer closures. If one wishes to close layers, take the tension off and evert the skin edges so as to obtain a satisfactory cosmetic result.

As the wound heals in the initial period postinjury, it will be virtually impossible to prevent some degree of stress being placed on the wound. The wound will naturally contract and loosen so that the edges are pulled down and away to flatten. If the edges are not everted in the initial closure, then it is likely that the wound will flatten and become concave, creating a depression.

Suturing Technique
There are advantages and disadvantages of both interrupted and continuous suturing techniques. Continuous (or running) sutures take less time to perform, leave less foreign body in tissue overall, may cause less tissue ischemia, and can be aesthetically better but have the disadvantage, in the event of infection, of disrupting the entire closure. Interrupted sutures, while more time consuming, should be used if there is concern of infection.

Take equal bites on each side.

With skin sutures and a two-layer closure, skin sutures can have 1- to 2-mm length from skin edges. With one-layer closure, sutures need to be 3 to 4 mm from skin edges.

Put the needle on the needle holder about 3/4 distance from needle point. Use the needle holder the way that is best for you, but practice not getting fingers locked into the needle holder holes to gain better control for placing sutures.

Instrument Tie: Hold needle holder parallel with incision; with long, free end of suture, make a loop around the end of the needle holder; grab the short end of the strand; pull through loop and bring end of strand to opposite side of wound; repeat this maneuver three to four times—always keep the instrument between the two ends of the suture while making loops; make square knots.

For specific considerations for facial lacerations see Chapter 10: Plastic and Reconstructive Surgery.

INDICATIONS

Primary repair can be performed in a clean, incised wound or in a clean contaminated wound if properly prepared.

Delayed primary repair of contaminated wounds can proceed safely if the potential for infection has been eliminated. Allows open wounds to mount sufficient resistance to infection.

Secondary closure or second intention is accomplished by closing the wound by contraction rather than primary union. Healing process is delayed and scar formation can be excessive and produce weak union of tissues.

CONTRAINDICATIONS

Primary repair in a contaminated wound, a facial laceration greater than 8 hours old (due to the risk of infection) should be treated by plastic surgery; significant associated injuries may delay primary laceration repair.

COMPLICATIONS

Infection, injury to underlying tissue (vascular, nervous), poor cosmetic result, pain, or keloid formation.

Further Readings

Ballweg R, Stolberg S, Sullivan E: Physician Assistant: A Guide to Clinical Practice. Philadelphia, W. B. Saunders, 1994.
Bryant W: Wound Healing. Clin Symp 29:1977.

Index

Note: Page numbers in *italics* refer to illustrations; page numbers followed by t refer to tables.